# Critical Care Nephrology and Renal Replacement Therapy in Children

Akash Deep • Stuart L. Goldstein
Editors

# Critical Care Nephrology and Renal Replacement Therapy in Children

Springer

*Editors*
Akash Deep
Paediatric Intensive Care Unit
King's College Hospital
London
United Kingdom

Stuart L. Goldstein
Center for Acute Care Nephrology
Cincinnati Children's
Hospital Medical Center
Cincinnati, OH
USA

ISBN 978-3-030-07981-9 ISBN 978-3-319-90281-4 (eBook)
https://doi.org/10.1007/978-3-319-90281-4



Printed on acid-free paper

This Springer imprint is published by the registered company Springer International Publishing AG part of Springer Nature.
The registered company address is: Gewerbestrasse 11, 6330 Cham, Switzerland

# Foreword 1

Perhaps no other area of pediatric intensive care medicine (PICM) has changed in the last decade as much as renal failure and its management: New definitions for acute kidney injury, biomarkers to define and guide treatment, and the normalization of safe and effective renal replacement therapy as a standard PICM therapy, rather than a rescue option. Children of all ages with severe sepsis, metabolic diseases, and intrinsic kidney disease together with those undergoing cardiac surgery or admitted with complications from stem cell transplant all benefit from this focus, and now with the prospect of long-term outcomes for affected children our knowledge base and concepts are expanded rapidly.

Textbooks from even a few years ago are now obsolete, and so this new textbook is necessary, relevant, and actually a very good read!

This book will serve as the current definitive textbook for intensivists and nephrologists dealing with acute kidney injury and diseases, including providing safe renal replacement therapies for critically ill children of all ages.

True world experts have provided chapters on the core areas of knowledge, meaning this work forms the ideal resource for those taking professional exams, such as the ESPNIC (European Society of Pediatric and Neonatal Intensive Care) diploma, and for the multidisciplinary teams caring for critically ill and injured children affected by renal failure and diseases, or needing renal replacement therapies in the intensive care environment.

Joe Brierley
Great Ormond St Hospital, London, UK

Past President, European Society of Pediatric and
Neonatal Intensive Care (ESPNIC)
Geneva, Switzerland

# Foreword 2

For the last 40 years, I have been trying to combine the fields of adult nephrology and intensive care studying the common ground of the critically ill patient with kidney problems. Indeed, such patients are too complex for a single specialist to deal with, and a common collaborative effort via a multidisciplinary task force is probably the solution for the multiple problems that we are facing in this setting. I also tried to take advantage of the bionic convergence and applied technology to create a new discipline called Critical Care Nephrology. It was in the early 1990s when Rinaldo Bellomo and I gave birth to Critical Care Nephrology as a new specialty combining the knowledge of dedicated intensivists and nephrologists focusing on the complex field of kidney disorders in critically ill patients. Our idea was that critical illness is a complex entity that may require more than one physician and more than one specialist at the bedside of the patient. A single musician can play a melody but it takes an orchestra to play a symphony. We can play different instruments but we must all be in the same key. Since then, the field Critical Care Nephrology has grown continuously as a result of studies and clinical trials, consensus conferences, and therapeutic innovation. In particular, new devices, biomaterials, and kidney support therapies have been developed and some of them have become a routine in clinical practice. The consequence of this process has been a progressive decrease in mortality of our patients in spite of a more complex and a sicker/older population. Since the early 1980s, I have had the chance to become interested in the pediatric application of adult techniques, and I discovered early on that there was a remarkable gap in translation of technology from adults to children and, in particular, neonates. New technologies are often tested in adults while technological knowledge in pediatric nephrology and intensive care is often insufficient due to limited number of procedures and cases. These factors, together with a limited engagement of industry in the pediatric field due to small size of the business and longer times for validation of dedicated technologies, explain the slow transfer of technological advances from adults to children. Nevertheless, there is a tremendous unmet need which can only be solved by dedicated physicians and passionate groups of investigators like the authors of many chapters of the present book. When I treated the first newborn with continuous arteriovenous hemofiltration in Vicenza in 1981, I discovered immediately that supplies were lacking and a dedicated technology was simply not available. Since then, I have spent a significant amount of my time to be an ambassador for the needs of children and neonates in the field of

Critical Care Nephrology. This led to a profound engagement in promoting the transition of adult technology into the pediatric field and even in designing from scratch new devices such as minifilters for CRRT or new equipment such as the CARPEDIEM device (Cardio Renal Pediatric Dialysis Emergency Machine). This endeavor begun several years ago and today we have outstanding physicians and investigators continuing the mission for an improved care of children and newborns. For this reason, I am particularly honored to open with my foreword the book on *Critical Care Nephrology and Renal Replacement Therapy in Children* edited by two outstanding authors and long lasting friends: Stuart Goldstein and Akash Deep. The book is a real compendium of information and current knowledge in the field, organized in two specific sections: Acute Kidney Injury and Renal Replacement Therapy. The first part describes the evolution of epidemiology, the understanding of pathophysiology, and the practice of monitoring of acute kidney disease in the last two decades, leading to the most recent advances in diagnosis and management of AKI in different settings using advanced tools such as the newest biomarkers. All chapters in this section pay particular attention to the collaborative effort between pediatric nephrology and pediatric intensive care for a better care of our small patients. The second part describes the most important aspects of renal replacement therapy in children and neonates with particular attention to the basic concepts, the optimal timing of application of extracorporeal techniques, the rationale for different modalities, and other practical issues such as prescription, monitoring, anticoagulation, and drug adjustments. Finally the book includes chapters on the use of CRRT and other techniques in special settings such as cardiac surgery, sepsis, liver failure, and exogenous intoxication.

I could not imagine a better organization of the table of contents that are so complete and exhaustive. I am gratified to see that the concept of critical care nephrology has crossed the line and barrier between adult and pediatric medicine. The authors of this book should be congratulated for the difficult but successful work they have done for the benefit of the scientific community and the patients and families we serve. Critical Care Nephrology in Children, the time has come!

**The First Patient treated with CAVH**
*(Vicenza-Italy, 1980)*

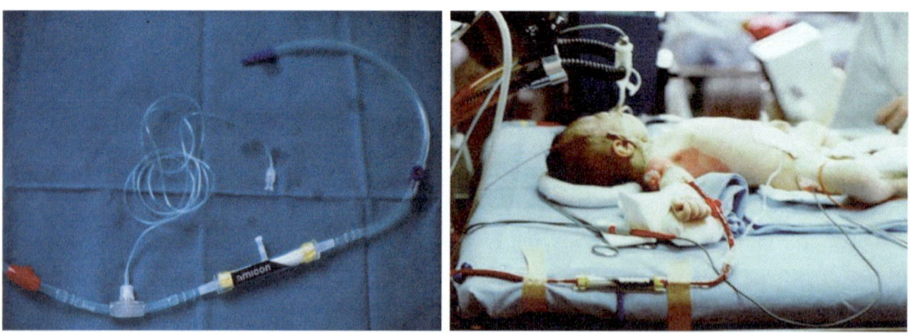

Renal function recovery after 96 hours of CAVH treatment
*Ronco C, Brendolan A, Bragantini L, et Al.* :Treatment of acute renal failure in newborns by Continuous Arterio-Venous Hemofiltration.
*Kidney International, 1984. Courtesy of C. Ronco*

**CAVH improves pulmonary exchanges and reduces the duration of mechanical ventilation**

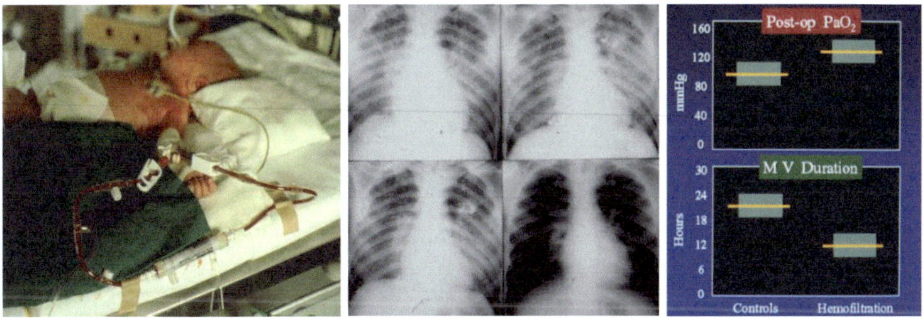


*Ronco C, Brendolan A, Bragantini L, et Al: Treatment of acute renal failure in the newborn by continuous arteriovenous hemofiltration. Trans ASAIO 1985;31:634-8. Courtesy of C. Ronco*

**CAVH efficiency and the hypercatabolic patient**

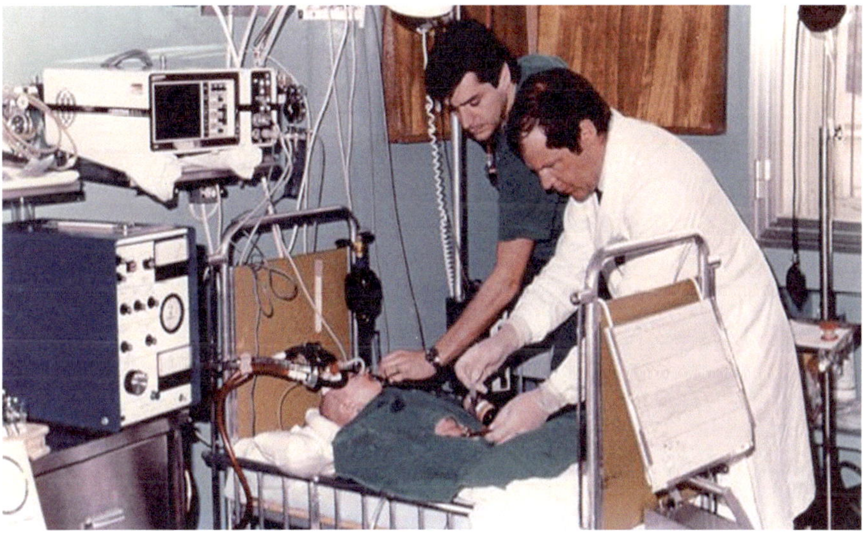

*Courtesy of C. Ronco*

## The birth of CVVHDF

*Ronco et Al, Int. J. Artif Organs, 1985*

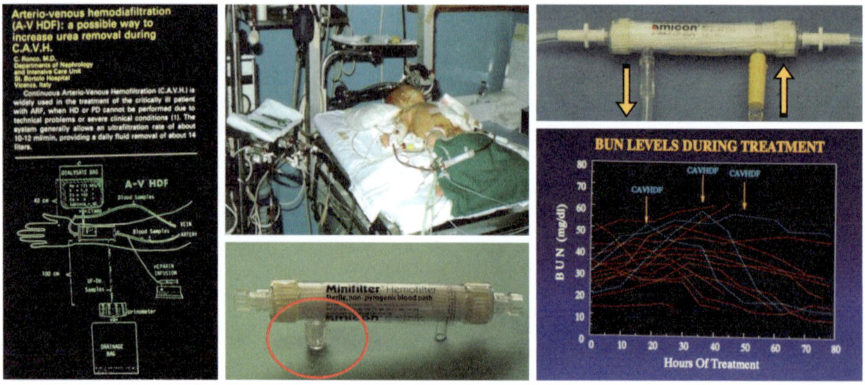


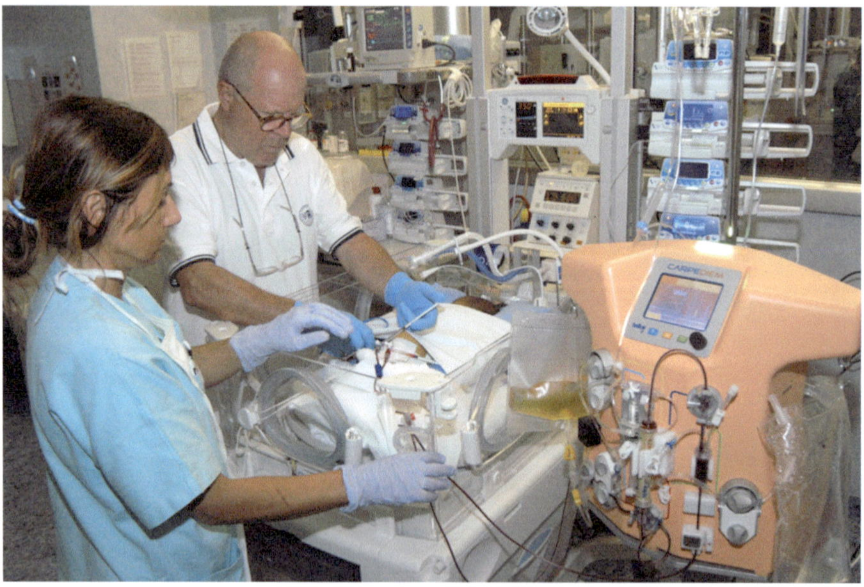
Courtesy of C. Ronco

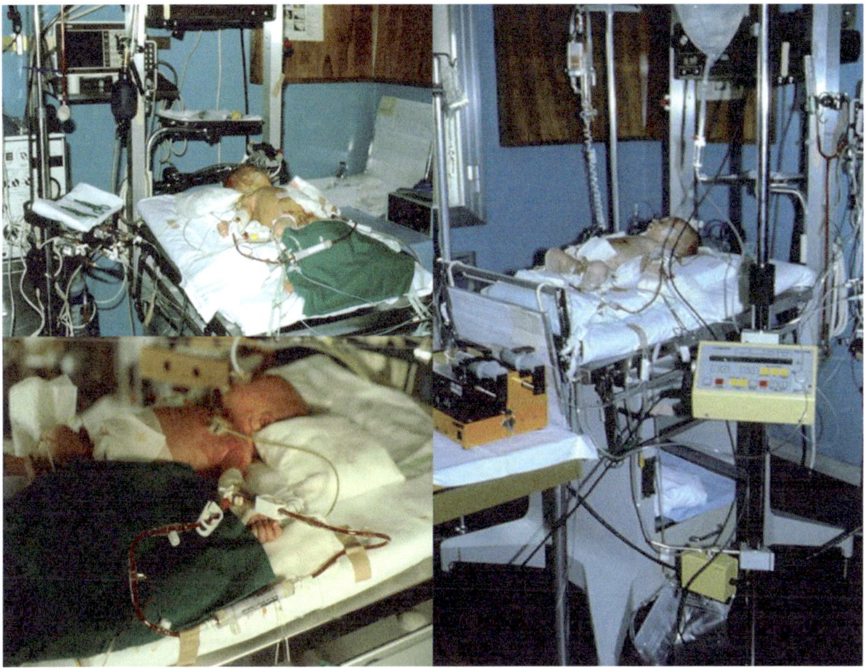

*Courtesy of C. Ronco*

Claudio Ronco
International Renal Research Institute of Vicenza (IRRIV),
San Bortolo Hospital
Vicenza, Italy

Department of Nephrology
San Bortolo Hospital
Vicenza, Italy

# Foreword 3

The care of the critically ill child and infant has evolved over the last 20 years, to a level where renal replacement therapy and care of the kidney has now become an integral part of the holistic care of the patient. While this may be seen as the "bread and butter" of intensive therapy, management of the kidney is often still relatively neglected, as management of "ABCD" may seem to take precedence. However, it has become increasingly clear that unless the kidneys are managed carefully and effectively, the patient will ultimately suffer—either by prolonged intensive care stay, increased morbidity, or even mortality.

I am honored to be asked to provide a foreword to the important work *Critical Care Nephrology and Renal Replacement Therapy in Children* edited by Akash Deep and Stuart Goldstein.

The editors are to be congratulated in assembling a complete and comprehensive anthology of important texts reviewing current state-of-the-art management and knowledge on a broad range of issues affecting the pediatric intensivist and nephrologist, when dealing with a neonate or child with critical illness.

I am particularly pleased to see that the editors have included chapters on nursing care, management of nephrotoxic medications, plasma exchange, metabolic and toxicological subjects, thus demonstrating the true multidisciplinary and multiprofessional nature of pediatric critical care medicine. It is also very helpful to have specific chapters on renal management in specific conditions such as the child on extracorporeal life support or with liver failure.

This book brings together current thinking from world experts on state-of-the-art management of all aspects of renal medicine in the critically ill child and is an important addition to our armory.

Simon Nadel

St Mary's Hospital and Imperial College
London, UK

Medical President, European Society of Neonatal and
Paediatric Intensive Care (ESPNIC)
Geneva, Switzerland

# Preface

The fields of pediatric acute kidney injury and renal replacement therapy provision for the critically ill child have undergone a clinical and research revolution over the past two decades, with advancements accelerating exponentially over the past 5 years. Small single-center studies have been supplanted by robust, multicenter and multinational epidemiological reports that clearly demonstrate that acute kidney injury is independently associated with child morbidity and mortality. Outcome assessment for the child with AKI has now been published repeatedly across the entire spectrum of pediatric critical illness, from neonates to young adults, and in every conceivable nonrenal system illness such as stem cell and solid organ transplantation, sepsis, heart and liver disease.

Provision of renal replacement therapy is no longer considered to be experimental or heroic—broad and detailed experiences have been published with respect to acute peritoneal dialysis, continuous renal replacement therapies, and integration of renal support with other advanced extracorporeal support. These publications and experiences form the foundation for a standard of care that can be provided by any intensive care unit focused on caring for the critically ill child.

In addition, many advancements in clinical and translational science have emanated from the pediatric experience. These include development of novel AKI risk stratification systems, discovery, validation, and clinical decision support integration of novel biomarkers to predict AKI development and severity and focus on fluid balance as an indication for renal replacement therapy initiation.

Previous compilations of the pediatric critical care nephrology literature have resided either as small components of larger pediatric nephrology, pediatric critical care, or critical care nephrology textbooks. Given the pediatric-specific advancements noted above, we felt strongly that a single volume dedicated to pediatric critical care nephrology and renal replacement therapy was needed to provide the appropriate space for detailed discussion about the field that is our professional passion. We are indebted to all the authors of the chapters contained herein, who are all international experts in their respective fields, and acknowledged as such in their own professional communities and in the critical care nephrology community as a whole. Their shared passion for our field is evident from the outstanding quality contained in each chapter. We are grateful to the European Society of Pediatric and Neonatal Intensive Care (ESPNIC) for all the support and endorsement of this book.

We are also greatly appreciative of our families Bonilla and Trisha Arora (Deep), and Elizabeth and Beau Goldstein, who suffer our long clinical hours and extensive professional commitments to serve as two of the pied pipers of our tightknit pediatric critical care nephrology community. Our time spent editing this unique textbook is just one of the many of our endeavors they have had to endure to support our careers. Neither of us would be able to achieve our goals without their support and patience.

Finally, in the words of one of the great leaders of pediatric nephrology, the late Dr. William Harmon, we are reminded that "it is a privilege that families allow us to care for their most precious children with kidney disease." This is especially true for families of children with critical illness who develop AKI. Most of these families meet us for the first time during one of the most stressful times of their lives, placing their faith and trust in us to provide expert care in the most complex of settings, and in many cases, agreeing to enroll their child in a research study which may not benefit their own but improve the outcomes for children in the future. We are a truly privileged group to work in this field.

London, UK — Akash Deep
Cincinnati, OH — Stuart L. Goldstein

# Contents

# About the Authors

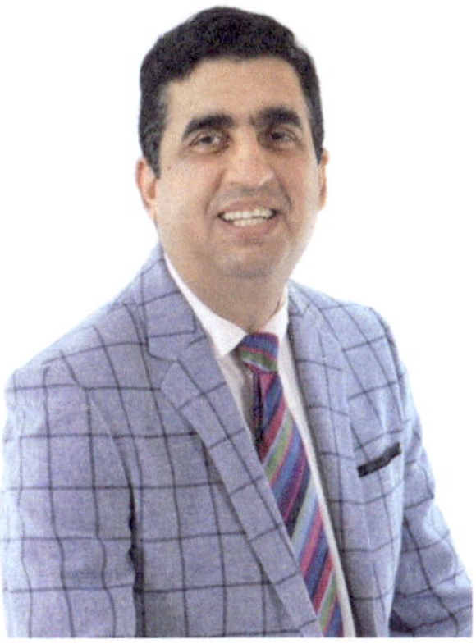

**Akash Deep** is the Director of the Paediatric Intensive Care Unit at King's College Hospital, London. He is also the Chair of the Renal/CRRT Section of the European Society of Paediatric and Neonatal Intensive Care (ESPNIC) and the Chair of the UK Paediatric Intensive Care Society's Science and Education Committee. Dr. Deep conducts workshops and seminars on AKI and CRRT in various parts of the world. He was the co-chairman of the 8th and 9th International conferences on pediatric CRRT hosted in London and Orlando, respectively. He regularly teaches on the winter and summer schools of the European Society of Paediatric and Neonatal Intensive Care (ESPNIC). His main interests include AKI in liver disease and RRT and other liver assist devices in liver failure, and he has published on both of these topics extensively.

Dr. Deep is a clinical expert on pediatric sepsis and an advisor for the UK Sepsis Trust. He works with a team of national and international experts who collaborate with the UK Sepsis Trust, Royal College of Paediatrics and Child Health, and NHS England.

Dr. Deep is the main author of the widely acclaimed "Paediatric sepsis toolkit" for emergency departments, which was launched at the House of Commons in 2015. He is a member of the most prestigious societies and author of several peer-reviewed articles and book chapters.

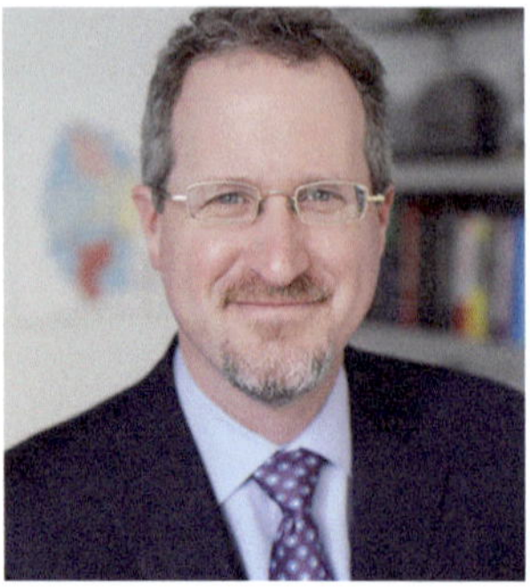

**Stuart L. Goldstein** is the Clark D. West Endowed Chair, director of the Center for Acute Care Nephrology, medical director of the Pheresis Service, co-medical director of the Heart Institute Research Core at Cincinnati Children's Hospital Medical Center, and Professor of Pediatrics at the University of Cincinnati College of Medicine, Cincinnati, Ohio, USA.

Dr. Goldstein has been an active investigator in the field of pediatric acute kidney injury (AKI) since 2000. His main research foci include AKI epidemiology and outcomes, acute renal replacement therapy provision, and investigation of novel urinary AKI biomarkers in the pediatric population. He has established a strong record of interdisciplinary and interinstitutional collaboration with cardiologists, intensivists, and emergency center physicians, which is evidenced by his establishment and directing of the Prospective Pediatric Continuous Renal Replacement Therapy Registry from 2001 to 2012 and the Prospective Pediatric AKI Research Group (ppAKI-RG) in 2012. Dr. Goldstein is also a respected educator; he has developed the only pediatric-specific acute care nephrology subspecialty fellowship with graduates who are now leaders in the field of pediatric AKI. He is a member of the most prestigious societies and has published 200 papers in international journals as well as 30 book chapters.

# Part I

# Acute Kidney Injury

# The Evolution of Acute Kidney Injury Research Over the Past Two Decades

1

Stuart L. Goldstein

## 1.1 Introduction

It is 5:30 in the morning, and the pediatric intensivist and critical care nephrologist log on to their computers to review the electronic health records of patients admitted to their pediatric intensive care unit (PICU).

**Case 1**

A 7-year-old male, with a baseline weight of 25 kg, was admitted to the PICU 5 days ago after resection of a liver mass in the left lobe. The patient is receiving invasive mechanical ventilation (respiratory rate 20 breaths/min, peak inspiratory pressure (30 cm$H_2O$), peak end expiratory pressure (10 cm$H_2O$), and fractional inspired oxygen (60%)). In the last 24 h, the urine output has decreased from 3200 mL from the previous day to 400 mL. The patient's serum creatinine has increased from 0.7 to 1.3 mg/dL.

**Case 2**

A 2-day-old (2.9 kg) neonate was admitted last night with poor feeding, lethargy, and respiratory distress. The infant is receiving invasive mechanical ventilation (respiratory rate 20 breaths/minute, peak inspiratory pressure (30 cm$H_2O$), peak end expiratory pressure (10 cm$H_2O$), and fractional inspired oxygen (30%). Serum ammonia was 879 µmol/L.

S. L. Goldstein
Center for Acute Care Nephrology, Cincinnati Children's Hospital Medical Center, Cincinnati, OH, USA
e-mail: Stuart.goldstein@cchmc.org



A. Deep, S. L. Goldstein (eds.), *Critical Care Nephrology and Renal Replacement Therapy in Children*, https://doi.org/10.1007/978-3-319-90281-4_1

**Case 3**

An 11-year-old (57 kg; BSA 1.7 $m^2$) presented to an outside hospital with history of an upper respiratory infection for 4–5 days manifested by sore throat and cough. He had decompensated with increased respiratory effort, mental status changes, and lethargy. He is transferred to the ICU for further management. In the ICU, he developed hypoxic respiratory failure, myocardial depression, and septic shock. He was noted to have persistent hypoxia despite high frequency oscillator requiring VA-ECMO support. He was subsequently determined to be positive for Influenza A, and then developed necrotizing pneumonia (S. aureus), sepsis, and DIC. He had an elevated creatinine (as high as 3.19 mg/dL) and decreased UOP in the setting of AKI and fluid overload.

**Case 4**

A 6-year-old male (22.4 kg, 118 cm, BSA 0.85 $m^2$) with a history of relapsing rhabdomyosarcoma received a stem cell transplant 17 days ago, and then developed fever, hypotension, and respiratory failure 3 days ago. He is receiving invasive mechanical ventilation (RR-20, 30/10, 60% $O_2$) and is receiving a continuous infusion of norepinephrine at 0.12 μg/kg/min. His PICU admission weight was 24.6 kg, and he developed a positive fluid balance of 3.8 L since admission.

These cases illustrate the current state of the patient epidemiology in terms of the care provided to infants, children, and adolescents with acute kidney injury (AKI) or who require some form of renal replacement therapy. Twenty years ago, the care of such patients was neither standardized nor based on published data from more than small single-center reports or case series. A search of the peer-reviewed literature using the terms "acute renal failure," "acute kidney injury," "pediatric," "children," "neonatal," "dialysis," and "renal replacement therapy" reveals not only an increasing volume of articles over the past two decades but also multiple systematic reviews of aspects of the entire spectrum of AKI components including assessment of different AKI definitions [1], specific disease populations, development of new AKI risk stratification systems [2, 3], and the performance of novel AKI biomarkers to predict AKI development and severity [4]. Furthermore, multiple studies have assessed the epidemiology and outcomes for neonates, children, and adolescents with AKI [5, 6] who receive acute renal replacement therapy, and recent years have observed the development and application or adaptation of novel devices to support the pediatric patient with AKI [7, 8]. What is especially remarkable about the pediatric AKI literature is that it has kept pace with adult AKI literature in many facets, and in some cases, pediatric AKI studies have been seminal and led the way in assessment of AKI, its sequelae, and associated outcomes. Fundamentally, children have fewer chronic comorbidities such as cirrhosis, metastatic malignancy, chronic heart failure, and diabetes that often impede the ability to assess for a direct association between AKI and outcomes in adult populations. Thus, it is not hyperbolic to state that the field of pediatric AKI has undergone a rapid and transformative evolution in the past two decades. This chapter will review the evolution of pediatric AKI research that forms the basis of current clinical care, with an attempt to highlight the seminal publications and essential factors that have led to the state of the art that exists in 2018. The main aim of this chapter is to create the background upon which subsequent chapters build their more comprehensive and detailed accounting of the field of AKI and renal replacement therapy in children.

## 1.2 Initial Focus on Acute Renal Replacement Therapy

The early pediatric AKI literature focused upon patients who received renal replacement therapy from single centers [6, 9], which resulted from the particular interest of pediatric nephrologists in providing dialysis therapy. As the cases above illustrate, AKI in the PICU is most often the result of some other systemic illness or its treatment [10], and therefore provision of expert critical care nephrology care requires an understanding of multi-organ failure and the underlying causes of AKI other than primary kidney disease. Furthermore the lack of a uniform definition for AKI and the view that AKI or acute renal failure (ARF) was most often a primary kidney disease relegated pediatric AKI research to the domain of the nephrologist.

### 1.2.1 Single-Center Studies

One of the first and most comprehensive single-center studies compared the outcomes of 226 children with AKI who received either acute intermittent hemodialysis, peritoneal dialysis, or continuous renal replacement therapy [6]. The primary outcome was survival to intensive care unit discharge. Children who received intermittent hemodialysis experienced better survival rates than those who received peritoneal dialysis or CRRT, yet the latter cohorts had higher illness severity as manifested by a greater pressor requirement. In addition, children with other primary illness such as stem cell transplantation or liver disease experienced lower survival than those with primary kidney disease. Subsequently other single-center studies of children with AKI receiving CRRT revealed a consistent association between the degree of fluid overload at CRRT initiation, based on ICU admission weight, and ICU mortality [9, 11, 12]. These studies, while provocative, were underpowered to conduct sophisticated multivariable analyses.

### 1.2.2 Multicenter Collaboration

In 2001, 13 pediatric institutions in the United States established the Prospective Pediatric Continuous Renal Replacement Therapy (ppCRRT) Registry Group [13]. The ppCRRT enrolled 340 patients over 5 years, and was constructed as a prospective observational cohort study aimed at identifying factors associated with patient outcomes and CRRT machine care delivery in children who received CRRT for any reason. The multitude of publications emanating from the ppCRRT dataset still serve as a benchmark for pediatric CRRT delivery and patient outcomes in terms of CRRT circuit functioning, vascular access, anticoagulation as well as sub-analyses of different patient populations and indications, and associations with patient mortality [5]. The results and conclusions will be discussed in great detail in subsequent chapters, so will not be addressed here. However, perhaps the most important outcome of the ppCRRT was the demonstration that pediatric investigators could collaborate successfully across multiple institutions to provide an epidemiological foundation upon which to base clinical practice recommendations which remain durable today.

## 1.3 Transition to Assessment of AKI Epidemiology Study

As with studies of renal replacement therapy, single-center studies predominated the adult and pediatric AKI literature until the mid-2000s. Prior to that time, there was a general consensus that patients died "with" and not "from" their AKI [14], since patients could receive dialysis and therefore not succumb to the imminent, life-threatening electrolyte disturbances such as hyperkalemia or hypophosphatemia that prompt similar thoughts for initiating dialysis therapy for patients progressing from chronic kidney disease to end-stage kidney disease. This "end-stage kidney disease mindset" and the term acute renal *failure* potentially also fostered a nihilistic attitude regarding potential interventions or systematic assessment of AKI epidemiology that could improve patient outcomes. A fundamental factor underlying this laissez-faire attitude was the lack of a consensus definition for AKI; improving patient outcomes in any field is impossible without a definition of disease. The AKI field experienced a seismic shift as a result of three publications. First, Chertow and colleagues demonstrated that a serum creatinine increase of 0.3 mg/dL over baseline was independently associated with mortality in hospitalized adult patients [15]. This finding is transformative because such a "small" creatinine increase is not associated with life-threatening hyperkalemia, hypocalcemia, fluid overload, or uremia that are, as mentioned above, the classic indications for initiating renal replacement therapy.

Second, the Acute Dialysis Quality Initiative (ADQI) convened a consensus panel to put forward a testable AKI definition and graded severity classification system term the RIFLE criteria (Risk, Injury, Failure, Loss, End-stage kidney disease) [16]. While RIFLE has been modified and calibrated with the Acute Kidney Injury Network (AKIN) [17] and Kidney Diseases Improving Global Outcomes (KDIGO) [18] AKI definition and classification systems, the importance of RIFLE was to standardize an AKI definition, and subsequently demonstrate independent graded associations between AKI development, severity, and morbidity and mortality. Third, Uchino performed a multinational observational study of critically ill adult patients who received renal replacement therapy and found that such patients exhibited increased mortality and a high rate of dialysis dependence at time of hospital discharge [19]. Taken together, these three studies have served as the convincing rationale to perform AKI directed research to identify novel AKI biomarkers, assess disease-specific AKI epidemiology, conduct prospective randomized trials of dialysis dose for AKI, and assess for the risk of chronic kidney disease in patients who survive an AKI episode.

### 1.3.1 Single-Center Pediatric Studies

Early pediatric single-center studies were descriptive, and generally focused on patients with AKI without a non-AKI control group to assess for an association between AKI and outcomes. However, these studies were important in that they demonstrated repeatedly that only a small fraction (7–10%) of AKI in children results from primary kidney disease [20–22], while the vast majority results from another system illness or its treatment. This epidemiology compelled pediatric AKI researchers to collaborate with other specialties to identify associations between AKI and outcomes in their patient populations, and if such associations exist, move forward with interventional studies to improve AKI outcomes. As AKI research field matured and the RIFLE, pediatric modified RIFLE [23], AKIN, and KDIGO criteria began to be tested in pediatric single center studies, the epidemiology showed that as in adults, AKI is associated with morbidity and mortality in critically ill children [1, 23–25]. However, these studies either relied on administrative datasets (which underestimate the true prevalence of AKI), or small patient populations. As such, their generalizability has been questioned.

### 1.3.2 Multicenter Collaboration

In 2014, 32 pediatric centers from nine countries in four continents undertook a prospective observational study of the association between AKI and outcomes in critically ill children [26]. The Assessment of Worldwide Acute kidney injury, Renal angina and Epidemiology (AWARE) represents the most comprehensive pediatric AKI study undertaken to date, with a detailed analysis of both the KDIGO serum creatinine and urine output AKI criteria in over 5000 patients [27]. AWARE will be discussed extensively in this book, but the main results show a high incidence of AKI (26.9%), an incremental risk of mortality for children with KDIGO Stage 2 or 3 AKI (odds ratio 1.77), a risk of missing AKI in a substantial proportion of children (67%) if only serum creatinine criteria are assessed and validation that AKI in critically ill children does not often result from primary kidney disease. Further output from AWARE will assess the relative contribution and outcomes of serum creatinine versus urine output AKI criteria in more detail, assessment of the performance of the renal angina index (see below) and novel urinary biomarkers to predict AKI development and severity, disease-specific epidemiology, and regional differences in AKI care. Finally, the AWARE cohort provides a virtually unique opportunity to follow up AKI survivors for the development of chronic kidney disease.

### 1.3.3 Neonatal Studies

The concept of AKI in the neonatal population has only received attention in the current decade [28]. Barriers to neonatal AKI study include the real and valid concern of multiple blood draws in small premature infants, the changing creatinine in the immediate postnatal period from maternal levels to infant levels and the normal increase in GFR over the first year of life leading to difficulty in the development of a standard definition. Similar to AWARE, a multicenter assessment of AKI in neonates was undertaken in 2014 [29]. The Assessment of Worldwide Acute Kidney injury Epidemiology in Neonates (AWAKEN) was a multinational retrospective study of more than 2000 neonates admitted to 24 neonatal ICUs across the world. Using a modified KDIGO AKI criteria, AWAKEN also demonstrated a high prevalence of AKI (30%) and an incremental association between AKI and poor outcomes in neonates [30]. Furthermore, AWAKEN observed AKI rates that varied with gestational age and AKI was associated with prolonged hospital stay. The data from AWAKEN clearly demonstrate that neonatal AKI is an area that requires study to develop interventions to prevent or mitigate AKI in this very vulnerable population.

### 1.3.4 Cardio-Renal Studies

Patients undergoing cardiac surgery, especially those who receive cardiopulmonary bypass (CPB), represent an important population for study. First and foremost, the timing of the kidney insult, namely cardiac surgery, is known. Second, congenital heart disease represents the most common congenital defect seen in humans, so the population available for study is relatively large. Finally, children with congenital heart disease rarely have other comorbidities, so the association between AKI and outcomes less confounded. When standardized AKI definitions are used, AKI after cardiac surgery occurs in over 50% of children, with independent associations between Stage 2 or 3 AKI and mortality [31–33]. Furthermore, this known AKI timing and high incidence has led to both preventive and early supportive interventions to improve outcomes in this population, which will be discussed later in this volume. Thus, the pediatric AKI research field will likely leverage the clinical infrastructure of cardiac surgery to further innovative developments in drugs and devices aimed at improving outcomes for children with or at risk for AKI.

## 1.4 Risk Stratification and Prevention: A Pediatric Mindset and AKI

The association between AKI and increased morbidity and mortality across the spectrum of pediatric critical illness compels us to identify patients at risk for AKI development. Such risk stratification is essential to design interventional studies to prevent AKI development or mitigate its severity, since once AKI develops, all current measures are aimed at providing supportive measures to treat AKI sequelae. Furthermore, while provision of acute renal replacement therapy has become more standardized and more commonplace, even for the most critically ill patient with multi-organ disease, acute dialysis remains an invasive and complex procedure. In the past few years, adult studies have strived to assess patient outcomes based on different "early *vs.* late" timing strategies, with conflicting results [34, 35]. The declination of early or late initiation has usually been based on KDIGO AKI stage or a chronological time from ICU admission. As noted above, the pediatric literature has repeatedly demonstrated, albeit in observational and not randomized studies, that relative fluid accumulation of 10–20% of ICU admission weight at CRRT initiation is independently associated with patient mortality. This concept of worsening fluid overload prevention fits with the pediatric mindset of harm prevention in our daily practice (vaccinations, bicycle helmets, etc.). Research in this decade has aimed at identifying AKI risk before it develops either using integration of patient demographics and signs of kidney dysfunction or novel biomarkers to identify structural kidney injury prior to functional loss manifest by increased serum creatinine or oliguria.

### 1.4.1 AKI Risk Stratification Systems

As noted previously, early pediatric AKI studies assessed the epidemiology of AKI in children who developed AKI, but little prospective study had been undertaken to compare children with vs. without AKI to ascertain the relative contribution of potential risk factors to the development of AKI. Since cardiac surgery associated AKI incidence is high, a number of risk factors including underlying surgical complexity, cardiopulmonary bypass duration, and patient age have been realized as risk factors for AKI development [36, 37]. Based on these factors, recent studies have randomized patients deemed at risk to fluid management by diuretics or peritoneal dialysis [38].

Acute kidney injury risk assessment in the nonsurgical critical care setting is made more difficult as the timing of kidney insult is not known and the causes of AKI are multifactorial. Recently, two renal-specific risk stratification systems for the pediatric ICU have been described: Renal Angina Index (RAI) and the Fluid Overload and Kidney Injury Score (FOKIS). The RAI integrates patient demographics and changes in creatinine or fluid accumulation thresholds within the first 24 h of ICU admission to predict KDIGO Stage 2 or 3 AKI at day three of ICU admission. Multiple studies have shown that children who do not meet the threshold of a RAI score of 8 or higher have a very low likelihood of developing persistent AKI [3, 39, 40]. The power of this negative predictive value resides in directing attention to the minority of patients (10–20%) who "rule-in" with an RAI of 8 or greater. The FOKIS combines AKI severity, fluid overload status, and nephrotoxin exposure burden to provide a multidimensional AKI kidney status measure throughout the PICU course [2]. An increasing FOKIS was associated with patient PICU morbidity and mortality. While both the RAI and FOKIS need to be validated in larger cohorts, extraction of the data from the electronic medical record in real time should be able to provide the bedside clinician with actionable data upon which to assess risk of AKI development and AKI-related outcomes.

### 1.4.2 AKI Biomarkers

The past 15 years has witnessed a translational research revolution with respect to the discovery, validation, and application of novel AKI structural biomarkers. The field's reliance on the functional biomarkers of serum creatinine increase and oliguria has limited the ability to provide more than supportive care. Not only are creatinine increase and oliguria late markers of AKI, they provide little insight into the nature or AKI or the underlying mechanism of injury, whether it be ischemic, toxic, or in some cases protective. Novel AKI biomarkers, as with similar markers in cardiac or oncological disease, have the potential benefit of identifying the precise nature of the injury, its severity, and, with repeated assessment, the time course. The seminal study demonstrating the potential utility of structural AKI biomarkers was undertaken in infants undergoing cardiac surgery [41]. In this study, 71 infants had serial assessments of urinary neutrophil gelatinase associated lipocalin (NGAL) starting at 2 h after initiation of cardiopulmonary bypass. Urinary NGAL was significantly elevated at 2 h in patients who developed serum creatinine-based AKI 36–48 h later, highlighting the potential for a therapeutic window between structural injury and kidney function change. Subsequent single-center study demonstrated the ability of NGAL and other novel markers (interleukin-18, kidney injury molecule-1, and liver-type fatty acid-binding protein) to predict not only AKI development prior to serum creatinine increase but also AKI severity [36]. In addition, another single-center study evaluated combination of NGAL and the functional marker Cystatin C to demonstrate the ability of these two markers to predict prolonged AKI (elevated NGAL/normal Cystatin C) versus rapidly reversible AKI (normal NGAL/elevated Cystatin C) [42]. Finally, the elevated cell cycle arrest AKI biomarker combination tissue inhibitor metalloproteinase-2/insulin-like growth factor binding protein-7 were integrated into clinical decision support in the adult cardiac surgery setting, directing an AKI bundle that led to reductions in AKI development and severity [43]. Taken together, these studies provide encouragement that we may be able to provide more personalized and directed care to improve outcomes for patients with or at-risk acute kidney injury.

## 1.5 A Vision for the Future of Pediatric AKI Research

The evolution of AKI research delineated in this chapter reflects a transformation in the mindset of the critical care nephrology community that AKI is an inevitable, non-modifiable, and unimportant consequence of caring for the critically ill patient. The strong and independent associations between AKI development, severity, and patient morbidity and mortality across the entire spectrum of pediatric critical illness is irrefutable. The potential to identify and stratify at-risk patients reliably, albeit imperfectly, provides the opportunity to focus diagnostic and therapeutic resources on patients who will benefit the most. The novel AKI biomarkers described briefly here and at length in the remainder of this textbook should not be used in isolation but rather integrated into the clinical decision support to improve prediction of risk and outcomes. Furthermore, we should listen to the mechanistic plausibility that each of these biomarkers provides for kidney injury, and use that understanding to develop therapeutic modalities to prevent or mitigate the effects of AKI. As in the fields of cardiology and oncology, we should not expect perfection from our risk stratification systems and biomarkers, but use them to improve our clinical practice even if only incrementally. If we take on this challenge, the time for nihilism will be over. Now, let's get to work.

## References


1. Sutherland SM, Byrnes JJ, Kothari M, Longhurst CA, Dutta S, Garcia P, et al. AKI in hospitalized children: comparing the pRIFLE, AKIN, and KDIGO definitions. Clin J Am Soc Nephrol. 2015;10(4):554–61.
2. Akcan-Arikan A, Gebhard DJ, Arnold MA, Loftis LL, Kennedy CE. Fluid overload and kidney injury score: a multidimensional real-time assessment of renal disease burden in the critically ill patient. Pediatr Crit Care Med. 2017;18(6):524–30.
3. Basu RK, Zappitelli M, Brunner L, Wang Y, Wong HR, Chawla LS, et al. Derivation and validation of the renal angina index to improve the prediction of acute kidney injury in critically ill children. Kidney Int. 2014;85(3):659–67.
4. Alge JL, Arthur JM. Biomarkers of AKI: a review of mechanistic relevance and potential therapeutic implications. Clin J Am Soc Nephrol. 2015;10(1):147–55.
5. Sutherland SM, Goldstein SL, Alexander SR. The prospective pediatric continuous renal replacement therapy (ppCRRT) registry: a critical appraisal. Pediatr Nephrol. 2014;29(11):2069–76.
6. Bunchman TE, McBryde KD, Mottes TE, Gardner JJ, Maxvold NJ, Brophy PD. Pediatric acute renal failure: outcome by modality and disease. Pediatr Nephrol. 2001;16(12):1067–71.
7. Ronco C, Garzotto F, Brendolan A, Zanella M, Bellettato M, Vedovato S, et al. Continuous renal replacement therapy in neonates and small infants: development and first-in-human use of a miniaturised machine (CARPEDIEM). Lancet. 2014;383(9931):1807–13.
8. Coulthard MG, Crosier J, Griffiths C, Smith J, Drinnan M, Whitaker M, et al. Haemodialysing babies weighing <8 kg with the Newcastle infant dialysis and ultrafiltration system (Nidus): comparison with peritoneal and conventional haemodialysis. Pediatr Nephrol. 2014;29(10):1873–81.
9. Goldstein SL, Currier H, Graf C, Cosio CC, Brewer ED, Sachdeva R. Outcome in children receiving continuous venovenous hemofiltration. Pediatrics. 2001;107(6):1309–12.
10. Symons JM, Chua AN, Somers MJ, Baum MA, Bunchman TE, Benfield MR, et al. Demographic characteristics of pediatric continuous renal replacement therapy: a report of the prospective pediatric continuous renal replacement therapy registry. Clin J Am Soc Nephrol. 2007;2(4):732–8.
11. Gillespie RS, Seidel K, Symons JM. Effect of fluid overload and dose of replacement fluid on survival in hemofiltration. Pediatr Nephrol. 2004;19(12):1394–9.
12. Foland JA, Fortenberry JD, Warshaw BL, Pettignano R, Merritt RK, Heard ML, et al. Fluid overload before continuous hemofiltration and survival in critically ill children: a retrospective analysis. Crit Care Med. 2004;32(8):1771–6.
13. Goldstein SL, Somers MJ, Brophy PD, Bunchman TE, Baum M, Blowey D, et al. The prospective pediatric continuous renal replacement therapy (ppCRRT) registry: design, development and data assessed. Int J Artif Organs. 2004;27(1):9–14.

14. Kellum JA, Angus DC. Patients are dying of acute renal failure. Crit Care Med. 2002;30(9):2156–7.
15. Chertow GM, Burdick E, Honour M, Bonventre JV, Bates DW. Acute kidney injury, mortality, length of stay, and costs in hospitalized patients. J Am Soc Nephrol. 2005;16(11):3365–70.
16. Bellomo R, Ronco C, Kellum JA, Mehta RL, Palevsky P. Acute renal failure – definition, outcome measures, animal models, fluid therapy and information technology needs: the second international consensus conference of the acute Dialysis quality initiative (ADQI) group. Crit Care. 2004;8(4):R204–12.
17. Mehta RL, Kellum JA, Shah SV, Molitoris BA, Ronco C, Warnock DG, et al. Acute kidney injury network: report of an initiative to improve outcomes in acute kidney injury. Crit Care. 2007;11(2):R31.
18. Kidney Disease: Improving Global Outcomes (KDIGO) Acute Kidney Injury Work Group. KDIGO clinical practice guideline for acute kidney injury. Kidney Int. 2012;2(Suppl 1):1–138.
19. Uchino S, Kellum JA, Bellomo R, Doig GS, Morimatsu H, Morgera S, et al. Acute renal failure in critically ill patients: a multinational, multicenter study. JAMA. 2005;294(7):813–8.
20. Hui-Stickle S, Brewer ED, Goldstein SL. Pediatric ARF epidemiology at a tertiary care center from 1999 to 2001. Am J Kidney Dis. 2005;45(1):96–101.
21. Vachvanichsanong P, Dissaneewate P, Lim A, McNeil E. Childhood acute renal failure: 22-year experience in a university hospital in southern Thailand. Pediatrics. 2006;118(3):e786–91.
22. Moghal NE, Brocklebank JT, Meadow SR. A review of acute renal failure in children: incidence, etiology and outcome. Clin Nephrol. 1998;49(2):91–5.
23. Akcan-Arikan A, Zappitelli M, Loftis LL, Washburn KK, Jefferson LS, Goldstein SL. Modified RIFLE criteria in critically ill children with acute kidney injury. Kidney Int. 2007;71(10):1028–35.
24. Plotz FB, Bouma AB, van Wijk JA, Kneyber MC, Bokenkamp A. Pediatric acute kidney injury in the ICU: an independent evaluation of pRIFLE criteria. Intensive Care Med. 2008;34(9):1713–7.
25. Slater MB, Anand V, Uleryk EM, Parshuram CS. A systematic review of RIFLE criteria in children, and its application and association with measures of mortality and morbidity. Kidney Int. 2012;81(8):791–8.
26. Basu RK, Kaddourah A, Terrell T, Mottes T, Arnold P, Jacobs J, et al. Assessment of worldwide acute kidney injury, renal angina and epidemiology in critically ill children (AWARE): study protocol for a prospective observational study. BMC Nephrol. 2015;16:24.
27. Kaddourah A, Basu RK, Bagshaw SM, Goldstein SL, Investigators A. Epidemiology of acute kidney injury in critically ill children and young adults. N Engl J Med. 2017;376(1):11–20.
28. Askenazi DJ, Ambalavanan N, Goldstein SL. Acute kidney injury in critically ill newborns: what do we know? What do we need to learn? Pediatr Nephrol. 2009;24(2):265–74.
29. Jetton JG, Guillet R, Askenazi DJ, Dill L, Jacobs J, Kent AL, et al. Assessment of worldwide acute kidney injury epidemiology in neonates: design of a Retrospective Cohort Study. Front Pediatr. 2016;4:68.
30. Jetton JG, Boohaker LJ, Sethi SK, Wazir S, Rohatgi S, Soranno DE, et al. Incidence and outcomes of neonatal acute kidney injury (AWAKEN): a multicentre, multinational, observational cohort study. Lancet Child Adolesc Health. 2017;1(3):184–94.
31. Blinder JJ, Goldstein SL, Lee VV, Baycroft A, Fraser CD, Nelson D, et al. Congenital heart surgery in infants: effects of acute kidney injury on outcomes. J Thorac Cardiovasc Surg. 2012;143(2):368–74.
32. Chiravuri SD, Riegger LQ, Christensen R, Butler RR, Malviya S, Tait AR, et al. Factors associated with acute kidney injury or failure in children undergoing cardiopulmonary bypass: a case-controlled study. Paediatr Anaesth. 2011;21(8):880–6.
33. Toth R, Breuer T, Cserep Z, Lex D, Fazekas L, Sapi E, et al. Acute kidney injury is associated with higher morbidity and resource utilization in pediatric patients undergoing heart surgery. Ann Thorac Surg. 2012;93(6):1984–90.
34. Zarbock A, Kellum JA, Schmidt C, Van Aken H, Wempe C, Pavenstadt H, et al. Effect of early vs delayed initiation of renal replacement therapy on mortality in critically ill patients with acute kidney injury: the ELAIN randomized clinical trial. JAMA. 2016;315(20):2190–9.

35. Gaudry S, Hajage D, Schortgen F, Martin-Lefevre L, Pons B, Boulet E, et al. Initiation strategies for renal-replacement therapy in the intensive care unit. N Engl J Med. 2016;375(2):122–33.
36. Krawczeski CD, Goldstein SL, Woo JG, Wang Y, Piyaphanee N, Ma Q, et al. Temporal relationship and predictive value of urinary acute kidney injury biomarkers after pediatric cardiopulmonary bypass. J Am Coll Cardiol. 2011;58(22):2301–9.
37. Kwiatkowski DM, Menon S, Krawczeski CD, Goldstein SL, Morales DL, Phillips A, et al. Improved outcomes with peritoneal dialysis catheter placement after cardiopulmonary bypass in infants. J Thorac Cardiovasc Surg. 2015;149(1):230–6.
38. Kwiatkowski DM, Goldstein SL, Cooper DS, Nelson DP, Morales DL, Krawczeski CD. Peritoneal Dialysis vs furosemide for prevention of fluid overload in infants after cardiac surgery: a randomized clinical trial. JAMA Pediatr. 2017;171(4):357–64.
39. Menon S, Goldstein SL, Mottes T, Fei L, Kaddourah A, Terrell T, et al. Urinary biomarker incorporation into the renal angina index early in intensive care unit admission optimizes acute kidney injury prediction in critically ill children: a prospective cohort study. Nephrol Dial Transplant. 2016;31(4):586–94.
40. Basu RK, Wang Y, Wong HR, Chawla LS, Wheeler DS, Goldstein SL. Incorporation of biomarkers with the renal angina index for prediction of severe AKI in critically ill children. Clin J Am Soc Nephrol. 2014;9(4):654–62.
41. Mishra J, Dent C, Tarabishi R, Mitsnefes MM, Ma Q, Kelly C, et al. Neutrophil gelatinase-associated lipocalin (NGAL) as a biomarker for acute renal injury after cardiac surgery. Lancet. 2005;365(9466):1231–8.
42. Basu RK, Wong HR, Krawczeski CD, Wheeler DS, Manning PB, Chawla LS, et al. Combining functional and tubular damage biomarkers improves diagnostic precision for acute kidney injury after cardiac surgery. J Am Coll Cardiol. 2014;64(25):2753–62.
43. Meersch M, Schmidt C, Hoffmeier A, Van Aken H, Wempe C, Gerss J, et al. Prevention of cardiac surgery-associated AKI by implementing the KDIGO guidelines in high risk patients identified by biomarkers: the PrevAKI randomized controlled trial. Intensive Care Med. 2017;43(11):1551–61.

# 2 Renal Function Monitoring in a Critically Sick Patient

Heather Lambert and Daljit Hothi

## 2.1 Introduction

Acute kidney insufficiency/injury (AKI) describes renal dysfunction from a wide spectrum of causes. AKI is increasingly common in children who are critically unwell, as survival from serious illness and major surgery, especially cardiac, improves. It is important to identify those at particularly high risk as there may be no clinical symptoms or signs of early AKI developing. Early recognition of deteriorating renal function may aid identification of underlying causes and enable prompt changes in management to avert or minimize AKI. Outcomes for children in paediatric intensive care (PICU) are worse in those with AKI [1] and particularly in those who require renal replacement therapy [2, 3] but even small changes in kidney function may represent significant renal damage and impact morbidity and mortality [4, 5]. Fluid overload is independently associated with poorer survival [6–9].

There is a greatly increased risk of chronic kidney disease in those who have had an episode of AKI even if there is recovery from the acute episode [10–12]. Thus, understanding renal function and interpretation of monitoring in the critically sick patient are central to improving outcomes in the short and long term, and failure to recognize AKI early and optimally intervene or alter management may contribute to significant kidney damage.

The incidence of AKI in critically ill children is high [13] but rates from different studies reflect different criteria used and different populations included. A large multinational prospective study [3] evaluated a total of 4683 patients

H. Lambert (✉)
The Great North Children's Hospital, Newcastle upon Tyne, UK
e-mail: heather.lambert@newcastle.ac.uk

D. Hothi
Great Ormond Street Hospital for Children, London, UK



A. Deep, S. L. Goldstein (eds.), *Critical Care Nephrology and Renal Replacement Therapy in Children*, https://doi.org/10.1007/978-3-319-90281-4_2

admitted to PICU; AKI developed in 1261 patients (27%), and severe AKI in 12%. Risk of death increased with severity of AKI. Outcomes are worse in children under 10 kg who receive renal replacement therapy [2]. AKI is associated with multi-organ failure, following cardiac and other major surgery [14, 15] and with sepsis [16]. Renal failure is most frequently secondary but in a small number of cases it is related to intrinsic renal disease as in acute glomerulonephritis and haemolytic uraemic syndrome (HUS), or to post-renal obstruction associated with congenital abnormalities like posterior urethral valves or neuropathic bladder. It is important that intrinsic nephro-urological disease is not overlooked as specific treatments may be possible. Patients, particularly those with other congenital conditions, may have underlying renal abnormalities that have been undiagnosed or undetected because they have not yet caused measurable changes in renal function. Even those with normal structural imaging and a normal plasma creatinine may have diminished renal reserve. In these patients, even mild kidney insults may precipitate profound changes in renal function.

Thus, predicting those at high risk of AKI, from taking a careful history and assiduous renal monitoring, is essential to detect development and progression of renal failure and to look for modifiable factors and underlying causes. The Renal Angina Index, a clinical scoring system, has been proposed to help stratification of risk [17, 18]. Multiple biomarkers have been studied but none have been clearly identified as reliable early predictors of AKI [19] Serum creatinine is a late marker of reduced glomerular filtration rate (GFR) rising only when 25–50% of GFR is lost. Various formulae exist for calculating GFR from serum creatinine but all are dependent on steady-state filtration and thus are much less useful in a rapidly changing situation. Formal GFR measurement using isotope or inulin clearance methods is not practically useful in intensive care.

## 2.2 Normal Kidney Function

Normal kidneys can be thought of as providing four main functions—glomerular function, tubular reabsorption, tubular secretion and urine excretion—which maintain homeostasis of fluids and electrolytes in the blood within a very narrow range despite wildly varying intake and production, by excreting or reabsorbing excessive fluid or solutes. Acid–base balance is maintained by several buffering systems with the kidney excreting excess bicarbonate or hydrogen ions to maintain stability. Thus, when the kidney sustains injury or insult, a wide array of biochemical and fluid derangements can result. The kidney has a role in maintaining blood pressure and AKI can result in hypertension which could be hormonally driven or resulting from salt and water retention. The kidney in addition has a significant role in regulating bone biochemistry, and producing erythropoietin; these have increasing importance if the renal impairment persists over a prolonged period. Even in an acute intensive care situation once renal failure has persisted for more than a week or two, the monitoring and management of chronic renal disease needs to be undertaken, closely with the nephrology team.

### 2.2.1 Glomerular Filtration Rate and Clearance

Glomerular filtration rate (GFR) is the volume of fluid filtered from the glomerular capillaries into the Bowman's capsule per unit time and represents the cumulative performance of all functioning nephrons. GFR is the most reliable marker of functioning renal mass but is influenced by age, sex, height and weight, as well as time of day, protein intake, pregnancy, extracellular fluid status, blood pressure extremes, and use of antihypertensive drugs. GFR cannot be measured directly. The most common method is based on the concept of clearance:

The renal clearance of substance $x$ ($C_x$) is calculated as:

$$C_X = U_X V / P_X$$

$V$ is the urine flow rate (mL/min)
$U_X$ is urine concentration of substance $x$
$P_X$ is the plasma concentration of substance $x$

If the substance is freely permeable across the glomerular capillary and is not synthesized, transported, or metabolized by the kidney, $C_X$ is equal to GFR.

Significant growth and developmental changes in childhood influence measurement of GFR. In a term baby at birth all nephrons are terminally differentiated, but only the juxtamedullary glomeruli are fully used. The term neonate has a GFR as low as 20 mL/min/1.73 $m^2$. Additionally, due to immature tubular function, neonates have reduced concentrating capacity, and reduced ability to conserve sodium and they are prone to dehydration and hyponatremia. Nephrogenesis is not complete until 35–36 weeks' gestation, so preterm babies born before this have incomplete nephron development. There is continuous development and maturation of glomerular and tubular function until around 18–24 months of age, but the kidney of a young child remains particularly vulnerable to injury and insult.

Growth spurts during the first year of life and during puberty are associated with rapid increase of muscle mass which have significant impact on plasma creatinine and GFR estimation. Measuring GFR by renal clearance of creatinine (or other substance) requires timed urine collection and thus is practically challenging in uncatheterized children, not toilet trained or with incomplete bladder emptying.

The ideal substance for measuring GFR is freely filtered at the glomeruli, neither secreted nor reabsorbed by the renal tubules. Renal clearance of *inulin* remains the gold standard in children and adults. Inulin is not protein bound, freely filtered by the glomerulus and not secreted, metabolized, or reabsorbed by the renal tubules. However, the need for continuous infusion and multiple blood and urine samples makes it difficult and time consuming. Alternative exogenous markers include $^{51}$Cr EDTA, $^{99m}$Tc-DTPA radioisotopes, and iohexol. None of these are useful in acute intensive care. Clearance of aminoglycoside can be used to measure GFR in an acute situation [20].

### 2.2.2 Estimated GFR (eGFR)

Creatinine is derived from creatine and phosphocreatine in the muscle, is freely filtered, not reabsorbed or metabolized but there is significant proximal tubular secretion which increases with lower GFR. Proximal tubular creatinine secretion equates to 10–20% of the excreted load and can reach up to 50% when GFR is reduced, resulting in overestimation of GFR. Age and muscle mass dependency of serum creatinine creates challenges in measuring GFR in children with co-morbidities like spina bifida, neuromuscular disease, anorexia nervosa, mitochondrial disease and liver cirrhosis.

### 2.2.3 Specific eGFR Challenges in PICU

Serum creatinine is not in a steady state in critically ill children admitted to the PICU. A positive fluid balance and increased volume of distribution dilutes serum creatinine concentration and may delay diagnosis of AKI. Rapidly fluctuating renal haemodynamics may cause changes in GFR and serum creatinine. A low protein/meat intake results in a lower plasma creatinine. There may be interference with serum creatinine from a variety of causes including inhibition of secretion by the renal tubule, for example, by trimethoprim, and interference with standardized assays from substances such as ketones. Though extra-renal excretion through degradation of creatinine by bacterial overgrowth in the gut is minimal in people with normal kidney function, it is increased in those with reduced renal function. Broad spectrum antibiotics may alter gut flora.

In children, a number of different formulae exist for estimating GFR.

The *Schwartz* formula is most commonly used clinically.

$$\text{eGFR} = k \times L / S_{\text{cr}}$$

$L$ is height in cms
$S_{\text{cr}}$ is serum creatinine
$k$ is an empirical constant

The *Cockroft–Gault equation* gives an appropriate estimate of creatinine clearance in children >12 years of age.

*Modification of Diet in Renal Disease* (MDRD) formula widely used in adults is more accurate than Cockroft–Gault equation but grossly inaccurate in children and underestimates GFR.

*The CKD-Epidemiology Collaboration* equation performs better than MDRD especially at GFR above 60 mL/min per 1.73 $m^2$.

However, in PICU where there is no steady state, these calculations are particularly inaccurate.

Aminoglycoside clearance can provide an estimation of renal function and may give a better estimate of creatinine clearance in some situations [20].

### 2.2.4 Cystatin C

Cystatin C is a non-glycosylated protein produced by all nucleated cells. It is freely filtered, reabsorbed and completely metabolized in tubular cells.

However, cystatin C only offers an estimation of GFR as it is catabolized and almost completely reabsorbed by renal proximal tubular cells. Cystatin C has a more stable rate of production and eGFR from cystatin C is less influenced by race and ethnicity than eGFR calculated from serum creatinine. Serum cystatin C levels are also influenced by non-GFR determinants—uncontrolled thyroid disease, corticosteroid use, age, sex and adipose tissue. In chronic kidney disease, eGFR by combining cystatin C, creatinine and demographic-based formulas have been proposed [e.g. CKiD study].

Cystatin C has 1/3rd the volume of distribution of creatinine and reaches a new steady state three times faster than creatinine. An increase in plasma cystatin C precedes plasma creatinine and subtle decrements in GFR may be more readily detected by changes in serum cystatin C than by serum creatinine partly due to the shorter half-life of cystatin C. However, the effect of acute illnesses on cystatin C production rate is unknown, there is considerable variation among cystatin C assays and it is more costly than serum creatinine measurements.

## 2.3 Acute Kidney Injury

There are no specific symptoms or signs of AKI, which may produce high urine output or low urine output renal failure and resultant fluid overload and hypertension if fluid intake cannot be reduced sufficiently. Biochemical disturbance may rapidly evolve—hyperkalaemia and resultant cardiac dysrhythmias may require urgent treatment; hypocalcaemia may affect myocardial contractility or precipitate fitting and there may be metabolic acidosis.

A rising plasma creatinine is a late marker of poor glomerular function but is not intrinsically harmful whereas a high plasma urea can cause nausea and affect level of consciousness. Definitions and severity of AKI are discussed in a subsequent chapter. There is no absolute consensus but the pRIFLE and KDIGO definitions are widely used and are dependent on finding a significantly increasing plasma creatinine, or oliguria of 0.5 or 1 mL/kg hourly. There are inherent issues with serum creatinine which have been described before. In addition, many children have not had a baseline plasma creatinine measured before they become ill, and there is considerable variation in baseline as it is related to age, sex and muscle mass, so rise from baseline is difficult to calculate.

KDIGO staging of AKI

| Stage | Serum creatinine | Urine output |
|---|---|---|
| 1. | 1.5–1.9 times baseline, OR<br>≥0.3 mg/dL (≥26.5 mol/L) increase | <0.5 mL/kg/h for 6–12 h |
| 2. | 1.0–2.9 times baseline | <0.5 mL/kg/h for ≥12 h |

| KDIGO staging of AKI | | |
|---|---|---|
| Stage | Serum creatinine | Urine output |
| 3. | 3.0 times baseline, OR<br>$S_{cr}$ ≥4.0 mg/dL (≥353.6 μmol/L), OR<br>Initiation of renal replacement therapy, OR<br>eGFR <35 mL/min per 1.73 m$^2$ (<18 years) | <0.3 mL/kg/h for ≥24 h<br>OR<br>Anuria for ≥12 h |

### 2.3.1 Early Recognition of AKI May Aid Early Intervention

It can be useful in monitoring to think of AKI as belonging to one of the three categories: Functional (previously termed as pre-renal), intrinsic or established and post-renal AKI.

*Functional AKI*—essentially a reversible renal dysfunction due to the kidneys being underperfused, in which there has not yet been structural changes within the renal tissue. Hypotension or lack of fluid in the vascular compartment leads to decreased renal blood flow. Renal autoregulation preserves glomerular filtration rate by increased renal sympathetic tone, activation of the renin-angiotensin-aldosterone system and hormones like vasopressin and endothelin which enhance proximal tubular sodium and water reabsorption, decreasing sodium and water loss and maintaining intravascular volume and blood pressure. Interventions to increase intravascular volume, e.g. fluid or albumin infusion, at this stage may be effective.

Any urine passed should be sent for biochemistry and if furosemide has not yet been given, the fractional excretion of sodium (FENa) is typically very low, indicating that the tubules are still functioning and able to respond by reabsorbing sodium avidly.

*In established AKI*, there is acute parenchymal damage to the kidneys. This may be secondary to hypoperfusion and involve the tubules in which case renal recovery may take place. But if there is more parenchymal and glomerular involvement, irreversible cortical necrosis may occur. Distinguishing between these and prognosticating whether recovery will take place is only really possible by renal biopsy which is seldom indicated in this situation as it is unlikely to change management in the acute phase. If renal tubules are damaged, then their ability to reabsorb sodium will be impaired and FENa will rise (>3%).

Whilst most children in critical care will have underlying normal kidneys, some will be receiving critical care because of their kidney failure, for example, in those with acute glomerulonephritis or haemolytic uraemic syndrome (HUS). A blood count and film should always be performed. Renal failure may be part of multisystem disease such as in SLE or disseminated angiopathies as described in subsequent chapters. Monitoring of those patients should follow the same principles but close collaboration with nephrologists and other specialist teams is essential. Renal biopsy may be indicated if clinically there is an active glomerulonephritis or nephrotic syndrome. Specific and effective therapies may be available.

*Post-renal* causes are due to obstruction of the urinary flow, and are less commonly seen in intensive care. Causes include renal stones, tumours and congenital abnormalities such as posterior urethral valve which may present late. It is important that these diagnoses are not missed as there are potential treatments.

## 2.4 Assessment and Monitoring of Renal Function

Good monitoring of renal function starts with the history and examination of the patient and charts. The purpose is to identify risk of AKI, underlying causes and ongoing factors with the aim of changing the course and preventing secondary insults.

### 2.4.1 Review of clinical history

This is to establish a history of potential renal insults—hypotension in theatre, bleeding, systemic insults, severe sepsis with evidence of multi-organ failure. These insults may have been "one-off" as in perioperative events or may be continuing as in hypotension or poor vascular filling. There may be a history of preexisting renal disease or associated conditions like rash or joint problems. It is not uncommon for children with congenital abnormalities to require intensive care and the incidence of renal anomalies is much higher in this population and this makes them at higher risk of AKI or acute on chronic renal failure.

### 2.4.2 Clinical examination

Clinical examination is important looking for rash, oedema, joint swelling, abdominal masses, bladder, bruits, uveitis as well as for assessing fluid status.

### 2.4.3 Review of medication

Review of medication for possible nephrotoxic drugs—commonly non-steroidal anti-inflammatory drugs, antibiotics or antifungals, but also immunosuppressants like tacrolimus, cyclosporine, and ACE inhibitors. Non-prescription drugs containing ibuprofen are frequently overlooked.

Assessment of renal function is also important to ensure appropriate dose change—often dose reduction or inter-dose interval increase, to ensure sufficient levels for efficacy whilst avoiding toxicity, is required.

### 2.4.4 Clinical Observations

Fluid and volume status assessment is key to understanding and appropriately managing AKI. Intravascular hypovolaemia is implicated in many cases of AKI and close monitoring is vital. Considering fluid in intra- and extra-vascular compartments may help in assessment.

(a) *Weight.* Assessment of weight is a useful starting point in assessing fluid overload—ideally compared with a previous clinic or community weight for new presentations but daily weight trends in PICU are also important for ongoing fluid status estimation.

(b) *Circulating blood volume.* Vital signs such as arterial blood pressure and CVP monitoring contribute to monitoring fluid and intravascular volume status. With all the associated fallacies of CVP, direct measurement of central venous pressure both in absolute terms and in trends can give a useful information on the fluid overload status. Clinical examination for peripheral temperature and capillary refill time is a useful skill particularly when repeated over a period of time whilst awaiting invasive monitoring or in the less unwell patient. Ideally in the sickest patients there should also be invasive monitoring for arterial blood pressure. Non-invasive cardiac output monitoring is gaining importance in intensive care units to measure important haemodynamic variables which might influence AKI.

(c) *Fluid balance.* Hourly accurate fluid intake and output recording is essential.

*Fluids in*

These will comprise intravenous fluids prescribed as well as enteral fluids and feeds. Non-prescribed fluids such as those given with and after medications are frequently overlooked in the intake assessment: for example, saline flushes with drug administration, central venous line (CVL) and arterial line flushes, enteral tube flushes—collectively these can contribute significant intake in small infants and should be recorded.

*Fluids out*

Losses need carefully monitoring with weighing of nappies or even bedding used to improve accuracy of estimations. Gut losses: vomit, tube aspirates, stool, and diarrhoea losses should be included.

For accurate measurement of urine output the patient should have a bladder catheterization, though weighing nappies can give good estimation in uncatheterized patients. Oliguria is defined as less than 0.5 mL/kg/h and anuria as <1 mL/kg/24 h.

Drain and other losses, for example, oozing wounds, need inclusion.

Insensible losses should be estimated—these will be higher when there is fever or in neonates receiving phototherapy.

### 2.4.5 Laboratory tests

Plasma biochemistry requires regular monitoring and should include sodium, potassium, chloride, bicarbonate, urea, creatinine, liver function tests, plasma protein and albumin, bone biochemistry, calcium phosphate, magnesium and glucose. Full blood count and film and clotting. Urinalysis, urine biochemistry (sodium, potassium, urea and creatinine), urine albumin or protein-to-creatinine ratio. Other tests will be indicated by the clinical picture such as blood cultures, clotting, complement C3 and C4, immunoglobulins and autoantibody screen.

Hyperkalaemia is common in AKI and is a potentially life-threatening electrolyte disturbance. A rising or elevated plasma potassium should be monitored frequently as hyperkalaemia has a depolarizing effect on cardiac conduction pathways and thus may produce disturbances of cardiac rhythm, with tall peaked T waves on ECG being an early sign. Cardiac effects are exacerbated by disturbances in acid–base balance and in the presence of hypocalcaemia.

Timely and repeated measurement of serum creatinine, recognition of normal ranges and its relationship to muscle mass and comparison to premorbid measurements are useful. However, serum creatinine is not a very sensitive measure of renal function nor a guide to impairment as >50% glomerular function may need to be lost for a rise in plasma creatinine. Calculations and equations to estimate GFR are also not very useful as they are dependent on a steady-state situation which is seldom the case in PICU. Estimating GFR is particularly challenging in extremes of body size, where muscles mass is abnormal (e.g., in mitochondrial disease), in neonates, where there is severe malnutrition (e.g. in liver cirrhosis), and where there is particularly high or low dietary creatinine intake.

However repeated measurements of plasma creatinine are useful to determine trends, plotting plasma creatinine (ideally on a logarithmic scale because doubling of creatinine is important rather than actual rise) is also of use in monitoring rate of decline of renal function. At lower GFR serum creatinine will lead to overestimation of renal function because of tubular secretion of creatinine. In neonates, serum creatinine reflects maternal renal function and rate of improvement is variable and influenced by gestational age. There are differences related to methods of creatinine measurement, which is particularly important when patients are referred from one centre to another. The enzymatic assay is most reliable and reproducible. Once dialysis has started, then some creatinine is removed and it no longer reflects renal function, but paired with dialysate can be useful to monitor efficiency and "dose" of dialysis.

Plasma albumin gives an indication of intravascular oncotic pressure and if low, investigations to determine if that is due to losses (as in nephrotic syndrome) or lack of production (as in liver disease) or related to poor nutrition should be carried out. A low plasma albumin is frequently accompanied by generalized oedema. Diuresis can sometimes be induced by careful infusion of albumin together with diuretic use.

Metabolic acidosis is common as production of acid may be increased in sepsis and shock but excretion is impaired when renal function is poor and there is impaired reabsorption and regeneration of bicarbonate.

Patients may develop hyperphosphataemia due to impaired excretion and hypocalcaemia. These need monitoring and adjustments made to reduce intake of phosphate and supplement calcium when needed.

If urinalysis reveals proteinuria, this should be quantified by measuring urine protein or albumin-to-creatinine ratio.

#### 2.4.5.1 Interpretation of Laboratory Results

Interpretation of laboratory results should be done in association with examination of the patient and their vital observations. In critical care when the clinical state is seldom static and responses to interventions are being assessed, serial clinical assessment together with serial biochemical blood and urine analysis are required.

The distribution of water in the body between intracellular and extracellular compartments is largely determined by osmotic forces, potassium being the principle solute for intracellular volume, sodium for extracellular and plasma proteins for intravascular component. Cell membrane pump activity, molecular size and charge contribute to maintenance of the differential composition.

Thus clinically, a low plasma sodium does not necessarily indicate sodium deficiency. Low, normal or high plasma sodium may occur with expansion or depletion of extracellular fluid volume. Changes in plasma sodium need to be interpreted in association with assessment of extracellular fluid volume and particularly intravascular fluid status.

The clinical finding of oedema should be interpreted along with laboratory results. Peripheral oedema can result from loss of intravascular oncotic pressure when albumin is lost in the urine as in nephrotic syndrome or in pleural effusion or chylothorax when significant albumin may be lost via drain fluid.

#### 2.4.5.2 Use of Fractional Excretion of Sodium

If any urine is being produced, functional and established renal failure may be differentiated by the fractional excretion of sodium (FENa), calculated from the sodium and creatinine concentrations of a plasma (P) and untimed urine (U) sample:

$$\mathrm{FE_{Na}}\,\% = U/P \text{ sodium} \times P/U \text{ creatinine} \times 100$$

A low $FE_{Na}$ indicates tubules are still capable of active sodium reabsorption; in functional renal failure, the value is typically less than 3%. $FE_{Na}$ is only really helpful when it is very low as it is an indicator of intravascular hypovolaemia that may respond to measures to increase intravascular volume, e.g. fluid or albumin infusion. Once parenchymal changes and tubular necrosis have occurred, the $FE_{Na}$ reaches much higher values and diuretic treatment (typically furosemide) makes $FE_{Na}$ unreliable.

### 2.4.6 Imaging

A renal ultrasound should be done at an early stage when there are any concerns about renal function—it is suitable to perform at the bedside in critical care and gives useful information about the presence of two kidneys, parenchymal appearance, Doppler blood flow, hydronephrosis and evidence of upper or lower renal tract obstruction.

Ultrasound may also be used to look for ascites, pleural and pericardial effusions and lung fluid.

### 2.4.7 Other

An ECG or continuous cardiac monitoring should be done; arterial blood pressure, CVP, blood gasses, $O_2$ saturation, should be monitored.

**Renal function monitoring in critical care**
Strict hourly fluid in & out—especially urine output
Volume status—passive leg raising, fluid responsiveness, CVP, non-invasive or invasive cardiac output monitoring
Arterial BP
Weight
ECG

**Bloods**
Plasma sodium, potassium, chloride, bicarbonate, urea, creatinine, calcium (ideally ionized calcium), phosphate, magnesium, liver enzymes, protein, albumin.
Cystatin C
FBC and film
Coagulation screen
Blood gases pH and acid-base

**Urine**
Urinalysis for blood & protein
Urine sodium, potassium, creatinine and urea, osmolality, protein to creatinine ratio, albumin to creatinine ratio. (RBP?)
Urine microscopy for glomerular RBCs & casts in glomerulonephritis, organisms and WBC in infection, urine culture and sensitivity
Other fluid losses
Eg Drain or Paracentesis fluid—biochemistry and albumin content of fluid lost

**Imaging**
Renal US—presence of two kidneys, Doppler blood flows arterial and venous, hydronephrosis, intrinsic renal diease, congenital renal disease. Ascites. Bladder pathology
Lung US—fluid in lungs or CXR
Cardiac ECHO—congenital cardiac disease, pump failure

## 2.5 Monitoring During Renal Replacement Therapy

Nephrologists should be involved in discussion at an early stage when renal function is impaired. The main function of renal replacement therapy is to maintain the stability of biochemistry and fluid volume whilst avoiding further renal insults. For this reason, peritoneal dialysis or continuous haemofiltration and dialysis are better suited to the critical care setting than intermittent haemodialysis as the need for rapid removal of fluid sometimes result in hypotension and rapid changes in biochemistry add further insults to the recovering kidney. Recent innovations in development of haemodialysis and filtration devices for small babies like NIDUS [21] and CARPEDIEM [22] offer the potential to treat infants without causing further hypotensive renal insult and, though still under clinical evaluation, may improve outcomes. Dialysis prescription and fluid removal prescription are important and require close and repeated assessment of the patient, fluid status and consideration of compartment fluid volumes. For example, ordering removal of large volumes of fluid from an oedematous patient may lead to harmful periods of hypoperfusion and hypotension if the fluid is not in the intravascular space.

### 2.5.1 Nutrition

Nutrition is very important in critical care and is too often compromised when there is oliguric AKI as there are conflicting needs to provide nutrition in the face of fluid restriction [23]. A multidisciplinary approach is essential and the dietician and pharmacist play an important role in maximizing nutrition whilst controlling biochemistry particularly when renal function is changing/deteriorating. The aim should be to provide the child with their normal calorie intake, whilst restricting fluids to minimize fluid overload and protein intake to around 1 g/kg/ day to minimize uraemia. Repeated biochemical monitoring and forward planning are required especially when individualized parenteral or enteral feeding prescriptions are required. Sometimes the need to provide adequate nutrition is the main indication for instituting dialysis or filtration. Nutritional requirements during AKI and whilst on renal replacement therapy are discussed in detail in a subsequent chapter.

### 2.5.2 Monitoring Renal Function in Recovery and Beyond PICU

Recovery from AKI may sometimes result in a period of diuresis, high urine output, poor tubular function and poor urinary concentration. This needs to be carefully monitored and appropriate changes made to fluids and electrolyte input to ensure adequate replacement.

Independence from renal replacement therapy is clearly not equivalent to normal renal function and plasma creatinine and biochemistry should be monitored longer term as renal recovery can continue for many months. Monitoring of ongoing phosphate and calcium as well as bicarbonate disturbance is important. It is not uncommon to find patients who have had severe renal impairment requiring some chronic renal management during a prolonged recovery phase. This may include use of therapies such as dietary restrictions, phosphate binders, calcium and vitamin D supplementation as well as erythropoietin. Joined up working with the clinical nephrology team is essential. What is less commonly recognized is that having a normal plasma creatinine does not equate to normal renal function and there is increasing recognition of post AKI chronic renal insufficiency [18].

There is a need to establish a prospective registry and long-term follow-up of PICU patients who have had significant AKI and particularly in those who required renal replacement therapy.

**Key Learning Points**

**Aims of renal function monitoring**

**Early awareness**

**Aim to avoid AKI**

- Identify high-risk patients
- Monitor renal function, risk stratification and use of biomarkers
- Early intervention—remove or modify contributing factors
- Early discussion with nephrology specialists

**Maintain intravascular blood volume and renal perfusion**

- Assessment of volume status
- Fluid challenge then monitor response: tailor intake to response and urine output
- Avoid overzealous fluid administration leading to fluid overload
- Manage blood pressure actively by supporting or reducing to optimize renal perfusion

**Prevent ongoing renal injury**

- **Avoid/Remove** nephrotoxic agents—non-steroidals; antibiotics, ACEi, calcineurin inhibitors, etc.
- Adjust dosage of drugs according to renal function to enable adequate therapeutic levels but minimize toxicity
- Maintain appropriate BP and renal perfusion

**The next stage**

- Make decisions regarding timing and need for renal replacement interventions.
- Long-term monitoring and follow-up

***Seek opportunity to modify the course of AKI***

## References


1. Alkandari O, Eddington KA, Hyder A, et al. Acute kidney injury is an independent risk factor for pediatric intensive care unit mortality, longer length of stay and prolonged mechanical ventilation in critically ill children: a two-center retrospective cohort study. Crit Care. 2011;15:R146.
2. Askenazi DJ, Goldstein SL, Koralkar R, Fortenberry J, Baum M, Hackbarth R, Blowey D, Bunchman T, Brophy PD, Symons J, Chua A, Flores F, Somers MJD. 2013 Continuous renal replacement therapy for children ≤10 kg: a report from the prospective pediatric continuous renal replacement therapy registry. J Pediatr. 2013;162:587–92.

3. Kaddourah A, Basu RK, Bagshaw SM, Goldstein SL, AWARE investigators. Epidemiology of acute kidney injury in critically ill children and young adults. N Engl J Med. 2017;376(1):11–20.
4. Zappitelli M, Bernier P-L, Saczkowski RS, et al. A small post-operative rise in serum creatinine predicts acute kidney injury in children undergoing cardiac surgery. Kidney Int. 2009;76:885–92.
5. Slater MB, Anand V, Uleryk EM, Parshuram CS. A systematic review of RIFLE criteria in children, and its application and association with measures of mortality and morbidity. Kidney Int. 2012;81(8):791–8. https://doi.org/10.1038/ki.2011.466. Epub 2012 Jan 18
6. Gillespie RS, et al. Effect of fluid overload and dose of replacement fluid on survival in hemofiltration. Pediatr Nephrol. 2004;19:1394–9.
7. Hayes LW, Oster RA, Tofil NM, Tolwani AJ. Outcomes of critically ill children requiring continuous renal replacement therapy. J Crit Care. 2009;2009:394–400.
8. Foland JA, Fortenberry JD, Warshaw BL, Pettignano R, Merritt RK, Heard ML, Rogers K, Reid C, Tanner AJ, Easley KA. Fluid overload before continuous hemofiltration and survival in critically ill children: a retrospective analysis. Crit Care Med. 2004;32:1771–6.
9. Sutherland SM, Zappitelli M, Alexander SR, et al. Fluid overload and mortality in children receiving continuous renal replacement therapy: the prospective pediatric continuous renal replacement therapy registry. Am J Kidney Dis. 2010;55:316–25.
10. Askenazi DJ, Feig DI, Graham NM, et al. 3–5 year longitudinal follow-up of pediatric patients after acute renal failure. Kidney Int. 2006;69:184–9.
11. Goldstein SL, Bertrand L, Jaber BL, Faubel S, Chawla LS, for the Acute Kidney Injury Advisory Group of the American Society of Nephrology. AKI transition of care: a potential opportunity to detect and prevent CKD. Clin J Am Soc Nephrol. 2013;8:476–83.
12. Greenberg JH, Coca S, Parikh CR. Long-term risk of chronic kidney disease and mortality in children after acute kidney injury: a systematic review. BMC Nephrol. 2014;15:184. https://doi.org/10.1186/1471-2369-15-184.
13. Sutherland SM. AKI in hospitalized children: epidemiology and clinical associations in a national cohort. Clin J Am Soc Nephrol. 2013;8(10):1661–9.
14. Lex DJ, et al. A comparison of the Systems for the Identification of postoperative acute kidney injury in pediatric cardiac patients. Ann Thorac Surg. 2014;97(1):202–10.
15. Li S, Krawczeski CD, Zappitelli M, et al. Incidence, risk factors, and outcomes of acute kidney injury after pediatric cardiac surgery – a prospective multicenter study. Crit Care Med. 2011;39(6):1493–9. https://doi.org/10.1097/CCM.0b013e31821201d3.
16. Fitzgerald JC, Basu R, Akcan-Arikan A, et al. Acute kidney injury in pediatric severe Sepsis, an independent risk factor for death and new disability. Crit Care Med. 2016;44(12):2241–50. https://doi.org/10.1097/CCM.0000000000002007.
17. Basu RK, Devarajan P, Wong H, Wheeler DS. An update and review of acute kidney injury in pediatrics. Pediatr Crit Care Med. 2011;12:339–47.
18. Goldstein SL. Renal angina. CJASM. 2010;5:943–9.
19. Goldstein SL, Devarajan P. 2011 acute kidney injury in childhood: should we be worried about progression to CKD? Pediatr Nephrol. 2011;26:509.
20. Jones TE, Peter JV, Field J. Aminoglycoside clearance is a good measure of creatinine clearance in intensive care unit patients. Anaesthesia and Intensive Care. 2009;37:944–52.
21. Coulthard MG, Crosier J, Griffiths C, Smith J, Drinnan M, Whitaker M, Beckwith R, Matthews JN, Flecknell P, Lambert HJ. Haemodialysing babies weighing <8 kg with the Newcastle infant dialysis and ultrafiltration system (Nidus): comparison with peritoneal and conventional haemodialysis. Pediatr Nephrol. 2014;29(10):1873–81. https://doi.org/10.1007/s00467-014-2923-3. Epub 2014 Aug
22. Ronco C, et al. Continuous renal replacement therapy in neonates and small infants: development and first-in-human use of a miniaturised machine (CARPEDIEM). Lancet. 2014;383:1807–13.
23. Kyle UG, Akcan-Arikan A, Orellana RA, et al. Nutrition support among critically ill children with AKI. Clin J Am Soc Nephrol. 2013;8:568–74.

# Acute Kidney Injury in Children: Definition and Epidemiology

# 3

Scott M. Sutherland and Stuart L. Goldstein

**Case Vignette**

An 8-year-old girl is admitted to the intensive care unit with sepsis related to a perforated appendix. A CT scan with contrast reveals an intra-abdominal abscess and she is started on vancomycin and piperacillin–tazobactam. Despite aggressive antimicrobial therapy, she experiences progressive hemodynamic instability, requiring intravenous fluid resuscitation and vasopressor support. Her creatinine, which was 0.9 mg/dL on admission, rises to 1.3 mg/dL 24 h later. Her urine output, which was robust initially, dwindles and she becomes anuric 48 h later. Her concerned parents ask what has happened and what they should expect? Additionally, they would like to know the cause of her kidney dysfunction and how often you see it.

## 3.1 Introduction

Acute kidney injury (AKI) has become a common complication in hospitalized patients that is associated with substantial morbidity and mortality [1, 2]. Our ability to recognize AKI and understand its consequences has increased, in large part, due to the establishment of a consensus definition [3–6]. Previously, epidemiologic analysis was hampered by inconsistent application of divergent classification systems. For instance, the incidence of AKI across studies ranged from 1 to 25%

S. M. Sutherland (✉)
Department of Pediatrics, Division of Nephrology, Stanford University, Stanford, CA, USA
e-mail: suthersm@stanford.edu

S. L. Goldstein
Center for Acute Care Nephrology, Cincinnati Children's Hospital Medical Center, Cincinnati, OH, USA



A. Deep, S. L. Goldstein (eds.), *Critical Care Nephrology and Renal Replacement Therapy in Children*, https://doi.org/10.1007/978-3-319-90281-4_3

and mortality rates varied from 30 to 90% [5]. The lack of standardized definitional criteria obscured risk factors and limited our capacity to investigate AKI across different populations and diseases. However, over the past 10–15 years, the nephrology and critical care communities have collaborated to develop a consensus approach to the diagnosis of AKI. This, in turn, has led to transformative epidemiologic advances in both adults and children. The objective of this chapter is to describe the evolution of AKI diagnosis and to illustrate our current understanding of AKI epidemiology in children.

## 3.2 Defining and Diagnosing Acute Kidney Injury: A Historical Account

Prior to 2004, studies in adults and children used widely disparate definitions for AKI. The vast majority relied on absolute creatinine thresholds or changes in values, decrements in urine output (UOP), or the receipt of dialysis. However, creatinine thresholds differed from study to study and oliguria was inconsistently defined; the Acute Dialysis Quality Initiative (ADQI) group estimated that over 30 different definitions had been applied in the literature up until that time [5]. This irregularity was exacerbated in children due to the normal age related variance in serum creatinine values; a creatinine of 1.2 mg/dL might be normal in an adolescent but markedly elevated in an infant. It was in this context that the ADQI developed the Risk, Injury, Failure, Loss, End Stage Renal Disease (ESRD) (RIFLE) criteria.

### 3.2.1 Risk, Injury, Failure, Loss, ESRD (RIFLE) Criteria

In 2004, to address concerns about many aspects of AKI research and care, ADQI convened the Second International ADQI Consensus Conference. They recognized that while creatinine and UOP were not idyllic indicators of renal injury, they were ubiquitously assessed and no other biomarker had been validated to replace them. However, in order to be optimally used to diagnose AKI, their relationship to AKI needed to be standardized. To this end, they developed the empiric RIFLE criteria [5]. The first three stages of the definition, "Risk," "Injury," and "Failure," corresponded to progressively more severe AKI as manifest by larger changes in serum creatinine and/or longer periods of oliguria. For example, to meet criteria for "Failure," a patient needed to have a larger increase in creatinine or more severe oliguria than a patient meeting criteria for "Risk." The last two stages, "Loss" and "ESRD," represented outcomes of progressive AKI. The complete RIFLE definitional criteria are shown in Table 3.1.

In addition to creating standard thresholds for the diagnosis and staging of AKI events, this ADQI conference introduced several complex concepts. The first is the concept of baseline creatinine or kidney function. The RIFLE definition relies on changes in creatinine *relative to baseline*. While some patients may have laboratory data from prior interactions with the medical establishment, many will present without having had a serum creatinine obtained in recent history. For these patients, they

**Table 3.1** Comparison of RIFLE and pediatric RIFLE (pRIFLE) AKI criteria [4, 5]

| | RIFLE criteria | | Pediatric RIFLE criteria[b] | |
|---|---|---|---|---|
| | Creatinine/GFR criteria[a] | Urine output criteria | Creatinine/GFR criteria | Urine output criteria |
| Risk | • SCr increase 1.5× baseline<br>• GFR decrease by 25% | • UOP < 0.5 mL/kg/h × 6 h | • GFR decrease by 25% | • UOP < 0.5 mL/kg/h × 8 h |
| Injury | • SCr increase 2× baseline<br>• GFR decrease by 50% | • UOP < 0.5 mL/kg/h × 12 h | • GFR decrease by 50% | • UOP < 0.5 mL/kg/h × 16 h |
| Failure | • SCr increase 3× baseline<br>• GFR decrease by 75%<br>• Creatinine >4 mg/dL | • UOP < 0.3 mL/kg/h × 24 h<br>• Anuria × 12 h | • GFR decrease by 75%<br>• GFR < 35 mL/min/1.73 m$^2$ | • UOP < 0.3 mL/kg/h × 24 h<br>• Anuria × 12 h |
| *Loss* | *Persistent AKI for > 4 weeks* | | | |
| *ESRD* | *ESRD (persistent for > 3 months)* | | | |

[a]ADQI recommends that all relative changes occur over a period of time not to exceed 7 days
[b]All thresholds for pRIFLE were assessed over a 14-day time frame

recommended extrapolating a baseline creatinine using the "modification of diet in renal disease" (MDRD) equation, assuming a normal eGFR of 75–100 mL/min/1.73 m$^2$. They also highlighted the need to separate true "acute" AKI from "acute on chronic" AKI ($AKI_C$). The ability to sub-designate these patients as having $AKI_C$ allows separate analysis of AKI and chronic kidney disease (CKD) exacerbations. Unfortunately, one concept the RIFLE criteria did not address was pediatric AKI; these criteria were not developed with children in mind, making them difficult to apply to pediatric populations.

### 3.2.2 Pediatric RIFLE (pRIFLE) Criteria

Following the development of the RIFLE criteria, a study by Akcan-Arikan *et al.* endeavored to modify them for use in the pediatric setting [4]. They investigated the modified RIFLE criteria, known as the Pediatric RIFLE (pRIFLE) criteria, in 150 critically ill children who were receiving invasive mechanical ventilation and one vasoactive medication. The diagnosis and staging of AKI were based only on changes in estimated GFR (eGFR) and duration/severity of oliguria; notably, they did not apply the relative changes in serum creatinine that the RIFLE criteria used. The full pRIFLE criteria are shown in Table 3.1. The investigators found that the incidence of AKI was 82% (123/150) and the incidence of severe (Stage I or F) AKI was 42%. AKI was associated with poorer outcomes including longer lengths of intensive care unit (ICU) stay and increased mortality. As a result, the authors suggested that the pRIFLE criteria were suitable for use in children and advocated for further studies using these criteria. They too addressed the concept of baseline creatinine; baseline data was even less prevalent in children than in adults. Their recommendation, similar to the ADQI group, was to back-calculate a baseline creatinine from an assumed eGFR of 100 mL/min/1.73 m$^2$ (using the Schwartz equation given the pediatric population).

### 3.2.3 Acute Kidney Injury Network (AKIN) Criteria

At nearly the same time as the pRIFLE study, the Acute Kidney Injury Network (AKIN) published their consensus statement on AKI [6]. One of the most formative recommendations was replacing the conventional, prevailing term, "acute renal failure (ARF)," with the more accurate term, "acute kidney injury (AKI)." Since publication of these guidelines, in almost every academic and clinical setting, AKI has been used to describe the phenomenon of an abrupt decline in kidney function hallmarked by reduced excretion of waste products, disordered electrolytes, and disrupted fluid homeostasis. The second substantial contribution of these guidelines was diagnostic and staging criteria for AKI that were essentially an evolution of the RIFLE criteria. They took the first three phases of RIFLE ("R," "I," and "F") and transformed them into Stages (R = Stage 1, I = Stage 2, and F = Stage 3); they converted the last two phases ("L" and "E") into post-AKI outcomes, eliminating them from the diagnostic concept. They recommended that patients be diagnosed with AKI when they met criteria for *at least* Stage 1 AKI and subsequently staged based on their highest creatinine or most significant decrement in urine output. Other changes included adding an absolute creatinine increase threshold to the RIFLE designated relative change thresholds and adding temporal constraints to all changes in creatinine and urine output (Table 3.2). The AKIN criteria, much like the RIFLE criteria, were not developed with applicability to children in mind.

**Table 3.2** Comparison of the AKIN and KDIGO AKI definitions [3, 6]

| | AKIN criteria | | KDIGO criteria | |
|---|---|---|---|---|
| | Creatinine/GFR criteria | Urine output criteria | Creatinine/GFR criteria | Urine output criteria |
| Stage 1 | • SCr increase 1.5× baseline<br>• SCr increase ≥0.3 mg/dL[a] | • UOP < 0.5 mL/kg/h × 6 h | • SCr increase 1.5× baseline<br>• SCr increase ≥0.3 mg/dL[a] | • UOP < 0.5 mL/kg/h × 6 h |
| Stage 2 | • SCr increase 2× baseline | • UOP < 0.5 mL/kg/h × 12 h | • SCr increase 2× baseline | • UOP < 0.5 mL/kg/h × 12 h |
| Stage 3 | • SCr increase 3× baseline\<br>• Creatinine >4 mg/dL (acute rise ≥0.5 mg/dL)<br>• Receipt of RRT | • UOP < 0.3 mL/kg/h × 24 h<br>• Anuria × 12 h | • SCr increase 3× baseline<br>• Creatinine >4 mg/dL (acute rise ≥0.5 mg/dL)<br>• Receipt of RRT<br>• In patients <18 y, decrease in eGFR to <35 mL/min/1.73 m$^2$ | • UOP < 0.3 mL/kg/h × 24 h<br>• Anuria × 12 h |

*RRT* renal replacement therapy, *GFR* glomerular filtration rate, *SCr* serum creatinine, *UOP* urine output

[a]While all relative changes must occur within 7 days, this absolute change must occur within 48 h

### 3.2.4 Kidney Disease: Improving Global Outcomes (KDIGO)

The most recent iteration of the consensus AKI diagnosis criteria are those created by the Kidney Disease: Improving Global Outcomes (KDIGO) Workgroup [3]. These criteria have been widely adopted and represent a harmonization of all previous consensus approaches (RIFLE, pRIFLE, and AKIN). The KDIGO criteria continue to diagnose and stage AKI based upon relative and absolute changes in serum creatinine as well as severity and duration of oliguria (Table 3.2). The most substantial change to the AKIN criteria was the addition of pediatric specific thresholds to the creatinine criteria. Thus, KDIGO is the first consensus AKI diagnosis/staging strategy which is applicable to both adults and children.

## 3.3 Defining and Diagnosing Acute Kidney Injury: The Current State

With the currently available data, application of the KDIGO AKI criteria is the most suitable approach to diagnose and stage AKI in children. The need to use one single definition is best illustrated by a study which compared the incidence of AKI in hospitalized children using the pRIFLE, AKIN, and KDIGO definitions [7]. In this study, AKI incidence ranged from 37 to 51% depending on the definition employed and inter-definitional agreement was as low as 77%. While each definitional iteration has theoretical pros and cons, KDIGO has harmonized those which came before, is applicable to both adults and children, and was employed by the Assessment of Worldwide AKI, Renal angina, and Epidemiology (AWARE) study, the largest and most comprehensive epidemiologic analysis of AKI in children performed to date [1]. The use of KDIGO criteria will allow the entire AKI community to apply the same definitional rigor to their populations, resulting in far more effective comparative studies. With that in mind, it is worthwhile to examine the two definitional characteristics of the KDIGO criteria, serum creatinine and urine output/oliguria.

### 3.3.1 Serum Creatinine

In clinical practice, the diagnosis of AKI is customarily made based upon the identification of increasing serum creatinine levels. Notably, several studies have demonstrated that creatinine is a functional biomarker which can be relatively insensitive to renal injury. It is not uncommon for significant elevations to only be detected 24–48 h after the inciting insult [8–10]. In pediatric patients, this is further complicated by the fact that many young children have low serum creatinine values at baseline; in chronically and critically ill children, this can be further exaggerated by malnutrition and fluid overload [11–13]. Thus, despite significant relative increases, the actual elevated values may not register as abnormally high; creatinine can double or triple and remain within the normal range. Nonetheless, better alternatives do not yet exist. Several serum and urinary biomarkers have shown promise, however, normative data are sparse, commercially available options are limited, and none are approved for use in children [14–22]. Thus, despite its limitations, a relative change in serum creatinine remains the principal method of diagnosing AKI in children. One aspect of the KDIGO definition which deserves special mention is the concept of baseline creatinine. While some children may have had a creatinine obtained in the months prior to admission, for many this will not be the case and no actual baseline will exist; for example, a measured baseline serum creatinine was unavailable 51.5% of the 5200 patient AWARE cohort [1]. In cases such as these, several approaches have been utilized [23–26]. One option is to define the admission creatinine as the baseline. This is simple and effective, however, it can misclassify and underestimate cases of AKI which are present upon admission [25]. A second option is to estimate a baseline creatinine by back-calculating from an assumed age- and sex-standard creatinine clearance [24–26]. The most common of these methods assumes a baseline creatinine clearance of 120 mL/min/1.73 $m^2$ [24]. This approach will capture AKI events present on admission, however, it will misclassify patients with CKD as having AKI; in adult patients, this approach can overestimate the incidence of AKI by 50% [25]. If baseline data are available, many studies have chosen the lowest creatinine obtained in the 3–6 months prior to hospitalization; other than in neonates and small infants, creatinine is unlikely to change physiologically in that time frame.

### 3.3.2 Urine Output and Oliguria

In addition to the creatinine-based AKI criteria, the KDIGO definition employs urine output (UOP) parameters. Until recently, the vast majority of pediatric AKI studies did not utilize these urinary criteria [7, 27]. This is likely related to a number of pediatric specific issues. The first is that many pediatric ICU patients and nearly all acute care patients do not have Foley catheters in place. There has been a push to avoid bladder catheter use in hospitalized children in order to prevent urinary tract infections; additionally, many practitioners are reluctant to place them in children given the invasive nature of the procedure. Secondly, especially in small children outside of the ICUs, UOP may be documented as a void count rather than volume. However, the more recently published AWARE study clearly demonstrated that disregarding the UOP criteria leads to an underdiagnosis of AKI. In this study, isolated use of the creatinine criteria would have missed nearly a third of AKI cases as they met only the UOP portion of the definition [1]. The potential ramifications of missing these patients are substantial as patients with Stage 3 AKI according to the UOP criteria exhibited the highest 28-day mortality rate (33%). Thus, despite the challenges, oliguria remains an integral part of AKI diagnosis in children and decreases in UOP should prompt evaluation of renal function and a search for injurious events.

## 3.4 Epidemiology of Pediatric AKI

Epidemiology is defined as "the study of the distribution (frequency and pattern) and determinants of health related states or events in specified populations" [28]. By this definition, the epidemiology of pediatric AKI should describe its incidence, demographics, and risk factors. While this seems straightforward, before the publication of the aforementioned consensus definitions, the application of widely divergent diagnostic strategies produced inconsistent descriptions of AKI epidemiology [4, 5]. Now that the majority of studies utilize one of the standard definitions, epidemiology data remains within a more confined range, though it has continued to be highly dependent on the population studied.

### 3.4.1 Incidence

Perhaps the most accurate assessment of pediatric AKI epidemiology, at least among critically ill children, is the recently published AWARE study, which examined 4683 children (ages 3 months to 25 years) admitted to 32 intensive care units. The overall incidence of AKI during the first week of hospitalization was 27% and 12% of children developed severe (KDIGO Stage 2/3) AKI [1]. This is slightly lower than seen in adults (Fig. 3.1); the similarly styled adult AKI-EPI analysis demonstrated that the incidence of AKI and severe AKI in critically ill adults is 57% and 27%, respectively [2].

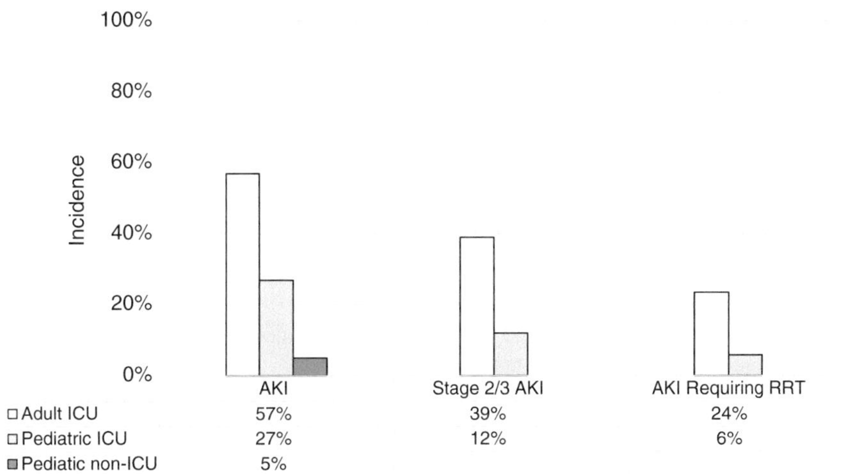


**Fig. 3.1** Incidence of AKI, severe AKI, and AKI requiring RRT in children and adults [1, 2, 29]. The incidence of AKI among non-critically ill children is approximately 5%. However, in children requiring critical care, this rate is significantly higher at 27%. Of note, 12% of critically ill children experience severe (KDIGO Stage 2/3) AKI and nearly 6% of those with any type of AKI require some form of renal replacement therapy. These rates are lower than those seen in adults, likely due to the fewer comorbidities seen in children

The need for renal replacement therapy (RRT) follows a similar trend as 23.5% of adults with AKI and 5.8% of children with AKI required RRT (Fig. 3.1) [1, 2]. These data suggest that children, likely due to the fact that they have fewer comorbidities on average, are less likely to develop AKI than hospitalized adults. However, as the demographics of pediatric AKI shift towards higher case complexity and greater underlying morbidity, these data imply that the incidence of AKI among hospitalized children is likely to rise. Outside of the ICU, AKI remains common; a retrospective single-center study suggested that at least 5% of hospitalized children will experience AKI during their acute-care stay (Fig. 3.1) [29]. The one area where pediatric AKI has not yet been well characterized is in the ambulatory setting. Several adult studies have examined hospital and community acquired AKI comparatively and while they suggest differences in incidence, risk factors, and outcomes, no such data yet exist in children [30, 31]. While these studies provide excellent general data regarding AKI incidence, it is important to remember that AKI rates are highly dependent on case mix and the population studied. In the previously described AWARE study, the rate of severe AKI varied from less than 5% to more than 30% across the 32 ICUs; this is likely related to variation in illness severity from unit to unit [1]. The incidence of AKI varies according to etiology as well. For example, AKI is seen in 10% of children receiving intravenous contrast, approximately 30% of those with sepsis, and over 70% of children receiving heart transplantation [32–35].

### 3.4.2 Demographics

Among hospitalized children, AKI occurs at extremes of age. One study found that the incidence of AKI increased in parallel with age, reaching its zenith in adolescents; however, approximately 20% of all AKI occurred in neonates and infants less than a month old [36]. AKI also seems to be more common in male children and those of African American ethnicity, findings which are echoed in adult studies [36–38]. From a causative standpoint, we have seen a dramatic shift. Though AKI due to primary renal disease was common historically, AKI is now due predominantly to systemic illnesses, multi-organ injury, and the treatments these conditions demand [36, 39, 40]. In developed countries, the most common causes of AKI are cardiopulmonary bypass, sepsis, heart failure, solid organ and stem cell transplantation, tumor lysis syndrome, and nephrotoxin exposure [1, 39, 41, 42]. In developing countries, on the contrary, primary kidney diseases are more prevalent with glomerulonephritis, toxin exposure, hypovolemia, and sepsis being the most common etiologies [43, 44]. Interestingly, there is striking center-to-center variation as well. For instance, a study from a single United States hospital found that oncologic disease was responsible for 40% of AKI [45]. Comparatively, a single-center study from Spain found that the most common underlying disease was cardiac, while oncologic disease only accounted for 3% of AKI [46].

### 3.4.3 Risk Factors

The determinants of AKI in children have varied based on underlying disease and etiology of AKI. However, some risk factors have proven to be generalizable and many underscore the impact of disease and illness severity; it is clear that children with greater illness burden are at higher AKI risk. For example, children who develop AKI following liver transplantation are more likely to have higher serum bilirubin levels and greater intraoperative blood loss, markers of disease severity and surgical complexity [47]. Those who develop AKI following venomous stings/bites are those with greater instability; following scorpion bites, children who experienced AKI were younger and more likely to have hemolytic anemia, thrombocytopenia, and fever [48–50]. In diabetic children admitted with diabetic ketoacidosis, those with acidosis and evidence of volume depletion (surrogates for more severe disease and inadequate tissue perfusion) had higher rates of AKI [51]. Children who require corrective surgery for congenital heart disease have strikingly high rates of AKI; risk factors in this population include longer cardiopulmonary bypass time (prolonged ischemia and more complex underlying disease), younger age, and greater surgical complexity [8, 52]. In more general pediatric populations, some of the more common risk factors for AKI include younger age, the need for vasopressors or respiratory support, multi-organ dysfunction syndrome (MODS), extracorporeal membrane oxygenation (ECMO), and preexisting chronic kidney disease [39, 53–56].

One of the more universal risk factors for AKI among hospitalized children is the administration of nephrotoxic medications. A number of studies in pediatric patients have demonstrated that administration of nephrotoxic medications increases the risk for AKI [30, 39, 55]. This has been corroborated by the study of several specific medications. The use of renin-angiotensin system (RAS) inhibitors in high-risk children can cause AKI in 14% of patients [57]. Vancomycin, one of the most ubiquitous antimicrobial agents used among pediatric inpatients, is associated with AKI in nearly 20% of cases [58]. Furthermore, 20% of non-critically ill children who receive aminoglycosides develop AKI [59]. As our understanding of nephrotoxicity has evolved, the pediatric community has moved away from the identification of individual nephrotoxic medications and towards the concept of nephrotoxin burden. For example, the concomitant administration of piperacillin/tazobactam and vancomycin is associated with significantly higher rates of AKI than administration of either medication alone [60]. Additionally, Rheault et al. examined AKI in children admitted with nephrotic syndrome and found that nephrotoxin exposure was one of the strongest AKI predictors; AKI risk increased by 38% for each nephrotoxic medication added [61]. This concept is perhaps best exemplified by the Nephrotoxic Injury Negated by Just-in-time Action (NINJA) project, which demonstrated that, when serum creatinine is assessed daily, 25% of children receiving three or more nephrotoxic medications develop AKI [40, 42].

## 3.5 Summary

Great strides have been made regarding our ability to diagnose AKI in a standard fashion using consensus definitions. The culmination of this process has been the establishment of the KDIGO AKI criteria which harmonize the previously existing approaches, creating a single method for diagnosing AKI in both adults and children. Although the majority of studies to date have employed the KDIGO creatinine criteria more universally, recent work has demonstrated that the urine output criteria are an integral part of the diagnostic algorithm; disregarding the urine criteria will lead to an underdiagnosis of AKI and a potentially incomplete understanding of AKI epidemiology. The work developing a consensus approach has allowed us to more accurately define the incidence of AKI and we now know that 27% of children receiving intensive care and at least 5% of those who are not critically ill will develop AKI, respectively. We have also found that children, especially in developed countries, are developing AKI due to systemic diseases and the treatments they require rather than primary, intrinsic renal disease. Risk factors for the development of AKI have tended to differ somewhat between patient populations; however, it is clear that AKI risk increases with case complexity and severity of illness. Hopefully, these definitional and epidemiologic advances will soon translate into therapeutic innovations, allowing us to improve outcomes in a similar fashion.

**Key Learning Points**

- While all of the recently developed consensus definitions are reasonable approaches to define AKI in children, we recommend the use of the KDIGO criteria since they harmonized all previous definitions and can be applied to both children and adults.
- While not as rigorously studied as the creatinine criteria, the KDIGO urine output criteria are an integral part of the AKI diagnostic strategy; disregarding them will result in an underdiagnosis of the overall AKI burden.
- AKI occurs in approximately 27% of children receiving intensive care and 5% of non-critically ill pediatric patients.
- While AKI risk factors vary between patient populations, certain risk factors have proven generalizable including younger age, case complexity, greater severity of illness, receipt of critical care, and nephrotoxin exposure.

## References

1. Kaddourah A, Basu RK, Bagshaw SM, Goldstein SL, Investigators A. Epidemiology of acute kidney injury in critically ill children and young adults. N Engl J Med. 2017;376(1):11–20.
2. Hoste EA, Bagshaw SM, Bellomo R, Cely CM, Colman R, Cruz DN, et al. Epidemiology of acute kidney injury in critically ill patients: the multinational AKI-EPI study. Intensive Care Med. 2015;41(8):1411–23.

3. Kidney Disease: Improving Global Outcomes (KDIGO) Acute Kidney Injury Work Group. KDIGO clinical practice guideline for acute kidney injury. Kidney Int. 2012;2:1–138.
4. Akcan-Arikan A, Zappitelli M, Loftis LL, Washburn KK, Jefferson LS, Goldstein SL. Modified RIFLE criteria in critically ill children with acute kidney injury. Kidney Int. 2007;71(10):1028–35.
5. Bellomo R, Ronco C, Kellum JA, Mehta RL, Palevsky P, Acute Dialysis Quality Initiative workgroup. Acute renal failure – definition, outcome measures, animal models, fluid therapy and information technology needs: the second international consensus conference of the acute Dialysis quality initiative (ADQI) group. Crit Care. 2004;8(4):R204–12.
6. Mehta RL, Kellum JA, Shah SV, Molitoris BA, Ronco C, Warnock DG, et al. Acute kidney injury network: report of an initiative to improve outcomes in acute kidney injury. Crit Care. 2007;11(2):R31.
7. Sutherland SM, Byrnes JJ, Kothari M, Longhurst CA, Dutta S, Garcia P, et al. AKI in hospitalized children: comparing the pRIFLE, AKIN, and KDIGO definitions. Clin J Am Soc Nephrol. 2015;10(4):554–61.
8. Li S, Krawczeski CD, Zappitelli M, Devarajan P, Thiessen-Philbrook H, Coca SG, et al. Incidence, risk factors, and outcomes of acute kidney injury after pediatric cardiac surgery: a prospective multicenter study. Crit Care Med. 2011;39(6):1493–9.
9. Blinder JJ, Goldstein SL, Lee VV, Baycroft A, Fraser CD, Nelson D, et al. Congenital heart surgery in infants: effects of acute kidney injury on outcomes. J Thorac Cardiovasc Surg. 2012;143(2):368–74.
10. Greenberg JH, Zappitelli M, Devarajan P, Thiessen-Philbrook HR, Krawczeski C, Li S, et al. Kidney outcomes 5 years after pediatric cardiac surgery: the TRIBE-AKI study. JAMA Pediatr. 2016;170:1071.
11. Hari P, Bagga A, Mahajan P, Lakshmy R. Effect of malnutrition on serum creatinine and cystatin C levels. Pediatr Nephrol. 2007;22(10):1757–61.
12. Basu RK, Andrews A, Krawczeski C, Manning P, Wheeler DS, Goldstein SL. Acute kidney injury based on corrected serum creatinine is associated with increased morbidity in children following the arterial switch operation. Pediatr Crit Care Med. 2013;14(5):e218–e24.
13. Viollet L, Gailey S, Thornton DJ, Friedman NR, Flanigan KM, Mahan JD, et al. Utility of cystatin C to monitor renal function in Duchenne muscular dystrophy. Muscle Nerve. 2009;40(3):438–42.
14. Krawczeski CD, Goldstein SL, Woo JG, Wang Y, Piyaphanee N, Ma Q, et al. Temporal relationship and predictive value of urinary acute kidney injury biomarkers after pediatric cardiopulmonary bypass. J Am Coll Cardiol. 2011;58(22):2301–9.
15. Bennett M, Dent CL, Ma Q, Dastrala S, Grenier F, Workman R, et al. Urine NGAL predicts severity of acute kidney injury after cardiac surgery: a prospective study. Clin J Am Soc Nephrol. 2008;3(3):665–73.
16. Wheeler DS, Devarajan P, Ma Q, Harmon K, Monaco M, Cvijanovich N, et al. Serum neutrophil gelatinase-associated lipocalin (NGAL) as a marker of acute kidney injury in critically ill children with septic shock. Crit Care Med. 2008;36(4):1297.
17. Hirsch R, Dent C, Pfriem H, Allen J, Beekman RH, Ma Q, et al. NGAL is an early predictive biomarker of contrast-induced nephropathy in children. Pediatr Nephrol. 2007;22(12):2089.
18. Mishra J, Ma Q, Kelly C, Mitsnefes M, Mori K, Barasch J, et al. Kidney NGAL is a novel early marker of acute injury following transplantation. Pediatr Nephrol. 2006;21(6):856–63.
19. Sirota JC, Walcher A, Faubel S, Jani A, McFann K, Devarajan P, et al. Urine IL-18, NGAL, IL-8 and serum IL-8 are biomarkers of acute kidney injury following liver transplantation. BMC Nephrol. 2013;14(1):17.
20. Meersch M, Schmidt C, Van Aken H, Rossaint J, Gorlich D, Stege D, et al. Validation of cell-cycle arrest biomarkers for acute kidney injury after pediatric cardiac surgery. PLoS One. 2014;9(10):e110865.
21. Gist KM, Goldstein SL, Wrona J, Alten JA, Basu RK, Cooper DS, et al. Kinetics of the cell cycle arrest biomarkers (TIMP-2*IGFBP-7) for prediction of acute kidney injury in infants after cardiac surgery. Pediatr Nephrol. 2017;32:1611.

22. Westhoff JH, Tönshoff B, Waldherr S, Pöschl J, Teufel U, Westhoff TH, et al. Urinary tissue inhibitor of metalloproteinase-2 (TIMP-2)• insulin-like growth factor-binding protein 7 (IGFBP7) predicts adverse outcome in pediatric acute kidney injury. PLoS One. 2015;10(11):e0143628.
23. James MT, Hobson CE, Darmon M, Mohan S, Hudson D, Goldstein SL, et al. Applications for detection of acute kidney injury using electronic medical records and clinical information systems: workgroup statements from the 15(th) ADQI consensus conference. Can J Kidney Health Dis. 2016;3:9.
24. Zappitelli M, Parikh CR, Akcan-Arikan A, Washburn KK, Moffett BS, Goldstein SL. Ascertainment and epidemiology of acute kidney injury varies with definition interpretation. Clin J Am Soc Nephrol. 2008;3(4):948–54.
25. Siew ED, Matheny ME, Ikizler TA, Lewis JB, Miller RA, Waitman LR, et al. Commonly used surrogates for baseline renal function affect the classification and prognosis of acute kidney injury. Kidney Int. 2010;77(6):536–42.
26. Bagshaw SM, Uchino S, Cruz D, Bellomo R, Morimatsu H, Morgera S, et al. A comparison of observed versus estimated baseline creatinine for determination of RIFLE class in patients with acute kidney injury. Nephrol Dial Transplant. 2009;24(9):2739–44.
27. Selewski DT, Cornell TT, Heung M, Troost JP, Ehrmann BJ, Lombel RM, et al. Validation of the KDIGO acute kidney injury criteria in a pediatric critical care population. Intensive Care Med. 2014;40(10):1481–8.
28. Last JM. Dictionary of epidemiology. New York: Oxford University; 2001.
29. McGregor TL, Jones DP, Wang L, Danciu I, Bridges BC, Fleming GM, et al. Acute kidney injury incidence in noncritically ill hospitalized children, adolescents, and young adults: a retrospective observational study. Am J Kidney Dis. 2016;67(3):384–90.
30. Hsu CN, Lee CT, Su CH, Wang YC, Chen HL, Chuang JH, et al. Incidence, outcomes, and risk factors of community-acquired and hospital-acquired acute kidney injury: a retrospective cohort study. Medicine. 2016;95(19):e3674.
31. Sawhney S, Fluck N, Fraser SD, Marks A, Prescott GJ, Roderick PJ, et al. KDIGO-based acute kidney injury criteria operate differently in hospitals and the community-findings from a large population cohort. Nephrol Dial Transplant. 2016;31(6):922–9.
32. Lopes JA, Jorge S, Resina C, Santos C, Pereira A, Neves J, et al. Acute kidney injury in patients with sepsis: a contemporary analysis. Int J Infect Dis. 2009;13(2):176–81.
33. Hollander SA, Montez-Rath ME, Axelrod DM, Krawczeski CD, May LJ, Maeda K, et al. Recovery from acute kidney injury and CKD following heart transplantation in children, adolescents, and young adults: a retrospective cohort study. Am J Kidney Dis. 2016;68(2):212–8.
34. MacDonald C, Norris C, Alton GY, Urschel S, Joffe AR, Morgan CJ, et al. Acute kidney injury after heart transplant in young children: risk factors and outcomes. Pediatr Nephrol. 2016;31(4):671–8.
35. Cantais A, Hammouda Z, Mory O, Patural H, Stephan JL, Gulyaeva L, et al. Incidence of contrast-induced acute kidney injury in a pediatric setting: a cohort study. Pediatr Nephrol. 2016;31(8):1355–62.
36. Sutherland SM. AKI in hospitalized children: epidemiology and clinical associations in a national cohort. J Pediatr. 2013;8(10):1661–9.
37. Xue JL, Daniels F, Star RA, Kimmel PL, Eggers PW, Molitoris BA, et al. Incidence and mortality of acute renal failure in Medicare beneficiaries, 1992 to 2001. J Am Soc Nephrol. 2006;17(4):1135–42.
38. Waikar SS, Curhan GC, Ayanian JZ, Chertow GM. Race and mortality after acute renal failure. J Am Soc Nephrol. 2007;18(10):2740–8.
39. Hui-Stickle S, Brewer ED, Goldstein SL. Pediatric ARF epidemiology at a tertiary care center from 1999 to 2001. Am J Kidney Dis. 2005;45(1):96–101.
40. Goldstein SL. Acute kidney injury in children: prevention, treatment and rehabilitation. Contrib Nephrol. 2011;174:163–72.
41. Williams DM, Sreedhar SS, Mickell JJ, Chan JC. Acute kidney failure: a pediatric experience over 20 years. Arch Pediatr Adolesc Med. 2002;156(9):893–900.

42. Goldstein SL, Kirkendall E, Nguyen H, Schaffzin JK, Bucuvalas J, Bracke T, et al. Electronic health record identification of nephrotoxin exposure and associated acute kidney injury. Pediatrics. 2013;132(3):e756–67.
43. Vachvanichsanong P, Dissaneewate P, Lim A, McNeil E. Childhood acute renal failure: 22-year experience in a university hospital in southern Thailand. Pediatrics. 2006;118(3):e786–91.
44. Sinha R, Nandi M, Tullus K, Marks SD, Taraphder A. Ten-year follow-up of children after acute renal failure from a developing country. Nephrol Dial Transplant. 2009;24(3):829–33.
45. Hayes LW, Oster RA, Tofil NM, Tolwani AJ. Outcomes of critically ill children requiring continuous renal replacement therapy. J Crit Care. 2009;24(3):394–400.
46. Santiago MJ, Lopez-Herce J, Urbano J, Solana MJ, del Castillo J, Ballestero Y, et al. Complications of continuous renal replacement therapy in critically ill children: a prospective observational evaluation study. Crit Care. 2009;13(6):R184.
47. Hamada M, Matsukawa S, Shimizu S, Kai S, Mizota T. Acute kidney injury after pediatric liver transplantation: incidence, risk factors, and association with outcome. J Anesth. 2017;31(5):758–63.
48. Valavi E, Amuri P, Ahmadzadeh A, Cheraghian B, Ahankoob E. Acute kidney injury in Hemiscorpius lepturus scorpion stung children: risk factors and clinical features. Saudi J Kidney Dis Transpl. 2016;27(5):936–41.
49. Jayakrishnan MP, Geeta MG, Krishnakumar P, Rajesh TV, George B. Snake bite mortality in children: beyond bite to needle time. Arch Dis Child. 2017;102(5):445–9.
50. Nishimura H, Enokida H, Kawahira S, Kagara I, Hayami H, Nakagawa M. Acute kidney injury and rhabdomyolysis after Protobothrops flavoviridis bite: a retrospective survey of 86 patients in a tertiary care center. Am J Trop Med Hyg. 2016;94(2):474–9.
51. Hursh BE, Ronsley R, Islam N, Mammen C, Panagiotopoulos C. Acute kidney injury in children with type 1 diabetes hospitalized for diabetic ketoacidosis. JAMA Pediatr. 2017;171(5):e170020.
52. Hirano D, Ito A, Yamada A, Kakegawa D, Miwa S, Umeda C, et al. Independent risk factors and 2-year outcomes of acute kidney injury after surgery for congenital heart disease. Am J Nephrol. 2017;46(3):204–9.
53. Alkandari O, Eddington KA, Hyder A, Gauvin F, Ducruet T, Gottesman R, et al. Acute kidney injury is an independent risk factor for pediatric intensive care unit mortality, longer length of stay and prolonged mechanical ventilation in critically ill children: a two-center retrospective cohort study. Crit Care. 2011;15(3):R146.
54. Bailey D, Phan V, Litalien C, Ducruet T, Merouani A, Lacroix J, et al. Risk factors of acute renal failure in critically ill children: a prospective descriptive epidemiological study. Pediatr Crit Care Med. 2007;8(1):29–35.
55. Slater MB, Gruneir A, Rochon PA, Howard AW, Koren G, Parshuram CS. Risk factors of acute kidney injury in critically ill children. Pediatr Crit Care Med. 2016;17(9):e391–8.
56. Hsu CN, Chen HL, Tain YL. Epidemiology and outcomes of community-acquired and hospital-acquired acute kidney injury in children and adolescents. Pediatr Res. 2018, 83(3):622–9.
57. Terano C, Ishikura K, Miura M, Hamada R, Harada R, Sakai T, et al. Incidence of and risk factors for severe acute kidney injury in children with heart failure treated with renin-angiotensin system inhibitors. Eur J Pediatr. 2016;175(5):631–7.
58. Totapally BR, Machado J, Lee H, Paredes A, Raszynski A. Acute kidney injury during vancomycin therapy in critically ill children. Pharmacotherapy. 2013;33(6):598–602.
59. Zappitelli M, Moffett BS, Hyder A, Goldstein SL. Acute kidney injury in non-critically ill children treated with aminoglycoside antibiotics in a tertiary healthcare Centre: a retrospective cohort study. Nephrol Dial Transplant. 2011;26(1):144–50.
60. Downes KJ, Cowden C, Laskin BL, Huang YS, Gong W, Bryan M, et al. Association of Acute Kidney Injury with Concomitant Vancomycin and Piperacillin/Tazobactam treatment among hospitalized children. JAMA Pediatr. 2017;171:e173219.
61. Rheault MN, Zhang L, Selewski DT, Kallash M, Tran CL, Seamon M, et al. AKI in children hospitalized with nephrotic syndrome. Clin J Am Soc Nephrol. 2015;10(12):2110–8.

# Biomarkers in AKI

# 4

Kelly R. McMahon and Michael Zappitelli

**Case Vignette**

A 4-year-old girl is admitted to the intensive care unit (ICU) with bacteremia and is prescribed gentamicin. Within 48 h, her infection parameters improve, though she requires vasopressors. Her serum creatinine (SCr) level appears normal. On day 4 of receiving gentamicin, her SCr concentration rises and aminoglycoside-induced acute kidney injury (AKI) is suspected. AKI management strategies are attempted (e.g., reducing gentamicin dosage, stopping other nephrotoxins, judicious fluid management). She progresses on to require dialysis. The gentamicin is changed to another antibiotic. The possibility of using an earlier diagnostic test for AKI than SCr would have led to more expeditious management (e.g., gentamicin stopped), renal injury mitigated and dialysis might have been avoided. In cases with multifactorial AKI causes, a tool to determine the cause of renal injury as it occurred would have been useful to manage this patient.

## 4.1 Introduction

This chapter provides a broad overview of research on new AKI biomarkers in children. Current AKI diagnosis is suboptimal, relying on detecting decline in kidney function or glomerular filtration rate (GFR), using SCr (rise) and urine output (decrease). SCr rise is often delayed, occurring *after* renal tissue injury has

K. R. McMahon
Department of Pediatrics, Division of Pediatric Nephrology, Montreal Children's Hospital, McGill University Health Centre, Montreal, QC, Canada
e-mail: kelly.mcmahon@mail.mcgill.ca

M. Zappitelli (✉)
Department of Pediatrics, Division of Nephrology, Toronto Hospital for Sick Children, University of Toronto, Toronto, ON, Canada
e-mail: mzaprdr@yahoo.ca



A. Deep, S. L. Goldstein (eds.), *Critical Care Nephrology and Renal Replacement Therapy in Children*, https://doi.org/10.1007/978-3-319-90281-4_4

occurred, hindering ability to treat AKI. A driving rationale for studying new AKI biomarkers is for early AKI diagnosis, before substantial GFR decline occurs, to allow developing and testing of new treatments, and enabling early conservative AKI management to avoid serious AKI complications. Different AKI mechanisms cause damage to different renal tissue compartments. There has been a goal to also use new biomarkers to inform on renal tissue injury *location* (proximal vs. distal tubule versus glomerulus). Such an application would have implications in providing injury-specific AKI treatments.

### 4.1.1 AKI Pathophysiology and Biomarker Utility

The most common causes of AKI in the pediatric intensive care unit (PICU) are ischemia, nephrotoxic drugs, and sepsis. Ischemic AKI may often coexist with other injury mechanisms and is often more complex than appreciated. With cardiopulmonary bypass (CPB), hypoxia/ischemia is well known to cause AKI; however, other injuries including oxidative stress and the pro-inflammatory nature of CPB might occur. With sepsis, inflammation or toxin-mediated injury occurs, however, hemodynamic changes may cause ischemia as well. Nephrotoxic AKI is a more specific injury, usually causing direct tubular injury, often to the proximal tubule. These injury mechanisms may cause renal tubular cell death (acute tubular necrosis (ATN)). Other renal injuries include glomerular (e.g., glomerulonephritis) or interstitial (e.g., some nephrotoxins), but may also include concomitant tubular injury. In patients with AKI, it is worthwhile thinking about injury origin (*what part* of renal tissue was injured). This helps understand the clinical picture and how best to utilize new AKI biomarkers when they become available. AKI in the ICU setting is often multifactorial (see Clinical Vignette). For successful clinical application of new AKI biomarkers, selecting time points where the clinical profile indicates a high risk of having renal injury, despite lack of SCr rise or urine output drop is key. Clinical scenarios where biomarkers would be useful are depicted in Fig. 4.1. Most novel biomarkers are not widely clinically available today. However, thinking about how they may help identify AKI (Fig. 4.1), may encourage clinicians to appreciate that renal tissue injury may be occurring despite lack of SCr rise and how early management may alter the course of AKI, avoiding complications. Figure 4.2 displays another potential biomarker utility in patients with established SCr rise. Biomarkers of kidney tissue damage may inform clinicians on whether patients truly have AKI or simply an adaptive GFR decrease due to hypovolemia or what is now termed functional AKI.

### 4.1.2 SCr Is a Poor AKI Diagnostic Test

Current AKI diagnosis is based on SCr rise or decreased urine output [1]. This definition has limitations. As described above, SCr and urine output are *delayed* kidney *function* markers, not direct markers of tissue damage. SCr is influenced by factors other than GFR (e.g., muscle mass, diet, age, sex, volume status, medications). Accurate urine output collection is challenging, especially without a urinary catheter.

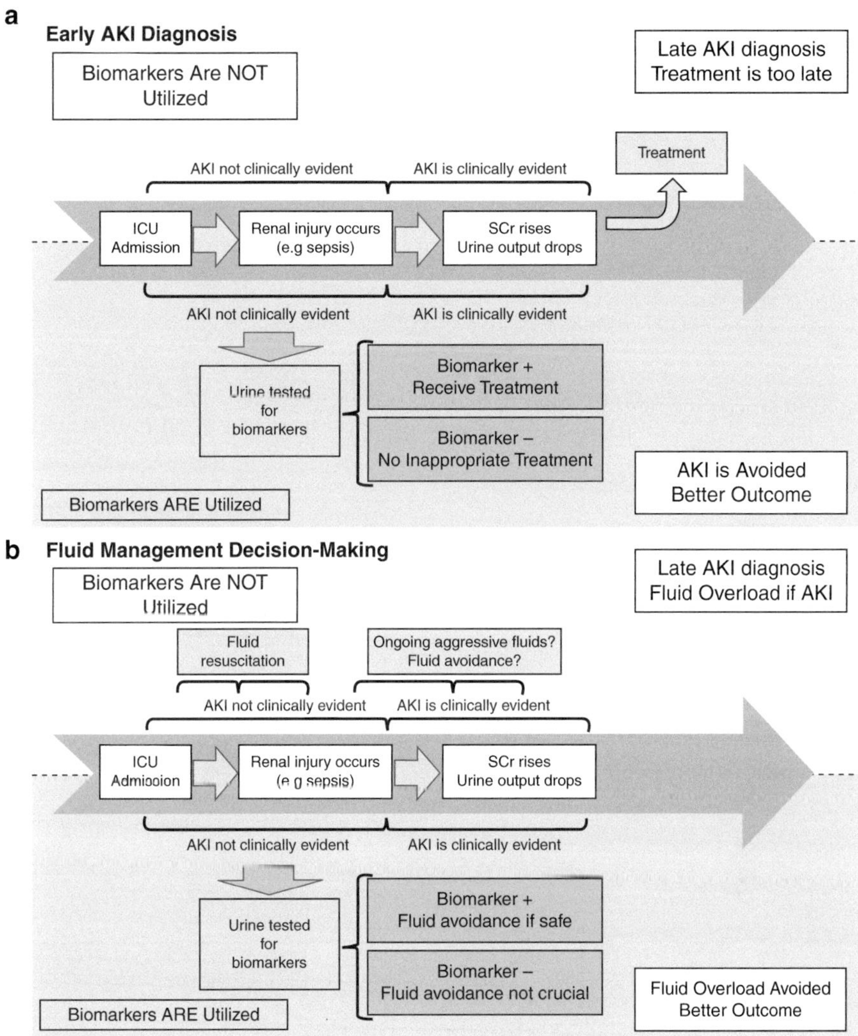


**Fig. 4.1** Utility of biomarkers in different clinical scenarios. All panels: top portion depicts when biomarkers are not used; bottom portion depicts when biomarkers are used. Panel **A**: biomarkers in early AKI diagnosis. Panel **B**: biomarkers' utility in fluid management. Panel **C**: biomarker for nephrotoxic AKI decision-making. Abbreviations: *AKI* Acute kidney injury, *ICU* Intensive care unit, *SCr* Serum creatinine, *CKD* Chronic kidney disease

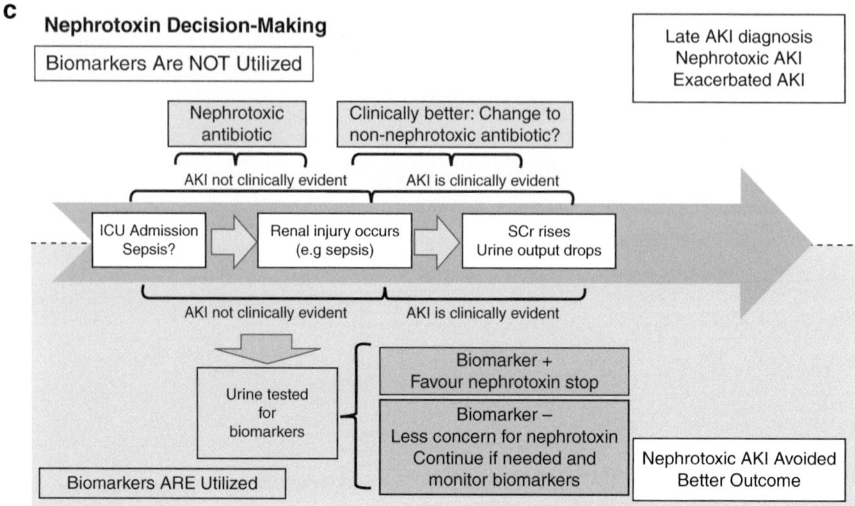


**Fig. 4.1** (continued)

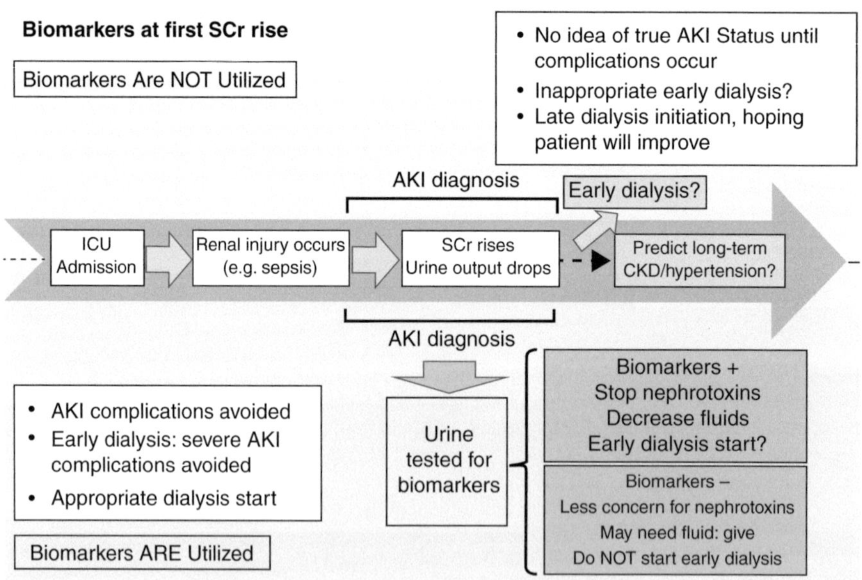


**Fig. 4.2** Biomarkers in patients with established AKI. Biomarker use for predicting/avoiding AKI complications and guide timing of early dialysis. Abbreviations: *AKI* Acute kidney injury, *ICU* Intensive care unit, *SCr* Serum creatinine, *CKD* Chronic kidney disease

Non-AKI factors affect urine output (e.g., diuretics). Adequate urine output does not exclude renal injury. For example, medications toxic to renal tubules can cause concentration defects, so urine output may appear adequate, despite significant tubular injury. Renal tissue injury biomarkers may provide a new window into the kidney, informing on tissue damage before GFR declines and help better interpret changes in traditional function markers.

### 4.1.3 The Ideal AKI Biomarker and Studying Biomarkers

An ideal biomarker should be easily measurable, and the assay to measure it should be reliable, reproducible, and inexpensive. Urine provides an ideal noninvasive fluid. The biomarker should have good diagnostic characteristics (sensitivity/specificity) to detect AKI, usually summarized using area under the receiver operating characteristic curve ((AUC-ROC); 0.50 indicates the test is no better than chance or "guessing" alone, 1.00 is perfect). The biomarker should be associated with a clinical outcome (e.g., AKI severity in terms of SCr or urine output change, ICU length of stay or mortality). The ideal AKI biomarker will not only diagnose the *presence* of AKI (referred to as *discrimination)* but also do so early, *predicting* function change. Other potentially desirable characteristics include: informing on severity of injury; predicting AKI progression and recovery, identifying the site of renal injury/etiology and applicability in many clinical settings. Different biomarkers may be more useful for specific use cases.

## 4.2 Overview of Specific AKI Biomarkers

Most AKI biomarkers are proteins that are measurable in blood or urine. One helpful manner by which to classify AKI biomarkers is listed below.

1. *Functional markers:* inform on GFR (filtration markers). Examples: SCr and serum cystatin C (CysC).
2. *Tubular damage biomarkers:* proteins released from damaged cells into urine when renal tubules are injured (e.g., N-acetyl-β-(D)-glucosaminidase (NAG)).
3. *Biomarkers induced in response to AKI*: protein products of genes that are upregulated in response to kidney tissue injury (e.g., neutrophil gelatinase-associated lipocalin (NGAL)), often associated with injury/repair processes.

Table 4.1 provides a summary of recently studied biomarkers. Although not reviewed in this chapter, new methodologies like proteomics and metabolomics are actively being investigated for AKI biomarker discovery. The description of biomarkers below includes a brief summary of data mostly about early AKI diagnosis, with an attempt to differentiate data regarding AKI discrimination versus prediction.

**Table 4.1** Non-exhaustive summary of AKI biomarkers

| Biomarker | Nephron localization | AKI pathophysiology role/reason for change with AKI | Preclinical studies | Pediatric AKI studies | Clinical approval status |
|---|---|---|---|---|---|
| Kidney function | | | | | |
| Serum CysC | Glomerulus | Rises when GFR drops | Ischemia; sepsis; nephrotoxic | ICU; CS; sepsis; nephrotoxic; contrast; cancer; KT | Approved |
| Tubular damage | | | | | |
| NAG | PT | Lysosomal enzyme; extruded in PT injury | Nephrotoxic; contrast | CS; nephrotoxic; contrast | |
| AAP | PT | PT brush border enzyme; released with injury | Nephrotoxic; contrast | Nephrotoxic; contrast | |
| AP | PT | PT brush border enzyme | Ischemia; nephrotoxic; contrast | Nephrotoxic | |
| GGT | PT | PT brush border enzyme | Ischemia; nephrotoxic; contrast | Nephrotoxic; cancer | |
| π-GST | DT | Detoxifying enzyme; extruded with injury | Nephrotoxic | Cancer; diabetes | Preclinical (ILSI/HESI) |
| α-GST | PT | Detoxifying enzyme; extruded with injury | Nephrotoxic | CS; neonates; cancer; diabetes | Preclinical (ILSI/HESI) |
| B2M | PT | Reduced PT reabsorption | Nephrotoxic | ICU; emergency; nephrotoxic; neonates; contrast | Preclinical |
| A1M | PT | Reduced PT reabsorption; antioxidant | Nephrotoxic | CS; nephrotoxic; diabetes | |
| Urine CysC | PT | Reduced PT reabsorption | Sepsis; nephrotoxic | ICU; sepsis; neonates | Preclinical |
| RBP | PT | Reduced PT reabsorption | Nephrotoxic | Nephrotoxic; neonates; tubular disorders | |
| Albumin | Glomerulus, PT | Reduced PT reabsorption; excess filtration with glomerular injury | Ischemia; nephrotoxic | CS; nephrotoxic; neonates; contrast; diabetes | Approved |

**Table 4.1** (continued)

| Biomarker | Nephron localization | AKI pathophysiology role/reason for change with AKI | Preclinical studies | Pediatric AKI studies | Clinical approval status |
|---|---|---|---|---|---|
| Induced with AKI | | | | | |
| NGAL | PT, DT | Injury/repair; iron transport; mitigates apoptosis/ necrosis | Ischemia; sepsis; nephrotoxic | ICU; CS; sepsis; emergency; nephrotoxic; neonates; contrast; KT; established AKI | Approved (Europe; FDA, preclinical) |
| KIM-1 | PT | Apoptotic/ necrotic bodies removal; cell regeneration | Sepsis; nephrotoxic; established AKI | ICU; CS; emergency; nephrotoxic; neonates; established AKI | Preclinical (Europe, Japan, USA) |
| IL-18 | PT | Mediates inflammation injury | Ischemia; sepsis; nephrotoxic | ICU; CS; sepsis; emergency; nephrotoxic; neonates; KT | |
| L-FABP | PT | Antioxidant | Ischemia; sepsis; nephrotoxic | ICU; CS | Approved (Japan) |
| TIMP-2 | DT | Cell cycle arrest, extracellular matrix degradation, fibrosis | Sepsis | CS; established AKI | Approved adult ICU (USA) |
| IGFBP7 | Tubules | Cell cycle arrest | Sepsis; nephrotoxic | CS; established AKI | Approved adult ICU (USA) |
| Osteopontin | Tubules | Epithelia regeneration | Ischemia; sepsis; nephrotoxic | Emergency; neonates | Preclinical (FDA, EMEA) |
| Clusterin | PT, DT | Apoptosis; tissue regeneration/ repair | Ischemia; sepsis; nephrotoxic | Neonates | Preclinical (USA, Japan, Europe) |
| VEGF | Tubules | Angiogenesis | Nephrotoxic | ICU; neonates; | |
| Calprotectin | CD | Calcium-binding protein; inflammation; repair | Ischemia | Established AKI; intrinsic AKI | |

(continued)

**Table 4.1** (continued)

| Biomarker | Nephron localization | AKI pathophysiology role/reason for change with AKI | Preclinical studies | Pediatric AKI studies | Clinical approval status |
|---|---|---|---|---|---|
| Downregulated with AKI | | | | | |
| Hepcidin-25 | Tubules | Iron homeostasis; upregulated with inflammation | Ischemia | | |
| UMOD | Thick ascending limb | Inflammation; renoprotective | Ischemia; nephrotoxic | Neonates; diabetes | |
| EGF | Henle's loop, DT | Cell repair | Nephrotoxic | Neonates; established AKI | |
| Other | | | | | |
| Trefoil Factor 3 | Tubules | Cell repair; may be downregulated with AKI | Nephrotoxic | Neonates | Preclinical (USA; Europe) |
| Cysteine-rich protein 61 | PT | Heparin-binding protein; tissue remodeling; apoptosis | Ischemia | | |
| RPA-1 | CD | Cell repair, regeneration | Nephrotoxic | | Preclinical (ILSI/HESI) |
| TIMP-1 | Glomerulus, PT | Extracellular matrix remodeling; inflammation | Ischemia; nephrotoxic | | |
| MMP-9 | Glomerulus, tubules | Extracellular matrix degradation; vascular remodeling | Ischemia; nephrotoxic | CS | |
| Calbindin | DT, CD | Calcium transport | Sepsis; nephrotoxic | | |

In this table, some biomarkers may be approved or not approved for clinical use in other countries

Abbreviations: *A1M* α1-microglobulin, *AAP* Alanine aminopeptidase, *AKI* Acute Kidney Injury, *AP* Alkaline phosphatase, *B2M* β2-microglobulin, CD Collecting duct, *CS* Cardiac surgery, *CysC* Cystatin C, *DT* Distal tubule, *EGF* Epidermal growth factor, *EMEA* European Medicines Agency, *FDA* Food and Drug Administration, *GFR* glomerular filtration rate, *GGT* γ-glutamyl transpeptidase, *GST* glutathione S-transferase, *ICU* intensive care unit, *IGFBP7* Insulin-like growth factor-binding protein 7, *IL-18* Interleukin-18, *ILSI/HESI* International Life Sciences Institute, Health and Environmental Sciences Institute, *KIM-1* Kidney injury molecule-1, *KT* Kidney transplant, *L-FABP* Liver-Type Fatty Acid Binding Protein, *MMP-9* Matrix metalloproteinase-9, *NAG* N-acetyl-β-(D)-glucosaminidase, *NGAL* Neutrophil gelatinase-associated lipocalin, *PT* Proximal tubule, *RBP* Retinol-binding protein, *RPA-1* Renal Papillary Antigen-1, *TIMP-1* Tissue inhibitor of metalloproteinase-1, *UMOD* Uromodulin, *VEGF* Vascular Endothelial Growth Factor

## 4.3 Functional Biomarkers

### 4.3.1 Serum CysC

CysC is a cysteine protease inhibitor filtered at the glomerulus. CysC concentration reflects GFR. In patients with chronic kidney disease (CKD), CysC is a more accurate marker of GFR than SCr [2, 3], likely because concentrations are less affected by age, sex, diet, and muscle mass. Hypo/hyperthyroidism lead to decreased/increased CysC concentrations, respectively. Steroids increase CysC concentrations. In AKI, CysC has mainly been evaluated in adults for earlier AKI diagnosis compared to SCr [4]. In critically ill children, CysC on the first day of PICU admission predicted SCr-defined AKI (AUC 0.71) and severe AKI (SCr doubling, AUC 0.80) within 48 h [5–7]. In children undergoing cardiac surgery, CysC 2 h after CPB initiation predicted AKI within 48 h (AUC 0.73) and CysC increased with worsening AKI severity [8]. CysC also rose before SCr in smaller nephrotoxic or sepsis AKI pediatric studies [9, 10]. Despite promising results that CysC is an earlier AKI biomarker than SCr, and that it is available in many clinical laboratories, it remains a marker of GFR change, and not direct tissue injury.

## 4.4 Tubular Damage Biomarkers

These biomarkers indicate tissue injury; they are released or have not been reabsorbed (as they normally would) by damaged cells. Success for AKI diagnosis using these markers has been variable. They likely rise rather late (i.e., not much earlier than SCr) with AKI, possibly because they indicate more severe cell damage.

### 4.4.1 NAG

NAG is a large enzyme not substantially filtered by the glomerulus. Though results are variable, studies in adults in ICU, cardiac surgery, sepsis, and nephrotoxicity have shown NAG discriminates for (identifies presence of) AKI, but lacks specificity [11–13]. NAG measured 4–12 h after pediatric CPB modestly predicted AKI (AUCs 0.69–0.75) but lacked specificity [14]. In children receiving aminoglycosides, NAG rose 3–5 days posttreatment [15].

### 4.4.2 Proximal Tubule Enzymes

Alanine aminopeptidase (AAP), alkaline phosphatase (AP), and γ-glutamyl transpeptidase (GGT) are proximal tubule brush border enzymes shed in urine with tubular injury. Adult studies have had varying results, but some have shown AAP, GGT, and AP rising with AKI and discriminating for AKI [11, 16]. Urine AAP and AP levels rose within 5 days of aminoglycoside infusion in children [15].

### 4.4.3 π-GST and α-GST

π-GST is found in distal tubular cells whereas α-GST in proximal cells. Following animal studies of nephrotoxicity showing GSTs rising before SCr with AKI, several adult studies were performed, with conflicting results. In ICU and cardiac surgery, π-GST and α-GST predicted AKI with AUCs as high as 0.93 [11, 16–18]. However, GSTs did not *predict* AKI in septic adults [19]. π-GST and α-GST have hardly been studied for AKI diagnosis in children. In neonates, peak α-GST modestly predicted AKI during early postnatal weeks (AUC 0.68) [20]. Despite limited data, GSTs appear to be early markers of AKI, but inconsistently.

### 4.4.4 Other Proximal Tubular Structural Damage Markers

Some urinary markers indicate proximal tubular damage, because they are normally filtered by the glomerulus and reabsorbed by proximal tubule cells. With AKI, urinary concentrations increase since tubular reabsorption is impaired.

Human studies demonstrated elevated urine β2-microglobulin (B2M) concentrations in adults with ATN, nephrotoxicity, cardiac surgery, and neonates [16, 20]. In the pediatric emergency room, urine B2M predicted AKI development (AUC 0.80) [21]. Few pediatric studies have adequately studied B2M as an early AKI biomarker. B2M concentrations may increase with malignancy or infection and is unstable in acidic urine [22].

α1-Microglobulin (A1M) and retinol-binding protein (RBP) are synthesized by the liver. In adults, A1M predicted renal replacement therapy (RRT) need [16]. Urine A1M predicted AKI (AUC 0.84) within 4 h after cardiac surgery in children [14]. RBP has been studied in adults and children with ATN and admitted to ICU [16, 23]. In a small cardiac surgery study, urine RBP at ICU admission predicted AKI (AUC 0.77) [24]. Urine RBP/creatinine detected AKI in a small study of asphyxiated infants [25].

Urine CysC was evaluated for early AKI diagnosis in adults in many settings with highly variable performance [4, 26]. Few pediatric studies exist; a small ICU study showed urine CysC was higher in children with vs. without AKI (discrimination) [9]. In neonates, two studies suggest it is an early AKI diagnostic test (AUCs: 0.70–0.82) [20, 27]. Urinary CysC 2 h post-cardiac surgery predicted poor outcomes in infants [28]. Urine CysC is attractive as an early AKI biomarker since clinical assays exist. However, more pediatric research is needed, especially given its variable performance in adults.

Although serum albumin is quite large, some is filtered at the glomerulus and reabsorbed by the proximal tubule. Albuminuria is traditionally a marker of glomerular damage, but may indicate proximal tubular injury due to that segment's role in reabsorbing albumin. Though results have been variable, urine albumin or albumin-to-creatinine ratio has been elevated and predicted AKI in adults and children with different forms of AKI (AUCs ~0.80) [14, 29, 30]. In neonates, urine albumin-to-creatinine ratio rose before SCr with AKI but moderately predicted AKI

(AUC ~0.65) [20]. Although urine albumin as an AKI biomarker is attractive since it is already measurable clinically, it will also be elevated at baseline in patients with CKD and may be difficult to differentiate tubular from glomerular damage.

## 4.5 Biomarkers Induced with AKI

These biomarkers have also shown variable results. However, overall, they are stronger and earlier AKI diagnostic tests, likely indicating subtler injury than markers described above.

### 4.5.1 NGAL

NGAL, the most studied novel AKI biomarker, is expressed in renal proximal and distal tubules. In adults, NGAL has been validated as an early AKI diagnostic test in various clinical settings [17, 31]. Initial studies of urine NGAL were in children undergoing cardiac surgery, showing AUCs >0.95 for predicting postoperative AKI, when measured shortly after surgery [32]. Subsequent single-center prospective studies demonstrated urine NGAL predicting AKI and AKI severity when measured as early as 2–4 h postoperatively, but with AUCs 0.75–0.95 [14, 33, 34]. Multicenter studies confirmed urine NGAL as an early post-cardiac surgery AKI predictor but with more modest AUCs ~0.70; serum NGAL did not predict AKI or poor outcomes [8, 35]. In infant cardiac surgery, urine NGAL 0–12 h postoperatively predicted risk for poor ICU outcomes (death, RRT need, prolonged time to extubation, longer ICU stay) [28]. In noncardiac surgery ICU, urinary NGAL predicted AKI 1–2 days before SCr (AUCs 0.68–0.82) and was associated with AKI severity [5, 36, 37]. In another ICU study, plasma NGAL predicted AKI whereas urine NGAL did not [6]. In infants, peak urine NGAL measured within 4 days post-birth predicted AKI within 2 weeks (AUC 0.67) [20]. Single-center studies in other settings (nephrotoxicity, emergency room) have shown urine NGAL was an early AKI diagnostic biomarker (AUCs 0.67–0.82) [21, 38]. Despite inconsistent findings, urine NGAL seems to be a better AKI marker than serum NGAL in children, overall. Meta-analyses including adult/pediatric studies showed NGAL was an early AKI diagnostic test (AUC 0.93, 24–48 h before SCr rise), predictor of mortality and RRT need, and that patients "positive" for NGAL (concentrations above a defined threshold) but "negative" for SCr rise were at higher mortality risk than NGAL "negative" patients [39, 40]. A special population is that of sepsis. Serum NGAL predicted AKI in septic children [41], but NGAL was higher in those with sepsis (or systemic inflammation/infections). One study found serum NGAL could not diagnose AKI in septic children, whereas urine NGAL could, perhaps because urine NGAL characterizes renal cell injury [9]. Research on NGAL has demonstrated key points in interpreting biomarker studies: it is important to understand a biomarker's origin and what other disease processes may impact its concentrations; validation in multicenter studies and different settings is crucial.

### 4.5.2 Kidney Injury Molecule 1 (KIM-1)

KIM-1 is a cell-adhesion molecule upregulated in injured proximal tubular cells. KIM-1 was shown to be elevated in biopsy-proven ATN [42]. In adults, KIM-1 has been validated as an AKI biomarker in ICU, cardiac surgery, sepsis, emergency and hospitalized settings [12, 17, 31]. In pediatrics, urine KIM-1 discriminated for AKI in chemotherapy and cardiac surgery [12, 43]. In both pediatric cardiac surgery and noncardiac surgery ICU patients, single- and multicenter studies have shown controversial results, with some studies showing KIM-1 to be an early diagnostic biomarker and a marker of AKI severity and some not [6, 8, 31, 33, 37]. In the emergency room, urine KIM-1 predicted AKI (AUC 0.77) [21]. In neonates, urine KIM-1 was elevated with gentamycin nephrotoxicity [44]. However, other studies in infants did not find urine KIM-1 diagnostic of AKI or predictive of outcomes [20, 28]. Overall, KIM-1 appears to rise with injury later than NGAL does, which may explain the variable results described above. Studies may not have considered most ideal *timing* of KIM-1 measurement.

### 4.5.3 Interleukin-18 (IL-18)

In humans, IL-18, a pro-inflammatory cytokine, predicted AKI development in various contexts: critical illness, ATN, sepsis, and cardiac surgery (AUCs ~0.74) [31, 45]. Pediatric studies show that urine IL-18 measured 0–12 h after cardiac surgery predicts AKI (AUCs 0.72–0.86), AKI severity, and poor outcomes [14, 31, 33, 35]. In pediatric ICU, urine IL-18 detected AKI approximately 2 days before SCr rise and correlated with AKI severity and mortality [46]. Urine IL-18 also predicted AKI in a small child study of nephrotoxic chemotherapy (highest AUC: 0.74), but not in pediatric emergency setting [21, 38]. Because IL-18 is an inflammatory marker, concentrations may be elevated in inflammatory states or infections.

### 4.5.4 Liver-Type Fatty Acid-Binding Protein (L-FABP)

Originally discovered in hepatocytes, L-FABP is an antioxidant involved in fatty acid transport. With AKI, L-FABP is upregulated and binds reactive oxygen species. After preclinical studies showing increased L-FABP expression with AKI, several adult studies in various settings showed that urinary L-FABP measured within 0–18 h of admission discriminated for AKI (AUCs 0.61–0.66) and predicted mortality [17, 31, 47]. In children, L-FABP measured 0–12 h after CPB predicted AKI and AKI severity (highest AUCs 0.78–0.89) [8, 33]. In a multicenter pediatric cardiac surgery study, urine L-FABP 0–6 h postoperatively was diagnostic of AKI (AUC 0.70) [31]. Urine L-FABP measured on first PICU day used in combination with the renal angina index ((RAI)—detailed below) predicted AKI in critically ill children (AUC 0.82) [48]. L-FABP needs further study in different pediatric populations and in multicenter studies.

### 4.5.5 Cell Cycle Arrest Biomarkers

Tissue inhibitor of metalloproteinase 2 (TIMP-2) and insulin-like growth factor-binding protein 7 (IGFBP7) are markers of G1 cell cycle arrest, important in tubular cell death. TIMP-2 and IGFBP7 were discovered and validated as AKI biomarkers in a large adult ICU study; their multiplication (TIMP-2*IGFBP7) predicted severe AKI (AUC 0.80 [0.75–0.84]) [17]. They were further validated as AKI diagnostic tests and associated with increased odds for developing AKI in adult ICU, sepsis, emergency room, and CPB [49–52]. In children, urine TIMP-2*IGFBP7 diagnosed AKI 4 h post-cardiac surgery (AUC: 0.85) [34]. Furthermore, urine TIMP-2*IGFBP7 discriminated for established AKI and predicted mortality in hospitalized children [53]. Despite good AKI diagnostic properties, TIMP-2-IGFBP7 need further validation in larger cohorts and in other clinical settings, especially in children.

### 4.5.6 Other Biomarkers Induced with AKI

Many other injury-induced biomarkers have been studied. Some seem involved in tubular damage pathophysiology in preclinical studies; others have been found elevated in patients with AKI serendipitously or are known to be abnormal in patients with non-AKI renal disease. These biomarkers require much further study and validation but are interesting, since they have all been linked to specific tubular injury mechanisms. *Osteopontin* is a phosphoprotein, involved in bone mineralization, apoptosis, and cell regeneration. Some studies have evaluated osteopontin for AKI diagnosis in adult CPB, emergency room, and neonates, with modest AUCs to predict AKI at best [20, 21, 29]. *Clusterin* is involved in cell adhesion, apoptosis, and tissue remodeling, and is upregulated with tubular injury. Other than modest AKI diagnostic performance in low-birth-weight infants, few human AKI validation studies have been performed [20]. *Vascular Endothelial Growth Factor (VEGF)* is involved in angiogenesis and induced by renal ischemia. In adult ischemic AKI setting, increased urinary VEGF predicted AKI non-recovery [54]. In infants, peak urine VEGF/creatinine measured within 4 days of birth predicted AKI development (AUC 0.68) [20]. *Calprotectin* is secreted by neutrophils and involved in kidney inflammation and repair. In single-center adult/pediatric studies, calprotectin was highly discriminatory for intrinsic AKI (likely ATN) versus controls/pre-renal AKI [55, 56]. In children with established AKI, urine calprotectin moderately predicted RRT need (AUC 0.72) [57].

### 4.5.7 Biomarkers Downregulated with AKI

These urinary biomarkers are different since their proposed use is to predict non-AKI. They are downregulated with AKI. In general, few pediatric studies exist. *Hepcidin-25* (Hep25) functions in regulating iron homeostasis. In adults undergoing cardiac surgery, urine Hep25 discriminated for AKI, followed by prospective studies showing prediction of non-AKI after cardiac surgery [58, 59]. *Uromodulin*

(UMOD, or Tamm-Horsfall protein) is involved in inflammation and may be protective for ischemic AKI. Lower preoperative urine UMOD/creatinine was associated with higher odds of AKI after adult cardiac surgery [60]. In neonates, two studies have shown urine UMOD discrimination and prediction for AKI [20, 27]. Kidney *epidermal growth factor* (EGF) may function in kidney tissue repair. In adult ischemic AKI, increased urine EGF predicted renal recovery [54]. Small studies in ICU children/neonates suggest that urine EGF discriminates for AKI [20, 27, 61].

### 4.5.8 Maximizing AKI Biomarker Performance: Biomarker Combinations

One biomarker will not perform outstandingly in all settings, reflecting complex AKI pathophysiology. Many AUCs for AKI diagnosis have been modest, especially in larger studies. This stimulated searching for best biomarker *combinations* (or panel) to predict AKI, identify AKI severity, and predict outcomes. Different biomarkers may capture different AKI mechanisms (e.g., nephrotoxic versus sepsis), tubular injury location (e.g., π-GST: distal tubule) and delineate AKI timing. Although cause-specific biomarker panels may be validated (e.g., a gentamicin nephrotoxicity panel), ideally a group of biomarkers (highly specific and sensitive) that predict AKI in various clinical settings will be validated. TIMP-2-IGFBP7 is an example of such a panel. Many biomarker combinations have been studied. For example, in pediatric cardiac surgery combining NAG, KIM-1, and MMP-9 was most diagnostic of AKI versus each alone [12]. However, other studies have shown moderate AKI diagnostic abilities for biomarker panels in different settings [31]. Biomarker panels will need to include what threshold concentration to consider "positive" for each biomarker. Some biomarker panels may be useful to inform on *timing* of AKI (where in AKI pathophysiology the patient is). For example, urine NGAL rises about 2 h after pediatric CPB, IL-18 and L-FABP about 6–8 h, and KIM-1 about 12–24 h [31, 33]. If urine is measured for biomarkers 12 h postoperatively, KIM-1 or L-FABP might be better at predicting or confirming AKI presence than NGAL.

### 4.5.9 Maximizing AKI Biomarker Performance: Adding Biomarkers to Clinical Risk Data

Moving towards clinical application, one must consider which patients will most benefit from AKI biomarker measurement. If AKI biomarkers were measured in everyone, regardless of their AKI risk, all biomarkers would have poor diagnostic characteristics. The common corollary used is measuring cardiac enzymes in patients with chest pain. These biomarkers are most useful in patients with signs and symptoms of myocardial infarction, or a high disease pre-probability. Aiming to optimize AKI biomarker utility, the renal angina concept was developed. It consists in using a combination of risk factors and AKI symptoms to guide biomarker evaluation at ICU admission [62]. A RAI equation was developed which includes *Risk of AKI* (known AKI clinical risk factors)**Evidence of AKI* (information on fluid overload and small

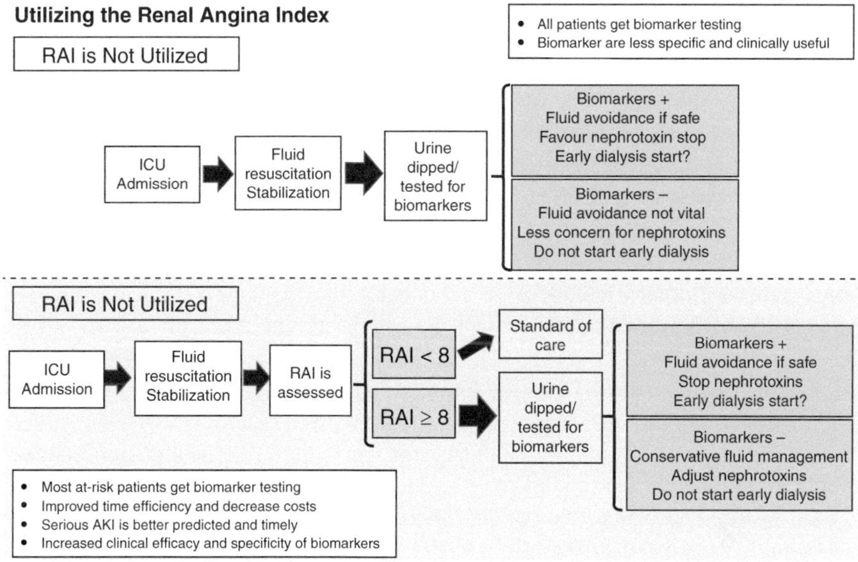


**Fig. 4.3** Potential use of biomarkers in combination with the RAI. Biomarkers used in combination with the RAI will be most clinically useful and improve AKI patient management. Similar methods could be utilized in clinical trials. Abbreviations: *AKI* Acute kidney injury, *ICU* Intensive care unit, *RAI* Renal angina index

SCr rises) [63]. The RAI score ranges from 1 to 40; a cutoff ≥8 is highly predictive of severe AKI (SCr doubling) and outcomes. A RAI ≥8 suggests renal angina; these are patients in whom it makes most sense to measure AKI biomarkers [63–65]. Studies show that RAI is effective for directing biomarker work in ICU children with heterogeneous causes of AKI. Single- and multicenter studies in ICU and septic children show that biomarkers measured at ICU admission predict AKI with AUCs around 0.70–0.80; the RAI predicts severe AKI with AUCs ~0.80. When biomarkers *and* the RAI threshold are used conjointly, AUC to predict severe AKI increases >0.95 [48, 66]. Figure 4.3 depicts how the RAI may be used in combination with biomarkers.

### 4.5.10 Conclusions: Bringing AKI Biomarker Research to Bedside and Future Research

AKI biomarker discovery and validation will continue for many years. More research in specific patient groups (e.g., sepsis) is needed. However, the tools for biomarker clinical application are there: several potential candidate biomarkers and a way of thinking on how best to use these biomarkers (e.g., the RAI). More knowledge on critical biomarker concentration thresholds is needed. AKI biomarker "positivity thresholds" have been proposed for some biomarkers (π/α-GST, NGAL, L-FABP, TIMP-2-IGFBP7, KIM-1, and others) [34, 48, 66]. But these need testing in different clinical populations. Pertinent to pediatrics, the neonatal/infant population is important to consider. Glomerular and tubular function development continues until about 2 years old and young children appear to have physiologically higher urine biomarker concentrations than older children. They will require different "positive thresholds" for AKI diagnosis [67]. Other areas of AKI biomarker research not discussed at length are their use for predicting long-term renal and other outcomes and their role in differential AKI diagnosis (e.g., the way we might use renal biopsies or ultrasounds). More research on these biomarker utilities in children is likely to emerge in the next 5 years [68]. As mentioned, the reference standard AKI definition is flawed (SCr rise; urine output drop). There is international consensus that biomarkers of tissue/structural damage should be *incorporated* with the current functional AKI definition, another area of research likely emerging shortly [68].

The role of clinicians in directing future utility of new AKI biomarkers is invaluable. It is worthwhile *now* to think of AKI not only as a rise in SCr (i.e., functional change) but also as injury/cell death within the kidney due to clinical/treatment events; to appreciate that acting early to modify AKI complications, severity and natural history could improve patient outcomes; and that patients at high *risk* for AKI should be treated differently and judiciously. With these concepts in mind, application of new biomarkers when they are available will be more natural and seem rational. When a new AKI biomarker is clinically available within your institution, if clinicians never use it, it will not help patients. Despite all the research out there, it is up to clinicians to appreciate new AKI biomarker utilities and try using them to help decision-making.

**Key Learning Points**

- New urine AKI biomarkers are indicative of direct kidney tissue (structural) *injury* whereas serum creatinine and urine output reflect impaired kidney *function*
- New AKI biomarkers allow early detection of kidney damage (before severe damage has occurred), before SCr rises substantially ("early AKI diagnosis")
- Pediatric studies show that several novel urinary AKI biomarkers (e.g., NGAL, KIM-1, IL-18, L-FABP) may predict AKI, but these must now be tested in different and specific patient populations. Moreover, children must be studied separately from adults in AKI biomarker validation studies
- Novel AKI biomarkers expressed in specific nephron segments may be useful to determine location of renal tissue injury and disease pathophysiology
- New AKI biomarkers will likely be most useful when (a) applied to patients at highest risk for developing AKI, as measured using risk scores (e.g., renal angina index) and (b) when combined with other biomarkers, to form a high diagnostic AKI biomarker panel

## References


1. Kidney Disease: Improving Global Outcomes (KDIGO) Acute Kidney Injury Work Group. KDIGO clinical practice guideline for acute kidney injury. Kidney Int. 2012;2(1):1–138.
2. Zappitelli M, Parvex P, Joseph L, Paradis G, Grey V, Lau S, et al. Derivation and validation of cystatin C-based prediction equations for GFR in children. Am J Kidney Dis. 2006;48(2):221–30.
3. Hoek FJ, Kemperman FA, Krediet RT. A comparison between cystatin C, plasma creatinine and the Cockcroft and gault formula for the estimation of glomerular filtration rate. Nephrol Dial Transplant. 2003;18(10):2024–31.
4. Zhang Z, Lu B, Sheng X, Jin N. Cystatin C in prediction of acute kidney injury: a systemic review and meta-analysis. Am J Kidney Dis. 2011;58(3):356–65.
5. Lagos-Arevalo P, Palijan A, Vertullo L, Devarajan P, Bennett MR, Sabbisetti V, et al. Cystatin C in acute kidney injury diagnosis: early biomarker or alternative to serum creatinine? Pediatr Nephrol. 2015;30(4):665–76.
6. McCaffrey J, Coupes B, Chaloner C, Webb NJ, Barber R, Lennon R. Towards a biomarker panel for the assessment of AKI in children receiving intensive care. Pediatr Nephrol. 2015;30(10):1861–71.
7. Volpon LC, Sugo EK, Carlotti AP. Diagnostic and prognostic value of serum cystatin C in critically ill children with acute kidney injury. Pediatr Crit Care Med. 2015;16(5):e125–31.
8. Peco-Antic A, Ivanisevic I, Vulicevic I, Kotur-Stevuljevic J, Ilic S, Ivanisevic J, et al. Biomarkers of acute kidney injury in pediatric cardiac surgery. Clin Biochem. 2013; 46(13–14):1244–51.
9. Di Nardo M, Ficarella A, Ricci Z, Luciano R, Stoppa F, Picardo S, et al. Impact of severe sepsis on serum and urinary biomarkers of acute kidney injury in critically ill children: an observational study. Blood Purif. 2013;35(1–3):172–6.
10. Lau L, Al-Ismaili Z, Harel-Sterling M, Pizzi M, Caldwell JS, Piccioni M, et al. Serum cystatin C for acute kidney injury evaluation in children treated with aminoglycosides. Pediatr Nephrol. 2017;32(1):163–71.
11. Westhuyzen J, Endre ZH, Reece G, Reith DM, Saltissi D, Morgan TJ. Measurement of tubular enzymuria facilitates early detection of acute renal impairment in the intensive care unit. Nephrol Dial Transplant. 2003;18(3):543–51.
12. Han WK, Waikar SS, Johnson A, Betensky RA, Dent CL, Devarajan P, et al. Urinary biomarkers in the early diagnosis of acute kidney injury. Kidney Int. 2008;73(7):863–9.
13. Liangos O, Tighiouart H, Perianayagam MC, Kolyada A, Han WK, Wald R, et al. Comparative analysis of urinary biomarkers for early detection of acute kidney injury following cardiopulmonary bypass. Biomarkers. 2009;14(6):423–31.
14. Zheng J, Xiao Y, Yao Y, Xu G, Li C, Zhang Q, et al. Comparison of urinary biomarkers for early detection of acute kidney injury after cardiopulmonary bypass surgery in infants and young children. Pediatr Cardiol. 2013;34(4):880–6.
15. Mohammadi-Karakani A, Asgharzadeh-Haghighi S, Ghazi-Khansari M, Seyed-Ebrahimi A, Ghasemi A, Jabari E. Enzymuria determination in children treated with aminoglycosides drugs. Hum Exp Toxicol. 2008;27(12):879–82.
16. Herget-Rosenthal S, Poppen D, Husing J, Marggraf G, Pietruck F, Jakob HG, et al. Prognostic value of tubular proteinuria and enzymuria in nonoliguric acute tubular necrosis. Clin Chem. 2004;50(3):552–8.
17. Kashani K, Al-Khafaji A, Ardiles T, Artigas A, Bagshaw SM, Bell M, et al. Discovery and validation of cell cycle arrest biomarkers in human acute kidney injury. Crit Care. 2013;17(1):R25.
18. Koyner JL, Vaidya VS, Bennett MR, Ma Q, Worcester E, Akhter SA, et al. Urinary biomarkers in the clinical prognosis and early detection of acute kidney injury. Clin J Am Soc Nephrol. 2010;5(12):2154–65.
19. Walshe CM, Odejayi F, Ng S, Marsh B. Urinary glutathione S-transferase as an early marker for renal dysfunction in patients admitted to intensive care with sepsis. Crit Care Resusc. 2009;11(3):204–9.

20. Askenazi DJ, Koralkar R, Patil N, Halloran B, Ambalavanan N, Griffin R. Acute kidney injury urine biomarkers in very low-birth-weight infants. Clin J Am Soc Nephrol. 2016;11(9):1527–35.
21. Du Y, Zappitelli M, Mian A, Bennett M, Ma Q, Devarajan P, et al. Urinary biomarkers to detect acute kidney injury in the pediatric emergency center. Pediatr Nephrol. 2011;26(2):267–74.
22. Bernard AM, Moreau D, Lauwerys R. Comparison of retinol-binding protein and beta 2-microglobulin determination in urine for the early detection of tubular proteinuria. Clin Chim Acta. 1982;126(1):1–7.
23. du Cheyron D, Daubin C, Poggioli J, Ramakers M, Houillier P, Charbonneau P, et al. Urinary measurement of Na+/H+ exchanger isoform 3 (NHE3) protein as new marker of tubule injury in critically ill patients with ARF. Am J Kidney Dis. 2003;42(3):497–506.
24. Che M, Xie B, Xue S, Dai H, Qian J, Ni Z, et al. Clinical usefulness of novel biomarkers for the detection of acute kidney injury following elective cardiac surgery. Nephron Clin Pract. 2010;115(1):c66–72.
25. Roberts DS, Haycock GB, Dalton RN, Turner C, Tomlinson P, Stimmler L, et al. Prediction of acute renal failure after birth asphyxia. Arch Dis Child. 1990;65(Spec 10):1021–8.
26. Aydogdu M, Gursel G, Sancak B, Yeni S, Sari G, Tasyurek S, et al. The use of plasma and urine neutrophil gelatinase associated lipocalin (NGAL) and cystatin C in early diagnosis of septic acute kidney injury in critically ill patients. Dis Markers. 2013;34(4):237–46.
27. Askenazi DJ, Koralkar R, Hundley HE, Montesanti A, Parwar P, Sonjara S, et al. Urine biomarkers predict acute kidney injury in newborns. J Pediatr. 2012;161(2):270–5.e1.
28. Hazle MA, Gajarski RJ, Aiyagari R, Yu S, Abraham A, Donohue J, et al. Urinary biomarkers and renal near-infrared spectroscopy predict intensive care unit outcomes after cardiac surgery in infants younger than 6 months of age. J Thorac Cardiovasc Surg. 2013;146(4):861–7.e1.
29. Schley G, Koberle C, Manuilova E, Rutz S, Forster C, Weyand M, et al. Comparison of plasma and urine biomarker performance in acute kidney injury. PLoS One. 2015;10(12):e0145042.
30. Ware LB, Johnson AC, Zager RA. Renal cortical albumin gene induction and urinary albumin excretion in response to acute kidney injury. Am J Physiol Renal Physiol. 2011;300(3):F628–38.
31. Parikh CR, Thiessen-Philbrook H, Garg AX, Kadiyala D, Shlipak MG, Koyner JL, et al. Performance of kidney injury molecule-1 and liver fatty acid-binding protein and combined biomarkers of AKI after cardiac surgery. Clin J Am Soc Nephrol. 2013;8(7):1079–88.
32. Mishra J, Dent C, Tarabishi R, Mitsnefes MM, Ma Q, Kelly C, et al. Neutrophil gelatinase-associated lipocalin (NGAL) as a biomarker for acute renal injury after cardiac surgery. Lancet. 2005;365(9466):1231–8.
33. Krawczeski CD, Goldstein SL, Woo JG, Wang Y, Piyaphanee N, Ma Q, et al. Temporal relationship and predictive value of urinary acute kidney injury biomarkers after pediatric cardiopulmonary bypass. J Am Coll Cardiol. 2011;58(22):2301–9.
34. Meersch M, Schmidt C, Van Aken H, Rossaint J, Gorlich D, Stege D, et al. Validation of cell-cycle arrest biomarkers for acute kidney injury after pediatric cardiac surgery. PLoS One. 2014;9(10):e110865.
35. Parikh CR, Devarajan P, Zappitelli M, Sint K, Thiessen-Philbrook H, Li S, et al. Postoperative biomarkers predict acute kidney injury and poor outcomes after pediatric cardiac surgery. J Am Soc Nephrol. 2011;22(9):1737–47.
36. Zappitelli M, Washburn KK, Arikan AA, Loftis L, Ma Q, Devarajan P, et al. Urine neutrophil gelatinase-associated lipocalin is an early marker of acute kidney injury in critically ill children: a prospective cohort study. Crit Care. 2007;11(4):R84.
37. Zwiers AJ, de Wildt SN, van Rosmalen J, de Rijke YB, Buijs EA, Tibboel D, et al. Urinary neutrophil gelatinase-associated lipocalin identifies critically ill young children with acute kidney injury following intensive care admission: a prospective cohort study. Crit Care. 2015;19:181.
38. Sterling M, Al-Ismaili Z, McMahon KR, Piccioni M, Pizzi M, Mottes T, et al. Urine biomarkers of acute kidney injury in noncritically ill, hospitalized children treated with chemotherapy. Pediatr Blood Cancer. 2017;64:10.
39. Haase M, Bellomo R, Devarajan P, Schlattmann P, Haase-Fielitz A, Group NM-aI. Accuracy of neutrophil gelatinase-associated lipocalin (NGAL) in diagnosis and prognosis in acute kidney injury: a systematic review and meta-analysis. Am J Kidney Dis. 2009;54(6):1012–24.

40. Haase M, Devarajan P, Haase-Fielitz A, Bellomo R, Cruz DN, Wagener G, et al. The outcome of neutrophil gelatinase-associated lipocalin-positive subclinical acute kidney injury: a multicenter pooled analysis of prospective studies. J Am Coll Cardiol. 2011;57(17):1752–61.
41. Wheeler DS, Devarajan P, Ma Q, Harmon K, Monaco M, Cvijanovich N, et al. Serum neutrophil gelatinase-associated lipocalin (NGAL) as a marker of acute kidney injury in critically ill children with septic shock. Crit Care Med. 2008;36(4):1297–303.
42. Han WK, Bailly V, Abichandani R, Thadhani R, Bonventre JV. Kidney Injury Molecule-1 (KIM-1): a novel biomarker for human renal proximal tubule injury. Kidney Int. 2002;62(1):237–44.
43. Carvalho Pedrosa D, Macedo de Oliveira Neves F, Cavalcante Meneses G, Pinheiro Gomes Wirtzbiki G, da Costa Moraes CA, Costa Martins AM, et al. Urinary KIM-1 in children undergoing nephrotoxic antineoplastic treatment: a prospective cohort study. Pediatr Nephrol. 2015;30(12):2207–13.
44. McWilliam SJ, Antoine DJ, Sabbisetti V, Turner MA, Farragher T, Bonventre JV, et al. Mechanism-based urinary biomarkers to identify the potential for aminoglycoside-induced nephrotoxicity in premature neonates: a proof-of-concept study. PLoS One. 2012;7(8):e43809.
45. Parikh CR, Abraham E, Ancukiewicz M, Edelstein CL. Urine IL-18 is an early diagnostic marker for acute kidney injury and predicts mortality in the intensive care unit. J Am Soc Nephrol. 2005;16(10):3046–52.
46. Washburn KK, Zappitelli M, Arikan AA, Loftis L, Yalavarthy R, Parikh CR, et al. Urinary interleukin-18 is an acute kidney injury biomarker in critically ill children. Nephrol Dial Transplant. 2008;23(2):566–72.
47. Doi K, Noiri E, Maeda-Mamiya R, Ishii T, Negishi K, Hamasaki Y, et al. Urinary L-type fatty acid-binding protein as a new biomarker of sepsis complicated with acute kidney injury. Crit Care Med. 2010;38(10):2037–42.
48. Menon S, Goldstein SL, Mottes T, Fei L, Kaddourah A, Terrell T, et al. Urinary biomarker incorporation into the renal angina index early in intensive care unit admission optimizes acute kidney injury prediction in critically ill children: a prospective cohort study. Nephrol Dial Transplant. 2016;31(4):586–94.
49. Bihorac A, Chawla LS, Shaw AD, Al-Khafaji A, Davison DL, Demuth GE, et al. Validation of cell-cycle arrest biomarkers for acute kidney injury using clinical adjudication. Am J Respir Crit Care Med. 2014;189(8):932–9.
50. Hoste EA, McCullough PA, Kashani K, Chawla LS, Joannidis M, Shaw AD, et al. Derivation and validation of cutoffs for clinical use of cell cycle arrest biomarkers. Nephrol Dial Transplant. 2014;29(11):2054–61.
51. Mayer T, Bolliger D, Scholz M, Reuthebuch O, Gregor M, Meier P, et al. Urine biomarkers of tubular renal cell damage for the prediction of acute kidney injury after cardiac surgery-a pilot study. J Cardiothorac Vasc Anesth. 2017;31:2072.
52. Kimmel M, Shi J, Latus J, Wasser C, Kitterer D, Braun N, et al. Association of renal stress/damage and filtration biomarkers with subsequent AKI during hospitalization among patients presenting to the emergency department. Clin J Am Soc Nephrol. 2016;11(6):938–46.
53. Westhoff JH, Tonshoff B, Waldherr S, Poschl J, Teufel U, Westhoff TH, et al. Urinary tissue inhibitor of Metalloproteinase-2 (TIMP-2) * insulin-like growth factor-binding protein 7 (IGFBP7) predicts adverse outcome in pediatric acute kidney injury. PLoS One. 2015;10(11):e0143628.
54. Kwon O, Ahn K, Zhang B, Lockwood T, Dhamija R, Anderson D, et al. Simultaneous monitoring of multiple urinary cytokines may predict renal and patient outcome in ischemic AKI. Ren Fail. 2010;32(6):699–708.
55. Seibert FS, Pagonas N, Arndt R, Heller F, Dragun D, Persson P, et al. Calprotectin and neutrophil gelatinase-associated lipocalin in the differentiation of pre-renal and intrinsic acute kidney injury. Acta Physiol (Oxf). 2013;207(4):700–8.
56. Westhoff JH, Fichtner A, Waldherr S, Pagonas N, Seibert FS, Babel N, et al. Urinary biomarkers for the differentiation of prerenal and intrinsic pediatric acute kidney injury. Pediatr Nephrol. 2016;31(12):2353–63.

57. Westhoff JH, Seibert FS, Waldherr S, Bauer F, Tonshoff B, Fichtner A, et al. Urinary calprotectin, kidney injury molecule-1, and neutrophil gelatinase-associated lipocalin for the prediction of adverse outcome in pediatric acute kidney injury. Eur J Pediatr. 2017;176(6):745–55.
58. Ho J, Lucy M, Krokhin O, Hayglass K, Pascoe E, Darroch G, et al. Mass spectrometry-based proteomic analysis of urine in acute kidney injury following cardiopulmonary bypass: a nested case-control study. Am J Kidney Dis. 2009;53(4):584–95.
59. Ho J, Reslerova M, Gali B, Gao A, Bestland J, Rush DN, et al. Urinary hepcidin-25 and risk of acute kidney injury following cardiopulmonary bypass. Clin J Am Soc Nephrol. 2011;6(10):2340–6.
60. Garimella PS, Jaber BL, Tighiouart H, Liangos O, Bennett MR, Devarajan P, et al. Association of Preoperative Urinary Uromodulin with AKI after cardiac surgery. Clin J Am Soc Nephrol. 2017;12(1):10–8.
61. Wai K, Soler-Garcia AA, Perazzo S, Mattison P, Ray PE. A pilot study of urinary fibroblast growth factor-2 and epithelial growth factor as potential biomarkers of acute kidney injury in critically ill children. Pediatr Nephrol. 2013;28(11):2189–98.
62. Goldstein SL, Chawla LS. Renal angina. Clin J Am Soc Nephrol. 2010;5(5):943–9.
63. Basu RK, Chawla LS, Wheeler DS, Goldstein SL. Renal angina: an emerging paradigm to identify children at risk for acute kidney injury. Pediatr Nephrol. 2012;27(7):1067–78.
64. Basu RK, Zappitelli M, Brunner L, Wang Y, Wong HR, Chawla LS, et al. Derivation and validation of the renal angina index to improve the prediction of acute kidney injury in critically ill children. Kidney Int. 2014;85(3):659–67.
65. Basu RK, Kaddourah A, Goldstein SL. Assessment of a renal angina index for prediction of severe acute kidney injury in critically ill children: a multicentre, multinational, prospective observational study. Lancet Child Adolesc Health. 2017;2:112–20.
66. Basu RK, Wang Y, Wong HR, Chawla LS, Wheeler DS, Goldstein SL. Incorporation of biomarkers with the renal angina index for prediction of severe AKI in critically ill children. Clin J Am Soc Nephrol. 2014;9(4):654–62.
67. Zappitelli M, Coca SG, Garg AX, Krawczeski CD, Thiessen Heather P, Sint K, et al. The association of albumin/creatinine ratio with postoperative AKI in children undergoing cardiac surgery. Clin J Am Soc Nephrol. 2012;7(11):1761–9.
68. McCullough PA, Bouchard J, Waikar SS, Siew ED, Endre ZH, Goldstein SL, et al. Implementation of novel biomarkers in the diagnosis, prognosis, and management of acute kidney injury: executive summary from the tenth consensus conference of the acute Dialysis quality initiative (ADQI). Contrib Nephrol. 2013;182:5–12.

# Neonatal Critical Care Nephrology

# 5

David Askenazi and Vesna Stojanović

**Case Vignette**

An infant is born to a 21-year-old mother at 27 weeks post conception with a birthweight of 900 g. His serum creatinine concentration increases over the coming days from 0.8 to 1.0 mg/dL and then improves over the coming weeks to 0.3 mg/dL at 3 weeks of age. The infant develops apnea and bradycardia, sepsis and has necrotizing enterocolitis by abdominal X-ray. His enteral feeding is discontinued and interventions are started including multiple blood product transfusions, intravenous vasoactive medication infusions, and invasive mechanical ventilator support. Over the following week, he develops progressive abdominal distension, hypoalbuminemia, decreased urine output, and edema. His serum creatinine concentration has increased to 1.3 mg/dL and he now weighs 1350 g.

This chapter provides insights to understand the physiology and management of neonates at risk for acute kidney injury (AKI) during the neonatal intensive care units (NICU) course. We will review renal physiology and evaluation of the glomerular filtration rate in the neonate. We will also provide a review of the assessment, diagnosis, risk factors, and outcomes of neonatal AKI. Medical management and strategies for renal support, including a review of novel machines designed for neonates, will be discussed. Finally, outcome data on the long-term consequences of kidney disease in NICU graduates are presented.

D. Askenazi (✉)
Division of Pediatric Nephrology, Department of Pediatrics, Pediatric and Infant Center for Acute Nephrology, University of Alabama at Birmingham, Birmingham, AL, USA
e-mail: daskenazi@peds.uab.edu

V. Stojanović
Medical Faculty, Department of Pediatrics, Novi Sad, Serbia

Intermediate Intensive Care Unit, Institute of Child and Youth Health Care of Vojvodina, Novi Sad, Serbia

 
A. Deep, S. L. Goldstein (eds.), *Critical Care Nephrology and Renal Replacement Therapy in Children*, https://doi.org/10.1007/978-3-319-90281-4_5

Extraordinary advancements in neonatal care have markedly reduced the mortality rates of infants hospitalized in NICU. Over the last decade, studies show that neonatal AKI is common and those with AKI have higher mortality and prolonged length of stay. Premature infants are born with low nephron numbers which predisposes them to AKI and chronic kidney disease (CKD). Despite recent insights that substantiate the impact of poor kidney health on outcomes in sick neonates, significant critical gaps in our understanding of the antenatal and postnatal factors exist. The global burden of AKI and CKD in NICU graduates need to be better understood. Fortunately, progress is being made as investigators are performing large observational studies, and randomized clinical trials that evaluate risk factors, outcomes, and interventions. In addition, novel devices designed specifically to provide renal support for neonates are currently in use in a few centers around the world.

## 5.1 Neonatal Renal Physiology

Nephrogenesis starts in the 5th and ends in the 34th–36th gestational week, although kidney maturation continues in the postnatal period (until the 40th postnatal day) [1].

*Renal Blood Flow* (RBF) in neonates during the first week of life is only 10% of the cardiac output (2.5–4% on birth), and it reaches the adult rate (25%) by 2 years of age. This increase of RBF occurs due to a combination of an increase of renal perfusion pressure, increase of systemic vascular resistance, and a reduction of renal vascular resistance via angiotensin II (AT II), prostaglandin, and other physiologic changes [2].

*Glomerular filtration rate* (GFR) is a measure of kidney function. In a healthy term newborn, the GFR at birth is 10–20 mL/min/1.73 m$^2$, rises to 30–40 mL/min/1.73 m$^2$ in the second week, and reaches the adult clearance of 100–120 mL/min/1.73 m$^2$ by the age of 2 years. In the first weeks of life, GFR is even lower in preterm neonates compared with term neonates as a result of renal immaturity, difference in renal blood flow, and distinct vascular resistance. Rigorous studies to estimate serum creatinine (SCr) clearance using SCr in neonates have not been performed recently. Older studies suggest that using SCr measured by Jaffe enzymatic reaction, that eGFR could be estimated using the following equation [3, 4].

Estimated creatinine clearance (mL/min/1.73 m$^2$) = k * BH/sCr

(k—constant—0.33; BH—height in cm; sCr—serum creatinine in mg/dL (mg/dL × 88.4 = μmol/L)).

Studies in children suggest that when using the enzymatic SCr to estimate GFR, the coefficient is about 10% lower than when using the Jaffe reaction. More data are needed, but it is possible that the correct coefficient when using the enzymatic reaction should be 10% lower than above, or 0.3 [5].

The maximal *urine concentration capacity* in the term neonate is 500–700 mOsm. The adult level (1400 mOsm) is reached between the 6th and 12th month of life. This relatively lower urinary concentration ability increases the risks of fluid loss, decreased reabsorption of substances and electrolyte imbalance.

In newborns, water makes 80% of the body weight (BW) of the newborn. Soon after birth, there is a redistribution of body fluids, with an early postnatal BW loss of up to 5–10% in healthy term infants. Very low birthweight (VLBW) infants need intravenous support of fluids to prevent dehydration. As VLBW infants may have very high insensible losses due to very thin skin, their fluid loss may be significantly higher than healthy term neonates. It is not uncommon for VLBW infant to lose up to 15% in VLBW neonates due to isotonic contraction of extracellular water through disposal of excess sodium and water through kidneys. Studies to optimize fluid delivery in this vulnerable cohort are greatly needed.

The most significant site of sodium exchange is distal tubule. If the term neonate can successfully feed from the breast or formula, he/she can maintain the positive sodium balance. However, it is not uncommon for a newborn less than 35 weeks gestation to be at risk for negative sodium balance in the first 3 months of life which could lead to hyponatremia. This is due to increased delivery of sodium and its reduced absorption in the distal tubule. This is important to consider when testing for prerenal azotemia. In term newborns, the fractional excretion of sodium (FENa) is highest during the first 10 days of life and can decrease to below 0.4% by 1 month of age, an ultimate threshold that is similar to adults. Due to inability to reabsorb sodium avidly during prerenal azotemia states, VLBW infants will have much higher FENa than term counterparts. FENa can also be increased in hypoxia, respiratory distress, hyperbilirubinemia, and in neonates taking diuretics and increased intake of fluids and salts [3, 6, 7].

The renin-angiotensin-aldosterone system (RAAS) is responsible for regulation of blood pressure, renal hemodynamics, and maintenance of fluid and electrolytes balance. Plasma renin activity is increased after birth and stays increased during infancy until it is reduced to adult levels by the age of 6–9 years. Angiotensin stimulates the secretion of aldosterone which regulates the reabsorption of sodium in kidneys. The fetal response to secrete aldosterone is less than that seen in adults [8].

On the other hand, prostaglandins represent the most important counter regulatory molecules in neonatal period and they lead to the dilation of afferent arteriole. Atrial natriuretic peptide (ANP) is a vasodilator and is significantly increased in the first days of life and then reduced by the 2nd week. It also reduces extracellular volume [3].

## 5.2 Evaluation of Neonatal Acute Kidney Injury (AKI)

Acute kidney injury (AKI) is a complex pathology characterized by a sudden reduction of kidney function caused by a heterogeneous group of underlying causes. Clinically, AKI is manifested by minimal kidney damage up to the complete kidney failure that requires renal replacement therapy.

### 5.2.1 History and Physical Examination

Previous reports suggest that neonatal AKI is due to: inadequate renal blood flow (previously referred to as prerenal—85%), intrarenal pathology—11%, and then obstruction of the urinary tract—3%. In newborns with AKI, it is very important to examine all the possible causes that could have led to AKI. The most causes of inadequate renal perfusion are: hypovolemia, hypotension, hypoxemia, heart failure, dehydration, septicemia, hypoalbuminemia, perinatal asphyxia, respiratory distress syndrome, congenital heart disease, cardiac surgery, polycythemia, and nephrotoxic drugs (e.g., indomethacin, captopril, vasodilators). The most common causes of intrarenal AKI are: acute tubular necrosis, corticomedullary necrosis, renal venous and arterial thrombosis, acute pyelonephritis, disseminated vascular coagulation, isoimmune hemolytic disease, congenital renal anomalies, systemic infections, intrauterine infections, and nephrotoxic drug exposure (aminoglycosides, radiocontrast agents). The most common causes of postrenal AKI are: posterior urethral valves, bilateral obstructive uropathy, neurogenic bladder, and blockade from fungal collections [9].

*The clinical history* should include data regarding gestational age, birthweight, antenatal ultrasound (renal anomalies, abdominal mass, oligohydramnios), the mother's exposure to nephrotoxic drugs during pregnancy (nonsteroidal anti-inflammatory drugs, ACE inhibitors and antibiotics), birth history (vital parameters on birth, reanimation, Apgar score), as well as the usage of nephrotoxic drugs in newborns during birth, hypotension, sepsis, congenital heart disease, ECMO support, and vasoactive drug use.

*The physical examination* should include the assessment of volume status. Signs of dehydration include tachycardia, hypotension, sunken fontanelle, and dry mucous membranes; signs of fluid overload include tachypnea, edemas, elevated blood pressure, escalating oxygen requirement and ventilator support. Careful attention to vital signs, daily weights, intake and output and cumulative fluid balance will help direct fluid provision goals and rates.

### 5.2.2 Laboratory and Radiology Examination

Laboratory parameters including electrolytes calcium, magnesium, phosphorous, complete blood cell count, blood urea nitrogen, serum creatinine, albumin, blood gas, and urinalysis should be measured in infants with or at risk of AKI. A random urine sodium and creatinine to calculate FENa can determine if there is intact tubular function in context of a rising creatinine caused by poor renal perfusion.

Based on the parameters given in Table 5.1, prerenal AKI can be differentiated from the acute tubular necrosis (ATN).

**Table 5.1** Differential diagnosis of prerenal and renal AKI

| Test | Prerenal AKI | ATN |
|---|---|---|
| $U_{osm}$(mOsm/L) | >400 | <400 |
| Urinary Na (mmol/L) | <20–30 | >30–40 |
| FENa | <2.5 (<1[a]) | >2.5 (>1[a]) |

[a]Term neonates

FENa—fractional sodium excretion $\left(\frac{U_{Na} \times P_{Cr}}{U_{Cr} \times P_{Na}} \times 100\right)$

An ultrasound of the bladder and kidneys should be performed if there is a suspicion for congenital renal abnormality and to rule out obstruction. Doppler assessment of renal vessels (to evaluate the blood flow) should be considered if renal vein or artery thrombosis is suspected. Additional test may include chest X-ray to assess lung volumes and heart size and a voiding cystourethrogram in infants with hydronephrosis demonstrated on ultrasound.

### 5.2.3 Neonatal AKI Definition

The most common accepted definition of neonatal AKI is based on a rise in SCr and/or decrease in urine output (UO). The worse of the two parameters is used to make the AKI diagnosis and classify the AKI stage (Table 5.2) [10, 11].

It is important to recognize the limitation of this definition and staging system. Unfortunately, SCr is a suboptimal biomarker for AKI as: (1) SCr is a marker of kidney function, not injury, (2) SCr may not change until 25–50% of the kidney function has been lost, (3) at a lower GFR, SCr will overestimate kidney function due to tubular secretion of creatinine, (4) SCr varies by muscle mass, hydration status, sex, age, and gender, (5) once a patient receives renal replacement therapy, SCr can no longer be used to assess kidney function since it is easily dialyzed, and (6) certain medications and bilirubin can affect SCr measurements by the Jaffe method. A most pertinent neonatal limitation is that the SCr level is high after birth, as it reflects maternal SCr concentration. After 36–96 h of life, the SCr concentration gradually decreases. In neonates with a lower gestational age, the initial values of SCr are higher and the subsequent decrease is more gradual. SCr levels do not differentiate causes of AKI: prerenal causes, timing of the kidney insult, nephrotoxic drug exposure, and ischemic acute tubular necrosis [10].

Most cases of AKI in neonates are nonoliguric, which may be due to the inherent poor tubular function of premature infants who will be challenged to hold on to fluid in states of decreased vascular volume. Also, newborns, especially preterm, have significantly higher total body water content than older children and adults. This, combined with immature tubules, can explain why the urine output may be higher in newborns with AKI. Although there are not tremendous data available to determine the optimal cutoff for UOP, more recent studies suggest that a UO < 1.5 mL/kg/h is associated with poor outcomes [12–14].

**Table 5.2** SCr and UO staging system for AKI diagnosis and severity

| | Serum creatinine criteria (SCr) | Urine output (UO) criteria |
|---|---|---|
| Stage 0 | No change or rise <0.3 mg/dL | UO > 1.0 mL/kg/h for 24 h |
| Stage I | ↑SCr 0.3 mg/dL or ↑150–200% from previous trough value | UO < 1.0 mL/kg/h for 24 h |
| Stage II | ↑SCr 200–300% from previous trough value | UO < 0.5 mL/kg/h for 24 h |
| Stage III | ↑SCr 300% from previous trough value or 2.5 mg/dL or receiving dialysis | UO < 0.3 mL/kg/h for 24 h or anuric for 12 h |

Zappitelli M et al. Pediatric Research 4: 569, 2017

### 5.2.4 Novel Biomarkers for AKI

Due to insufficient reliability on SCr for early AKI diagnosis, numerous studies to improve the ability to identify neonates with kidney injury have been performed in neonates. The ideal biomarker should rise early in the disease course, is noninvasive and sensitive indicator of AKI, and can specify different etiologies of neonatal AKI.

The most promising noninvasive early biomarkers of neonatal AKI are serum and urinary neutrophil gelatinase-associated lipocalin (NGAL), urinary interleukin-18, kidney injury molecule-1, serum cystatin C, osteopontin (OPN), and beta-2 microglobulin. For some of them there are established normal values in dependence of GA and BW. These biomarkers promise to improve our ability to identify AKI early in the course of disease and help to differentiate the etiology of a rising SCr and/or drop in UO [15].

### 5.2.5 Incidence and Outcomes of Neonatal AKI

While the study of AKI in critically ill neonates has lagged behind studies in pediatric and adult populations, the last 5 years have seen an intensification of research in this area. Small, single-center studies in select patient groups such as those with congenital heart disease [16], sepsis [17], hypoxic ischemic injury [18–20], infants who receive extracorporeal membrane oxygenation [21], and very low birthweight infants [11, 22–24] suggest that AKI is common, and that those with AKI have worse outcomes.

In 2014, a group of neonatologists and nephrologists formed the Neonatal Kidney Collaborative. The inaugural project of the Neonatal Kidney Collaborative, the Assessment of Worldwide Assessment of Kidney Epidemiology in Neonates (AWAKEN) was a retrospective cohort study that screened 4273 infants who were admitted to level 2–3 NICU across 24 sites in 4 countries. 2022 infants met inclusion and exclusion criteria (most were excluded due to not being on intravenous fluid for 48 h). Neonatal AKI occurred in 30% of those enrolled with differences in AKI rates in those who were born at less than 29 weeks (46%), 29–36 weeks (18%), and >36 weeks (46%). Those with AKI had about 10% mortality rate compared to 1.5% in those without AKI. Even after adjusting for potential confounders, those with AKI had 4.6 times higher odds of death and 8.8 more hospitalized days compared to neonates without AKI. These associations remained when these analysis were performed for individual GA groups [25].

### 5.2.6 Risk Factors of Neonatal AKI

The risk for neonatal AKI can be attributed to four broad factors [3]. The first is the state of the infant's kidneys at the time of birth. If an infant is born with a paucity of nephron numbers, the kidneys will lack the potential reserve necessary to overcome a stressful event, leading a reduction in kidney function. Reasons that can lead to a paucity of nephron numbers prior to birth include maternal disease such as diabetes, maternal exposure to nephrotoxic and teratogenic substances, prematurity as renal development continues until 34 weeks gestational age, and congenital anomalies of the kidneys.

The second set of risk factors for the development of neonatal AKI are centered on the hemodynamic and metabolic physiologic demands which occur around the time of birth. Studies consistently show that Apgar scores, receipt of interventions around the time of birth, birth lactate levels, and CRIB 2 scores are risk factors for AKI [26]. Depending on the degree of kidney damage, disruption of the normal physiologic process can result in transient or permanent kidney damage.

The third set of factors of neonatal AKI are secondary to events that may occur during the neonatal time frame. These include episodes of shock (cardiogenic, hypovolemic, or ischemic shock) that can occur during cardiopulmonary bypass surgery, sepsis, and other neonatal conditions. The risk factors for neonatal AKI during cardiopulmonary bypass include preoperative factors (such as degree of hypotension), intraoperative factors (such as aortic bypass time), and post-op factors such as cardiac performance. The risk factors to develop AKI during episodes of sepsis, necrotizing enterocolitis, or wide patent ductus arteriosus have not been fully examined.

The fourth set of risk factors for neonatal AKI development are the iatrogenic medications that are used to treat the infant. Studies in premature infants suggest that most infants admitted to the NICU receive multiple nephrotoxic medications. Indeed the potential impact of nephrotoxic medications on the development of AKI is likely very substantial [11, 24]. Strategies to limit high nephrotoxic exposure and reduce AKI in those who are exposed to nephrotoxic medications could have a tremendous impact on the long-term outcomes.

Strategies to identify AKI in the most premature infants, around the time of birth in infants with difficult delivery, during high-risk events, and while nephrotoxic medications are being given may help prevent AKI and its consequences. The need for a more comprehensive evaluation of the risk factors associated with AKI during these four broad risk factors will be helpful in developing clinical guidelines for clinicians [3].

## 5.3 Interventions to Prevent/Treat AKI

Several therapeutic options have been used to prevent and/or mitigate AKI. In patients with perinatal asphyxia, four randomized clinical trials show that theophylline given in the first hours of life to neonates with asphyxia decrease the rates and severity of AKI. Theophylline is an adenosine receptor agonist which can prevent AKI by inhibiting adenosine-induced vasoconstriction [27]. Dopamine leads to vasodilation of the renal vasculature. However, regardless of encouraging results on animal models, it is not proven that there is a benefit in prevention or treatment of AKI with it [28]. On the other hand, fenoldopam, high selective dopamine type 1 receptor agonist which leads to the dilation of renal vasculature, showed some modest benefit in a small, single-center study of infants undergoing cardiopulmonary bypass for congenital heart disease repair [29].

Diuretics are commonly given in order to maintain urine output in the neonates with AKI. There are only a few of studies reporting the use of diuretics in neonates with oliguric AKI, and long-term outcomes have not been reported. The loop diuretics should not be used to prevent AKI, although in cases of fluid overload with oliguria/anuria they do provide a reasonable therapeutic option [30]. The studies haven't shown a better outcome in adults who have been receiving diuretics [31]. The use of recombinant urate oxidase (rasburicase) in the context of hyperuricemia has been shown to reduce SCr levels and improve UOP in a case series of term infants with AKI [32].

## 5.4 Supportive Medical Management

Supportive care to help achieve electrolyte and fluid homeostasis should be started as soon as possible in order to prevent the development of sequelae. Close attention to detail and serial monitoring of urine output and kidney function in neonates is paramount. The keys to supportive management include: (a) identification and correction of risk factors when able, (b) identification and treatment of the cause, (c) prevent further kidney injury by maintaining kidney perfusion with adequate oncotic pressure, intravascular volume, and cardiac contractility, (d) avoidance and unnecessary and appropriate dosing of nephrotoxic drugs, (e) prevention of fluid overload, (f) maintenance of electrolyte balance, and (g) placement of a urinary catheter if obstruction is documented or suspected.

Close attention to fluid status (measure weight, fluid intake and output, serum electrolytes twice a day) is imperative. In a case of oliguria or anuria, one strategy to determine fluid intake is to calculate and only replace the estimated fluid losses: diuresis + insensible losses + extra losses (chest tube losses + gastrointestinal losses, etc.) Depending on the environment of the neonate (incubator vs. open crib vs. warmer) insensible losses may vary. The full term neonate may have insensible losses of 300–400 mL/m$^2$ = 25 mL/kg/day but this can be significantly higher for preterm newborns—40–100 mL/kg/day due to excess fluid losses via their very thin skin. In the first week after birth, >10% weight loss is excessive and should be avoided.

Strategies for fluid balance maintenance of in the neonate should be optimized based on the stage of fluid provision. In the resuscitative stage, a fluid challenge of 10–20 mL/kg should be provided, and possibly repeated depending on the hemodynamic changes seen. Once the resuscitative phase in complete, a strategy to prevent further fluid accumulation should be instituted. Maximizing concentration of fluids (including nutrition) and avoiding excess fluid provision will minimize fluid overload. Diuretics can be given to help achieve euvolemia, recognizing that a failed response to diuretic challenge suggests that AKI will progress. Repeated attempts to escalate diuretics can delay appropriate renal support therapy (dialysis). Surgical decompression of the abdomen in cases of high abdominal pressures should be considered.

Close monitoring of electrolytes is critical, electrolytes should be replaced as needed. Discontinuation of infusions of phosphorous and potassium-containing solutions may be critical. Metabolic acidosis can be due to premature tubular function or other reasons and for the most part should be corrected.

It is important to follow the serum level of drugs the patient is getting which could potentially damage the kidney function. If there is no vital indication, nephrotoxic drugs should be avoided. If, however they must be given, they should be given at the proper interval and dosage based on the estimated creatinine clearance [20, 33, 34].

## 5.5 Renal Support Therapy for Neonates

Renal support therapy in the form of hemodialysis, peritoneal dialysis (PD), or continuous renal replacement therapy (CRRT) is rarely used in the NICU, even in high volume NICUs in large tertiary hospitals. One of the reasons is that until recently, CRRT machines have not been designed for neonates, thus the risk of the procedure push the balance toward watchful waiting to initiate therapy. In the AWAKEN cohort, neonatal RRT was performed on 25/4273 (0.5%) of neonates admitted to 24 tertiary NICUs during the 3 months period. The types of RRT included peritoneal dialysis alone ($N = 9$), continuous renal replacement therapy (CRRT) ($N = 4$), CRRT + ECMO ($n = 11$), and peritoneal dialysis + CRRT ($n = 1$). No infants were dialyzed with intermittent hemodialysis or slow low efficiency dialysis. Of those who received RRT, 19/25 (76%) survived [25].

*Indications for renal replacement therapy*: Absolute indications include hypervolemia resistant to diuretics, congestive cardiac failure, severe hypertension with high intravascular volume, hyperkalemia (>8 mmol/L), metabolic acidosis (pH < 7.20, or $HCO_3$ < 12 mmol/L), other symptomatic electrolyte disorders (hypo or hypernatremia, hypocalcemia, hyperphosphatemia), rapid increase of urea, and creatinine concentrations (uremic symptoms). Relative indications for dialysis are inability to provide adequate nutrition in context of fluid restriction, prevention of further fluid overload. In addition, HD or CRRT with high clearance rates are first line therapies for infants born with specific inborn errors of metabolism with high ammonia levels.

## 5.6 Peritoneal Dialysis (PD)

Peritoneal dialysis is a method of choice for kidney function replacement in newborns, and especially in ELBW newborns. Advantages of PD come from its technical simplicity without the need for vascular access or blood prime of an extracorporeal circuit, no need for systemic heparinization, and slow continuous fluid removal. In infants, the peritoneal surface area per unit weight is approximately twice that of an adult and, overall, it shows more efficiency in both urea clearance and ultrafiltration. Disadvantages of PD are: slower correction of metabolic parameters; lower clearance of small molecules; PD is less effective than other modalities in pulmonary edema, poisoning, or drug overdose, hypercatabolic states, and hyperkalemia. The main risks of the procedure are peritonitis, catheter/exit-site infection, and electrolyte abnormalities. Also, as compared to CRRT, PD does not allow precision in the net fluid removal rates, instead one can only increase or decrease the dextrose concentration in hopes of achieving ultrafiltration goals [35].

The use of PD after cardiopulmonary bypass surgery to prevent fluid accumulation has been shown to improve outcomes [36, 37] and is discussed fully in Chap. 15.

Relative *contraindications* for acute PD are: recent abdominal surgery, pleuroperitoneal communication, diaphragmatic hernia, severe respiratory failure, life-threatening hyperkalemia, extremely hypercatabolic state, severe volume overload in a patient not on a ventilator, severe gastroesophageal reflux disease, low peritoneal clearance, fecal or fungal peritonitis, and abdominal wall cellulitis.

There are two types of peritoneal catheters. The *semirigid acute catheter*—the advantages of this kind of catheter are that they can be placed bedside under a local anesthesia and they do not need any surgical help. The disadvantages are: higher risk of infection, bowel perforation risk, and they cannot be left in place for more than 72 h. The *Cuffed permanent catheter*—the most popular and the most used one is a Tenckhoff catheter. The advantages are: lower risk of infection and bowel perforation; can be used immediately after insertion. The disadvantage is that it requires a surgical insertion, and ideally these catheters are left to heal and optimize the tunnel for 2–3 weeks prior to use.

Due to the limited space in the peritoneal cavity in neonates especially in ELBW neonates, it is very difficult to place a rigid peritoneal catheter, which is why the alternatives are exploited, such as the suction catheter tip, plastic catheter, angiocath, neonatal chest drain, IV cannula, femoral vein catheter, Wallace catheter, and Cook 5F catheter.

A downward pointing exit site (outside the diaper area and stomas) is recommended for peritoneal access. Catheters can be inserted either through the linea alba or laterally or paramedially through the rectus muscle directly into the peritoneum. For permanent catheters, the catheter is tunneled under the skin. For very small neonates, the PD catheter is inserted directly through the abdominal wall, without tunneling. If the insertion is done surgically, it is recommended to do an omentectomy, at the time of PD catheter insertion. After implantation, the catheters are flushed with 10 mL/kg of dialysis solution until the effluent is clear. Perioperative it is recommended to give an antibiotic prophylaxis, mostly given as a single dose of a first- or second-generation cephalosporin or vancomycin. After inserting the catheter, heparin in the dialysate fluid (250–500 units/L) is used to prevent clot formation [35, 38, 39].

### 5.6.1 Acute PD Prescription for Neonates

Continuous PD is performed in newborns. The initial volume of fluid should ideally be 10 mL/kg per exchange for at least 1 week. Exchanges can be done every 20–30 min, although most of the time, hourly cycles are sufficient, especially if the procedure is performed 24 h a day. After 1 week, the PD fluid volume is increased slowly over a course of weeks toward the maximum of 40 mL/kg. As the volume is increased, the total cumulative duration of the exchanges is decreased toward 8–12 h per day [35].

Potassium can be added to the PD fluid in hypokalemic patients. Usually 3–4 meq/L is added to maintain normal potassium levels. Fluid removal will be driven by the dextrose concentration in the fluids. A higher dextrose concentration will lead to a higher total fluid removal or ultrafiltration.

#### 5.6.1.1 Complications of PD

*Infectious complications include:* exit-site infection (flare, suppurative secretion, granulation) or peritonitis. *Staphylococcus aureus* is the most common causative agent. *Noninfectious complications include:* migration of the catheter, perforation, blood in dialysate, dialysate leakage, respiratory insufficiency, extravasation of fluid in tissue compartments, hernias, and hydrothorax. Metabolic complications include *fluid,* electrolyte, and acid base disturbances. It is important to recognize that up to 1.5 g/kg/day of protein can be lost during peritoneal dialysis.

#### 5.6.1.2 Bacterial Peritonitis

The main symptoms of peritonitis are: cloudy peritoneal fluid, feeding intolerance, irritability, pain, and fever although the latter two may be difficult to manifest in an infant on a warmer. It is diagnosed based on peritoneal fluid cell count, differential count, gram stain, and culture. A presumptive diagnosis of peritonitis can be made when there are more than 100 leukocytes/mm$^3$, with more than 50% polymorphonuclear cells. Bacterial peritonitis often is caused by a tunnel infection or an inadvertent break in the sterile handling of the PD catheter tubing set or transfer set. Therapy of bacterial peritonitis includes either systemic or intraperitoneal antibiotics. For intraperitoneal antibiotics, two or three rapid PD exchanges are performed initially, followed by a loading dose of intraperitoneal antibiotics (vancomycin 500 mg/L, ceftazidime 250 mg/L) in the abdomen for 4 h. After that the antibiotic doses are reduced (vancomycin 30 mg/L, ceftazidime 125 mg/L) and the patient is maintained on continuous (24 h/day) dialysis, often with longer exchange times. Intraperitoneal antibiotics are continued for 2–3 weeks after obtaining fluid for cell count, differential count, Gram stain, and culture.

#### 5.6.1.3 Leaking of Peritoneal Fluid Around the PD Catheter

Incidence of pericatheter leaks can vary from 0 to 40%. PD catheters with fluid leak pose a significant risk for peritonitis, and continuation of PD with a leak is not recommended. Management strategies include: temporary discontinuation of PD (2–7 days) in favor of hemodialysis, placement of a new PD catheter (rare), or decrease of the PD fill volume. Surgical glue has been used successfully in combination with the above maneuvers [40].

## 5.7 Continuous Renal Replacement Therapy (CRRT)—Novel Machines to Provide Renal Support for Neonates

As mentioned above, continuous renal replacement therapy (CRRT) is rarely used in the NICU, and when it is used, it is usually performed in neonates who have contraindications for peritoneal dialysis or have failed PD. CRRT is used over PD in most ICUs due to its more reliable access, and its ability to ultrafilter a precise amount of fluid; however it is not the primary modality in neonates because CRRT poses additional challenges and risks in this population. The technical challenges of traditional machines make CRRT initiation very difficult, even at experienced tertiary children's hospitals. Until recently, the volume needed to prime the CRRT circuit varied between 92 and 165 mL. In the United States, the smallest CRRT circuit is around 92 mL (Prismaflex™ M60), and no circuits are FDA approved for use in children <20 kg. In Canada, Europe, and many other countries, the Prismaflex™ HF20 (extracorporeal volume (ECV) = 60 mL) is available. When used, these larger machines necessitate that small children receive CRRT with proportionally larger filters, higher blood flows, massive clearance rates, and big vascular catheters compared to bigger children [41]. The relative large ECV require larger vascular access and make the CRRT initiation procedure higher risk. For these reasons, many centers do not offer CRRT to any infant, especially very small infants and those who are too critically ill to tolerate CRRT initiation.

Initiation of neonatal CRRT therapy has historically been fraught with anxiety, and hemodynamic compromise when initiating the therapy in small infants. In our experience, the higher the % ECV and the more critically ill the patient is before initiation, the more likely problems will arise as a consequence to CRRT initiation. Using the pediatric prospective continuous renal replacement therapy (ppCRRT) registry, which included 13 centers and over 350 children on CRRT, we showed that children <10 kg have lower survival than children >10 kg (33 vs. 67%; $p < 0.05$) [41]. The lower rates of survival are perhaps due to patient selection, initiation of CRRT only as "last resort," the added risks of circuit initiation, or a combination of these factors.

Priming the CRRT circuit with packed red blood cells (pRBC) reduces morbidity; however, it is important to recognize that compared to physiologic blood, pRBC are cold, very concentrated, acidic, hyperkalemic, and hypocalcemic. Most centers that perform neonatal CRRT have protocols in place to buffer the acidic environment, reverse hypocalcemia, and dilute the higher hematocrit of pRBCs. Even with these measures, blood primes are not without risk, as blood primes can cause hypothermia, acidosis, hypocalcemia, hyperkalemia, thrombocytopenia, hypotension, and coagulopathy. These risks increase exponentially with smaller sized infants, those who are hemodynamically unstable and with frequent repeated initiation. These complications and the need to alter the CRRT prescription stem from the markedly large ECV inherent to available machinery.

CRRT machines with smaller ECV could reduce the risks associated with the therapy and improve outcomes. For these reasons, several groups have developed or adapted dialysis and convective clearance devices which use a smaller size circuit. What is common to all of these machines is that the smaller ECV of these machines allows for adequate flows with much smaller diameter catheters. In addition, initiation of CRRT circuit with much lower ECV is for the most part uneventful, even in very small and very critically ill infants [42].

The Newcastle Infant Dialysis Ultrafiltration System (NIDUS) [43] has an ECV of around 10 mL and can provide continuous or intermittent dialysis with the use of a 4F single lumen catheter. The circuit uses automated syringe pumps to accomplish four separate steps: (a) remove a volume of blood from the patient, (b) send blood through a dialysis filter that has countercurrent dialysis running, (c) return the blood back to the initial syringe pump, and (d) return that volume of blood (now cleaned) back to the patient.

The Cardiac And Renal Pediatric Dialysis Emergency (CARPEDIEM™) has available circuits of 27, 34, and 45 mL [42] for filters of 0.075; 0.15, and 0.25 $m^2$). By using smaller blood pump with a unique design, it is able to reduce the peak pressure for a given blood volume, reducing the need for a very wide catheter. A 4.5 F double lumen catheter can be used to accomplish the needed flows for this machine. The circuit has to be changed out daily. The blood flow can be titrated from 2 to 40 mL/min and it has very precise fluid scales available.

To mitigate concerns posed by CRRT machines with large ECV in relation to blood volume size, Askenazi adapted the Aquadex™ machine (a machine designed for ultrafiltration in adults with heart failure) to provide convective clearance by using an independent IV pump to deliver the replacement fluid. The machine can ultrafilter up to 500 mL/h. It has an integrated hematocrit detector that guide ultrafiltration by detecting abrupt changes in blood volume, which is inversely proportional to hematocrit. This system can provide adequate clearance, adequate electrolyte balance and fluid ultrafiltration, with minimal need for interventions during circuit initiation. The biggest drawback to this system is that the replacement pump is not directly in communication with the blood flow pump [44].

Clearly, as these devices become more widely accepted, there will be lower risk in performing this procedure. The risk/benefit ratio will allow for more judicious use, earlier intervention and will likely serve as a profound improvement in critically ill neonates.

## 5.8 Follow-Up After Neonatal AKI

*Long-term risk of CKD in premature infants*—Nephrogenesis begins at the fifth week of gestation and continues until 34–36 weeks. Nephron endowment and kidney function is determined by genetics and the intrauterine environment and varies across individuals. In term neonates and healthy adults, nephron numbers vary from 200,000 to 1.2 million per kidney—which also correlates closely with kidney mass and function in an individual. Prenatal factors (i.e., prenatal delivery, maternal diabetes, and intrauterine growth restriction) are factors which lead to impaired nephrogenesis [45].

The epidemiology of CKD in NICU graduates was recently reviewed by our group [3] and others [46]. The exact incidence of CKD in NICU graduates is not known. Based on a meta-analysis published by White et al. [47] in 2009, moderately premature infants (those with birthweight <2500 g) have a 70% higher risk of CKD during childhood than term infants. This meta-analysis likely underestimated the current CKD risk of premature infants, as it studied infants with birthweight <2500 g who were born in the 1980s. Now that many NICUs successfully support and graduate many more extremely premature infants (<24 weeks GA, and with birthweights <500 g) compared with 20 years ago, the magnitude of the problem is likely more substantial.

*Long-term risk of CKD after AKI in NICU graduates*—Previously it was assumed that those who survived an episode of AKI would recover kidney function without long-term effects. Recent data from animals, critically ill children [48], and adults with AKI suggest that survivors are at risk for the development of CKD. The impact of prematurity, intrauterine growth failure, and AKI on nephrogenesis has not been fully delineated but small studies suggest that the extrauterine environment and AKI are detrimental to nephrogenesis and in turn lead to CKD in adult life. Recent studies in term and preterm NICU graduates that evaluate the impact of AKI on the development of CKD are listed in Table 5.3. Acknowledging that these were small single-center studies with a potential risk of selection bias due to relatively low follow-up rates, the prevalence of CKD in these studies in aggregate was 31% (range of 9–83%). Importantly, the studies found that those with neonatal AKI had higher composite CKD rates, low estimated GFR, smaller total kidney volume (TKV), and abnormal urine kidney damage markers. An adequately powered prospective cohort study using a formal GFR metric with iohexol is greatly needed to evaluate the impact AKI has on CKD in NICU graduates.

**Table 5.3** Long-term studies on CKD in term and preterm NICU graduates

| | N (etiology) | Mean years at f/up (range) | CKD rate | Method to assess CKD | Differences AKI vs. no AKI |
|---|---|---|---|---|---|
| Term neonates | | | | | |
| Polito, 1998 | 6 (asphyxia) | 8.0 (6.5–19) | 83% | eGFR <90 mL/min/1.73 m$^2$, BP > 95% tile | N/A |
| Zwiers, 2014 | 169 (ECMO) | 8.2 (5.2–12.1) | 32% | eGFR <90 mL/min/1.73 m$^2$, BP > 95% tile, proteinuria | More CKD |
| Cooper, 2016 | 51 (CHD) | 8.0 (6.9–9.6) | 9% | eGFR <90 mL/min/1.73 m$^2$ | Biomarkers |
| Premature infants | | | | | |
| Abitbol, 2003 | 20 (ELBW) | 7.5 (3.2–18.5) | 45% | eGFR <75 mL/min/1.73 m$^2$ | N/A |
| Bruel, 2016 | 77 (<33 GA) | 6.6 (5–8) | 30% | eGFR <90 mL/min/1.73 m$^2$, BP > 95% tile, albuminuria | Lower TKV |
| Harer, 2017 | 34 (VLBW) | 5.0 (4–6) | 44% | eGFR <90 mL/min/1.73 m$^2$ BP > 95% tile, albuminuria | More CKD |

*ECMO* extracorporeal membrane oxygenations, *CHD* congenital heart disease, *ELBW* birthweight <1000 g, *VLBW* birthweight <1500 g

**Key Learning Points**

- The most common accepted definition of the neonatal AKI is based on a rise in serum creatinine (SCr) and/or decrease in urine output (UO).
- Most cases of AKI in neonates are nonoliguric.
- The most promising noninvasive early biomarkers of neonatal AKI are serum and urinary neutrophil gelatinase-associated lipocalin (NGAL), urinary interleukin-18, kidney injury molecule-1, serum cystatin C, osteopontin (OPN), and beta-2 microglobulin.
- The keys to supportive management include: (a) identify and correct risk factors when able, (b) identify and treat the cause, (c) prevent further kidney injury by maintaining kidney perfusion with adequate and avoidance oncotic pressure, blood pressure and intravascular volume, and contractility, (d) avoid and appropriately dose nephrotoxic drug, (e) prevent fluid overload, (f) maintain electrolyte balance, and (g) placement of a urinary catheter if obstruction is documented or suspected
- Peritoneal dialysis is a method of choice for kidney function replacement in newborns, and especially in ELBW newborns.
- CRRT machines with smaller extracorporeal volume could reduce the risks associated with the therapy and improve outcomes. Currently, Newcastle Infant Dialysis Ultrafiltration System (NIDUS), cardiac And Renal Pediatric Dialysis Emergency (CARPEDIEM™), and the Aquadex™ are being used to provide CRRT in small children.

## References


1. Hinchliffe SA, Sargent PH, Howard CV, Chan YF, van Velzen D. Human intrauterine renal growth expressed in absolute number of glomeruli assessed by the disector method and Cavalieri principle. Lab Investig. 1991;64(6):777–84.
2. Saint-Faust M, Boubred F, Simeoni U. Renal development and neonatal adaptation. Am J Perinatol. 2014;31(9):773–80.
3. Selewski DT, Charlton JR, Jetton JG, Guillet R, Mhanna MJ, Askenazi DJ, et al. Neonatal acute kidney injury. Pediatrics. 2015;136(2):e463–73.
4. Abitbol CL, Seeherunvong W, Galarza MG, Katsoufis C, Francoeur D, Defreitas M, et al. Neonatal kidney size and function in preterm infants: what is a true estimate of glomerular filtration rate? J Pediatr. 2014;41(3):487–502.
5. Schwartz GJ, Gauthier B. A simple estimate of glomerular filtration rate in adolescent boys. J Pediatr. 1985;106(3):522–6.
6. Sulemanji M, Khashayar V. Neonatal renal physiology. Semin Pediatr Surg. 2013;22:195–8.
7. Gubhaju L, Sutherland MR, Horne RSC, Medhurst A, Kent AL, Ramsden A, et al. Assessment of renal functional maturation and injury in preterm neonates during the first month of life. Am J Physiol Renal Physiol. 2014;307:F149–58.
8. Kobori H, Nangaku M, Navar LG, Nishiyama A. The intrarenal renin-angiotensin system: from physiology to the pathobiology of hypertension and kidney disease. Pharmacol Rev. 2007;59(3):251–87.

9. Ottonello G, Dessi A, Neroni P, Trudu ME, Fanos V. Acute kidney injury in neonatal age. J Pediatr Neonat Individual Med. 2014;3(2):e030246.
10. Askenazi DJ, Ambalavanan N, Goldstein LS. Acute kidney injury in critically ill newborns: what do we know? What do we need to learn? Pediatr Nephrol. 2009;24(2):265–74.
11. Koralkar R, Ambalavanan N, Levitan EB, McGwin G, Goldstein S, Askenazi D. Acute kidney injury reduces survival in very low birth weight infants. Pediatr Res. 2011;69(4):354–8.
12. Bezerra CT, Van Cunha LC, Liborio AB. Defining reduced urine output in neonatal ICU: importance for mortality and acute kidney injury classification. Nephrol Dial Transplant. 2013;28(4):901–9.
13. Ricci Z, Ronco C. Neonatal RIFLE. Nephrol Dial Transplant. 2013;28(9):2211–4.
14. Stojanović V, Barišić N, Radovanović T, Bjelica M, Milanović B, Doronjski A. Acute kidney injury in premature newborns-definition, etiology, and outcome. Pediatr Nephrol. 2017;32(10):1963–70.
15. Askenazi DJ, Montesanti A, Hunley H, Koralkar R, Pawar P, Shuaib F, et al. Urine biomarkers predict acute kidney injury and mortality in very low birth weight infants. J Pediatr. 2011;159:907–12.
16. Wong JH, Selewski DT, Yu S, Leopold KE, Roberts KH, Donohue JE, et al. Severe acute kidney injury following stage 1 Norwood palliation: effect on outcomes and risk of severe acute kidney injury at subsequent surgical stages. Pediatr Crit Care Med. 2016;17(7):615–23.
17. Mathur NB, Agarwal HS, Maria A. Acute renal failure in neonatal sepsis. Indian J Pediatr. 2006;73(6):499–502.
18. Sarkar S, Askenazi DJ, Jordan BK, Bhagat I, Bapuraj JR, Dechert RE, et al. Relationship between acute kidney injury and brain MRI findings in asphyxiated newborns after therapeutic hypothermia. Pediatr Res. 2014;75(3):431–5.
19. Selewski DT, Jordan BK, Askenazi DJ, Dechert RE, Sarkar S. Acute kidney injury in asphyxiated newborns treated with therapeutic hypothermia. J Pediatr. 2013;162(4):725–9.e1.
20. Askenazi DJ, Koralkar R, Hundley HE, Montesanti A, Patil N, Ambalavanan N. Fluid overload and mortality are associated with acute kidney injury in sick near-term/term neonate. Pediatr Nephrol. 2013;28(4):661–6.
21. Askenazi DJ, Ambalavanan N, Hamilton K, Cutter G, Lancy D, Kaslow R, et al. Acute kidney injury and renal replacement therapy independently predict mortality in neonatal and pediatric noncardiac patients on extracorporeal membrane oxygenation. Pediatr Crit Care Med. 2011;12(1):e1–6.
22. Askenazi DJ, Griffin R, McGwin G, Carlo W, Ambalavanan N. Acute kidney injury is independently associated with mortality in very low birthweight infants: a matched case-control analysis. Pediatr Nephrol. 2009;24(5):991–7.
23. Carmody JB, Swanson JR, Rhone ET, Charlton JR. Recognition and reporting of AKI in very low birth weight infants. Clin J Am Soc Nephrol. 2014;9(12):2036–43.
24. Stojanovic V, Barisic N, Milanovic B, Doronjski A. Acute kidney injury in preterm infants admitted to a neonatal intensive care unit. Pediatr Nephrol. 2014;29(11):2213–20.
25. Jetton JG, Boohaker LJ, Sethi SK, Wazir S, Rohatgi S, Soranno DE, et al. Incidence and outcomes of neonatal acute kidney injury (AWAKEN): a multicentre, multinational, observational cohort study. Lancet. 2017;1(3):184–94.
26. Weintraub AS, Connors J, Blanco V, Green RS. The spectrum of onset of acute kidney injury in premature infants less than 30 weeks gestation. J Perinatol. 2016;36:474–80.
27. Bakr AF. Peophylactic theophylline to prevent renal dysfunction in newborns exposed to perinatal asphyxia – a study in a developing country. Pediatr Nephrol. 2005;20:1249–52.
28. Friedrich JO, Adhikari N, Herridge MS, Beyene J. Metaanalysis: low-dose dopamine increase urine output but does not prevent renal dysfunction or death. Ann Intern Med. 2005;142:510–24.
29. Ricci Z, Luciano R, Favia I, Gariso G, Muraca M, Morelli S, et al. High-dose fenoldopam reduces postoperative neutrophil gelatinase-associated lipocaline and cystatin C levels in pediatric cardiac surgery. Crit Care. 2015;15(3):R160.

30. Pandey V, Dummula K, Go M, Parimi P. Bumetanide use in the management of oliguric preterm infants with acute kidney injury–a single center experience. J Clin Pediatr Nephrol. 2015. https://doi.org/10.15401/jcpn/2014/v2i2/66346.
31. Ho KM, Sheridan D. Meta-analysis of furosemide to prevent or treat acute renal failure. BMJ. 2006;333:420–3.
32. Hobbs DJ, Steinke JM, Chung JY, Barletta GM, Bunchman TE. Rasburicase improves hyperuricemia in infants with acute kidney injury. Pediatr Nephrol. 2010;25(2):305–9.
33. Pandey V, Kumar D, Vijayaraghavan P, Chaturvedi T, Raina R. Non-dialytic management of acute kidney injury in newborns. J Renal Inj Prev. 2017;6(1):1–11.
34. Gouyon JB, Guignard JP. Management of acute renal failure in newborns. Pediatr Nephrol. 2000;14:1037–44.
35. Alparslan C, Yavascan O, Bal A, Kanik A, Kose E, Kasap Demir B, et al. The performance of acute peritoneal dialysis treatment in neonatal period. Ren Fail. 2012;34(8):1015–20.
36. Sasser WC, Dabal RJ, Askenazi DJ, Borasino S, Moellinger AB, Kirklin JK, et al. Prophylactic peritoneal dialysis following cardiopulmonary bypass in children is associated with decreased inflammation and improved clinical outcomes. Congenit Heart Dis. 2014;9(2):106–15.
37. Kwiatkowski DM, Menon S, Krawszeski CD, Goldstein SL, Morales LSD, Philips A, et al. Improved outcomes with peritoneal dialysis catheter placement after cardiopulmonary bypass in infants. J Thorac Cardiovasc Surg. 2015;149:230–6.
38. Stojanović V, Bukarica S, Antić J, Doronjski A. Peritoneal dialysis in very low birth weight neonates. Perit Dial Int. 2017;37(4):389–96.
39. Stojanović V, Bukarica S, Doronjski A, Marinković S. Peritoneal dialysis in neonates with extremely low body weight at birth: new modality of using IV cannula for peritoneal access. Iran J Pediatr. 2013;23(6):718–20.
40. Unal S, Bilgin L, Gunduz M, Uncu N, Azili MN, Tiryaki T. The implementation of neonatal peritoneal dialysis in a clinical setting. J Matern Fetal Neonatal Med. 2012;25:2111–4.
41. Askenazi DJ, Goldstein SL, Koralkar R, Fortenberry J, Baum M, Hackbarth R, et al. Continuous renal replacement therapy for children </=10 kg: a report from the prospective pediatric continuous renal replacement therapy registry. J Pediatr. 2013;162(3):587–92.e3.
42. Ronco C, Garzotto F, Brendolan A, Zanella M, Bellettato M, Vedovato S, et al. Continuous renal replacement therapy in neonates and small infants: development and first-in-human use of a miniaturised machine (CARPEDIEM). Lancet. 2014;383(9931):1807–13.
43. Coulthard MG, Crosier J, Griffiths C, Smith J, Drinnan M, Whitaker M, et al. Haemodialysing babies weighing <8 kg with the Newcastle infant dialysis and ultrafiltration system (Nidus): comparison with peritoneal and conventional haemodialysis. Pediatr Nephrol. 2014;29(10):1873–81.
44. Askenazi D, Ingram D, White S, Cramer M, Borasino S, Coghill C, et al. Smaller circuits for smaller patients: improving renal support therapy with Aquadex™. Pediatr Nephrol. 2016;31(5):853–60.
45. Bertram JF, Douglas-Denton RN, Diouf B, Hughson MD, Hoy WE. Human nephron number: implications for health and disease. Pediatr Nephrol. 2011;26(9):1529–33.
46. Levin A, Tonelli M, Bonventre J, Coresh J, Donner JA, Fogo AB, et al. Global kidney health 2017 and beyond: a roadmap for closing gaps in care, research, and policy. Lancet. 2017;390(10105):1888–917.
47. White SL, Perkovic V, Cass A, Chang CL, Poulter NR, Spector T, et al. Is low birth weight an antecedent of CKD in later life? A systematic review of observational studies. Am J Kidney Dis. 2009;54(2):248–61.
48. Askenazi DJ, Feig DI, Graham NM, Hui-Stickle S, Goldstein SL. 3–5 year longitudinal follow-up of pediatric patients after acute renal failure. Kidney Int. 2006;69(1):184–9.

# Sepsis-Associated Acute Kidney Injury: Making Progress Against a Lethal Syndrome

6

Rajit K. Basu

## 6.1 Introduction

*What we think, we become—Gautama Buddha.*

Sepsis and acute kidney injury (AKI) are epidemic problems in hospitalized patients. Together, sepsis-associated AKI (S-AKI) is a syndrome carrying lethal downstream sequelae. Epidemiologic data indicate sepsis increases the rate of AKI, AKI increases the rate of sepsis, and together, S-AKI increases the rates of morbidity and mortality significantly above baseline. Evidence from small and large biological models of sepsis and AKI describes considerable overlap between the pathophysiologic drivers of both processes. These are recapitulated in models of S-AKI. Unfortunately, a significant proportion of published literature focuses either on associative population data or the complex minutiae underpinning the mechanistic drivers of the syndrome. Very few reports attempt to connect the dots and describe how the bench and the bedside can be understood together and even fewer describe how this connection can be leveraged. This chapter takes a progress-driven approach to S-AKI. The existing perspective and *status quo* of epidemiology, understanding of pathophysiology, diagnostic tools, and management options will be described. Assumptions regarding S-AKI will be discussed. The chapter will then describe how these assumptions should be challenged and how challenging opens the door to making actual progress. Using collaboration, innovation, and a more contemporary approach, it will be possible to refine and improve the understanding of disease epidemiology, untangle the syndrome pathophysiology, increase the sophistication of diagnostics, and facilitate the targeting of putative therapy.

R. K. Basu
Division of Pediatric Critical Care, Children's Healthcare of Atlanta, Department of Pediatrics, Emory University, Atlanta, GA, USA
e-mail: Rajit.basu@choa.org



A. Deep, S. L. Goldstein (eds.), *Critical Care Nephrology and Renal Replacement Therapy in Children*, https://doi.org/10.1007/978-3-319-90281-4_6

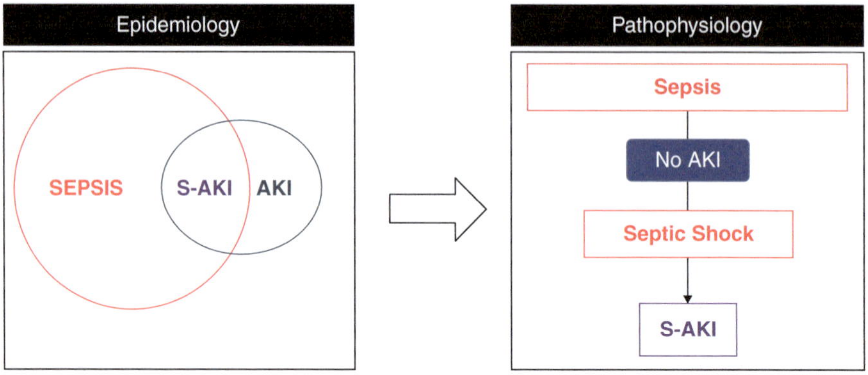


**Fig. 6.1** Current perspective—epidemiology drives physiology. The status quo for how sepsis-associated acute kidney injury (S-AKI) is depicted above. The epidemiology for the disease process is entirely contained within the scope of both sepsis and AKI. Sepsis is the predominant driver of AKI. The findings clinically drive research strategy in the laboratory, where the pathophysiology is studied by examining the kidney in models of sepsis and septic shock

The understanding of how sepsis-associated AKI occurs, is diagnosed, and is managed has been fueled by clinical incidence and prevalence data. Epidemiology has driven, and biased, study of pathophysiology and impacted the ability to identify options for effective management (Fig. 6.1).

### 6.1.1 Existing Perspective: Epidemiology

The incidence of sepsis or septic shock has increased over the past two decades. Prior to the most recent reports, the population incidence for sepsis was 22 to 240 per 100,000 and 13–300 per 100,000 for severe sepsis [1]. A 22-year retrospective analysis of hospitalization records in the United States found an 8.7% annual increase for sepsis diagnosis [2]. The incidence of severe sepsis from 2004 to 2009 demonstrated an average annual increase of 13% [3]. Global estimates suggested significant associations with sepsis encompassing all aspects of ICU-related morbidity—including prolonged length of stay, ventilation, secondary infections, and mortality along with long-term survival [4–7]. Meanwhile, integration of consensus AKI criteria definitions of RIFLE, AKIN, and most recently KDIGO has facilitated identification of AKI incidence in intensive care unit (ICU) settings. Adult reports ranged between 16 and 67% [8–18] while scattered pediatric ICU studies reported similarly high incidence rates [19, 20]. Like sepsis, mounting evidence has indicated a rise in AKI incidence. In a large 10-year cohort that included more than 90,000 from more than 20 ICUs, AKI incidence increased by 2.8% per year [10]. A longitudinal pediatric study demonstrated a parallel rise in reported AKI incidence [21]. Also, like sepsis, the presence of AKI has been consistently associated with increased morbidity and mortality for both adults and children. The epidemiologic data for AKI has created paradigm shift, suggesting people are no longer just dying with AKI, but *from* AKI [22].

Sepsis-associated AKI (S-AKI) occurs at a high incidence rate in critically ill patients. A large adult ICU study from Australia and New Zealand identified S-AKI in 11.7% of 120,123 patients [23]. Sepsis is the leading predominant condition associated with AKI; the BEST kidney study reported an AKI incidence of 5.7% in 29,000 patients with sepsis being the highest associated etiology (47.5%) [24]. Analysis of 276,731 admissions to 170 adult critical care units of the Intensive Care National Audit and Research Center in the United Kingdom (ICNARC) identified concurrent sepsis and AKI in 8246 ICU admissions in first 24 h [25]. Meanwhile, in another cohort, AKI was present in 17.7% of 722 patients admitted to an ICU specific for infectious disease [26]. Infection was identified as an independent predictor of AKI in large pediatric cohort of 2106 critically ill children (18% AKI incidence) [27]. A 10-year longitudinal retrospective analysis reported sepsis as a leading cause of AKI in 180 children [28]. A prospective multicenter study from Turkey reported sepsis as a leading cause of AKI in 18% of 472 patients [29]. Similarly, sepsis was an independent risk factor for the development of AKI in a retrospective observation study from India [30]. Thus, S-AKI is a global health care issue in adults and children.

Sepsis-associated AKI is strongly associated with a poor prognosis. Observational studies consistently report significantly worse outcome with S-AKI versus non-septic AKI or sepsis alone. Length of stay (LOS) is longer in patients with S-AKI versus AKI without sepsis or sepsis alone. Septic patients developing AKI were found to have twice the duration of ICU stay compared to septic patients without AKI [23]. Similar findings from a larger cohort found S-AKI patients to have longer ICU and hospital stay compared to non-septic AKI or sepsis alone. Recovery of renal function is similar for patients with S-AKI versus AKI without sepsis. Complete renal function recovery occurred in 95.7% of 315 S-AKI patients, with mean time for complete recovery of 10.1 ± 8 days [31]. Both ICU and inhospital mortality were significantly higher for patients with S-AKI compared to AKI without sepsis (ICU mortality: 19.8 vs. 13.4% and inhospital mortality: 29.7 vs. 21.6%). Mortality was significantly higher in S-AKI for AKI-AKIN stage 3 (64.1%) compared with AKI-AKIN stage 1 (34.6%). Very little data have been published focused on S-AKI in pediatrics. A small, single-center study identified a mortality rate of 57.1% in children with septic shock and acute renal failure compared to 6.7% in septic shock without ARF [32]. Prior to the past 3 years, extrapolations are made from adult studies and applied to children and neonates.

In total, the epidemiology of S-AKI has suggested that the injury is entirely a subset of sepsis and AKI (Fig. 6.1).

### 6.1.2 Existing Perspective: Pathophysiology

Current understanding of S-AKI pathophysiology is based on the predominant systemic effects (and understanding) of septic shock [33, 34]. The argument created is that the disease process in S-AKI is linear, occurring in stepwise series fashion from sepsis to septic shock to S-AKI (Fig. 6.1). Understanding sepsis, therefore, would facilitate a complete understanding of S-AKI.

Sepsis is, in simplistic terms, an infection leading to a dysregulated host immune response. This dysregulation is manifest by aberrancies in pro- and anti-inflammatory mediators. Septic shock is the sequelae of sepsis, wherein a host suffers from the imbalance of oxygen supply and demand. Oxygen demand increases as utilization can increase at the tissue level and supply decreases secondary to issues with cardiovascular efficiency. The relationship between cardiac output and systemic vascular resistance in sepsis is, however, highly variable by age. Adult septic shock is generally characterized by high cardiac output and low systemic vascular resistance (SVR), also known as "warm shock." Conversely, most children with septic shock have low cardiac output and high SVR, or "cold shock" [35]. Myocardial function varies considerably in children—and varies from infancy to adolescence. Regulation of myocardial excitation-contraction coupling is incomplete in the neonatal period and is further characterized by a relatively greater sensitivity and dependence of neonates on calcium and β-adrenergic stimuli compared with older children or adults. Endothelial disruption is a hallmark of sepsis in adults. Alterations in adult endothelial homeostasis include leukocyte adhesion, vasodilation, creation of a pro-coagulant milieu, and loss of the capillary brush border. As endothelium covers the lining of essentially all vital organs, these perturbations in sepsis lead to end-organ effects secondarily. Epithelial changes also occur in sepsis and organ epithelial tissue (e.g., lung and gut epithelia) becomes more friable and leaky. Organ epithelia and the vascular endothelium in children is highly reactive and, in an effort to compensate for changes in cardiac output, switches rapidly to a vasoconstricted or high resistance state in septic shock [35]. Due to both the fragility of the myocardium and vascular integrity, children are much more vulnerable to the end-organ effects of shock from sepsis than adults.

Dysregulation of the innate and adaptive immune responses in sepsis leads to injury. The dysregulation is not consistent from patient to patient and neither is the degree of injury. Sepsis leads to wide variations in the host immune response, with early pro-inflammatory effects predominating and later predominating anti-inflammatory or immunosuppressive effects. Both cytokines and chemokines involved in direct inflammation mediation or cellular recruitment are dysregulated in sepsis. End-organ effects of sepsis are highly variable based on age of the patient and degree of systemic comorbidities. Adults with chronic heart disease, diabetes, and autoimmune or immunosuppressive conditions are highly susceptible to damage from inflammatory dysregulation. While children with similar comorbidities are also at higher risk, the average child has a baseline increased risk. Maturation of the immune system, both adaptive and innate, is incomplete until toddler age, explaining why neonates and children have marked heterogeneity in inflammatory response. In general, inflammatory dysregulation (particularly the immunosuppressive effects of sepsis) plays a greater role in septic shock in children than in adults [36]. Taken together, sepsis leads to host homeostatic imbalance starting from the microscopic and cellular level, cascading into significant host dysregulation with deleterious end-organ impact. Significant differences exist in the pathophysiology of sepsis between adults, children, and neonates.

Per traditional thinking, S-AKI is the net result of septic shock on the kidneys. As sepsis progresses, systemic vascular resistance shifts from low to high, spurred by neurohormonal-mediated vasoconstriction, thereby heightening end-organ vascular tone. This model may not be entirely recapitulated in young patients. Unfortunately, an age-specific adjustment (or model), appropriate for cardiovascular effects on the kidney in sepsis, has not been reported. Inflammation of the nephron, hypoxic and/or oxidant stress, cytokine and chemokine driven direct tubular injury, and tubular and mesenchymal apoptosis have all been linked in the process of S-AKI. Strong associations exist between pro-inflammatory cytokines TNF-α, IL-6, and IL-10 and S-AKI. Additionally, interactions between pathogens and pathogen receptors such as toll-like receptors (TLRs), pathogen-associated molecular patterns (PAMPs), and damage-associated molecular patterns (DAMPs) have all been implicated in S-AKI [37]. Pro-inflammatory cytokines, DAMPs, and PAMPs directly and indirectly induce tubular damage, proximal to renal tubular epithelium, and contribute to loss of function. Oxidative stress is associated with renal tubular damage. Mainly secondary to ischemia-reperfusion or neutrophil burst, oxidative stress can affect the balance of cell survival, arrest, necrosis, or programmed cell death (apoptosis). Bioenergetic failure, mitochondrial arrest, occurs during sepsis and has been implicated in S-AKI [38]. The combination of findings is a laundry list of putative intracellular mechanisms that induce damage independently and synergistically. How the pieces fit together remains a mystery [39]. Even more of a mystery is how the pieces fit together differently for a child versus an adult. Despite the uncertainty, the "given" is that S-AKI pathophysiology is driven in a linear manner by sepsis, is a natural consequence of septic shock, and leads to severe, persistent tubular cell death.

### 6.1.3 Existing Perspective: Diagnostics and Management

To date, no effective singular therapy for AKI exists, so management of S-AKI is predicated on recognition of AKI and management of sepsis. What follows is management "in series" (Fig. 6.2). Standardized criteria (RIFLE, pRIFLE, AKIN, and KDIGO) have facilitated description of AKI epidemiology based on creatinine and urine output changes from baseline. Therefore, recognition of S-AKI is also based on these parameters. Some of these data were discussed earlier. In the context of sepsis, many clinicians will institute the parameters of goal-directed therapy

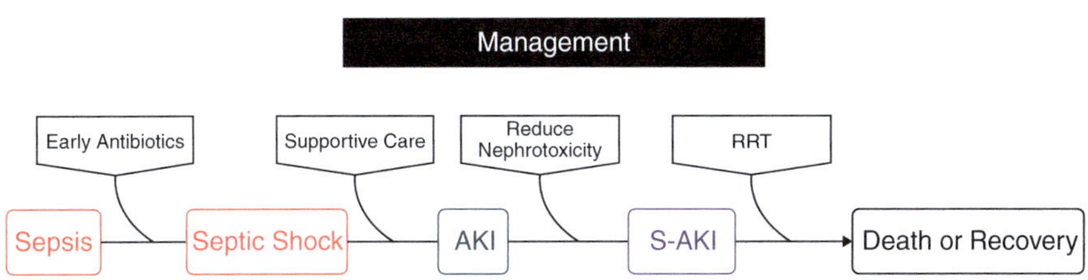


**Fig. 6.2** Current perspective—management in series. The status quo for how sepsis-associated acute kidney injury (S-AKI) is treated is depicted above. Sepsis is managed initially and support is escalated when shock is manifest. When end-organ effects on the kidney are detected by changes in creatinine, kidney-specific "management" is incorporated. Renal replacement therapy is incorporated as a "last line" intervention in the case of life-threatening S-AKI

including stabilization and optimization of fluid status, mean perfusion pressure, and oxygen delivery. Source control of the infectious agent (s) is paramount as delayed antimicrobial therapy is associated with increased mortality in septic shock, every hour without coverage increases mortality by nearly 10% [40]. Randomized controlled trials testing the effects of other interventions have failed to demonstrate consistent efficacy in sepsis. When AKI is recognized in the context of sepsis, management of sepsis is combined with adapted KDIGO AKI guidelines to include: minimization of unnecessary nephrotoxins and adjustment of nephrotoxic medications based on renal clearance (as estimated by creatinine), conservative resuscitation (with regards to administration of intravenous fluids), and consideration of renal replacement therapy. Indications for the initiation of RRT in adult patients with S-AKI have included "life-threatening AKI complications" and "aberrant fluid balance" [41] but RRT therapy for critically ill septic patients is controversial. Timing and modality are uncertain although evidence suggests initiation of support before significant fluid accumulation may be associated with improved patient outcomes. Additionally, recent data have suggested that initial support with CRRT may better facilitate recovery of kidney function to RRT independence and reduce the long-term risk of incident CKD [42, 43]. Despite early data by Ronco et al. suggesting potential benefit from higher intensity dose dialysis (35–45 mL/kg/h) [44], subsequent evidence from two large multicenter randomized trials (RENAL: randomized evaluation of normal versus augmented level renal replacement therapy and ATN: Veterans Affairs/National Institutes of Health Acute Renal Failure Trial Network Study) showed no added benefit of higher intensity-dose RRT compared to lower intensity-dose RRT with fewer metabolic complications [45, 46]. Additionally, in both the RENAL and ATN studies, there were no significant difference in the odds ratios (OR) for mortality in patients with sepsis who received higher versus lower intensity RRT. In the RENAL study, high versus low intensity RRT conferred an OR for death by 90 days of 0.84 (0.62–1.12) while in the ATN study intensive versus less intensive therapy conferred an OR for death at 60 days of 1.19 (0.88–1.62) [45, 46]. Although some data suggest that CRRT might have potential immunomodulatory effect in sepsis, the IVOIRE study investigated high volume hemofiltration in septic shock patients with AKI and found no survival or clinical benefits [47]. Very little published data discusses the diagnostics or management of S-AKI in children.

### 6.1.4 Interlude—Challenging the Givens

*When there is a problem, always identify and evaluate your underlying assumptions that may be contributing to the problem or preventing you from seeing the problem clearly—Elizabeth Thornton*

In total, the existing paradigm of sepsis-associated AKI is driven by the influence and understanding of sepsis. Epidemiology of sepsis governs the epidemiology of S-AKI. Sepsis pathophysiology drives the pathophysiology of S-AKI. Diagnostics are based on recognition of sepsis and signs of severe sepsis or septic shock while creatinine change is used to identify AKI in the context of sepsis unless fluid accumulation becomes clinically significant. Management of S-AKI is governed

**Table 6.1** Assumptions to challenge for sepsis-associated AKI

| |
|---|
| • S-AKI is the result of a construct in "series" |
| – Sepsis is the pathophysiologic driver of S-AKI |
| – S-AKI morbidity and mortality is driven by the sepsis |
| – S-AKI epidemiology is contained entirely within sepsis epidemiology |
| – S-AKI management is governed by the principles of sepsis management |
| • Creatinine is a sufficient marker of incipient S-AKI and to direct guide S-AKI management |
| • "Life-threatening" AKI is an indication for initiation of RRT |
| • The phenotype of S-AKI is similar in adults, children, and neonates |

primarily by the management of sepsis (source control, optimization of oxygen delivery and utilization) while the management AKI in S-AKI approximates the Hippocratic Oath ("*primum non nocere*") applied to the kidneys. Adults and children and neonates are not differentiated with regards to diagnostics or management strategies. Meanwhile, outcomes for these patients (all ages) are ominous and significantly worse both in the short and long term compared to patients without sepsis or AKI, with sepsis and no AKI, or AKI and no sepsis. The question that must be asked by all is simply—is the *status quo* adequate? The answer is no.

In order to move past the existing paradigm and the twentieth century approach to S-AKI, "givens" must be challenged, a comprehensive reevaluation must be performed, and innovation must be leveraged (Table 6.1).

### 6.1.5 Contemporary Approach to Sepsis-Associated AKI

The contemporary approach to understanding sepsis-associated AKI, particularly in children, requires a return to the biology of the syndrome. It is not by accident that the second half of this chapter begins with a discussion regarding pathophysiology. The existing dogma must be challenged. In the text that follows, the central role of the kidney in pathophysiology will be described and a modified view of S-AKI constructed, careful to delineate the findings that can and cannot be extrapolated to pathophysiology in children and neonates. An adjusted understanding of S-AKI epidemiology will be detailed, including newer large, multicenter population data. The necessary approach created will be pathophysiology driving the understanding of epidemiology. A new diagnostic framework will be illustrated—incorporating risk and context and novel biomarker approaches to refine and improve the precision of diagnosis. Finally, the options for management will be shifted to a contemporary, personalized approach, targeting S-AKI phenotypes.

### 6.1.6 Contemporary Approach: Pathophysiology

The kidney is a central mediator of host homeostasis and aberrant kidney function impacts systemic health. Responsible for not only solute and fluid clearance, the kidney governs vascular stability, neurohormonal response to stress, calcium–phosphorus balance, regulates acid–base control, and modulation of erythropoietin in states of marrow suppression and/or anemia. Recent evidence from both animal and human models indicates an even more expansive set of distant organ molecular checks and balances controlled by kidney function [48]. Aside from propagating injury in endocrine fashion, that is isolated models of AKI triggering a cascade of localized injury in the glomerulus, renal mesenchyme, and tubular epithelium, AKI models also result in distal organ injury [48, 49]. Isolated models of AKI induce host vasomotor instability secondary to changes in the vascular endothelial response to catecholamines, loss of vascular and epithelial integrity in the lung and brain, myocardial dysfunction by myocyte apoptosis, and aberrant T-cell trafficking [50]. In two-stage models, a primary AKI leads to a far worse secondary injury phenotype (sepsis, lung injury, hemorrhagic shock). In a majority of these models, the distal organ effects on the host occur before changes in creatinine or urine output and end-stage renal failure—pointing to early and notably *independent* effects of AKI on the host. Finally, although not yet studied extensively, pediatric-aged animal models of AKI demonstrate a different injury pattern than adult-aged models [51]. The cumulative evidence suggests not only does an isolated injury to the kidney trigger a continuous propagation of renal injury in multiple areas of the nephron but also impacts host homeostasis, varied by age. AKI contributes to adverse systemic pathophysiology including propagation of infections and sepsis [52].

The effects of sepsis on renal perfusion in the kidney vary based on context. Sepsis inconsistently leads to aberrant renal perfusion. Multivariate analysis in a systematic review of 159 animal studies, a majority of which (62%) reported decreased renal blood flow during sepsis, demonstrated that RBF is only predicted by sepsis induced changes to cardiac output (i.e., low cardiac output) [53]. In an ovine model of *E. coli* sepsis, sepsis conferred a period of *hyper-dynamic* RBF for 48-h after *E. coli* infusion, attributed to increased cardiac output and renal vasodilatation [54]. Overall RBF seems to be less contributory to renal perfusion during sepsis unless cardiac output is affected. This dynamic has not been studied in relationship to host age, however. As described earlier, pediatric septic shock is more often associated with low cardiac output (myocardial stun) than adult septic shock. Further decreasing age is associated with less myocardial functional reserve and less myocyte actin-myosin cross-bridging, ultimately leading to higher myocardial oxygen consumption for the same level of myocardial demand. Neonates are particularly vulnerable to the effects of septic shock and impaired end-organ effects are commonly seen in the neonate (necrotizing enterocolitis, cerebral ischemic-hypoxic injury in meningitis). Intravascular capacitance, combining both the amount of functional vascular reserve and endothelial integrity, is compromised in pediatric models of sepsis. Together, the hemodynamic effects of sepsis on the kidney in the younger patient may actually be more contributory to S-AKI than in adults. An adjudicated understanding of renal perfusion in sepsis needs to be taken—in adults, the primary effects on the kidney occurring during the early stages of sepsis may not be related to hemodynamics, while in children and neonates, the effects on renal perfusion may be more significant.

The contribution of inflammation in the propagation of AKI during sepsis is highly variable from host to host. In fact, when attempting to understand the rationale behind the long list of failed sepsis therapeutics treating inflammation (e.g., steroids) a major rationale is now absent or insufficient patient stratification. Therefore, a substantial amount of data describes serum-based sepsis genotypes or endotypes in both adults and children [55, 56]. These data suggest both from the laboratory and from the bedside that distinct patient phenotypes correspond with different pathophysiology and different patient outcome. These findings also support the hypothesis that the influence of sepsis-mediated inflammation on renal function and tubular integrity may also be highly variable. The variability in turn should lead us to challenge the dogma regarding S-AKI. Tubular necrosis, traditionally cited as the major cellular switch for injury, is not supported by the available experimental evidence [57]. Renal tubular *apoptosis* may be a significant contributing mechanism of injury in SA-AKI [58]. In a side-by-side experimental comparison of murine models of SA-AKI versus ischemia-reperfusion (using cecal ligation puncture model), renal cell apoptosis was more prominent on renal histology in the SA-AKI mice with minimal tubular injury or inflammation [58]. In a porcine model of fecal peritonitis, renal tubular cells demonstrated vacuolization and injury to cellular brush borders but no evidence of necrosis [59]. In a model of lipopolysaccharide (LPS) induced endotoxemic AKI, reactive nitrogen species (RNS) and reactive oxygen species (ROS) were over-expressed in the renal cytosolic compartment, implicating mitochondrial and oxidative dysfunction during sepsis. Direct bacterial instillation leads to a polymicrobial inflammatory response—varied by organism used in the slurry. The net result is the importance of limiting extrapolation, as the type of inflammatory dysregulation depends on the type of sepsis model used. Genetic predisposition to injury is also varied in animals secondary to selective inbreeding, an allelic characteristic obviously not present in the majority of available human data [60].

AKI and sepsis contribute individually and synergistically to the pathophysiologic derangements evident in patients with S-AKI. Sepsis can drive AKI, but AKI can also drive sepsis (Fig. 6.3). Different aspects of each drive S-AKI, and importantly these vary from patient to patient. Additionally, S-AKI may actually be a distinct clinical entity from both sepsis and AKI individually, displaying a unique genetic, proteomic, and phenotypic signature. Finally, the drivers of S-AKI pathophysiology in adults should not be assumed to be consistent in children and neonates. The pathophysiology of S-AKI in the pediatric patient is unique as the pathophysiology of both sepsis and AKI in children is unique. Very little formalized and focused data describes the pathophysiology of S-AKI in a pediatric patient or young animal models, but this is essential to properly characterize and ultimately treat these patients.

### 6.1.7 Contemporary Approach: Epidemiology

Context must be incorporated to understand the epidemiology of sepsis-associated AKI. The varied pathophysiology of sepsis would suggest that stratification systems for studying the epidemiology of S-AKI are needed. Not all sepsis-associated

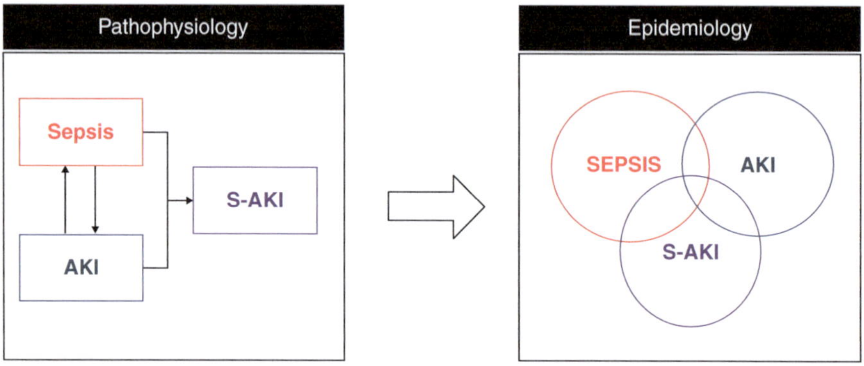


**Fig. 6.3** Modern approach—physiology drives epidemiology. Recent evidence indicates that sepsis drives acute kidney injury (AKI) but AKI also drives sepsis. They synergistically can lead to sepsis-associated AKI (S-AKI). This appreciation should lead us to examine newer, large datasets in varied populations from the perspective of S-AKI as perhaps its own unique entity. S-AKI remains an overlap with sepsis and AKI but perhaps there are aspects of S-AKI unique and separate from either of the two processes. Genomic, proteomic, and phenotypic evidence support this hypothesis

AKI is created equal! Risk factors for AKI both in adults and children have been identified. Using these risk factors, a parallel to Prinzmetals' angina for identification/prediction of acute coronary syndrome has been developed for AKI. Named "renal angina," Chawla and Goldstein identified the risk factors associated with the development of severe AKI. Importantly, the risk criteria were dichotomized into adult- and pediatric-specific factors [61]. The importance of the risk stratification system is to identify patients at high risk of severe AKI *early* in their ICU course. The system smooths out the heterogeneity of patient illness severity by creating an objective scoring system (the renal angina index) for the hierarchy of risk [62]. This methodology may enable a more targeted approach to disease diagnostics.

New epidemiologic data may facilitate a more accurate understanding of disease prevalence. A recent worldwide meta-analysis of adult and pediatric datasets identified AKI rates of 21.6% and 33.7%, respectively, and pointed to the need for data from developing nations. The adult AKI-EPI study identified an AKI incidence of 21% in septic patients (vs. 8% in non-septic patients) [63]. The young adult and pediatric AWARE study identified a sepsis prevalence of 14.6% in close to 5000 patients with an AKI incidence rate of 41% in the septic population [64]. The point prevalence SPROUT study identified an AKI prevalence of 21% in septic children with a significant association between severe AKI and death or long-term disability [65]. Finally, the neonatal AWAKEN study reports a sepsis evaluation was less common in babies with AKI (45 vs. 52% in babies without AKI). These large studies multicenter, multinational, collaborative studies on critically ill patients from all agents will facilitate the identification of the true epidemiologic associations with sepsis and AKI as they were designed to study AKI itself rather than AKI being studied in post hoc analysis.

**Past and Present**

| Time Frame | Marker |
|---|---|
| 1960-1980s | Creatinine |
| 1980s-1990s | Creatinine |
| 2000s-2010s | Creatinine |

| Location | Marker |
|---|---|
| "Renal" | Creatinine |

| Population Age | Marker |
|---|---|
| Adults | Creatinine |
| Children | Creatinine |
| Neonates | Creatinine (or nothing) |

| Etiology | Marker |
|---|---|
| Ischemic | Creatinine |
| Septic | Creatinine |
| Nephrotoxic | Creatinine |
| Hypoxic | Creatinine |
| Obstructive | Creatinine |

| Severity/Progression | Marker |
|---|---|
| Low | Creatinine |
| High | Creatinine |

**Future**

| Time Frame | Marker |
|---|---|
| 2020-2025 | Creatinine, Urine Output & Biomarkers |
| 2025-2030 | Dynamic Biomarker Combinations |
| Beyond | Real-time functional tests & endotyping |

| Location | Marker |
|---|---|
| Glomerulus | Real-time GFR |
| Tubular Epithelium | Urine biomarker panel |
| Vasa recta | Renal oximetry |
| Collecting Duct | Kinetic Urine Output |

| Population Age | Marker |
|---|---|
| Variable | Age Specific Marker Panels |

| Etiology | Marker |
|---|---|
| Perfusion/Reperfusion | Real-time GFR |
| Apoptosis/Necrosis/Autophagy | Biomarker profile |
| Inflammation/Oxidative Stress | Bioenergetics panel |
| Chloride Transport | Furosemide Stress Test |

| Severity/Progression | Marker |
|---|---|
| Low | Negative renal angina |
| Moderate | Renal angina+/Stable Biomarkers |
| Progressive/High | Renal angina+/Rising biomarkers |

**Fig. 6.4** Modernization of diagnostics. The side-by-side comparison of markers for acute kidney injury (AKI) depicts the stark contrast of the past and present construct and the potential of the future. Creatinine is the beginning, middle, and end of diagnostics—even for S-AKI. The future opens the door to possibilities of advances in diagnostics—able to identify the what, when, why, and how of AKI. (*GFR* glomerular filtration rate)

Reliance on creatinine and urine output for diagnostics limits the ability to accurately identify the S-AKI epidemiologic signal. Although imminently useful for standardizing AKI diagnosis for the purposes of getting comparable data across institutions, nations, and populations, these markers have significant, recognized limitations. Aside from being highly varied by age and gender and delayed in response to injury, referenced normative values for creatinine are measured in steady state, a situation diametrically opposed to that for a patient suffering sepsis or AKI. Creatinine itself offers very little insight into the "who, what, where, when, and why" of AKI (Fig. 6.4). Meanwhile, although urine output is a vital sign indicative of a multitude of normal physiologic processes (tubular epithelial integrity and function, juxtaglomerular apparatus sensing, collecting duct aquaporin channel function, sodium–potassium ATPase function, oxygen tension in the vasa recta, just to name a few), it is generically only used to signify "adequate renal perfusion." Current diagnostic strata include urine output but only as a static index in a designated period of time (mL/kg/h). Unfortunately, clinicians generally disregard urine output as a marker of AKI, placing primacy on creatinine changes. The ability to quantify urine output is impeded when priority is placed on removing indwelling bladder catheters (to prevent catheter-associated infections) or when patients wear diapers—obviously a significant problem for the pediatric patient population.

When urine output is not included in the assessment of AKI severity, a significant proportion of AKI is missed. Recent data indicates accounting for UOP in AKI recognition along with creatinine pathways actually identifies a unique subset of AKI patients in adults (vs. either criteria alone) [66]. The AWARE study reports that failure to account for UOP in children misses 20% of AKI cases [64]. Although an imperfect index, failure to even account for urine output in the assessment of AKI is a mistake. A new analysis of creatinine suggests that static measures of creatinine are less indicative of glomerular filtration, instead supporting the case for a kinetic GFR based on change in creatinine over time [67]. In parallel fashion, urine output should be tracked and should likely be tracked in a dynamic state, flow rate change as a function of time.

Novel biomarkers and functional tests of the kidney offer a diagnostic advancement. Novel biomarkers have already demonstrated an ability to identify S-AKI before changes in serum creatinine. Plasma and urine neutrophil gelatinase-associated lipocalin (NGAL) levels were significantly higher at 0, 12, and 24 h in 83 patients with SA-AKI compared with non-septic AKI [68]. Though plasma NGAL increases in patients with sepsis, levels were significantly associated with the renal subscore of the sequential organ failure assessment score (SOFA) in critically ill adults [69]. In a separate, prospective evaluation of 150 septic patients, urinary netrin-1 and KIM-1 were increased within 3 h of admission for patients with AKI [70]. Recent studies demonstrate the ability of NGAL to improve the prediction of severe AKI afforded by the clinical context model of the renal angina index (AUC increased from 0.72 to 0.86, 0.80 to 0.97) [71]. Elevation of E-selectin, typical of inflammatory and endothelial activation, is associated with future AKI in a longitudinal evaluation of patients after sepsis [72]. In a large multicenter study of critically ill adults, cell-cycle arrest markers tissue inhibitor of matrix metalloproteinase-2 (TIMP-2) and insulin-like growth factor binding protein 7 (IGFB7) demonstrated superior discrimination for AKI compared to other novel biomarkers such as NGAL, interleukin-18, liver type-fatty acid binding protein, and kidney injury molecule-1 (KIM-1) (AUC of 0.80 for TIMP-2/IGFBP7 vs. <0.72 for the others) [73]. In this study, the predictive performance of TIMP-2/IGFBP7 for AKI was further increased in patients with sepsis (AUC 0.82). Genomic and proteomic expression also varies in models of AKI [74]. Gene expression in models of S-AKI demonstrates some overlap with both sepsis and AKI models, but also unique characteristics, supporting the notion that S-AKI is an independent, unique disease process.

Functional tests of renal reserve can be performed. The recently described furosemide stress test objectively quantifies the urine flow rate response to a standardized dose of furosemide [75]. The results not only are predictive of AKI progression but also provide information on the health of numerous segments of the kidney (function of the glomerulus, proximal tubule, and loop of Henle are all requisite for furosemide effect). Meanwhile, newer technology being developed may facilitate the tracking of real-time GFR, using fluorescent probes detected by transdermal sensors, real-time GFR monitoring is capable of responding instantaneously to changes in GFR induced by stressors to the kidney [76].

Taken together the field of S-AKI diagnostics requires advancement. The assessment of a patient must begin with a risk assessment, inclusive of patient age. Patients demonstrating greater than low risk merit AKI biomarker assessment and follow up, with functional testing to determine a more precise S-AKI phenotype (Fig. 6.4).

### 6.1.8 Moving Forward: Management and Targeted Therapeutics

Management of S-AKI can be improved. To date, no singular therapy for S-AKI has been identified and the mainstays of "therapy" are supportive care, removal or reduction of nephrotoxic agents, and renal replacement therapy. As mentioned earlier, RRT initiation is controversial, but post hoc analysis of two large adult studies investigating the effect of "early" initiation of RRT are currently being conducted to determine population-based differences (i.e., sepsis vs. no sepsis) [77–79]. Additionally, ongoing studies (STARRT-AKI) will examine this question further. As S-AKI is a multifactorial process involving a number of molecular switches (programmed cell survival or death, inflammatory and counter inflammatory signaling, hypoxia and oxidative stress to name a few), countering these pathways with novel adjuncts may be beneficial. Targeting the apoptotic pathway with caspase inhibitors and suppressing inflammatory cascades have shown some promising results in experimental models [80, 81]. Other therapeutic agents such as Ghrelin [82], low dose vasopressin [83], adenosine receptor agonists [84], and erythropoietin [85] have shown some renal anti-inflammatory and apoptosis suppressing qualities. Modulation of mitochondrial oxidative phosphorylation through antioxidants also may be of benefit in S-AKI as hypoxia-induced ROS and NOS during sepsis may contribute to renal tubular injury [86]. Recent experimental data demonstrates the potential for the enzyme alkaline phosphatase to improve outcome in S-AKI by favorably modulating the immune response [87].

A novel approach to managing S-AKI will facilitate identification of effective therapy. This approach contrasts starkly with the uniform approach currently in place. The traditional pathway of management has occurred "in series." The number of problems in this approach includes: lack of stratification, lack of early appreciation of AKI effects, reliance on a delayed marker of injury, and a paucity of options for treatment. A novel and more appropriate approach treats S-AKI "in parallel" (Fig. 6.5). Sepsis is treated but incorporated early in the algorithm for AKI risk stratification. Patients with high risk are delineated from those at low risk although both receive supportive care and an AKI prevention bundle (based on KDIGO management guidelines). The high-risk patients then have a series of tests done to phenotype their injury pattern including a panel of urine and serum biomarkers specific for timing, location, and mechanism of injury. A furosemide stress test is performed to determine tubular function and reserve. A real-time GFR monitor is placed to track filtration on a more constant basis and determine kinetic changes in GFR. A combination of these results yields specific, individual phenotypes for AKI or S-AKI. Targeted therapies are then instituted for the specific phenotypes.

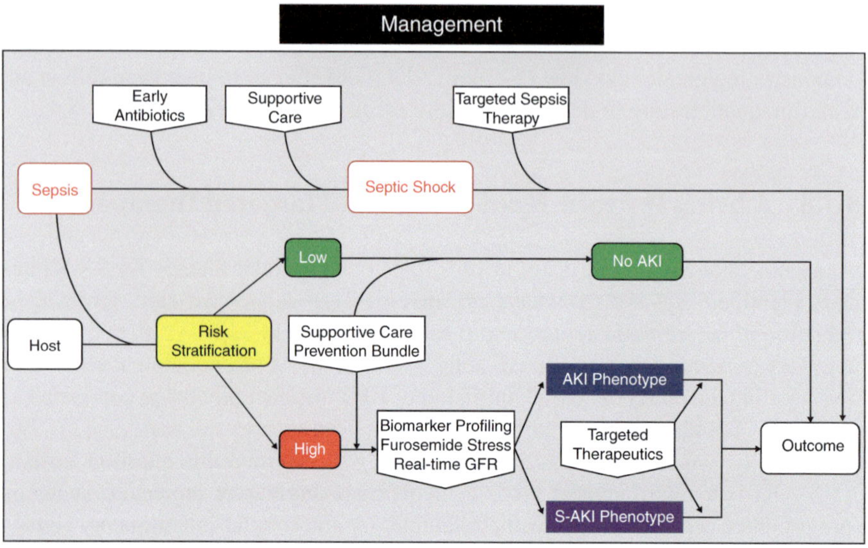


**Fig. 6.5** Modern approach—management in parallel. Sepsis and AKI should be recognized and managed from the beginning, starting with appreciation of risk. The complexity of newer sepsis management strategies are not shown here but involve potential to target therapy based on sepsis signatures. Patients can be risk stratified for AKI and then assessed at an early stage, with concurrent supportive care and AKI prevention in place, using urinary and serum biomarkers and real-time outputs of glomerular and tubular function yielding specific phenotypes of injury. Targeted therapies (including early renal replacement therapy initiation) can be tested in this context and specific phenotype and therapy-based outcomes determined

## 6.1.9 Conclusion: The Path Forward

Sepsis-associated AKI is a significant problem in critically ill patients. The past and present paradigm of how this syndrome-like injury is understood needs to be changed, updated, and refined. An analytical, objective evaluation of the strengths and weaknesses of the S-AKI paradigm can be created using a "SWOT" (Fig. 6.6). The strengths of the current paradigm include, most importantly, a growing appreciation of the S-AKI, not just in the critical care and nephrology community. The weaknesses have been described in this chapter and cumulatively lead to a black box and one-size-fits-all approach S-AKI. Epidemiologic data from developing nations is infrequent yet sepsis and AKI are undoubtedly common in these parts of the world (notably Southeast Asia, most of sub-Saharan Africa, and Central America). This data is needed to fully understand the scope of disease. Opportunities exist and must be leveraged, including utilization of the electronic medical record (EMR) while simultaneously paying appropriate respect to factors that imperil progress (threats). Diagnostic modernization is possible with technology that currently exists and would lead to a more precise understanding of the disease. Ultimately, these combined approaches and efforts on all aspects of S-AKI disease should facilitate improvements in management and ultimately improve outcomes for patients of all ages.

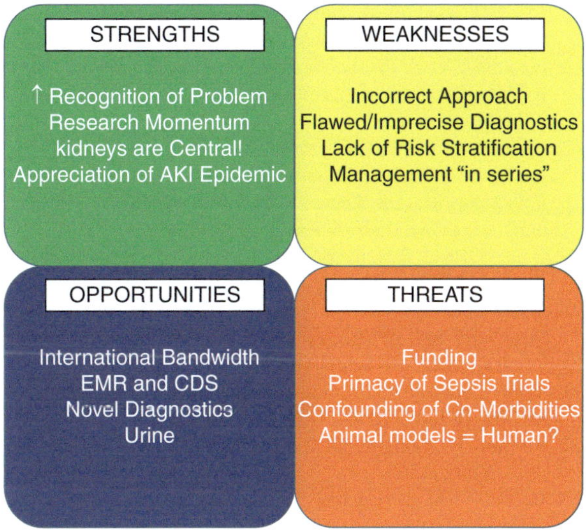


**Fig. 6.6** Sepsis-associated AKI—A SWOT approach. Depicted above are the strengths (S), weaknesses (W), opportunities (O), and threats (T) in the past, present, and future paradigm of S-AKI. (*EMR* electronic medical record, *CDS* clinical decision support)

## References


1. Jawad I, Luksic I, Rafnsson SB. Assessing available information on the burden of sepsis: global estimates of incidence, prevalence and mortality. J Glob Health. 2012;2(1):010404.
2. Martin GS, et al. The epidemiology of sepsis in the United States from 1979 through 2000. N Engl J Med. 2003;348(16):1546–54.
3. Gaieski DF, et al. Benchmarking the incidence and mortality of severe sepsis in the United States. Crit Care Med. 2013;41(5):1167–74.
4. Annane D, et al. Current epidemiology of septic shock: the CUB-Rea network. Am J Respir Crit Care Med. 2003;168(2):165–72.
5. Angus DC, et al. Epidemiology of severe sepsis in the United States: analysis of incidence, outcome, and associated costs of care. Crit Care Med. 2001;29(7):1303–10.
6. Martin CM, et al. A prospective, observational registry of patients with severe sepsis: the Canadian Sepsis treatment and response registry. Crit Care Med. 2009;37(1):81–8.
7. Karlsson S, et al. Incidence, treatment, and outcome of severe sepsis in ICU-treated adults in Finland: the Finnsepsis study. Intensive Care Med. 2007;33(3):435–43.
8. de Mendonca A, et al. Acute renal failure in the ICU: risk factors and outcome evaluated by the SOFA score. Intensive Care Med. 2000;26(7):915–21.
9. Uchino S, et al. Acute renal failure in critically ill patients: a multinational, multicenter study. JAMA. 2005;294(7):813–8.
10. Bagshaw SM, et al. Changes in the incidence and outcome for early acute kidney injury in a cohort of Australian intensive care units. Crit Care. 2007;11(3):R68.
11. Ostermann M, Chang RW. Acute kidney injury in the intensive care unit according to RIFLE. Crit Care Med. 2007;35(8):1837–43. quiz 1852
12. Bagshaw SM, et al. A multi-Centre evaluation of the RIFLE criteria for early acute kidney injury in critically ill patients. Nephrol Dial Transplant. 2008;23(4):1203–10.
13. Andrikos E, et al. Epidemiology of acute renal failure in ICUs: a multi-center prospective study. Blood Purif. 2009;28(3):239–44.
14. Thakar CV, et al. Incidence and outcomes of acute kidney injury in intensive care units: a veterans administration study. Crit Care Med. 2009;37(9):2552–8.

15. Medve L, et al. Epidemiology of acute kidney injury in Hungarian intensive care units: a multicenter, prospective, observational study. BMC Nephrol. 2011;12:43.
16. Piccinni P, et al. Prospective multicenter study on epidemiology of acute kidney injury in the ICU: a critical care nephrology Italian collaborative effort (NEFROINT). Minerva Anestesiol. 2011;77(11):1072–83.
17. Nisula S, et al. Incidence, risk factors and 90-day mortality of patients with acute kidney injury in Finnish intensive care units: the FINNAKI study. Intensive Care Med. 2013;39(3):420–8.
18. Poukkanen M, et al. Acute kidney injury in patients with severe sepsis in Finnish intensive care units. Acta Anaesthesiol Scand. 2013;57(7):863–72.
19. Bailey D, et al. Risk factors of acute renal failure in critically ill children: a prospective descriptive epidemiological study. Pediatr Crit Care Med. 2007;8(1):29–35.
20. Schneider J, et al. Serum creatinine as stratified in the RIFLE score for acute kidney injury is associated with mortality and length of stay for children in the pediatric intensive care unit. Crit Care Med. 2010;38(3):933–9.
21. Vachvanichsanong P, et al. Childhood acute renal failure: 22-year experience in a university hospital in southern Thailand. Pediatrics. 2006;118(3):e786–91.
22. Kellum JA, Angus DC. Patients are dying of acute renal failure. Crit Care Med. 2002;30(9):2156–7.
23. Bagshaw SM, et al. Early acute kidney injury and sepsis: a multicentre evaluation. Crit Care. 2008;12(2):R47.
24. Bagshaw SM, et al. Septic acute kidney injury in critically ill patients: clinical characteristics and outcomes. Clin J Am Soc Nephrol. 2007;2(3):431–9.
25. Kolhe NV, et al. Case mix, outcome and activity for patients with severe acute kidney injury during the first 24 hours after admission to an adult, general critical care unit: application of predictive models from a secondary analysis of the ICNARC case mix Programme database. Crit Care. 2008;12(Suppl 1):S2.
26. Daher EF, et al. Acute kidney injury in an infectious disease intensive care unit – an assessment of prognostic factors. Swiss Med Wkly. 2008;138(9–10):128–33.
27. Alkandari O, et al. Acute kidney injury is an independent risk factor for pediatric intensive care unit mortality, longer length of stay and prolonged mechanical ventilation in critically ill children: a two-center retrospective cohort study. Crit Care. 2011;15(3):R146.
28. Pundziene B, Dobiliene D, Rudaitis S. Acute kidney injury in pediatric patients: experience of a single center during an 11-year period. Medicina (Kaunas). 2010;46(8):511–5.
29. Duzova A, et al. Etiology and outcome of acute kidney injury in children. Pediatr Nephrol. 2010;25(8):1453–61.
30. Mehta P, et al. Incidence of acute kidney injury in hospitalized children. Indian Pediatr. 2012;49(7):537–42.
31. Lopes JA, et al. Acute kidney injury in patients with sepsis: a contemporary analysis. Int J Infect Dis. 2009;13(2):176–81.
32. Plotz FB, et al. Effect of acute renal failure on outcome in children with severe septic shock. Pediatr Nephrol. 2005;20(8):1177–81.
33. Parrillo JE. Pathogenetic mechanisms of septic shock. N Engl J Med. 1993;328(20):1471–7.
34. Schrier RW, Wang W. Acute renal failure and sepsis. N Engl J Med. 2004;351(2):159–69.
35. Ceneviva G, et al. Hemodynamic support in fluid-refractory pediatric septic shock. Pediatrics. 1998;102(2):e19.
36. Riley C, et al. Pediatric sepsis: preparing for the future against a global scourge. Curr Infect Dis Rep. 2012;14(5):503–11.
37. Gotts JE, Matthay MA. Sepsis: pathophysiology and clinical management. BMJ. 2016;353:i1585.
38. Gomez H, et al. A unified theory of sepsis-induced acute kidney injury: inflammation, microcirculatory dysfunction, bioenergetics, and the tubular cell adaptation to injury. Shock. 2014;41(1):3–11.
39. Chawla LS. Disentanglement of the acute kidney injury syndrome. Curr Opin Crit Care. 2012;18(6):579–84.

40. Liu VX, et al. The timing of early antibiotics and hospital mortality in Sepsis. Am J Respir Crit Care Med. 2017;196(7):856–63.
41. Prowle JR. Sepsis-associated AKI. Clin J Am Soc Nephrol. 2018;13(2):339–42.
42. Schneider AG, et al. Choice of renal replacement therapy modality and dialysis dependence after acute kidney injury: a systematic review and meta-analysis. Intensive Care Med. 2013;39(6):987–97.
43. Wald R, et al. The association between renal replacement therapy modality and long-term outcomes among critically ill adults with acute kidney injury: a retrospective cohort study*. Crit Care Med. 2014;42(4):868–77.
44. Ronco C, et al. Effects of different doses in continuous veno-venous haemofiltration on outcomes of acute renal failure: a prospective randomised trial. Lancet. 2000;356(9223):26–30.
45. Network, V.N.A.R.F.T, et al. Intensity of renal support in critically ill patients with acute kidney injury. N Engl J Med. 2008;359(1):7–20.
46. Investigators, R.R.T.S, et al. Intensity of continuous renal-replacement therapy in critically ill patients. N Engl J Med. 2009;361(17):1627–38.
47. Joannes-Boyau O, et al. High-volume versus standard-volume haemofiltration for septic shock patients with acute kidney injury (IVOIRE study): a multicentre randomized controlled trial. Intensive Care Med. 2013;39(9):1535–46.
48. Feltes CM, Van Eyk J, Rabb H. Distant-organ changes after acute kidney injury. Nephron Physiol. 2008;109(4):p80–4.
49. Shiao CC, et al. Long-term remote organ consequences following acute kidney injury. Crit Care. 2015;19:438.
50. Yap SC, Lee HT. Acute kidney injury and extrarenal organ dysfunction: new concepts and experimental evidence. Anesthesiology. 2012,116(5):1139–48.
51. Shin YJ, et al. Age-related differences in kidney injury biomarkers induced by cisplatin. Environ Toxicol Pharmacol. 2014;37(3):1028–39.
52. Vandijck DM, et al. Severe infection, sepsis and acute kidney injury. Acta Clin Belg. 2007;62(Suppl 2):332–6.
53. Langenberg C, et al. Renal blood flow in sepsis. Crit Care. 2005;9(4):R363–74.
54. Langenberg C, et al. Renal blood flow in experimental septic acute renal failure. Kidney Int. 2006;69(11):1996–2002.
55. Scicluna BP, et al. Classification of patients with sepsis according to blood genomic endotype: a prospective cohort study. Lancet Respir Med. 2017;5(10):816–26.
56. Wong HR, et al. Improved risk stratification in pediatric septic shock using both protein and mRNA biomarkers. PERSEVERE-XP. Am J Respir Crit Care Med. 2017;196(4):494–501.
57. Langenberg C, et al. The histopathology of septic acute kidney injury: a systematic review. Crit Care. 2008;12(2):R38.
58. Zarbock A, Gomez H, Kellum JA. Sepsis-induced acute kidney injury revisited: pathophysiology, prevention and future therapies. Curr Opin Crit Care. 2014;20(6):588–95.
59. Chvojka J, et al. Renal haemodynamic, microcirculatory, metabolic and histopathological responses to peritonitis-induced septic shock in pigs. Crit Care. 2008;12(6):R164.
60. Doi K, et al. Animal models of sepsis and sepsis-induced kidney injury. J Clin Invest. 2009;119(10):2868–78.
61. Goldstein SL, Chawla LS. Renal angina. Clin J Am Soc Nephrol. 2010;5(5):943–9.
62. Basu RK, et al. Derivation and validation of the renal angina index to improve the prediction of acute kidney injury in critically ill children. Kidney Int. 2014;85(3):659–67.
63. Hoste EA, et al. Epidemiology of acute kidney injury in critically ill patients: the multinational AKI-EPI study. Intensive Care Med. 2015;41(8):1411–23.
64. Kaddourah A, et al. Epidemiology of acute kidney injury in critically ill children and young adults. N Engl J Med. 2017;376(1):11–20.
65. Fitzgerald JC, et al. Acute kidney injury in pediatric severe Sepsis: an independent risk factor for death and new disability. Crit Care Med. 2016;44(12):2241–50.
66. Kellum JA, et al. Classifying AKI by urine output versus serum creatinine level. J Am Soc Nephrol. 2015;26(9):2231–8.

67. Chen S. Retooling the creatinine clearance equation to estimate kinetic GFR when the plasma creatinine is changing acutely. J Am Soc Nephrol. 2013;24(6):877–88.
68. Bagshaw SM, et al. Plasma and urine neutrophil gelatinase-associated lipocalin in septic versus non-septic acute kidney injury in critical illness. Intensive Care Med. 2010;36(3):452–61.
69. Kim H, et al. Plasma neutrophil gelatinase-associated lipocalin as a biomarker for acute kidney injury in critically ill patients with suspected sepsis. Clin Biochem. 2013;46(15):1414–8.
70. Tu Y, et al. Urinary netrin-1 and KIM-1 as early biomarkers for septic acute kidney injury. Ren Fail. 2014;36(10):1559–63.
71. Basu RK, et al. Incorporation of biomarkers with the renal angina index for prediction of severe AKI in critically ill children. Clin J Am Soc Nephrol. 2014;9(4):654–62.
72. Powell TC, et al. Association of inflammatory and endothelial cell activation biomarkers with acute kidney injury after sepsis. Spring. 2014;3:207.
73. Kashani K, et al. Discovery and validation of cell cycle arrest biomarkers in human acute kidney injury. Crit Care. 2013;17(1):R25.
74. Devarajan P. Genomic and proteomic characterization of acute kidney injury. Nephron. 2015;131(2):85–91.
75. Chawla LS, et al. Development and standardization of a furosemide stress test to predict the severity of acute kidney injury. Crit Care. 2013;17(5):R207.
76. Solomon R, Goldstein S. Real-time measurement of glomerular filtration rate. Curr Opin Crit Care. 2017;23(6):470–4.
77. Gaudry S, et al. Initiation strategies for renal-replacement therapy in the intensive care unit. N Engl J Med. 2016;375(2):122–33.
78. Zarbock A, et al. Effect of early vs delayed initiation of renal replacement therapy on mortality in critically ill patients with acute kidney injury: the ELAIN randomized clinical trial. JAMA. 2016;315(20):2190–9.
79. Smith OM, et al. Standard versus accelerated initiation of renal replacement therapy in acute kidney injury (STARRT-AKI): study protocol for a randomized controlled trial. Trials. 2013;14:320.
80. Lee SY, et al. Distinct pathophysiologic mechanisms of septic acute kidney injury: role of immune suppression and renal tubular cell apoptosis in murine model of septic acute kidney injury. Crit Care Med. 2012;40(11):2997–3006.
81. Homsi E, Janino P, de Faria JB. Role of caspases on cell death, inflammation, and cell cycle in glycerol-induced acute renal failure. Kidney Int. 2006;69(8):1385–92.
82. Wang W, et al. Ghrelin protects mice against endotoxemia-induced acute kidney injury. Am J Physiol Renal Physiol. 2009;297(4):F1032–7.
83. Simon F, et al. Comparison of cardiac, hepatic, and renal effects of arginine vasopressin and noradrenaline during porcine fecal peritonitis: a randomized controlled trial. Crit Care. 2009;13(4):R113.
84. Lee HT, et al. A3 adenosine receptor activation decreases mortality and renal and hepatic injury in murine septic peritonitis. Am J Physiol Regul Integr Comp Physiol. 2006;291(4):R959–69.
85. Bahlmann FH, Fliser D. Erythropoietin and renoprotection. Curr Opin Nephrol Hypertens. 2009;18(1):15–20.
86. Pathak E, MacMillan-Crow LA, Mayeux PR. Role of mitochondrial oxidants in an in vitro model of sepsis-induced renal injury. J Pharmacol Exp Ther. 2012;340(1):192–201.
87. Pickkers P, et al. Alkaline phosphatase for treatment of sepsis-induced acute kidney injury: a prospective randomized double-blind placebo-controlled trial. Crit Care. 2012;16(1):R14.

# Post Cardiac Surgery Acute Kidney Injury and Cardiorenal Syndromes

7

David S. Cooper and Zaccaria Ricci

## 7.1 Acute Kidney Injury Following Cardiac Surgery

Acute kidney injury (AKI) is a frequent complication of pediatric cardiac surgery affecting 40–60% of high-risk cohorts [1, 2] and is becoming increasingly recognized as a major health concern within pediatric patients [3]. AKI is associated with increased durations of mechanical ventilation, inotropic support and ICU stay, and increased mortality, even among patients with only minor creatinine changes [1, 2, 4, 5]. The fluid overload caused by AKI is furthermore associated with mortality and worse clinical outcomes [6, 7]. Increased awareness of this complication has spurred research devoted to improved diagnostics, potential therapeutics, an understanding of the long term significance of AKI, and the scope of AKI within nonsurgical cardiac cohorts. This review intends to be an overview of AKI and its management within this vulnerable population.

## 7.2 Pathophysiology of AKI After Cardiac Surgery

The etiology of cardiac surgery-associated AKI is multifactorial and incompletely understood, extending beyond low cardiac output and impaired renal blood flow [8]. The primary driving mechanisms include ischemia-reperfusion injury, mechanical

D. S. Cooper (✉)
Cardiac Intensive Care Unit and Center for Acute Care Nephrology, The Heart Institute, Cincinnati Children's Hospital Medical Center, Cincinnati, OH, USA
e-mail: David.Cooper@cchmc.org

Z. Ricci
Department of Cardiology and Cardiac Surgery, Pediatric Cardiac Intensive Care Unit, Bambino Gesù Children's Hospital, Rome, Italy



A. Deep, S. L. Goldstein (eds.), *Critical Care Nephrology and Renal Replacement Therapy in Children*, https://doi.org/10.1007/978-3-319-90281-4_7

blood trauma, oxidative stress, venous congestion, and pro-inflammatory cytokine activation [9–13]. A reduction in mean arterial pressure and non-pulsatile flow during cardiopulmonary bypass (CPB) result in activation of apoptotic and necrotic pathways of tubule and endothelial cell death [12, 14]. The kidney is able to tolerate up to 60 min of ischemia with only mild structural changes and no loss of function [15], but with release of vascular clamps subsequent reperfusion injury results in activation of the oxidative pathways that exacerbate tubular and microvascular injury [12, 14]. Red cell hemolysis due to the CPB circuit releases free hemoglobin and catalytic iron, which exacerbates oxidant-mediated injury, resulting in release of pro-inflammatory cytokines from injured tubules and endothelial cells. Contact of the blood with the artificial surfaces of the CPB circuit exacerbates injury via activation of neutrophils, platelets, and pro-inflammatory cytokines. Perioperative nephrotoxic medication use may increase the severity of existing injury.

## 7.3 Incidence and Risk Factors for AKI

Acute kidney injury occurs in approximately 40% of children following cardiac surgery [1]. An in-depth discussion of the methods and challenges of diagnosing AKI in children, especially neonates, can be found in Chaps. 3 and 5. AKI has consistently been associated with increased morbidity and mortality, including prolonged length of stay, prolonged need for mechanical ventilation, fluid and electrolyte disturbances, and drug metabolism [1, 16]. The incidence of AKI is similar among those with congestive heart failure (CHF) and receiving extracorporeal therapies [17–19]. Adults with congenital heart disease (CHD) may have other renal comorbidities, including diabetes and hypertension and are at significant risk for postoperative AKI and chronic kidney disease (CKD) [20, 21]. In fact, nearly 50% of adults with CHD have some degree of renal dysfunction, and approximately 20% of those patients have moderate CKD [22]. Compared to the general population, the incidence of renal dysfunction has been found to be 18-times higher in acyanotic adult patients, and 35-times higher in cyanotic patients [22]. Additionally, renal function in CHD patients is also found to decline at a faster rate than the general population [23].

Although perioperative risk factors for the development of AKI have been identified, few of them are modifiable. Younger age, longer CPB duration, higher surgical complexity, and preoperative ventilator support are risk factors for the development of AKI, but also correlate with a sick patient substrate [1, 2, 4, 5]. Intraoperative risk factors include low blood pressure and hemoglobin during CPB, need for emergent intervention, and need for thoracic aortic surgery [24]. After controlling for age and surgical severity, bypass times >180 min had an odds ratio of 7.6 for the development of AKI [1]. Postoperative risk factors include volume overload, preexisting CKD, nephrotoxin use, and use of mechanical circulatory support [1, 8].

In patients with acute heart failure, age, inotrope use, and higher admission creatinine and blood urea nitrogen were associated with severe AKI, in-hospital mortality, and need for mechanical circulatory support [17, 18]. Lesions with a high postoperative central venous pressure (CVP) also have high incidence of AKI. This includes lesions with residual right ventricular hypertrophy and diastolic dysfunction, such as tetralogy of Fallot, and lesions with obligate CVP elevation due to surgical palliation, such as the Fontan surgery [25].

More recently, novel serum and urinary biomarkers have been used to diagnose and prognosticate AKI and is discussed in Chap. 4. Given the same set of risk factors and a similar renal insult, there will be some patients who develop AKI and others who do not. While some of this may be due to chance or differences in surgical or bypass techniques, there is growing evidence that there may be genetic variations that either predispose patients to or protect them from the development of AKI. Given the common mechanisms of postoperative AKI, polymorphisms associated with renal inflammatory, oxidative stress, or vasoconstrictor responses have been of highest interest [26, 27]. A study among adult patients undergoing aortic-coronary surgery found two alleles (interleukin 6 – 572C and angiotensinogen 842C) associated with AKI in Caucasians [26]. The ability to predict AKI increased fourfold when genetic polymorphism use was added to clinical risk factors.

## 7.4 Prevention and Treatment of AKI

The majority of AKI occurs in the perioperative period and therefore this constitutes a primary research focus. Postoperative AKI is generally self-limited, and consequently much of the management is focused on a major sequela of AKI—fluid overload. Although the essence of preventing fluid overload requires avoiding volume input in excess of output, this is often impossible. Fluids for nutritional demands, resuscitation, essential blood products, and medications are given during a period in which patients have AKI-induced oliguria. Loop diuretics are the mainstay of treatment for oliguria, although the effectiveness of aggressive diuretic use among AKI patients is controversial [28]. Ricci and colleagues demonstrated that utilization of ethacrynic acid versus furosemide was effective and safe in neonates and infants undergoing cardiac surgery [29]. Ethacrynic acid resulted in an optimized fluid balance in the first postoperative day resulting in shorter ventilation time and improved cardiac output, without increasing creatinine levels with respect to furosemide.

Intraoperative factors influence the predilection of postoperative AKI. Since longer bypass times and the use of circulatory arrest are associated with higher incidence of AKI, both should be limited as possible [1]. Modified ultrafiltration after CPB has been shown to reduce fluid overload, decrease postoperative blood loss and the need for transfusion, and improve postoperative systolic ventricular function [30, 31]. Unnecessary blood transfusion may mediate AKI by multiple mechanisms including inflammatory changes and hemolysis causing release of free iron [32].

The use and timing of postoperative renal replacement therapy via peritoneal dialysis varies between centers. Recent studies have demonstrated that earlier use of peritoneal dialysis in infants after CPB is associated with shorter duration of mechanical ventilation and ICU stay, less inotropic medication use, and lower mortality [33–35]. Although mechanisms are incompletely understood, peritoneal dialysis decreases edema, which allows improved renal perfusion and also is thought to clear pro-inflammatory cytokines. Future delivery of renal replacement therapy is likely to be revolutionized by the miniaturization of continuous renal replacement therapies already common in larger patients [36].

Although a fair amount of research has been devoted to finding a therapeutic agent for postoperative AKI, there have been no consistently successful agents. Because AKI has multiple mechanisms, proposed therapies have focused on several different pathways, including vasoconstriction, ATP depletion, oxidative stress, free-iron, inflammatory response, and apoptosis. The most common mechanism of attempted renal protection is via medications that augment renal perfusion, often via afferent glomerular arteriole dilation or efferent constriction. This is the concept behind the popularized "renal dose dopamine," which has not been shown effective [37]. Many agents have been used within pediatrics with mixed results, including fenoldopam, aminophylline, nesiritide, and dexmedetomidine [38–42]. Several medications, including glucocorticoids and pentoxifylline, have been proposed to address inflammatory pathways mediated by CPB, but have also yet to show evidence of efficacy [42, 43]. N-Acetylcysteine has demonstrated potential utility preventing AKI through anti-oxidative and anti-inflammatory mechanisms [44]. Bronicki and colleagues conducted a retrospective study of nesiritide therapy in children with CHD who showed resistance to diuretic therapy and pulmonary congestion [45]. Nesiritide was able to significantly decrease central venous pressure and heart rate and increase urine output with concomitant decrease in serum creatinine and stage of AKI. Interestingly, intraoperative infusion of dexmedetomidine has been associated with attenuation of the renal dysfunction after pediatric cardiac surgery [40, 46]. Novel therapeutic pathways are being investigated but likely many years from being part of mainstream care.

There is little research focused on renal protection in pediatric patients outside of the postoperative period. The use of N-acetylcysteine has been well studied for prevention of contrast-induced AKI, although is not well studied in pediatric populations [47]. The use of theophylline or aminophylline had been studied for prevention of calcineurin-induced AKI and has some pediatric evidence [48].

## 7.5 Outcomes After AKI

AKI after CPB is often a self-limited complication, occurring in the first 24–48 h postoperatively. In the Translational Research Investigation Biomarker Endpoints in AKI (TRIBE-AKI) consortium, almost half of patients met AKI diagnostic criteria for just 1 day and only 1 of 9 patients still met the definition by the fourth postoperative day [1]. For this reason the importance of postoperative AKI has historically been minimized. However, recent research has emphasized the strong association of AKI with worse postoperative and long-term outcomes.

AKI has been shown to be an independent risk factor for prolonged duration of mechanical ventilation, longer ICU and hospital stays, and mortality [1, 2, 4]. In the TRIBE-AKI consortium, 30% of patients with AKI were mechanically ventilated at

48-h postoperative as opposed to 8% of those without AKI [1]. Blinder and colleagues studied 430 infants after bypass finding that 52% developed AKI. Stage 2 AKI was associated with a 5-times risk of death, and stage 3 AKI was associated with nearly a 10-times risk. These were stronger predictors of death than having single ventricle physiology or needing mechanical circulatory support [4].

Even small increases in creatinine are important. Compared to those with no change in creatinine, adults after cardiac surgery with a creatinine increase of just 0.1–0.5 mg/dL had a threefold increase in the rate of mortality, and this association worsened with larger creatinine changes [49]. There are also data among pediatric patients after cardiac surgery that small early changes in creatinine predict later development of AKI [5]. A large multinational study of critically ill children demonstrated that AKI was common and associated with worse outcomes [3]. In addition, use of urine output criteria uncovered additional cases of AKI that would have been missed by using serum creatinine alone. The development of standardized AKI definitions has allowed for a more complete understanding of pediatric AKI epidemiology, but long-term clinical outcomes after AKI in critically ill children and neonates have not been well established. The damage induced by subclinical or manifested episodes of AKI may produce irreversible loss of renal mass with deleterious effects on overall renal function and predispose to an increased risk of developing CKD.

It previously was assumed that patients with a single episode of AKI would recover kidney function without long-term consequence. However, during the last decade, epidemiologic data from critically ill children and adults suggest that AKI survivors are at considerable risk of developing CKD [50–52]. Coca and colleagues demonstrated that adults who experienced AKI have a ninefold increased risk of developing CKD, a threefold increased risk of developing end-stage kidney disease, and a twofold increased risk of long-term mortality risk as compared to those without AKI [53]. Mammen and colleagues found that 10% of previously critically ill children (including postoperative cardiac patients) had developed CKD 1–3 years following AKI, and almost half were considered at risk of CKD development (mildly decreased GFR, hypertension, and/or hyperfiltration) [54]. Wong and colleagues described the incidence and significance of AKI throughout the three stages of palliation for hypoplastic left heart syndrome and its variants [55]. AKI was common among these high-risk patients and the sequelae of severe AKI as a neonate was substantial, predisposing patients to death or need for ECMO after stage 1 palliation, and despite normalization of creatinine, subsequent risk of severe AKI after stage 2 was elevated. Morgan and colleagues followed a cohort of neonates after cardiac surgery and found that 2–4 years later, those who developed AKI were at higher risk of growth impairment, cardiac-related hospitalization, and increased health care utilization, even when controlling for gestational age, surgical type, preoperative ventilation, lactate elevation, and use of mechanical circulatory support [2]. With regard to adults with CHD, Dimopoulos and colleagues revealed that 50% of young adults with CHD have impaired GFR, even those with "simple" defects [22]. Given the known limitations of traditional biomarkers to detect AKI early, attention has been focused on the utility of novel urinary biomarkers to follow and predict rapid CKD progression in both pediatric and adult CKD populations. Cooper and colleagues evaluated patients 7 years following CPB, and although there was no conventional evidence of CKD there was evidence of novel renal urinary biomarker elevation consistent with ongoing subclinical injury [56]. These data highlight the importance of following AKI survivors throughout adulthood to understand the long-term implications of AKI.

## 7.6 Pediatric Cardiorenal Syndromes

Renal injury occurs commonly in patients with heart failure. Diminished cardiac function coupled with renal dysfunction has been defined as Cardiorenal syndrome (CRS). This reciprocal pathogenic relation between worsening kidney function and deteriorating heart function was described about 30 years ago but is a concept reinvigorated recently. Ronco and colleagues [57] have divided cardiorenal syndrome into five types depending on the whether the symptoms are "driven" by the kidney or heart and whether it is acute or chronic in nature (Table 7.1). Cardiorenal syndrome has been associated with poor prognosis, with the occurrence of worsening renal function strongly associated with mortality in this setting [58]. The most common types seen in the pediatric intensive care unit are acute cardiorenal syndrome (CRS Type I—acute decompensation of cardiac function leading to acute renal failure) and secondary CRS (CRS Type V—systemic illness leading to simultaneous organ dysfunction). As management of patients with chronic cardiac failure (cardiomyopathy, failing Fontan physiology, or heart transplant graft dysfunction) has improved, the frequency of CRS Type 2 has increased. In any of these settings, however, decreased urine output and resultant fluid retention can aggravate heart failure symptoms and contribute to clinical deterioration.

**Table 7.1** Types of cardiorenal syndromes

| Type of cardiorenal syndrome | Description |
|---|---|
| Type I—Acute cardiorenal syndrome | Abrupt worsening of cardiac function (e.g., acute cardiogenic shock or acutely decompensated CHF) leading to acute kidney injury |
| Type II—Chronic cardiorenal syndrome | Chronic abnormalities in cardiac function (e.g., chronic CHF) causing progressive and potentially permanent chronic kidney disease |
| Type III—Acute renocardiac syndrome | Abrupt worsening of renal function (e.g., acute kidney ischemia or glomerulonephritis) causing acute cardiac disorder (e.g., heart failure, arrhythmia, ischemia) |
| Type IV—Chronic renocardiac syndrome | Chronic kidney disease (e.g., chronic glomerular or interstitial disease) contributing to decreased cardiac function, cardiac hypertrophy and/or increased risk of adverse cardiovascular events |
| Type V—Secondary cardiorenal syndrome | Systemic condition (e.g., diabetes mellitus, sepsis) causing both cardiac and renal dysfunction |

Among patients hospitalized for acute decompensated heart failure, CRS is associated with longer length of stay, higher inhospital costs, and an increased risk of inhospital mortality [59]. Even a modest increase in serum creatinine (i.e., >0.3 mg/dL) can predict mortality in patients hospitalized for heart failure [60]. Similarly, asymptomatic patients with renal injury and left ventricular dysfunction are also at risk of cardiac systolic failure and death [61]. The relationship of renal function and heart failure in children has not been as well examined. Price and colleagues described the prevalence of worsening renal function (WRF) in 73 consecutive patient hospitalizations with a primary diagnosis of acute decompensated heart failure [18]. WRF was defined as an increase in serum creatinine of ≥0.3 mg/dL at any time during hospitalization. Renal failure at the time of admission was uncommon in this cohort but serum creatinine subsequently increased in 82% and WRF occurred during 48% of hospitalizations. These data are consistent with reports in adults with left ventricular systolic dysfunction and congestive heart failure [62, 63] and, in all cohorts, patients with WRF had a worse outcome.

Use of a ventricular assist device (VAD) as a bridge to transplant or destination therapy has become more common in children with end-stage heart disease (ESHD). In this context, renal function during VAD therapy has been assessed because, importantly, as mechanical support evolves in the pediatric community, candidate selection should also be based on end organ assessment. However, renal recovery is challenging to predict and several studies in adults have reported improved kidney function both in the short and long term after VAD implantation. VAD implantation can also improve short- and long-term renal function in children with ESHD [64]. Children with advanced heart failure commonly have renal dysfunction at the time of VAD placement. As reported by May and colleagues, more than 50% of this population has a baseline estimated glomerular filtration rate (eGFR) below 90 mL/min/1.73 m$^2$; the median eGFR in these children is 64 mL/min/1.73 m$^2$, consistent with stage 2 CKD. In this observational study, AKI occurred in 60% of children after VAD implantation, but renal function recovered relatively quickly, returning to or exceeding baseline by the end of the first week after VAD implant. Patients with intact pre-VAD renal function maintained renal function throughout the study period. More impressively, patients with pre-VAD renal dysfunction experienced a significant improvement in eGFR as early as postoperative day 4 and sustained this improvement through day 180 [64].

Heart transplantation is lifesaving treatment for end-stage heart failure, however, the impact of heart transplant on renal function is large. Previous analyses of renal function in pediatric heart and lung transplant recipients have shown conflicting results [65, 66]. Pradhan and colleagues evaluated renal function following thoracic organ transplantation in 46 children (32 heart, 9 lung, 5 heart-lung) with a median age of 4.1 years. Twenty-two percent of transplant recipients had an abnormal GFR prior to thoracic organ transplantation, which was likely related to HF. In the first 2 years posttransplant, the percentage of recipients with normal renal function declined from 78 to 29%. Younger age at transplant was associated with a greater decline in GFR%, and this decline persisted after adjustment for nutritional status with body mass index or weight-for-length z-scores, that reflects loss of renal function rather than improved muscle mass. The prevalence of renal insufficiency (GFR < 75%) increased from 22% at transplant to 55% and 85% at 1 and 5 years posttransplant, respectively, while 15% had a GFR% < 50 at 5 years post transplantation. The nephrotoxicity of calcineurin inhibitors may be particularly important in the youngest transplant recipients [67].

The physiologic interaction of the heart and kidney is complex and not well understood. Renal insufficiency occurring in heart failure patients is usually attributed to diminished cardiac output causing decreased renal perfusion, or a pre-renal state. This explanation of concomitant cardiorenal dysfunction oversimplifies the complex interrelationship of these two organs and fails to acknowledge the neurohormonal and vasoreactive elements in the setting of heart failure. Over time these adaptive mechanisms become maladaptive, leading to elevated systemic vascular resistance, fluid overload, and decreased renal perfusion. Additional factors such as persistent or elevated systemic vasoconstriction, use of nephrotoxic drugs, contrast agents, infection, or renal vein hypertension can lead to AKI during the treatment of heart failure [68]. Elevated central venous pressure also plays an important role as it is associated with reduced glomerular filtration rate even while other hemodynamic measurements (cardiac output and mean arterial pressure) are preserved.

Early recognition of CRS and better understanding of its pathophysiology are critical to guide therapy and hopefully improve outcome of affected patients. Among the promising emerging methods to recognize risk for CRS may be the use of novel renal biomarkers, possibly for more accurate early diagnosis and risk stratification. Use of biomarkers has an advantage in that they provide important pathophysiologic understanding.

## Conclusions

The reduction of morbidity following cardiac surgery remains challenging. Recent insights have allowed us to recognize the impact of perioperative acute kidney injury as a significant contributor to morbidity and mortality. Adopting a strategy of anticipation, early recognition and aggressive prevention and/or treatment of AKI and fluid overload should result in a decline in morbidity. Medical therapies for the prevention and treatment of AKI and fluid overload continue to evolve. Although the presence of negative cardiorenal interactions may not be avoidable, diagnostic and therapeutic innovation may help minimize the adverse outcomes associated with cardiorenal disease. There is growing evidence showing a strong association between AKI and CKD dispelling the previous notion that survivors of AKI fully recover renal function without subsequent consequence. The long-term follow-up of AKI survivors throughout adulthood is necessary to understand its ongoing implications on outcome.

**Key Learning Points**

- Acute kidney injury (AKI) is associated with significant morbidity and mortality in pediatric cardiac surgical patients.
- Fluid overload, as a consequence of AKI, is associated with morbidity and mortality.
- Cardiorenal syndromes describe an interdependent relationship between the heart and kidneys that becomes pathologic in the setting of acute cardiac and/or kidney disease.
- Previous conventional wisdom that survivors of AKI fully recover renal function without subsequent consequences is flawed.

## References


1. Li S, Krawczeski CD, Zappitelli M, et al. Incidence, risk factors, and outcomes of acute kidney injury after pediatric cardiac surgery–a prospective multicenter study. Crit Care Med. 2011;39(6):1493.
2. Morgan CJ, Zappitelli M, Robertson CM, et al. Risk factors for and outcomes of acute kidney injury in neonates undergoing complex cardiac surgery. J Pediatr. 2013;162(1):120–7.e1.
3. Kaddourah A, Basu RK, Bagshaw SM, Goldstein SL. Epidemiology of acute kidney injury in critically ill children and young adults. N Engl J Med. 2017;376(1):11–20.
4. Blinder JJ, Goldstein SL, Lee V-V, et al. Congenital heart surgery in infants: effects of acute kidney injury on outcomes. J Thorac Cardiovasc Surg. 2012;143(2):368–74.
5. Zappitelli M, Bernier P-L, Saczkowski RS, et al. A small post-operative rise in serum creatinine predicts acute kidney injury in children undergoing cardiac surgery. Kidney Int. 2009;76(8):885–92.
6. Hassinger AB, Wald EL, Goodman DM. Early postoperative fluid overload precedes acute kidney injury and is associated with higher morbidity in pediatric cardiac surgery patients. Pediatr Crit Care Med. 2014;15(2):131–8.
7. Seguin J, Albright B, Vertullo L, et al. Extent, risk factors, and outcome of fluid overload after pediatric heart surgery*. Crit Care Med. 2014;42(12):2591–9.
8. Jefferies JL, Devarajan P. Early detection of acute kidney injury after pediatric cardiac surgery. Prog Pediatr Cardiol. 2016;41:9–16.
9. Dupont M, Mullens W, Tang WH. Impact of systemic venous congestion in heart failure. Curr Heart Fail Rep. 2011;8(4):233–41.
10. Holdsworth SR, Gan PY. Cytokines: names and numbers you should care about. Clin J Am Soc Nephrol. 2015;10(12):2243–54.
11. Axelrod DM, Sutherland SM. Acute kidney injury in the pediatric cardiac patient. Paediatr Anaesth. 2014;24(9):899–901.
12. Devarajan P. Update on mechanisms of ischemic acute kidney injury. J Am Soc Nephrol. 2006;17(6):1503–20.
13. Thiele RH, Isbell JM, Rosner MH. AKI associated with cardiac surgery. Clin J Am Soc Nephrol. 2015;10(3):500–14.
14. Devarajan P. Cellular and molecular derangements in acute tubular necrosis. Curr Opin Pediatr. 2005;17(2):193–9.
15. Parekh DJ, Weinberg JM, Ercole B, et al. Tolerance of the human kidney to isolated controlled ischemia. J Am Soc Nephrol. 2013;24(3):506–17.

16. Watkins SC, Williamson K, Davidson M, Donahue BS. Long-term mortality associated with acute kidney injury in children following congenital cardiac surgery. Paediatr Anaesth. 2014;24(9):919–26.
17. Medar SS, Hsu DT, Lamour JM, Aydin SI. Acute kidney injury in pediatric acute decompensated heart failure. Pediatr Crit Care Med. 2015;16(6):535–41.
18. Price JF, Mott AR, Dickerson HA, et al. Worsening renal function in children hospitalized with decompensated heart failure: evidence for a pediatric cardiorenal syndrome? Pediatr Crit Care Med. 2008;9(3):279–84.
19. Rajagopal SK, Yarlagadda VV, Thiagarajan RR, et al. Pediatric heart failure and worsening renal function: association with outcomes after heart transplantation. J Heart Lung Transplant. 2012;31(3):252–8.
20. Cohen SB, Ginde S, Bartz PJ, Earing MG. Extracardiac complications in adults with congenital heart disease. Congenit Heart Dis. 2013;8(5):370–80.
21. Kwiatkowski DM, Price E, Axelrod DM, et al. Incidence, risk factors, and outcomes of acute kidney injury in adults undergoing surgery for congenital heart disease. Cardiol Young. 2016;27(6):1068–75.
22. Dimopoulos K, Diller GP, Koltsida E, et al. Prevalence, predictors, and prognostic value of renal dysfunction in adults with congenital heart disease. Circulation. 2008;117(18):2320–8.
23. Buelow MW, Dall A, Bartz PJ, et al. Renal dysfunction is common among adults after palliation for previous tetralogy of Fallot. Pediatr Cardiol. 2013;34(1):165–9.
24. Parolari A, Pesce LL, Pacini D, et al. Risk factors for perioperative acute kidney injury after adult cardiac surgery: role of perioperative management. Ann Thorac Surg. 2012;93(2):584–91.
25. Algaze CA, Koth AM, Faberowski LW, et al. Acute kidney injury in patients undergoing the Extracardiac Fontan operation with and without the use of cardiopulmonary bypass. Pediatr Crit Care Med. 2017;18(1):34–43.
26. Stafford-Smith M, Podgoreanu M, Swaminathan M, et al. Association of genetic polymorphisms with risk of renal injury after coronary bypass graft surgery. Am J Kidney Dis. 2005;45(3):519–30.
27. Cardinal-Fernández P, Ferruelo A, Martín-Pellicer A, et al. Genetic determinants of acute renal damage risk and prognosis: a systematic review. Med Intensiva (English Edition). 2012;36(9):626–33.
28. Sampath S, Moran JL, Graham PL, et al. The efficacy of loop diuretics in acute renal failure: assessment using Bayesian evidence synthesis techniques. Crit Care Med. 2007;35(11):2516–24.
29. Ricci Z, Haiberger R, Pezzella C, et al. Furosemide versus ethacrynic acid in pediatric patients undergoing cardiac surgery: a randomized controlled trial. Crit Care. 2015;19:2.
30. Naik SK, Knight A, Elliott M. A prospective randomized study of a modified technique of ultrafiltration during pediatric open-heart surgery. Circulation. 1991;84(5 Suppl):III422–31.
31. Davies MJ, Nguyen K, Gaynor JW, Elliott MJ. Modified ultrafiltration improves left ventricular systolic function in infants after cardiopulmonary bypass. J Thorac Cardiovasc Surg. 1998;115(2):361–9. discussion 9–70
32. Haase M, Bellomo R, Story D, et al. Effect of mean arterial pressure, haemoglobin and blood transfusion during cardiopulmonary bypass on post-operative acute kidney injury. Nephrol Dial Transplant. 2012;27(1):153–60.
33. Bojan M, Gioanni S, Vouhé PR, et al. Early initiation of peritoneal dialysis in neonates and infants with acute kidney injury following cardiac surgery is associated with a significant decrease in mortality. Kidney Int. 2012;82(4):474–81.
34. Kwiatkowski DM, Menon S, Krawczeski CD, et al. Improved outcomes with peritoneal dialysis catheter placement after cardiopulmonary bypass in infants. J Thorac Cardiovasc Surg. 2015;149(1):230–6.
35. Kwiatkowski DM, Goldstein SL, Cooper DS, et al. Peritoneal dialysis vs furosemide for prevention of fluid overload in infants after cardiac surgery: a randomized clinical trial. JAMA Pediatr. 2017;171(4):357–64.

36. Ronco C, Ricci Z, Goldstein SL. (R)evolution in the Management of Acute Kidney Injury in newborns. Am J Kidney Dis. 2015;66(2):206–11.
37. Kellum JA. Use of dopamine in acute renal failure: a meta-analysis. Crit Care Med. 2001;29(8):1526–31.
38. Ricci Z, Luciano R, Favia I, et al. High-dose fenoldopam reduces postoperative neutrophil gelatinase-associated lipocaline and cystatin C levels in pediatric cardiac surgery. Crit Care. 2011;15(3):R160.
39. Axelrod DM, Sutherland SM, Anglemyer A, et al. A double-blinded, randomized, placebo-controlled clinical trial of aminophylline to prevent acute kidney injury in children following congenital heart surgery with cardiopulmonary bypass. Pediatr Crit Care Med. 2016;17(2):135–43.
40. Kwiatkowski DM, Axelrod DM, Sutherland SM, et al. Dexmedetomidine is associated with lower incidence of acute kidney injury after congenital heart surgery. Pediatr Crit Care Med. 2016;17(2):128–34.
41. Costello JM, Thiagarajan RR, Dionne RE, et al. Initial experience with fenoldopam after cardiac surgery in neonates with an insufficient response to conventional diuretics. Pediatr Crit Care Med. 2006;7(1):28–33.
42. Ejaz AA, Martin TD, Johnson RJ, et al. Prophylactic nesiritide does not prevent dialysis or all-cause mortality in patients undergoing high-risk cardiac surgery. J Thorac Cardiovasc Surg. 2009;138(4):959–64.
43. Graham EM, Atz AM, Butts RJ, et al. Standardized preoperative corticosteroid treatment in neonates undergoing cardiac surgery: results from a randomized trial. J Thorac Cardiovasc Surg. 2011;142(6):1523–9.
44. Aiyagari R, Gelehrter S, Bove EL, et al. Effects of N-acetylcysteine on renal dysfunction in neonates undergoing the arterial switch operation. J Thorac Cardiovasc Surg. 2010;139(4):956–61.
45. Bronicki RA, Domico M, Checchia PA, et al. The use of Nesiritide in children with congenital heart disease. Pediatr Crit Care Med. 2017;18:151–8.
46. Jo YY, Kim JY, Lee JY, et al. The effect of intraoperative dexmedetomidine on acute kidney injury after pediatric congenital heart surgery: a prospective randomized trial. Medicine (Baltimore). 2017;96(28):e7480.
47. Kelly AM, Dwamena B, Cronin P, et al. Meta-analysis: effectiveness of drugs for preventing contrast-induced nephropathy. Ann Intern Med. 2008;148(4):284–94.
48. McLaughlin GE, Abitbol CL. Reversal of oliguric tacrolimus nephrotoxicity in children. Nephrol Dial Transplant. 2005;20(7):1471–5.
49. Lassnigg A, Schmid ER, Hiesmayr M, et al. Impact of minimal increases in serum creatinine on outcome in patients after cardiothoracic surgery: do we have to revise current definitions of acute renal failure? Crit Care Med. 2008;36(4):1129–37.
50. Askenazi D, Feig D, Graham N, et al. 3–5 year longitudinal follow-up of pediatric patients after acute renal failure. Kidney Int. 2006;69(1):184–9.
51. Lo LJ, Go AS, Chertow GM, et al. Dialysis-requiring acute renal failure increases the risk of progressive chronic kidney disease. Kidney Int. 2009;76(8):893–9.
52. Ishani A, Nelson D, Clothier B, et al. The magnitude of acute serum creatinine increase after cardiac surgery and the risk of chronic kidney disease, progression of kidney disease, and death. Arch Intern Med. 2011;171(3):226–33.
53. Coca SG, Yusuf B, Shlipak MG, et al. Long-term risk of mortality and other adverse outcomes after acute kidney injury: a systematic review and meta-analysis. Am J Kidney Dis. 2009;53(6):961–73.
54. Mammen C, Al Abbas A, Skippen P, et al. Long-term risk of CKD in children surviving episodes of acute kidney injury in the intensive care unit: a prospective cohort study. Am J Kidney Dis. 2012;59(4):523–30.
55. Wong JH, Selewski DT, Yu S, et al. Severe acute kidney injury following stage 1 Norwood palliation: effect on outcomes and risk of severe acute kidney injury at subsequent surgical stages. Pediatr Crit Care Med. 2016;17(7):615–23.

56. Cooper DS, Claes D, Goldstein SL, et al. Follow-up renal assessment of injury long-term after acute kidney injury (FRAIL-AKI). Clin J Am Soc Nephrol. 2016;11(1):21–9.
57. Ronco C, Haapio M, House A, et al. Cardiorenal syndrome. J Am Coll Cardiol. 2008;52:1527–39.
58. Legrand M, Mebazaa A, Ronco C, et al. When cardiac failure, kidney dysfunction, and kidney injury intersect in acute conditions: the case of Cardiorenal syndrome. Crit Care Med. 2014;42:2109–17.
59. Krumholtz HM, Chen YT, Vaccarino V, et al. Correlates and impact on outcomes of worsening renal function in patients ≥65 years of age with heart failure. Am J Cardiol. 2000;85:1110–3.
60. Smith GL, Vaccarino V, Kosiborod M, et al. Worsening renal function: what is a clinically meaningful change in creatinine during hospitalization with heart failure? J Card Fail. 2003;9:13–25.
61. Dries DL, Exner DV, Domanski MJ, et al. The prognostic implications of renal insufficiency in asymptomatic and symptomatic patients with left ventricular systolic dysfunction. J Am Coll Cardiol. 2000;35:681–9.
62. Bibbins-Domingo K, Lin F, Vittinghoff E, et al. Renal insufficiency as an independent predictor of mortality among women with heart failure. J Am Coll Cardiol. 2004;44:1593–600.
63. McAlister FA, Ezekowitz J, Tonelli M, et al. Renal insufficiency and heart failure: prognostic and therapeautic implications from a prospective cohort study. Circulation. 2004;109:1004–9.
64. May LJ, Montez-Rath ME, Yeh J, et al. Impact of ventricular assist device placement on longitudinal renal function in children with end-stage heart failure. J Heart Lung Transplant. 2016;35:449–56.
65. Starnes V, Bernstein D, Oyer P, et al. Heart transplantation in children. J Heart Transplant. 1989;8:20–6.
66. Pradhan M, Leonard MB, Bridges ND, et al. Decline in renal function following thoracic organ transplantation in children. Am J Transplant. 2002;2:652–7.
67. Heywood JT. The cardiorenal syndrome: lessons from the ADHERE database and treatment options. Heart Fail Rev. 2004;9:195–201.
68. Cagli K, Ulas MM, Ozisik K, et al. The intraoperative effect of pentoxifylline on the inflammatory process and leukocytes in cardiac surgery patients undergoing cardiopulmonary bypass. Perfusion. 2005;20(1):45–51.

# Acute Kidney Injury in Stem Cell Transplant Recipients

# 8

Daniella Levy-Erez, Sangeeta Hingorani, and Benjamin Laskin

**Case Vignette**

A 7-year-old boy with a history of severe aplastic anemia received a stem cell transplant from an unrelated donor 2 months ago. Prior to transplant, his aplastic anemia was treated with 2 years of cyclosporine. He received transplant conditioning with fludarabine, cyclophosphamide, and antithymocyte globulin. His posttransplant course has been notable for graft-versus-host disease of the skin, requiring tacrolimus and oral corticosteroid treatment. He continues on acyclovir prophylaxis, but has not received any recent treatment course antibiotics. He has now developed acute kidney injury, with a serum creatinine of 1.3 mg/dL, increased over the past week from his baseline serum creatinine of 0.6 mg/dL. He maintains good urine output, has a blood pressure of 128/85 mm Hg, and has developed proteinuria but no hematuria. His complete blood count is notable for persistent anemia and thrombocytopenia that has gradually improved since transplant. An ultrasound shows echogenic and slightly enlarged kidneys without hydronephrosis and a normal bladder. Over the course of the following week, his blood pressure worsens, serum creatinine rises to 2.1 mg/dL, and he requires transfer to the intensive care unit for hypertension management.

D. Levy-Erez · B. Laskin (✉)
Division of Nephrology, The Children's Hospital of Philadelphia, Philadelphia, PA, USA
e-mail: laskinb@email.chop.edu

S. Hingorani
Division of Nephrology, Seattle Children's Hospital, Seattle, WA, USA



A. Deep, S. L. Goldstein (eds.), *Critical Care Nephrology and Renal Replacement Therapy in Children*, https://doi.org/10.1007/978-3-319-90281-4_8

## 8.1 Introduction

Although hematopoietic cell transplantation (HCT) treats life-threatening disorders in children, the transplant process is associated with very high rates of morbidity affecting multiple organ systems [1–3]. Outcomes for patients treated with HCT, including mortality rates, have improved in recent years, but the risk of death from relapse of primary disease or transplant-related complications remains high [4].

The kidney is commonly affected in children and adults who have received an HCT [1, 2, 5]. In adults, acute kidney injury (AKI) occurs frequently [6–8]. Less data are available regarding the incidence of AKI in children after HCT, although the risks are likely comparable. The causes of AKI among this unique population are often multifactorial and depend on the timing of kidney injury in relation to the transplant; AKI may occur during conditioning, before or after engraftment, or even years later [1, 9]. Patients can be susceptible to developing AKI from preexisting kidney disease or secondary to the complex treatments and side effects that occur as a result of the HCT process.

Patients undergoing HCT are exposed to multiple potential nephrotoxins including chemotherapy and radiation used for conditioning, antimicrobials to prevent or treat infections, and calcineurin inhibitors and other medications to prevent or treat graft-versus-host disease (GVHD) [10, 11]. Additional causes of AKI include sepsis leading to hemodynamic instability, resulting in acute tubular necrosis (ATN). Endothelial injury causing sinusoidal obstruction syndrome (SOS) or thrombotic microangiopathy (TMA) are other significant mechanisms for AKI after HCT [3, 12].

While targeted therapies for AKI are limited, management includes close attention to fluid and electrolyte balance and the correct dosing of medications. Severe volume overload or dangerous electrolyte abnormalities may necessitate renal replacement therapy, which itself has been associated with very high mortality rates after HCT [13–15]. We review the most current data on the risk of AKI in children after HCT, the presumed causes, and the approach to diagnosing and managing these complex patients.

## 8.2 Epidemiology of AKI in Children After HCT

AKI occurs commonly in adults undergoing HCT. Among 147 mostly adults followed prospectively, Hingorani found that 36% of patients had a doubling of their baseline serum creatinine by a median of 33 days after transplant, and risk factors for AKI included amphotericin and SOS [10]. Kersting retrospectively analyzed 363 adult patients after allogeneic myeloablative HCT and found that half had severe AKI [16]. In one of the largest studies to date, Gooley analyzed over 2500 patients receiving their first allogeneic HCT from 1993 to 2007 and found that over 33% of patients doubled their creatinine in the first 100 days and >5% of patients needed acute dialysis [4].

There are fewer data regarding the risk of AKI in children after HCT. Raina reviewed four studies describing the risk of AKI in 237 children from 1992 to 2008 [9]. The incidence of AKI was 17–29% within the first 100 days after transplant, with 2% of patients needing acute dialysis. Risk factors for AKI were cyclosporine, foscarnet, SOS, sepsis, GVHD, gentamicin, and amphotericin. A separate systematic review by Didsbury including some but not all of the studies described by Raina, summarized 5 studies of 571 total children undergoing HCT [1].The reported risk of AKI varied from 9.6 to 42% in these studies, and only 14 patients received dialysis.

Two studies from the University of Minnesota have identified the prevalence of AKI in a large cohort of children after HCT. Rajpal examined 1431 patients <21 years of age receiving HCT from 1990 to 2009 and focused on those needing dialysis in the first 100 days after transplant [17]. About 10% of patients required acute dialysis, with only 23% surviving to 1 year in the most recent era (2000–2009) (Fig. 8.1). In a more recent study from the same center, AKI was identified using the pRIFLE criteria in 205 consecutive patients. Over 80% of patients were found to have AKI in the first 100 days after transplant, and mortality was increased with

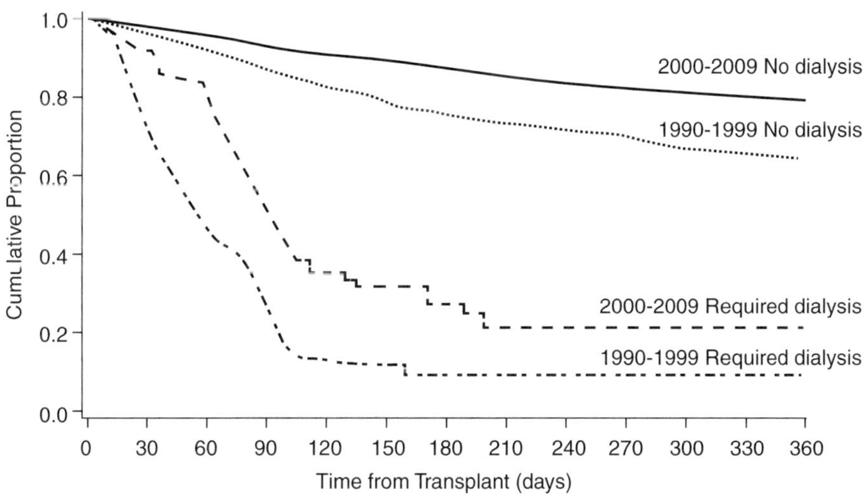


**Fig. 8.1** Overall survival for children receiving hematopoietic cell transplantation by era and need for acute dialysis. Overall, 1-year survival among 1305 children and adolescents who did not need dialysis in the first 100 days after hematopoietic cell transplant, as compared to 122 children and adolescents needing acute dialysis, at the University of Minnesota from 1990 to 2009. While survival improved over time for both groups of patients, those requiring dialysis had markedly higher mortality, with survival rates <25%. Above figure originally published in Rajpal JS, Patel N, Vogel RI, Kashtan CE, Smith AR. Improved survival over the last decade in pediatric patients requiring dialysis after hematopoietic cell transplantation. Biol Blood Marrow Transplant. 2013 Apr;19 (4):661–5. doi: https://doi.org/10.1016/j.bbmt.2012.12.012. Copyright 2013 American Society for Blood and Marrow Transplantation, published by Elsevier Inc. Used with permission under the Creative Commons Attribution-Non-Commercial-No Derivatives License (CC BY NC ND)

greater severity of AKI [18]. In summary, these studies suggest that AKI is common in children after HCT, survival is poor for those needing dialysis, and risk factors and incidences vary on the population studied.

## 8.3 Evaluation of the Child with AKI After HCT

The evaluation of a child with AKI after HCT includes a careful review of the medical history, current and past medication exposures, a physical exam focused on the patient's volume status (including attention to the heart rate, blood pressure, and weight trends), and laboratory and radiological examinations.

### 8.3.1 Urinalysis

Hematuria is common in HCT recipients and typically indicates a lower urinary tract process such as hemorrhagic cystitis, either from viral infection or medications, which can lead to AKI if obstruction is present. Hematuria could also suggest acute viral damage to the bladder and kidney, as reported for adenovirus after cord blood transplant [19]. Hematuria may indicate an acute glomerulonephritis, which is much less common after HCT. Micro- or macroalbuminuria can also signify glomerular involvement, either from acute glomerulonephritis, tubulointerstitial inflammation, or TMA. Macroalbuminuria should be assessed in the context of the urine specific gravity, as dilute urine may be falsely negative for proteinuria. Measuring the spot urine albumin to creatinine ratio can be helpful in these situations. A low specific gravity can be seen in patients with drug-induced interstitial nephritis whereas a very concentrated urine could point to volume depletion as a cause for AKI. However, a low urine specific gravity is common after HCT due simply to the large amount of intravenous fluids patients receive.

### 8.3.2 Blood Work

Reviewing the patient's baseline serum creatinine, both before HCT and before the episode of AKI, is important. Those with decreased kidney function prior to transplant may be at greater risk for posttransplant AKI [10]. While the changes in serum creatinine and urine output define AKI, creatinine has limitations, especially in the HCT population. Creatinine measurements are influenced by fluid status and volume overload can dilute the serum creatinine and underestimate the risk of AKI [20]. Creatinine measurements are also influenced by muscle mass, which can be altered in HCT recipients from corticosteroid use, poor nutrition, chronic inflammation, and prolonged admissions to the hospital [21]. Newer markers of kidney function such as cystatin C are increasingly being utilized in clinical care, although cystatin C-based definitions of AKI are not yet available. Cystatin C levels are also increased in patients receiving corticosteroids, so this may not be a reliable marker of kidney function in this situation.

### 8.3.3 Imaging

A renal/bladder ultrasound can provide valuable information on the size and echogenicity of the kidneys, presence of obstruction, or bladder pathology. The kidneys can be enlarged with acute interstitial nephritis, and can have loss of corticomedullary differentiation and altered echogenicity with almost any type of renal injury, and demonstrate hydronephrosis in the presence of obstruction. Renal enlargement is common in children after HCT and should not necessarily prompt further evaluation in the absence of other markers of kidney disease. Chapman examined 450 renal ultrasounds from 101 children receiving HCT from 2006 to 2010 and found transient renal enlargement in the first 90 days after transplant which later resolved [22]. If the differential of AKI includes SOS, attention to the abdominal ultrasound and vascular flow to the liver is also important [23].

### 8.3.4 Kidney Biopsy

A kidney biopsy may be helpful in determining the cause of AKI in children after HCT. Due to the risk of bleeding from low platelets and elevated blood pressures, both of which are common after HCT, a kidney biopsy can be high-risk in the acute setting and the benefits of diagnosis must be carefully weighed against these risks [24]. Nevertheless, in the appropriate clinical setting, a kidney biopsy may be needed to diagnose TMA if the laboratory findings are not typical, or in patients with concern for interstitial nephritis whose creatinine does not improve after removal of potentially causative agents, or in those with nephrotic syndrome or acute glomerulonephritis [11]. Specific clinical situations in which a biopsy may be useful are discussed in more detail in the following sections.

## 8.4 Contribution of the HCT Procedure to the Risk of AKI

Depending on the patient's primary disease, donor type, and source of cells, different conditioning regimens are used to treat children undergoing HCT, each with different associated risk factors for the development of AKI (Table 8.1). Autologous HCT involves harvesting a patient's peripheral stem cells, using myeloablative chemotherapy to treat the underlying malignancy, and then reinfusing collected stem cells to allow for hematopoiesis. Importantly, patients do not require potentially nephrotoxic GVHD prophylaxis because they receive their own cells. Nevertheless, children undergoing autologous HCT, especially those with high-risk neuroblastoma, remain at very high risk for developing AKI. The mechanisms of AKI in patients treated for neuroblastoma are not completely understood but likely involve a combination of decreased renal reserve in those requiring partial or total nephrectomy and endothelial injury from abdominal radiation and the use of cis-retinoic acid for treatment [25].

**Table 8.1** Types of hematopoietic cell transplant procedures and associated exposures and complications [57]

| Conditioning | Donor | Potential exposure to radiation | Exposure to calcineurin inhibitors | Risk of acute graft-versus-host disease | Risk of infection and sepsis | Risk of thrombotic microangiopathy | Risk of sinusoidal obstruction syndrome |
|---|---|---|---|---|---|---|---|
| Myeloablative | Allogeneic | Yes | Yes | Yes | Yes | Yes | Yes |
| | Autologous | Yes | No | No | Lower | Yes | Yes |
| Reduced intensity | Allogeneic | No | Yes | Yes | Yes | Yes | Less common |

Allogeneic HCT treats patients with malignancies affecting hematopoietic cells or those with immune deficiencies and other genetic conditions where replacement of dysfunctional stem cells can be corrected by donor cells. Allogeneic HCT involves a process of preconditioning with myeloablative chemotherapy and/or radiation or reduced intensity regimens that are non-myeloablative. Patients are admitted to the hospital days to weeks before the infusion of donor stem cells in order to receive the conditioning regimen. Donor cells can derive from human-leukocyte antigen (HLA) matched-related family members (typically siblings), haplotype donors (such as parents), or unrelated persons. The stem cells are obtained from bone marrow aspirate, peripheral blood harvest after mobilization, or stored cord blood.

Total body radiation and many of the chemotherapeutic agents used for conditioning can lead to AKI. Nephrotoxic chemotherapy includes platinum agents and ifosfamide. High-dose etoposide phosphate was associated with a 57% incidence of AKI in 21 children receiving HCT for lymphoblastic leukemia [26]. After stem cell infusion (known as day zero in the transplant process), patients are significantly immunocompromised and therefore require frequent doses of nephrotoxic antimicrobials including vancomycin, piperacillin/tazobactam, and aminoglycosides. Infectious prophylaxis causes further nephrotoxin exposure due to the need to protect against viruses, bacteria, and fungi. Those requiring treatment for infection may need to receive additional nephrotoxic medications including cidofovir, foscarnet, and amphotericin [27].

Finally, patients receiving an allogeneic transplant must be prescribed medications to prevent GVHD [28]. Medications used for the prevention and treatment of GVHD, including methotrexate and calcineurin inhibitors, are associated with AKI after HCT and careful attention to drug levels is therefore important. Although calcineurin inhibitors cause acute decreases in renal blood flow and can lead to AKI, especially in patients with volume depletion, studies after HCT have not found a significant association between the dose or trough levels of calcineurin inhibitors and the risk of AKI [3].

In summary, patients undergoing HCT are exposed to multiple nephrotoxins during the transplant process including chemotherapy, radiation, antimicrobials, and GVHD prophylaxis (Table 8.2). In patients developing AKI, it is common to dose-adjust or even withhold these essential medications. This potentially has important consequences on patient outcomes, including survival, if, for example, chemotherapy (i.e., cis-retinoic acid in neuroblastoma) or calcineurin inhibitors (i.e., impacting the course of GVHD) are discontinued due to renal dysfunction. In these cases, it is important to balance the risks to the kidney against the potential benefit to patient survival to guide individual treatment decisions.

## 8.5 Contribution of Transplant Complications to the Risk of AKI After HCT

Children undergoing HCT can develop AKI from many potential mechanisms, including transplant-related complications such as sepsis, hemorrhage, endothelial injury, or GVHD. These mechanisms can be divided into classic categories

**Table 8.2** Medications associated with acute kidney injury after hematopoietic cell transplant

| Medication | Presumed mechanisms of acute kidney injury | Additional renal adverse reactions |
|---|---|---|
| **Conditioning therapy** | | |
| Busulfan | Sinusoidal obstruction syndrome | Hypertension, edema, hypokalemia, hypophosphatemia, hypomagnesemia |
| Cyclophosphamide | Urine obstruction from hemorrhagic cystitis | Hematuria |
| Cisplatin/carboplatin | Tubular cell injury | Hypokalemia, hypophosphatemia, hypomagnesemia |
| Etoposide | | Metabolic acidosis |
| Ifosfamide | Proximal tubular injury | Metabolic acidosis, hypophosphatemia, nephrogenic diabetes insipidus |
| Melphalan | Sinusoidal obstruction syndrome | |
| **Antiviral agents** | | |
| Acyclovir/ganciclovir | Direct tubular toxicity/crystal production | |
| Cidofovir | Direct tubular toxicity | Proteinuria |
| Foscarnet | Crystallization in glomeruli | Proteinuria |
| **Antifungal agents** | | |
| Amphotericin | Tubular cell damage, renal vasoconstriction | Hypertension, hematuria, hypokalemia, hypomagnesemia, hypocalcemia, hyponatremia |
| Caspofungin | | Edema, hypokalemia |
| **Antibacterial** | | |
| Aminoglycosides | Direct tubular toxicity | Hypomagnesemia, hypokalemia, hypocalcemia, hyponatremia, proteinuria |
| Vancomycin | Inflammation, mitochondrial dysfunction and cellular apoptosis | Hyperkalemia |
| Trimethoprim-sulfamethoxazole | Interstitial nephritis | Hyperkalemia, proteinuria |
| Piperacillin-tazobactam | Interstitial nephritis | |
| **GVHD prophylaxis** | | |
| Calcineurin inhibitors | Arteriolar vasoconstriction, endothelial injury | Hypertension, hyperkalemia, hypokalemia, metabolic acidosis, hypomagnesemia |
| Methotrexate | Tubular precipitation | Hyperuricemia |
| **Other** | | |
| Contrast | Vasoconstriction, direct tubular toxicity | |

**Table 8.3** Potential risk factors, mechanisms, and locations of injury for patients with acute kidney injury after hematopoietic cell transplant [3]

| Mechanism/histological location of kidney injury | |
|---|---|
| Intravascular volume depletion | Vomiting and diarrhea with or without associated acute gastrointestinal graft-versus-host disease<br>Decreased intake from mucositis |
| Systemic vasodilation | Sepsis |
| Renal arteriolar vasoconstriction | Sinusoidal obstruction syndrome<br>Calcineurin inhibitors |
| Endothelial injury to glomerulus or other small vessels | Thrombotic microangiopathy<br>Calcineurin inhibitors<br>Sinusoidal obstruction syndrome<br>Acute graft-versus-host disease<br>Total body radiation |
| Tubular injury | Medications including conditioning chemotherapy, amphotericin, antiviral, additional antimicrobials such as vancomycin and aminoglycosides |
| Obstruction to urine flow | Hemorrhagic cystitis with clots from viral infections (BK virus or adenovirus) or medications such as cyclophosphamide |

including prerenal, intrinsic renal, and post-renal causes and can also be categorized by mechanisms and location of injury (Table 8.3).

### 8.5.1 Prerenal Injury

Volume depletion is common after HCT related to poor intake from chemotherapy and mucositis-related complications, diarrhea from infectious causes or GVHD, and hemorrhage from thrombocytopenia or GVHD-related gastrointestinal bleeding [2, 9]. Careful attention to a patient's weight is important to assess prerenal azotemia. Inpatient, many children are treated with intravenous fluids, which can make volume depletion less of a concern. However, among patients admitted from outpatient care after HCT, acute gastrointestinal or other volume depleting illnesses can be a common cause of AKI in this population, especially among those taking concomitant calcineurin inhibitors.

### 8.5.2 Intrinsic Renal Injury

Direct injury to the renal parenchyma can be caused by prolonged hypoperfusion leading to ATN, nephrotoxic medications, or inflammation/endothelial damage. Intrinsic renal damage can occur to the glomeruli, the endothelial cells of other small vessels, the tubular epithelium, or the interstitium. ATN is common after HCT from decreased renal perfusion resulting in ischemia or nephrotoxic injury from medications. Sepsis and the resulting hypotension from distributive shock can occur frequently in children after HCT and typically requires further exposure to nephrotoxic antibiotics, large volume fluid resuscitation, and vasoactive medications to support tissue perfusion. These patients often develop decreased urine output after the injury [1, 2]. Acute interstitial nephritis is an acute inflammatory process involving the interstitial space of the kidney which can be due to a wide variety of medications, especially antibiotics or to an underlying infection, such as viral infection after HCT, and possibly result from GVHD, as discussed below. Patients with interstitial nephritis typically maintain normal urine output, although may develop an abnormal ability to concentrate the urine and the resulting polyuria can lead to further AKI from dehydration. Infections directly affecting the kidney as a cause of AKI are less common after HCT, but can occur in patients with acute pyelonephritis. Several viral infections such as adenovirus and CMV may also cause direct renal injury, while others such as BK virus cause chronic nephropathy [29, 30].

Sinusoidal obstruction syndrome (SOS), previously known as veno-occlusive disease of the liver, occurs in about 10% of recipients, and in severe cases, is associated with >90% mortality [23, 31]. Liver injury is from toxic agents used during conditioning such as busulfan, cyclophosphamide, or melphalan. SOS typically occurs early after transplantation. Patients with SOS can develop AKI from endothelial injury or a clinical picture similar to hepatorenal syndrome with accompanying volume overload and third spacing of intravascular fluid. Treatment includes close attention to fluid status to avoid volume overload and defibrotide, a drug with antithrombotic and anti-inflammatory properties that has been approved for the treatment of SOS with concomitant renal or pulmonary disease and may also be useful to prevent the disease [32]. Some have advocated early placement of peritoneal dialysis catheters to drain ascites and prevent fluid overload and subsequent AKI from abdominal compartment syndrome in children with SOS [31]. Others have added high-dose steroids to defibrotide treatment with good response rates [33].

Thrombotic microangiopathy (TMA), like SOS, is associated with endothelial injury and is a cause of AKI after HCT. TMA is a histological diagnosis which, after HCT, may be secondary to medications, infections, conditioning therapy, inflammation, or GVHD. Endothelial cell injury initiates a cascade of events leading to microangiopathic hemolytic anemia, thrombocytopenia, and subsequent vessel damage leading to end-organ dysfunction. For unclear reasons, the kidney is most commonly affected in patients with TMA after HCT, although histological findings and clinical disease can also be found in the lung (pulmonary hypertension), bowel (gastrointestinal bleeding often difficult to distinguish clinically from GVHD), heart (pericardial effusion), and brain (seizures and altered mental status) [34]. TMA after HCT has typically been reported in children with malignancies, immune deficiencies, or bone marrow failure syndromes, but is increasingly being noted in other conditions requiring HCT, such as hemoglobinopathies, possibly from pretransplant endothelial dysfunction related to the underlying disease [35].

Evidence suggests that complement dysregulation may be involved in the pathogenesis of TMA after HCT, similar to what occurs in patients with inherited complement abnormalities with atypical hemolytic uremic syndrome. Children developing AKI with evidence of TMA can have abnormalities in the alternative pathway of complement including factor H autoantibodies and deletions in factor H related genes [36], signs of classical pathway activation with C4d deposition on kidney biopsy [37], and mutations in complement genes previously identified in patients with atypical hemolytic uremic syndrome [38]. Conversely, markers of coagulation activation including plasminogen activator inhibitor (PAI-1) and tissue plasminogen activator have not been associated with AKI after HCT [39]. The diagnosis of TMA as a cause of AKI in children undergoing HCT requires a high index of suspicion because anemia and thrombocytopenia are common. In patients with unexplained AKI, hypertension, or proteinuria, a lactic dehydrogenase, haptoglobin, and peripheral smear for schistocytes should be checked. Those with severe AKI and laboratory findings of TMA should be assessed for evidence of complement activation by measuring C3, C4, a CH50/AH50 level, and the soluble membrane attack complex (sC5b-9), which may justify using the complement inhibitor eculizumab [40]. HCT recipients with severe AKI and TMA, especially those with gastrointestinal bleeding, may require higher and more frequent doses of eculizumab than is currently prescribed for patients with atypical hemolytic uremic syndrome. In such situations, the frequency of dosing with eculizumab can be adjusted by measuring CH50 levels to assess for complement blockade (low levels associated with successful blockade) [12, 40]. Although eculizumab is associated with improved response rates in children with AKI and TMA after HCT compared to historical controls, its impact on long-term survival is less clear, and clinical trials are needed to determine exactly which patients may benefit from therapy and the optimal duration of treatment [41].

GVHD is one of the most common complications of HCT and classically involves epithelial cell injury to the skin or gastrointestinal tract. Increasing evidence suggests that the kidney may also be a target of GVHD, either through epithelial or endothelial damage. In fact, TMA may represent a form of "endothelial GVHD." A study of 103 consecutive children receiving an allogeneic HCT found that elevated levels of double-stranded DNA, an extracellular marker of neutrophil and complement activation, were apparent by 2 weeks after transplant and predicted later TMA. Increased double-stranded DNA levels in the first 3 months after transplant were associated with GVHD [42]. In one of the largest histological studies to date, Changsirikulchai evaluated 314 autopsy specimens from patients who died after HCT from 1992 to 1999 and found that TMA was associated with higher grade acute GVHD [11]. However, in their study of 147 mostly adults after HCT, Hingorani et al. did not find that acute GVHD or cyclosporine levels were associated with AKI [10]. A more recent analysis included 205 mostly adults receiving transplant from 2003 to 2010 to test the association between urinary elafin, a known marker for skin GVHD, and kidney disease in the first year after transplant [43]. Urinary elafin levels were associated with an increased risk of proteinuria (both microalbuminuria and macroalbuminuria), AKI, later CKD, and death. Those with proteinuria also had a higher risk of GVHD, confirming previous observations from the same group [44]. Interestingly, kidney biopsy specimens also showed staining for elafin, supporting the hypothesis that GVHD affects the kidney. An increase in inflammatory cytokines including urinary interleukin-6, interleukin-15, and MCP-1 was also associated with proteinuria in a cohort including primarily adults after HCT [45]. In summary, recent data suggests that the kidney can be a target of GVHD, either alone or in combination with TMA. More research is needed to determine the exact mechanisms and how to best tailor treatment.

Finally, as mentioned, acute glomerulonephritis is an uncommon complication after HCT. Glomerular disease leading to nephrotic syndrome, with or without AKI, can occur after HCT and typically presents with findings of membranous nephropathy or minimal change disease on kidney biopsy, with case reports of membranoproliferative glomerulonephritis, focal segmental glomerulosclerosis, and IgA nephropathy. Therefore, biopsy should be considered in HCT recipients with nephrotic range proteinuria to help guide immunosuppressive treatment, especially if the renal findings are associated with acute GVHD [3]. Several of these case reports describing nephrotic syndrome developing after HCT have been in children [46–48].

### 8.5.3 Post-renal Injury

Urine obstruction is a reversible cause of AKI and can be identified by careful attention to the urine output and diagnosed radiographically by the presence of hydronephrosis on either abdominal ultrasonography or computed tomography. Hemorrhagic cystitis secondary to either medications such as cyclophosphamide or viral infection such as BK polyomavirus or adenovirus is common in HCT recipients, and when severe, can lead to obstruction and AKI [49, 50]. While detection of BK virus or adenovirus in the urine is a useful diagnostic test, the prognostic implications of viruria are less clear, given that viral shedding is very common after HCT, even in asymptomatic patients [29]. In a retrospective review of 221 children receiving allogeneic HCT over a 6-year period, BK viremia $\geq$10,000 copies/mL was associated with grade IV (severe) hemorrhagic cystitis requiring bladder catheterization or surgical intervention [51].

## 8.6 Management and Outcomes of Children Developing AKI After HCT

Children with AKI after HCT require collaboration from transplant providers, nephrologists, intensivists, infectious disease specialists, pharmacists, and dieticians. Initially, the treatment should focus on managing hypertension, correcting electrolyte derangements, monitoring, preventing, and treating volume overload, and addressing reversible causes of AKI such as obstruction and minimization of nephrotoxic agents [52], when feasible. The importance of close attention to daily weights, intake, and output cannot be overemphasized to prevent and detect volume overload early in the AKI course.

Renal replacement therapy may be needed to allow appropriate nutrition or if patients require frequent blood transfusions. Many children who develop severe AKI after HCT have multi-organ failure and are therefore best treated with continuous renal replacement therapy (CRRT). Michael et al. reported on their center's protocol to prevent and treat fluid overload in children after HCT [15]. Patients with AKI and >5% fluid overload were started on diuretic therapy and acute dialysis was started for those with >10% fluid overload. Among 272 transplant patients, 26 (10%) developed oliguric AKI, of whom 14 required dialysis, with only 4 (29%) surviving. Supporting the adverse consequences of fluid overload in this population, surviving patients were able to maintain <10% fluid overload, with either diuretic or dialysis therapy. A separate report from the prospective pediatric CRRT registry identified 51 children treated with CRRT after HCT, with >75% having multisystem organ failure [13]. Only 45% of patients survived and better survival was associated with using convective (hemofiltration) versus dialytic CRRT modalities and patients with respiratory failure had worse survival. While survival has improved over time for children requiring acute dialysis after HCT [17], mortality rates remain very high for this patient population [53, 54].

## 8.7 Conclusions and Future Directions

AKI is common in children undergoing HCT and associated with poor outcomes. While therapies such as eculizumab for TMA and defibrotide for SOS offer promise, more research is needed to understand the exact mechanisms of kidney injury for most children developing AKI after HCT. In recent years, novel structural biomarkers have allowed AKI to be detected earlier in the course of disease, prior to elevations in serum creatinine, potentially allowing a window for preventative or therapeutic strategies. Newer prediction models, such as the pediatric renal angina index, incorporate HCT as a risk factor for developing AKI, in addition to intensive care unit admission, need for mechanical ventilation or vasoactive support, change in estimated creatinine clearance and fluid overload, and elevations in biomarkers [55]. Animal models suggest that immune dysregulation may be involved in the pathogenesis of AKI outside the transplant setting, but limited data exists in humans [56]. Therefore, given the high incidence of AKI and the newly developing immune system, patients receiving HCT provide unique opportunities to better understand the mechanisms of injury and to test novel detection and treatment strategies, hopefully leading to better outcomes for both HCT recipients and for other patients with kidney injury.

**Key Learning Points**

- Acute kidney injury is common in children receiving a hematopoietic cell transplant and is associated with poor outcomes, especially among those needing acute dialysis.
- The evaluation of a child with acute kidney injury after hematopoietic cell transplant should include a comprehensive review of current and past medications, baseline kidney function, a physical examination focused on blood pressure and the patient's volume status, and laboratory and radiographic studies looking for evidence of infection, thrombotic microangiopathy, sinusoidal obstruction syndrome, and graft-versus-host disease, with consideration of renal biopsy as clinically indicated.

- Endothelial cell injury is common in children receiving hematopoietic cell transplant and can lead to acute kidney injury via graft-versus-host disease, thrombotic microangiopathy, or sinusoidal obstruction syndrome of the liver.
- Treatment of the child with acute kidney injury after hematopoietic cell transplant is typically supportive and involves correction of electrolyte abnormalities, close attention to fluid status to prevent volume overload, avoidance of nephrotoxic agents, when feasible, and consideration of targeted therapies such as eculizumab for thrombotic microangiopathy, defibrotide for sinusoidal obstruction syndrome, and urinary drainage for those with severe hemorrhagic cystitis.

## References

1. Didsbury MS, Mackie FE, Kennedy SE. A systematic review of acute kidney injury in pediatric allogeneic hematopoietic stem cell recipients. Pediatr Transplant. 2015;19(5):460–70.
2. DiCarlo J, Alexander SR. Acute kidney injury in pediatric stem cell transplant recipients. Semin Nephrol. 2008;28(5):481–7.
3. Hingorani S. Renal complications of hematopoietic-cell transplantation. N Engl J Med. 2016;374(23):2256–67.
4. Gooley TA, Chien JW, Pergam SA, Hingorani S, Sorror ML, Boeckh M, et al. Reduced mortality after allogeneic hematopoietic-cell transplantation. N Engl J Med. 2010;363(22):2091–101.
5. Ando M, Ohashi K, Akiyama H, Sakamaki H, Morito T, Tsuchiya K, et al. Chronic kidney disease in long-term survivors of myeloablative allogeneic haematopoietic cell transplantation: prevalence and risk factors. Nephrol Dial Transplant. 2010;25(1):278–82.
6. Lopes JA, Jorge S, Neves M. Acute kidney injury in HCT: an update. Bone Marrow Transplant. 2016;51(6):755–62.
7. Lopes JA, Jorge S, Silva S, de Almeida E, Abreu F, Martins C, et al. Acute renal failure following myeloablative autologous and allogeneic hematopoietic cell transplantation. Bone Marrow Transplant. 2006;38(10):707.
8. Krishnappa V, Gupta M, Manu G, Kwatra S, Owusu OT, Raina R. Acute kidney injury in hematopoietic stem cell transplantation: a review. Int J Nephrol. 2016;2016:5163789.
9. Raina R, Herrera N, Krishnappa V, Sethi SK, Deep A, Kao WM, Bunchman T, Abu-Arja R. Hematopoietic stem cell transplantation and acute kidney injury in children: a comprehensive review. Pediatr Nephrol. 2017;21(4):e12935.
10. Hingorani SR, Guthrie K, Batchelder A, Schoch G, Aboulhosn N, Manchion J, et al. Acute renal failure after myeloablative hematopoietic cell transplant: incidence and risk factors. Kidney Int. 2005;67(1):272–7.
11. Changsirikulchai S, Myerson D, Guthrie KA, McDonald GB, Alpers CE, Hingorani SR. Renal thrombotic microangiopathy after hematopoietic cell transplant: role of GVHD in pathogenesis. Clin J Am Soc Nephrol. 2009;4(2):345–53.
12. Jodele S, Dandoy CE, Myers KC, El-Bietar J, Nelson A, Wallace G, et al. New approaches in the diagnosis, pathophysiology, and treatment of pediatric hematopoietic stem cell transplantation-associated thrombotic microangiopathy. Transfus Apher Sci. 2016;54(2):181–90.
13. Flores FX, Brophy PD, Symons JM, Fortenberry JD, Chua AN, Alexander SR, et al. Continuous renal replacement therapy (CRRT) after stem cell transplantation. A report from the prospective pediatric CRRT registry group. Pediatr Nephrol. 2008;23(4):625–30.

14. Symons JM, Chua AN, Somers MJ, Baum MA, Bunchman TE, Benfield MR, et al. Demographic characteristics of pediatric continuous renal replacement therapy: a report of the prospective pediatric continuous renal replacement therapy registry. Clin J Am Soc Nephrol. 2007;2(4):732–8.
15. Michael M, Kuehnle I, Goldstein SL. Fluid overload and acute renal failure in pediatric stem cell transplant patients. Pediatr Nephrol. 2004;19(1):91–5.
16. Kersting S, Dorp SV, Theobald M, Verdonck LF. Acute renal failure after nonmyeloablative stem cell transplantation in adults. Biol Blood Marrow Transplant. 2008;14(1):125–31.
17. Rajpal JS, Patel N, Vogel RI, Kashtan CE, Smith AR. Improved survival over the last decade in pediatric patients requiring dialysis after hematopoietic cell transplantation. Biol Blood Marrow Transplant. 2013;19(4):661–5.
18. Kizilbash SJ, Kashtan CE, Chavers BM, Cao Q, Smith AR. Acute kidney injury and the risk of mortality in children undergoing hematopoietic stem cell transplantation. Biol Blood Marrow Transplant. 2016;22(7):1264–70.
19. Keddis M, Leung N, Herrmann S, El-Zoghby Z, Sethi S. Adenovirus-induced interstitial nephritis following umbilical cord blood transplant for chronic lymphocytic leukemia. Am J Kidney Dis. 2012;59(6):886–90.
20. Liu KD, Thompson BT, Ancukiewicz M, Steingrub JS, Douglas IS, Matthay MA, et al. Acute kidney injury in patients with acute lung injury: impact of fluid accumulation on classification of acute kidney injury and associated outcomes. Crit Care Med. 2011;39(12):2665–71.
21. Laskin BL, Nehus E, Goebel J, Furth S, Davies SM, Jodele S. Estimated versus measured glomerular filtration rate in children before hematopoietic cell transplantation. Biol Blood Marrow Transplant. 2014;20(12):2056–61.
22. Chapman T, Bodmer N, Benkeser DC, Hingorani SR, Parisi MT. Transient renal enlargement in pediatric hematopoietic cell transplant recipients. Pediatr Transplant. 2014;18(3):288–93.
23. Bajwa RPS, Mahadeo KM, Taragin BH, Dvorak CC, McArthur J, Jeyapalan A, et al. Consensus report by pediatric acute lung injury and Sepsis investigators and pediatric blood and marrow transplantation consortium joint working committees: supportive care guidelines for Management of Veno-Occlusive Disease in children and adolescents, part 1: focus on investigations, prophylaxis, and specific treatment. Biol Blood Marrow Transplant. 2017;23(11):1817–25.
24. Laskin BL, Goebel J, Davies SM, Jodele S. Small vessels, big trouble in the kidneys and beyond: hematopoietic stem cell transplantation-associated thrombotic microangiopathy. Blood. 2011;118(6):1452–62.
25. Laskin BL, Goebel J, Davies SM, Khoury JC, Bleesing JJ, Mehta PA, et al. Early clinical indicators of transplant-associated thrombotic microangiopathy in pediatric neuroblastoma patients undergoing auto-SCT. Bone Marrow Transplant. 2011;46(5):682–9.
26. Cordero C, Loboda C, Clerc-Urmes I, Clement L, Pochon C, Chastagner P. Unexpected acute renal injury after high-dose etoposide phosphate and total body irradiation in children undergoing hematopoietic stem cell transplantation. Pediatr Blood Cancer. 2017;64(12):e26669. https://doi.org/10.1002/pbc.26669. Epub 2017 Jul 11
27. Caruso Brown AE, Cohen MN, Tong S, Braverman RS, Rooney JF, Giller R, et al. Pharmacokinetics and safety of intravenous cidofovir for life-threatening viral infections in pediatric hematopoietic stem cell transplant recipients. Antimicrob Agents Chemother. 2015;59(7):3718–25.
28. Ferrara JL, Levine JE, Reddy P, Holler E. Graft-versus-host disease. Lancet. 2009;373(9674):1550–61.
29. Haines HL, Laskin BL, Goebel J, Davies SM, Yin HJ, Lawrence J, et al. Blood, and not urine, BK viral load predicts renal outcome in children with hemorrhagic cystitis following hematopoietic stem cell transplantation. Biol Blood Marrow Transplant. 2011;17(10):1512–9.
30. Sanchez-Pinto LN, Laskin BL, Jodele S, Hummel TR, Yin HJ, Goebel J. BK virus nephropathy in a pediatric autologous stem-cell transplant recipient. Pediatr Blood Cancer. 2011;56(3):495–7.

31. Parmar V, Lewis M, Shenoy M, Bonney D, Wynn R. Ascitic fluid drainage using a peritoneal dialysis catheter to prevent and treat multi-organ dysfunction in veno-occlusive disease in children undergoing hematopoietic stem cell transplantation. Pediatr Blood Cancer. 2017;64(9):e26469.
32. Corbacioglu S, Richardson PG. Defibrotide for children and adults with hepatic veno-occlusive disease post hematopoietic cell transplantation. Expert Rev Gastroenterol Hepatol. 2017;11(10):885–98.
33. Gloude NJ, Jodele S, Teusink-Cross A, Grimley M, Davies SM, Lane A, et al. Combination of high-dose methylprednisolone and defibrotide for veno-occlusive disease in pediatric hematopoietic stem cell transplant recipients. Biol Blood Marrow Transplant. 2018;24(1):91–5.
34. Jodele S, Laskin BL, Dandoy CE, Myers KC, El-Bietar J, Davies SM, et al. A new paradigm: diagnosis and management of HSCT-associated thrombotic microangiopathy as multi-system endothelial injury. Blood Rev. 2015;29(3):191–204.
35. Abusin GA, Abu-Arja R, Bajwa RPS, Horwitz EM, Auletta JJ, Rangarajan HG. Severe transplant-associated thrombotic microangiopathy in patients with hemoglobinopathies. Pediatr Blood Cancer. 2017;64:9. https://doi.org/10.1002/pbc.26503. Epub 2017 Mar 23
36. Jodele S, Licht C, Goebel J, Dixon BP, Zhang K, Sivakumaran TA, et al. Abnormalities in the alternative pathway of complement in children with hematopoietic stem cell transplant-associated thrombotic microangiopathy. Blood. 2013;122(12):2003–7.
37. Laskin BL, Maisel J, Goebel J, Yin HJ, Luo G, Khoury JC, et al. Renal arteriolar C4d deposition: a novel characteristic of hematopoietic stem cell transplantation-associated thrombotic microangiopathy. Transplantation. 2013;96(2):217–23.
38. Jodele S, Zhang K, Zou F, Laskin B, Dandoy CE, Myers KC, et al. The genetic fingerprint of susceptibility for transplant-associated thrombotic microangiopathy. Blood. 2016;127(8):989–96.
39. Hingorani SR, Seidel K, Pao E, Lawler R, McDonald GB. Markers of coagulation activation and acute kidney injury in patients after hematopoietic cell transplantation. Bone Marrow Transplant. 2015;50(5):715–20.
40. Jodele S, Davies SM, Lane A, Khoury J, Dandoy C, Goebel J, et al. Diagnostic and risk criteria for HSCT-associated thrombotic microangiopathy: a study in children and young adults. Blood. 2014;124(4):645–53.
41. Bohl SR, Kuchenbauer F, von Harsdorf S, Kloevekorn N, Schonsteiner SS, Rouhi A, et al. Thrombotic microangiopathy after allogeneic stem cell transplantation: a comparison of eculizumab therapy and conventional therapy. Biol Blood Marrow Transplant. 2017;23(12):2172–7.
42. Gloude NJ, Khandelwal P, Luebbering N, Lounder DT, Jodele S, Alder MN, et al. Circulating dsDNA, endothelial injury, and complement activation in thrombotic microangiopathy and GVHD. Blood. 2017;130(10):1259–66.
43. Hingorani S, Finn LS, Pao E, Lawler R, Schoch G, McDonald GB, et al. Urinary elafin and kidney injury in hematopoietic cell transplant recipients. Clin J Am Soc Nephrol. 2015;10(1):12–20.
44. Hingorani SR, Seidel K, Lindner A, Aneja T, Schoch G, McDonald G. Albuminuria in hematopoietic cell transplantation patients: prevalence, clinical associations, and impact on survival. Biol Blood Marrow Transplant. 2008;14(12):1365–72.
45. Hingorani S, Gooley T, Pao E, Sandmaier B, McDonald G. Urinary cytokines after HCT: evidence for renal inflammation in the pathogenesis of proteinuria and kidney disease. Bone Marrow Transplant. 2014;49(3):403–9.
46. Chien YH, Lin KH, Lee TY, Lu MY, Tsau YK. Nephrotic syndrome in a bone marrow transplant recipient without chronic graft-versus-host disease. J Formos Med Assoc. 2000;99(6):503–6.
47. Motoyama O, Takasu J, Kawamura T, Aikawa A, Shigetomi Y, Nara C, et al. A male patient with malignant lymphoma and thyroid papillary carcinoma after pediatric renal transplantation. Clin Exp Nephrol. 2010;14(1):94–6.
48. Walker JV, Morich D, Anasetti C. Minimal-change nephrotic syndrome after cyclosporine withdrawal in a marrow transplant recipient. Am J Kidney Dis. 1995;26(3):532–4.
49. Montaruli E, Wildhaber BE, Ansari M, Birraux J. Adenovirus-induced obstructive uropathy with acute renal failure in an immunodeficient child. Urology. 2014;83(1):217–9.

50. Haab AC, Keller IS, Padevit C, John H. BK virus associated pronounced hemorrhagic cysto-ureteritis after bone marrow transplantation. Can J Urol. 2015;22(5):8009–11.
51. Oshrine B, Bunin N, Li Y, Furth S, Laskin BL. Kidney and bladder outcomes in children with hemorrhagic cystitis and BK virus infection after allogeneic hematopoietic stem cell transplantation. Biol Blood Marrow Transplant. 2013;19(12):1702–7.
52. Goldstein SL, Mottes T, Simpson K, Barclay C, Muething S, Haslam DB, et al. A sustained quality improvement program reduces nephrotoxic medication-associated acute kidney injury. Kidney Int. 2016;90(1):212–21.
53. Zinter MS, Dvorak CC, Spicer A, Cowan MJ, Sapru A. New insights into multicenter PICU mortality among pediatric hematopoietic stem cell transplant patients. Crit Care Med. 2015;43(9):1986–94.
54. Chima RS, Daniels RC, Kim MO, Li D, Wheeler DS, Davies SM, et al. Improved outcomes for stem cell transplant recipients requiring pediatric intensive care. Pediatr Crit Care Med. 2012;13(6):e336–42.
55. Basu RK, Zappitelli M, Brunner L, Wang Y, Wong HR, Chawla LS, et al. Derivation and validation of the renal angina index to improve the prediction of acute kidney injury in critically ill children. Kidney Int. 2014;85(3):659–67.
56. Kinsey GR, Sharma R, Okusa MD. Regulatory T cells in AKI. J Am Soc Nephrol. 2013;24(11):1720–6.
57. Hingorani S. Chronic kidney disease in long-term survivors of hematopoietic cell transplantation: epidemiology, pathogenesis, and treatment. J Am Soc Nephrol. 2006;17(7):1995–2005.

# Hemolytic Uremic Syndrome

9

Uma Ali and Bradley P. Dixon

**Case Vignette**

A 15-month-old female infant presents to the emergency department with lethargy and pallor in the context of a gastrointestinal illness, with profuse vomiting for 2–3 days and 1 day of non-bloody diarrhea. Her past medical history is significant for a previous episode of unexplained thrombocytopenia in context of a febrile illness. Laboratory evaluation reveals mild anemia with schistocytes on her peripheral blood smear, thrombocytopenia, and acute kidney injury. She receives a diagnosis of Shigatoxin-producing *E. coli*-associated hemolytic uremic syndrome (STEC-HUS). Shortly after her admission to the hospital, seizures and altered mental status occur. A stool culture obtained on admission is negative for pathogenic organisms. Due to the neurological involvement and negative stool culture, the differential diagnosis is expanded to include thrombotic thrombocytopenic purpura (TTP) and atypical hemolytic uremic syndrome (aHUS). She is started on therapeutic plasma exchange until an ADAMTS13 activity obtained on admission is reported as normal (>67%). Complement studies performed reveal a low C3, the patient is diagnosed with aHUS, and eculizumab is initiated. However, her Shigatoxin PCR sent to a reference laboratory is subsequently found to be positive, confirming the ultimate diagnosis as STEC-HUS. Eculizumab is discontinued, and the patient makes a complete recovery of renal function and hematologic abnormalities.

U. Ali
Department of Pediatric Nephrology, Bai Jerbai Wadia Hospital and Institute of Child Health, Mumbai, Maharashtra, India

B. P. Dixon (✉)
Renal Section, Department of Pediatrics, University of Colorado School of Medicine, Aurora, CO, USA
e-mail: Bradley.dixon@childrenscolorado.org



A. Deep, S. L. Goldstein (eds.), *Critical Care Nephrology and Renal Replacement Therapy in Children*, https://doi.org/10.1007/978-3-319-90281-4_9

## 9.1 Thrombotic Microangiopathies

### 9.1.1 Definition of Thrombotic Microangiopathy

Hemolytic uremic syndrome (HUS) is one of several forms of thrombotic microangiopathy, a category of disease processes characterized by endothelial cell injury of the microvasculature, with subsequent aggregation and activation of platelets at the surface of the injured endothelium, activation of the coagulation cascade with fibrin deposition, mechanical hemolysis due to increased shear stress in the microvasculature, and tissue ischemia from occlusion by microthrombi in the vascular bed [1]. This pathological sequence leads to the hallmark clinical features of thrombotic microangiopathy (TMA), namely a consumptive thrombocytopenia, microangiopathic hemolytic anemia (MAHA), and organ dysfunction. As a multitude of pathomechanisms may ultimately cause endothelial cell injury, many disease processes can share the final common pathway of TMA and have overlapping clinical features.

### 9.1.2 Differential Diagnosis of Thrombotic Microangiopathy

The thrombotic microangiopathies may be separated into two broad subcategories: primary TMA syndromes, in which endothelial cell injury occurs as an inherent component of the disease process itself, and secondary TMA, in which a separate clinical condition or disease process causes endothelial cell injury with subsequent development of the TMA. The differential diagnosis of TMA is thus quite broad (Table 9.1).

**Table 9.1** Differential diagnosis of TMA

| | |
|---|---|
| **Primary TMA syndromes** | • TMA associated with malignant hypertension |
| • Shigatoxin-producing *E. coli*-associated HUS (STEC-HUS)<br>• Thrombotic thrombocytopenic Purpura (TTP)<br>• Atypical HUS<br>• Cobalamin C metabolism-associated HUS | • HELLP syndrome<br>• TMA associated with malignancy<br>• Hematopoietic stem cell transplant-associated TMA |
| **Secondary TMA syndromes** | • TMA associated with solid organ transplantation |
| • *Streptococcus pneumoniae*-associated HUS | • HIV-associated TMA |
| • Drug-induced TMA<br>– Cyclosporine and tacrolimus<br>– Sirolimus<br>– Gemcitabine<br>– Mitomycin C<br>– Anti-VEGF therapies<br>– Quinine<br>– Ticlopidine and clopidogrel | • TMA associated with collagen vascular disease<br>– SLE-related TMA<br>– Scleroderma renal crisis<br>– Catastrophic antiphospholipid syndrome |

### 9.1.3 Laboratory Evaluation of Thrombotic Microangiopathy

As the various forms of thrombotic microangiopathy share overlapping clinical features, ancillary laboratory testing is often vital to make an accurate diagnosis. Measurement of the activity of the von Willebrand Factor-cleaving protease ADAMTS13 in blood has been widely implemented as a screening test for TTP, as a severe deficiency (<5–10% activity) is relatively specific for this disease process. Infusions of fresh frozen plasma or plasmapheresis performed prior to obtaining a blood specimen for ADAMTS13 testing may lead to a partial correction of such a severe deficiency, and could obscure a diagnosis of TTP, and thus the timing of such a specimen is critical [2]. In the setting of gastrointestinal symptoms, which may be associated with either Shigatoxin-producing *E. coli*-associated HUS (STEC-HUS) or atypical HUS, investigation for the presence of Shigatoxin is needed. As stool culture on sorbitol MacConkey (SMAC) agar or other selective media may be insufficiently sensitive for the detection of Shigatoxin-producing organisms, especially serotypes other than *E. coli* O157:H7 [3], additional methods including serologies for Shigatoxin-producing serotypes [4] or direct molecular testing for the Shigatoxin by immunoassay or PCR are currently recommended [5]. When invasive pneumococcal disease is also evident, testing for the presence of circulating T antigen with peanut lectin agglutination of RBCs may be performed to investigate for *Streptococcus pneumoniae*-associated HUS. The presence of preformed IgM antibodies against the TF antigen, central to the pathogenesis of pneumococcal HUS, will also lead to a positive Coombs test, unlike in most other forms of TMA [6]. In infants presenting with TMA less than 1 year of age, evaluation of plasma homocysteine, methionine, and methylmalonic acid levels is important to evaluate for cobalamin C metabolism-associated HUS. Finally, if a diagnosis of atypical HUS is suspected, an interrogation of the complement system, including both quantitative and genetic investigations, is warranted to provide both added diagnostic clarity and prognostic understanding of the disease [7]. In addition to these laboratory studies, maintaining an index of suspicion for secondary forms of TMA and/or testing specifically for underlying disease processes that may cause secondary TMA is appropriate.

## 9.2 Infection-Associated Forms of Hemolytic Uremic Syndrome

Infections are the leading cause of hemolytic uremic syndrome worldwide. HUS is predominantly due to enterohemorrhagic Shigatoxin (*Stx*)-producing strains of *Escherichia coli* (STEC-HUS), occurring in 1 to 2 per 100,000 children between 3 and 5 years of age in Europe and North America [8], with serotype O157:H7 responsible for the majority of cases [9]. In a smaller number of cases, more than fifty other serotypes of *Stx*-producing *E. coli* have been implicated. In the recent German epidemic, *E. coli* O104:H4 was identified as the pathogenic strain that caused severe renal failure and neurological involvement in many [10]. Non-STEC organisms collectively are responsible for a small number of HUS (Table 9.2).

**Table 9.2** Non-STEC organisms associated with HUS

| Enteric organisms | Non-enteric organisms |
|---|---|
| • Bacteria<br>– *Shigella dysenteriae 1*<br>– *Citrobacter freundii*<br>• Viruses<br>– *Rotavirus* | • Bacteria<br>– *Streptococcus pneumoniae*<br>• Viruses<br>– *H1N1 influenza A*<br>– *Dengue viruses*<br>– *Hepatitis C, hepatitis A*<br>– *Parvovirus B19*<br>– *Adenovirus*<br>– *Epstein Barr virus* |

### 9.2.1 Shigatoxin-Producing *E. coli*-Associated HUS (STEC-HUS)

#### 9.2.1.1 Pathogenesis

HUS develops in 5–15% of children having diarrheal illness due to STEC infections. STEC are noninvasive strains that produce *Stx*1, *Stx2*, or both. Colonization of the gut, facilitated by the presence of the Locus of Enterocyte Effacement region (LEE) in *E. coli,* is followed by translocation of toxins from gastrointestinal tract into the blood stream [11].

Translocated toxins bind to the globotriaosylceramide (Gb3) receptors found on the cell surface of target organs. The toxins are endocytosed by the host cells where they irreversibly inactivate the ribosomes, inhibiting protein synthesis and leading to apoptosis. The bound *Stx* also induces cells to produce proinflammatory cytokines [12, 13].

*Stx* may also activate the alternate complement pathway by binding to and inactivating Factor H, the regulator of the alternate pathway. This activation generates the terminal complement complex producing endothelial injury [14, 15].

*Stx* has a high affinity for microvascular endothelial cells. The activated endothelium becomes thrombogenic causing platelet adhesion and aggregation leading to platelet microthrombi and consumptive thrombocytopenia. RBCs traversing these roughened narrow vascular channels undergo mechanical damage resulting in hemolysis and fragmentation. The kidney is the major target organ as it has the highest number of Gb3 receptors. Gb3 receptors are also found in the nervous system, colon, and other tissues. The kidney and brain are both highly flow-dependent and hence bear the brunt of this vascular damage.

#### 9.2.1.2 Clinical Features

STEC-HUS develops most commonly in young children, 2–8 days after a diarrheal illness that is often bloody. Forty percent of children may only have a watery diarrhea. STEC-HUS typically presents abruptly with oliguria, edema, and decreased urine output. Hypertension is common, and fever is usually absent. Extrarenal involvement is seen in 20% of cases. CNS involvement presents as irritability, lethargy, and seizures. Other systems affected occasionally are the myocardium and the pancreas. STEC-associated HUS may occur without diarrhea, and HUS following *E Coli* urinary tract infection has been reported [16].

In the acute phase, the patient's serum hemoglobin level usually drops to less than 8 gm/dL. The hemolytic anemia is Coombs negative with high reticulocyte count, markedly elevated LDH, and decreased haptoglobin levels. Peripheral smear shows frequent RBC fragments and schistocytes. The platelet counts are low, and leukocytosis may also be present. Coagulation studies are generally normal and there is no increase of fibrin degradation products, differentiating it from disseminated intravascular coagulation (DIC). Renal function is nearly universally abnormal with elevated blood urea nitrogen and serum creatinine, and accompanying electrolyte and acid base disturbances. Urinalysis generally reveals proteinuria and hematuria.

#### 9.2.1.3 Treatment

There is no specific therapy for STEC-HUS. The mainstay of treatment is judicious supportive therapy.

Restrictive fluid therapy to prevent fluid overload is needed in all oligoanuric children. However, children with STEC-HUS may be hypovolemic and hemoconcentrated due to the preceding diarrheal illness. This may reduce perfusion and promote the formation of microthrombi perpetuating organ dysfunction. A systematic review and meta-analysis of 1511 children with HUS suggested that children presenting with high hematocrit had a higher incidence of oligoanuric renal failure, greater need of renal replacement therapy (RRT), and higher mortality, suggesting an association between dehydration and adverse outcomes in children with HUS [17]. Volume expansion with isotonic fluids early during HUS reduced the need for RRT, incidence of CNS involvement, mortality, and improved long-term outcomes [18].

The role of antibiotics is controversial. Antibiotic usage during STEC diarrhea has been associated with increased incidence of HUS, particularly with antibiotics that damage bacterial DNA such as quinolones and trimethoprim-sulfamethoxazole. This has been attributed to a greater release of Shigatoxin in the gut as the organisms undergo lysis [19]. However, in a Japanese outbreak of HUS, early use of fosfomycin was associated with decreased incidence of HUS [20]. As evidence supporting the use of antibiotics in STEC diarrheal illness is lacking, antibiotics should be avoided [21]. Antimotility agents should be avoided as stagnation allows the toxin to remain longer in the gut leading to greater *Stx* translocation.

Packed red cell transfusions may be needed when hemoglobin is less than 6–7 gm/dL. Concurrent dialysis is needed in oliguric children needing transfusions to prevent fluid overload and hypertension. Platelet transfusion should be restricted and reserved for patients with active bleeding or prior to invasive procedures as it is widely believed that platelets may fuel the pathology by increasing formation of microthrombi [22, 23]. There is no evidence that *Stx* is removed by plasma exchange (PE). Plasma infusions or PE have not been consistently shown to be helpful in STEC-HUS [24].

Dialysis is required in 40% of children with STEC-HUS. The indications are not different for HUS than in any other AKI. As most children with STEC-HUS are young children, peritoneal dialysis is the most widely used modality worldwide. No single modality has been shown to be superior to the other and the choice of modality should be based on the patient's clinical status and institutional expertise.

Early reports of the use of eculizumab in some children with severe neurological involvement were associated with rapid improvement clinically and in laboratory markers of activity [25]. However, in the German HUS outbreak, use of eculizumab was largely ineffective in rapidly progressing HUS with multiorgan involvement and when given late during the disease [10, 26]. Follow-up of these patients over an intermediate term did not show any difference in renal sequelae between patients treated with eculizumab, plasmapheresis, and supportive care [27]. Prospective studies are needed to evaluate the efficacy of eculizumab therapy in STEC-HUS.

Orally administered *Stx* binding agent Synsorb PK failed to prevent progression of HUS. Studies are underway to assess the efficacy of monoclonal antibodies against toxins in preventing or treating HUS [12, 28], although these therapies will likely require administration early in the disease process.

#### 9.2.1.4 Prognosis

With improvements in supportive care such as dialysis, death occurs in only a small minority of patients (3–5%), typically as a result of neurological or cardiovascular sequelae of the disease rather than of renal failure. ESRD occurs in approximately 9% of children with STEC-HUS, although 25% may have long-term sequelae such as proteinuria, hypertension, or reduced renal function [29]. The duration of oligoanuria is the best predictor of long-term outcome, as oligoanuria lasting less than 2 weeks is generally considered to be associated with a favorable long-term outcome [12, 13].

### 9.2.2 Hemolytic Uremic Syndrome Due to *Streptococcus pneumoniae*

Hemolytic uremic syndrome may occur concurrently with invasive infections with *Streptococcus pneumoniae* (Pneumococcal HUS), including complicated pneumonia, meningitis, peritonitis, or disseminated infections, resulting in severe anemia with Coombs' positivity, thrombocytopenia, and AKI. Circulating neuraminidases derived from pneumococci unmask the normally hidden Thomsen-Friedenreich antigen (TF antigen) on RBCs, platelets, and endothelial cells leading to thrombotic microangiopathy. Plasma infusions and plasma exchange with fresh frozen plasma are contraindicated as they may provide more preformed antibodies against TF antigen, although plasma exchange using albumin as replacement fluid has demonstrated benefit in some patients [30]. Blood products should be avoided, and if needed, dextran-washed cells should be given. Up to 85% of children require dialysis with a mortality rate of 12%, and with 10% progressing to ESRD, 16% to CKD and/or hypertension [6].

## 9.3 Other Forms of Hemolytic Uremic Syndrome

### 9.3.1 Atypical Hemolytic Uremic Syndrome

Atypical hemolytic uremic syndrome (aHUS), more recently termed complement-mediated TMA [31], is a rare form of thrombotic microangiopathy, occurring in approximately 1–2 cases per one million population, although the precise incidence is unknown [32]. Earlier understanding of the epidemiology of aHUS is that it is largely a disease of childhood, although more recent registry data has demonstrated a substantial portion of patients presents in adulthood [33]. The disease is distributed evenly between males and females in childhood, and with a slight female predominance in adulthood due to the proportion of women in whom initial disease manifestations are triggered by pregnancy and the postpartum period [32].

#### 9.3.1.1 Pathogenesis

Dysregulation of the alternative pathway of the complement system with subsequent uncontrolled activation on the endothelial cell surface is the primary mechanism leading to thrombotic microangiopathy in aHUS. This dysregulation may occur due to genetic or acquired defects in the regulatory components of the alternative pathway, leading to prolonged stabilization of the C3 convertase C3bBb, through which additional molecules of C3b are generated to perpetuate the pathway activation. With the addition of a second molecule of C3b to this complex (C3bBb•C3b), a C5 convertase is created which cleaves C5 into C5a, a potent anaphylotoxin, and C5b-9, which serves as the nidus for the formation of the membrane attack complex C5b-9 (Fig. 9.1). Genetic defects of complement regulation may occur both as loss of function mutations in regulatory proteins (Factor H, Factor I, Membrane Cofactor Protein/CD46, thrombomodulin) [34, 35], and gain of function mutations in alternate pathway components C3 [36] and Factor B [37], generally present in the heterozygous state leading to autosomal dominant inheritance with incomplete penetrance. Acquired defects in alternative pathway regulation may also occur by neutralizing autoantibodies against Factor H [38], almost exclusively in the setting of homozygous deletion of the Factor H-related genes *CFHR1* and *CFHR3* [39].

The principle of aHUS as exclusively a disease of complement dysregulation has recently been challenged with the identification of mutations in genes that regulate the coagulation system in association with aHUS. Thrombomodulin serves a dual function of regulating both the coagulation and complement systems, and discovery of its association with aHUS led to identification of additional genes, notably diacylglycerol kinase ε (*DGKE*) [40] and plasminogen (*PLG*) [41], in association with aHUS but without known complement regulatory functions.

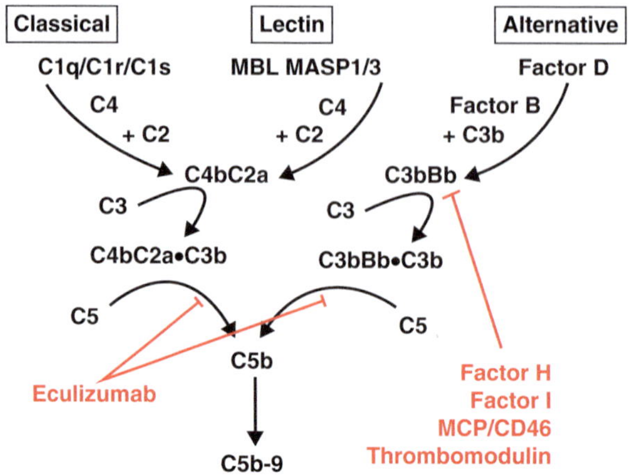


**Fig. 9.1** The complement cascade, in which activation of the classical, lectin, or alternative pathways leads to the formation of a C5 convertase. Dysregulation of the alternative pathway by loss of function mutations of Factor H, Factor I, MCP, or thrombomodulin (shown in red), or gain of function mutations of Factor B or C3, have been identified in patients with aHUS. The complement-targeted drug eculizumab (also shown in red), binds with high affinity to C5 and has been shown to be effective in suppressing the uncontrolled complement activation of aHUS

The complement system is a highly versatile component of the innate immune system, activated by a variety of microbial threats as well as immune complexes, lipopolysaccharide, and necrotic cells. This leads to complement activation accompanying a myriad of clinical conditions (upper respiratory infections, gastroenteritis, immunosuppressive or chemotherapeutic medications, pregnancy, collagen vascular diseases such as systemic lupus erythematosus and scleroderma, solid organ and hematopoietic stem cell transplantation, malignant hypertension, and others). In individuals harboring genetic defects in complement regulation, and therefore susceptible to developing aHUS, such complement activation can lead to the unmasking of disease. This is particularly problematic as many of these conditions may be associated with secondary forms of TMA distinct from aHUS (i.e., HELLP syndrome in pregnancy, lupus-associated TMA, drug-induced HUS, hematopoietic stem cell transplantation). Failure of the TMA to clinically improve in the expected timeframe despite appropriate management of the underlying condition should warrant suspicion for the unmasking of aHUS.

#### 9.3.1.2 Diagnosis

Clinical features of aHUS share substantial overlap with those of other primary and secondary TMA syndromes. The diagnosis of aHUS is often one of exclusion if Shigatoxin and ADAMTS13 activity testing are nondiagnostic and other conditions leading to secondary forms of TMA are clinically ruled out. This is perhaps most critically important in distinguishing between aHUS and TTP, as the treatment strategies for these diseases have become more divergent with the advent of complement-targeted therapies. Moderate thrombocytopenia and severe renal dysfunction have

**Table 9.3** Extrarenal manifestations of atypical hemolytic uremic syndrome

| | |
|---|---|
| Cardiovascular<br>• Myocardial infarction<br>• Pericardial effusion<br>• Cardiomyopathy<br>• Peripheral vascular disease | Gastrointestinal<br>• Diarrhea<br>• Colitis<br>• Elevated transaminases<br>• Pancreatitis |
| CNS<br>• Seizures<br>• Stroke<br>• Confusion, delirium<br>• Coma | Pulmonary<br>• Pulmonary hemorrhage<br>Ocular<br>• Retinal vessel occlusion |

been identified as being more commonly noted in aHUS [2], and these clinical distinctions coupled with ADAMTS13 activity testing may enhance diagnostic certainty and allow for earlier implementation of more specific management.

Atypical hemolytic uremic syndrome is frequently associated with extrarenal manifestations (Table 9.3), occurring in 8–25% of children and 16–29% of adults and predominantly of the neurological and cardiovascular systems. Involvement of the gastrointestinal tract in aHUS may cause diarrhea and colitis, ultimately leading to diagnostic uncertainty between this and STEC-HUS, and has led to waning use of the designations "D+ HUS" and "D-HUS".

A complete investigation of the complement system is warranted in the evaluation of a patient with suspected aHUS. This includes quantitative testing of individual complement factors in serum (C3, C4, Factor B, Factor H, and Factor I levels) and testing for Factor H autoantibodies, as well as a comprehensive genetic evaluation with both sequencing of the *CFH*, *CFI*, *MCP/CD46*, *CFB*, *C3*, *THBD*, and *DGKE* genes as well as copy number variant analysis of *CFH* and the *CFH*-related gene locus [7]. Low levels of C3 and/or Factor B with normal levels of C4 would be indicative of isolated activation of the alternative pathway, which suggests a diagnosis of aHUS in a patient with TMA. However, decreased C3 levels may only be identified in 30–40% of patients with aHUS [42]. Similarly, only ~60% of patients with aHUS may have an identifiable genetic or acquired complement regulatory defect, and thus a nondiagnostic genetic evaluation cannot exclude the diagnosis of aHUS. Complement fragments such as sC5b-9 and Bb have shown promise in characterizing dysregulated complement activation in patients with suspected aHUS [43], although these markers lack sufficient specificity to be widely implemented as diagnostic tools [15, 44]. Functional assays have also been described which may ultimately provide greater specificity for the complement dysregulation associated with aHUS but are technically challenging or require specialized reagents [45, 46], limiting their widespread use in the diagnostic evaluation of suspected aHUS.

#### 9.3.1.3 Treatment

Until recent advances in complement therapeutics, the standard of care for atypical hemolytic uremic syndrome was plasma infusion or plasma exchange based on the principle that these interventions could correct complement dysregulation by reconstituting nonmutant complement regulatory factors. Although ample anecdotal reports of its efficacy are published, a meta-analysis studying the use of plasma therapy in hemolytic uremic syndrome (both STEC-HUS and aHUS) did not demonstrate superiority over supportive care alone in avoiding long-term outcomes of ESRD, proteinuria, or hypertension [47]. More recently, a meta-analysis of case reports demonstrated no difference between plasma exchange and complement blockade in short-term outcomes of normalization of platelet count or renal function; however, higher mortality was noted in the group receiving plasma exchange [48]. A notable exception in which plasma exchange is considered first-line therapy is Factor H autoantibody-associated aHUS, for which plasma exchange is rated as a Category I recommendation in the 2014 American Society for Apheresis (ASFA) guidelines [49] in concert with immunosuppressive therapy.

The use of eculizumab was first reported in the treatment of aHUS in 2009 [50]. Eculizumab, a monoclonal antibody which binds with high affinity to the terminal complement protein C5 and thus prevents its cleavage to C5a and C5b, demonstrated efficacy in correcting the microangiopathic hemolysis, thrombocytopenia, and renal dysfunction in ~80% of adult patients with aHUS in two pivotal clinical trials [51], and continued to maintain this efficacy in treated patients over long-term follow-up [52]. Eculizumab has shown similar efficacy in children with aHUS, both in an uncontrolled retrospective case series [53] and in a prospective trial [54]. Despite its well-described safety and efficacy, the uncertain optimal duration of therapy and the cost of long-term treatment with eculizumab have led to individualization of dosing intervals with the use of complement biomarkers and functional testing [55], as well as study into the safety of discontinuation of eculizumab in select patients with favorable genetic and clinical risk factors [56].

#### 9.3.1.4 Prognosis

Compared to STEC-HUS, the prognosis of atypical hemolytic uremic syndrome has historically been poor, with substantially higher rates of ESRD and mortality [32]. This is particularly true in patients with mutations in *CFH* (Factor H), in whom progression to death or ESRD was noted in ~75% of individuals by 5 years of follow-up [34]. Patients with mutations in *CFB*, *CFI*, *C3*, and *THBD*, and those individuals in whom no mutations were identified, also tended to have poor outcomes with approximately 50–60% progressing to death or ESRD by 5 years of follow-up. Only patients with mutations in *MCP/CD46* had a more favorable outcome, with only 6% of patients progressing to death or ESRD in the same timeframe. With the advent of the use of eculizumab in aHUS, the prognosis has markedly improved as the vast majority of patients may remain free of disease manifestations while receiving complement blockade [52]. Due to concerns of the sustainability of indefinite therapy with eculizumab, there is growing recognition as to the need for tailoring length of therapy based on an individual's clinical and genetic risk factors, carefully monitoring such patients for relapse of their disease [7].

Kidney transplantation has historically had variable outcomes in patients with aHUS, owing largely to the risk of disease recurrence in the renal allograft in 50% of patients with 80–90% of patients with recurrence experiencing graft loss [32]. Use of eculizumab in the perioperative and posttransplant setting has markedly improved graft outcomes, although there is considerable debate on the length of therapy that is optimal in such patients. Combined liver-kidney transplantation has also been demonstrated in a growing series of patients to improve renal allograft outcomes, specifically performed in individuals with mutations in hepatically synthesized complement factors *CFH*, *CFI*, *CFB*, and *C3* [57].

### 9.3.2 Cobalamin C Metabolism Defect-Related HUS

Affected individuals typically present in early infancy with prominent neurological involvement (feeding difficulties, lethargy, hypotonia) as well as multiorgan dysfunction from TMA [31], although rarely individuals can present with a milder phenotype later in childhood [8]. This entity is due to homozygous or compound heterozygous mutations in the *MMAHAC* gene, leading to a defect in cobalamin C metabolism and causing hyperhomocysteinemia, hypomethioninemia, and methylmalonic aciduria. The precise mechanism by which this metabolism defect causes HUS is unknown; however, parenteral hydroxycobalamin, betaine, and folinic acid administration is the treatment of choice.

## 9.4 Secondary Forms of TMA

### 9.4.1 Drug-Induced TMA

A variety of medications may cause endothelial cell injury resulting in TMA, although the mechanisms by which these medications cause injury are diverse (Table 9.4). Generally, endothelial injury is either mediated by direct toxicity by the agent or immune-mediated injury. Typically, the treatment of choice is supportive care in which the suspected offending agent is discontinued with resolution of clinical features of TMA over several days. Drugs that cause direct endothelial toxicity may be rechallenged without recurrence of TMA, whereas immune-mediated drug-induced TMA is likely to recur with rechallenge [58].

**Table 9.4** Medications associated with drug-induced TMA

| Medication | Mechanism |
|---|---|
| Cyclosporine and tacrolimus | Direct endothelial toxicity |
| Sirolimus | Direct endothelial toxicity |
| Quinine | Immune (autoantibody formation against platelets, leukocytes, and endothelial cells) |
| Anti-VEGF therapies (e.g., bevacizumab, sorafenib) | Direct endothelial and podocyte toxicity |
| Gemcitabine | Immune (mechanism unknown) and direct endothelial toxicity |
| Mitomycin C | Direct endothelial toxicity |
| Ticlopidine and clopidogrel | Immune (autoantibodies against platelet antigens, ADAMTS13) and direct endothelial toxicity |

### 9.4.2 TMA Associated with Collagen Vascular Disease

Thrombotic microangiopathy is an uncommon disease manifestation of collagen vascular diseases (CVD) in adults and children, primarily attributed to endothelial injury from vasculitis and thrombosis of the microvasculature. The precise incidence may be difficult to assess, however, as CVD, and in particular systemic lupus erythematosus (SLE), are associated with complement activation and may serve to unmask aHUS in genetically susceptible individuals. SLE-associated TMA generally occurs in the setting of proliferative glomerulonephritis, with an incidence of 9–14% [59, 60] in patients with SLE nephritis. Generally, treatment focuses on aggressive immunosuppression with or without plasma exchange, and outcome is generally similar to SLE nephritis without TMA, with reported mortality in the largest series of ~4% and ESRD in 43% of patients [60]. Scleroderma renal crisis is another defined TMA syndrome in the context of CVD, which occurs in ~10–15% of adults with scleroderma and rarely (<5%) in children [61]. Scleroderma renal crisis is associated with severe hypertension, with its pathogenesis due to obliterative microvasculopathy of arterioles. The treatment of choice is blood pressure control specifically with ACE inhibitor therapy, although ESRD may still occur in 40–50% of individuals despite treatment [62]. Catastrophic antiphospholipid syndrome (CAPS) may also be associated with TMA, with multiorgan dysfunction from small vessel occlusion by microthrombi. Approximately 10% of patients with CAPS in one registry presented during childhood, with a tendency to present with CAPS as their initial manifestation of antiphospholipid syndrome, and frequently in association with another CVD such as SLE. The treatment of choice based on published consensus guidelines in adults is anticoagulation with heparin infusion and corticosteroids, with intravenous immune globulin and plasma exchange reserved for life-threatening manifestations [63].

### 9.4.3 TMA Associated with Malignant Hypertension

Thrombotic microangiopathy related to malignant hypertension is uncommon in children. The presumed pathogenesis is due to endothelial cell injury from shear stress from severe hypertension, with subsequent platelet activation and microvascular thrombosis. Treatment is rapid and sustained control of blood pressure, which generally leads to improvement in the hematological and renal sequelae. Both endothelial complement activation and ADAMTS13 deficiency have been implicated in disease pathogenesis, and thus complement blockade or plasma exchange may have an adjunctive role in this disease [64]. Recently, evidence has emerged that a subset of patients with TMA related to malignant hypertension may harbor genetic variants in complement regulatory factors [65], raising the possibility that some patients with presumed malignant hypertension-related TMA may actually have aHUS with accompanying severe hypertension, and in whom complement blockade may be particularly beneficial.

### 9.4.4 HELLP Syndrome

Although an uncommon consideration in pediatric patients, HELLP syndrome (*H*emolytic anemia, *E*levated *L*iver enzymes, and *L*ow *P*latelets) may also be considered in the pediatric patient with pregnancy and clinical evidence of TMA. The pathogenic mechanism is proposed to be due to endothelial injury by anti-angiogenic factors such as sFlt1 and endoglin [8], as an extreme form of pre-eclampsia. Clinically, this may be difficult to distinguish from aHUS and TTP, both of which also may occur in the later stages of pregnancy. The timeframe of onset may help distinguish these diseases, as TTP in pregnancy tends to manifest most commonly in the second and third trimesters, HELLP syndrome in the third trimester and peripartum periods, and aHUS in the peripartum and postpartum periods. ADAMTS13 activity testing may be a helpful adjunct in the setting of pregnancy-associated TMA. HELLP syndrome generally resolves with delivery, and prolonged findings of TMA following delivery may herald an alternate diagnosis of aHUS.

**Key Learning Points**

- Hemolytic uremic syndrome is one of many forms of thrombotic microangiopathy, with overlapping clinical features.
- Shigatoxin-producing *E. coli*-associated HUS (STEC-HUS) is the most common form of HUS in children, occurring 2–8 days after enterocolitis, and in which meticulous supportive care remains the standard of care.
- Pneumococcal HUS occurs in the setting of invasive *Streptococcus pneumoniae* infection, with higher rates of morbidity and mortality in comparison to STEC-HUS
- Atypical hemolytic uremic syndrome is due to genetic or acquired defects in complement regulation, with improved survival through the widespread use of eculizumab.
- Secondary forms of TMA may occur in children and may lead to diagnostic confusion with aHUS.

## References

1. Moake JL. Thrombotic microangiopathies. N Engl J Med. 2002;347(8):589–600.
2. Laurence J, et al. Atypical hemolytic uremic syndrome (aHUS): essential aspects of an accurate diagnosis. Clin Adv Hematol Oncol. 2016;14(Suppl 11(11)):2–15.
3. Gilmour MW, et al. Isolation and detection of Shiga toxin-producing Escherichia coli in clinical stool samples using conventional and molecular methods. J Med Microbiol. 2009;58(Pt 7):905–11.
4. Leszczynska B, et al. Diagnostic value of serological tests against verotoxigenic Escherichia coli in hemolytic uremic syndrome in children. Adv Clin Exp Med. 2015;24(6):1031–6.

5. Gould LH, et al. Recommendations for diagnosis of Shiga toxin--producing Escherichia coli infections by clinical laboratories. MMWR Recomm Rep. 2009;58(RR-12):1–14.
6. Copelovitch L, Kaplan BS. Streptococcus pneumoniae-associated hemolytic uremic syndrome. Pediatr Nephrol. 2008;23(11):1951–6.
7. Loirat C, et al. An international consensus approach to the management of atypical hemolytic uremic syndrome in children. Pediatr Nephrol. 2016;31(1):15–39.
8. Fakhouri F, et al. Haemolytic uraemic syndrome. Lancet. 2017;390(10095):681–96.
9. Mody RK, et al. Infections in pediatric postdiarrheal hemolytic uremic syndrome: factors associated with identifying Shiga toxin-producing Escherichia coli. Arch Pediatr Adolesc Med. 2012;166(10):902–9.
10. Kielstein JT, et al. Best supportive care and therapeutic plasma exchange with or without eculizumab in Shiga-toxin-producing E coli O104:H4 induced haemolytic-uraemic syndrome: an analysis of the German STEC-HUS registry. Nephrol Dial Transplant. 2012;27(10):3807–15.
11. Paton JC, Paton AW. Pathogenesis and diagnosis of Shiga toxin-producing Escherichia coli infections. Clin Microbiol Rev. 1998;11(3):450–79.
12. Thorpe CM. Shiga toxin-producing Escherichia coli infection. Clin Infect Dis. 2004;38(9):1298–303.
13. Andreoli SP, et al. Hemolytic uremic syndrome: epidemiology, pathophysiology, and therapy. Pediatr Nephrol. 2002;17(4):293–8.
14. Orth D, et al. Shiga toxin activates complement and binds factor H: evidence for an active role of complement in hemolytic uremic syndrome. J Immunol. 2009;182(10):6394–400.
15. Thurman JM, et al. Alternative pathway of complement in children with diarrhea-associated hemolytic uremic syndrome. Clin J Am Soc Nephrol. 2009;4(12):1920–4.
16. Starr M, et al. Hemolytic-uremic syndrome following urinary tract infection with enterohemorrhagic Escherichia coli: case report and review. Clin Infect Dis. 1998;27(2):310–5.
17. Grisaru S, et al. Associations between hydration status, intravenous fluid administration, and outcomes of patients infected with Shiga toxin-producing Escherichia coli: a systematic review and meta-analysis. JAMA Pediatr. 2017;171(1):68–76.
18. Ardissino G, et al. Early volume expansion and outcomes of hemolytic uremic syndrome. Pediatrics. 2016;137(1):e20152153.
19. Wong CS, et al. The risk of the hemolytic-uremic syndrome after antibiotic treatment of Escherichia coli O157:H7 infections. N Engl J Med. 2000;342(26):1930–6.
20. Ikeda K, et al. Effect of early fosfomycin treatment on prevention of hemolytic uremic syndrome accompanying Escherichia coli O157:H7 infection. Clin Nephrol. 1999;52(6):357–62.
21. Freedman SB, et al. Shiga toxin-producing Escherichia coli infection, antibiotics, and risk of developing hemolytic uremic syndrome: a meta-analysis. Clin Infect Dis. 2016;62(10):1251–8.
22. Goel R, et al. Platelet transfusions in platelet consumptive disorders are associated with arterial thrombosis and in-hospital mortality. Blood. 2015;125(9):1470–6.
23. Balestracci A, et al. Impact of platelet transfusions in children with post-diarrheal hemolytic uremic syndrome. Pediatr Nephrol. 2013;28(6):919–25.
24. Menne J, et al. Validation of treatment strategies for enterohaemorrhagic Escherichia coli O104:H4 induced haemolytic uraemic syndrome: case-control study. BMJ. 2012;345:e4565.
25. Lapeyraque AL, et al. Eculizumab in severe Shiga-toxin-associated HUS. N Engl J Med. 2011;364(26):2561–3.
26. Pape L, et al. Eculizumab in typical hemolytic uremic syndrome (HUS) with neurological involvement. Medicine (Baltimore). 2015;94(24):e1000.
27. Loos S, et al. Intermediate follow-up of pediatric patients with hemolytic uremic syndrome during the 2011 outbreak caused by E. Coli O104:H4. Clin Infect Dis. 2017;64(12):1637–43.
28. Trachtman H, et al. Effect of an oral Shiga toxin-binding agent on diarrhea-associated hemolytic uremic syndrome in children: a randomized controlled trial. JAMA. 2003;290(10):1337–44.
29. Garg AX, et al. Long-term renal prognosis of diarrhea-associated hemolytic uremic syndrome: a systematic review, meta-analysis, and meta-regression. JAMA. 2003;290(10):1360–70.
30. Weintraub L, et al. Management of streptococcal pneumoniae-induced hemolytic uremic syndrome: a case report. Clin Nephrol Case Stud. 2014;2:9–17.

31. George JN, Nester CM. Syndromes of thrombotic microangiopathy. N Engl J Med. 2014;371(7):654–66.
32. Loirat C, Fremeaux-Bacchi V. Atypical hemolytic uremic syndrome. Orphanet J Rare Dis. 2011;6:60.
33. Licht C, et al. The global aHUS registry: methodology and initial patient characteristics. BMC Nephrol. 2015;16:207.
34. Noris M, et al. Relative role of genetic complement abnormalities in sporadic and familial aHUS and their impact on clinical phenotype. Clin J Am Soc Nephrol. 2010;5(10):1844–59.
35. Delvaeye M, et al. Thrombomodulin mutations in atypical hemolytic-uremic syndrome. N Engl J Med. 2009;361(4):345–57.
36. Fremeaux-Bacchi V, et al. Mutations in complement C3 predispose to development of atypical hemolytic uremic syndrome. Blood. 2008;112(13):4948–52.
37. Goicoechea de Jorge E, et al. Gain-of-function mutations in complement factor B are associated with atypical hemolytic uremic syndrome. Proc Natl Acad Sci U S A. 2007;104(1):240–5.
38. Dragon-Durey MA, et al. Anti-factor H autoantibodies associated with atypical hemolytic uremic syndrome. J Am Soc Nephrol. 2005;16(2):555–63.
39. Jozsi M, et al. Factor H autoantibodies in atypical hemolytic uremic syndrome correlate with CFHR1/CFHR3 deficiency. Blood. 2008;111(3):1512–4.
40. Lemaire M, et al. Recessive mutations in DGKE cause atypical hemolytic-uremic syndrome. Nat Genet. 2013;45(5):531–6.
41. Bu F, et al. Comprehensive genetic analysis of complement and coagulation genes in atypical hemolytic uremic syndrome. J Am Soc Nephrol. 2014;25(1):55–64.
42. Nester CM, et al. Atypical aHUS: state of the art. Mol Immunol. 2015;67(1):31–42.
43. Cataland SR, et al. Biomarkers of the alternative pathway and terminal complement activity at presentation confirms the clinical diagnosis of aHUS and differentiates aHUS from TTP. Blood. 2014;123(24):3733–8.
44. Reti M, et al. Complement activation in thrombotic thrombocytopenic purpura. J Thromb Haemost. 2012;10(5):791–8.
45. Noris M, et al. Dynamics of complement activation in aHUS and how to monitor eculizumab therapy. Blood. 2014;124(11):1715–26.
46. Gavriilaki E, et al. Modified Ham test for atypical hemolytic uremic syndrome. Blood. 2015;125(23):3637–46.
47. Michael M, et al. Interventions for haemolytic uraemic syndrome and thrombotic thrombocytopenic purpura. Cochrane Database Syst Rev. 2009;1:CD003595.
48. Krishnappa V, et al. Atypical hemolytic uremic syndrome: a meta-analysis of case reports confirms the prevalence of genetic mutations and the shift of treatment regimens. Ther Apher Dial. 2018;22(2):178–88.
49. Schwartz J, et al. Guidelines on the use of therapeutic apheresis in clinical practice-evidence-based approach from the writing Committee of the American Society for apheresis: the seventh special issue. J Clin Apher. 2016;31(3):149–62.
50. Gruppo RA, Rother RP. Eculizumab for congenital atypical hemolytic-uremic syndrome. N Engl J Med. 2009;360(5):544–6.
51. Legendre CM, et al. Terminal complement inhibitor eculizumab in atypical hemolytic-uremic syndrome. N Engl J Med. 2013;368(23):2169–81.
52. Licht C, et al. Efficacy and safety of eculizumab in atypical hemolytic uremic syndrome from 2-year extensions of phase 2 studies. Kidney Int. 2015;87(5):1061–73.
53. Simonetti D, et al. Eculizumab therapy for atypical hemolytic uremic syndrome in pediatric patients: efficacy and safety outcomes from a retrospective study. Haematologica. 2011;96(Suppl 2):165.
54. Greenbaum LA, et al. Eculizumab is a safe and effective treatment in pediatric patients with atypical hemolytic uremic syndrome. Kidney Int. 2016;89(3):701–11.
55. Wehling C, et al. Monitoring of complement activation biomarkers and eculizumab in complement-mediated renal disorders. Clin Exp Immunol. 2017;187(2):304–15.

56. Ardissino G, et al. Discontinuation of eculizumab treatment in atypical hemolytic uremic syndrome: an update. Am J Kidney Dis. 2015;66(1):172–3.
57. Saland J. Liver-kidney transplantation to cure atypical HUS: still an option post-eculizumab? Pediatr Nephrol. 2014;29(3):329–32.
58. Masias C, Vasu S, Cataland SR. None of the above: thrombotic microangiopathy beyond TTP and HUS. Blood. 2017;129(21):2857–63.
59. Copelovitch L, Kaplan BS. The thrombotic microangiopathies. Pediatr Nephrol. 2008;23(10):1761–7.
60. Barrera-Vargas A, et al. Renal thrombotic Microangiopathy in proliferative lupus nephritis: risk factors and clinical outcomes: a case-control study. J Clin Rheumatol. 2016;22(5):235–40.
61. Torok KS. Pediatric scleroderma: systemic or localized forms. Pediatr Clin N Am. 2012;59(2):381–405.
62. Guillevin L, et al. Scleroderma renal crisis: a retrospective multicentre study on 91 patients and 427 controls. Rheumatology (Oxford). 2012;51(3):460–7.
63. Berman H, et al. Pediatric catastrophic antiphospholipid syndrome: descriptive analysis of 45 patients from the "CAPS registry". Autoimmun Rev. 2014;13(2):157–62.
64. Mathew RO, Nayer A, Asif A. The endothelium as the common denominator in malignant hypertension and thrombotic microangiopathy. J Am Soc Hypertens. 2016;10(4):352–9.
65. Timmermans S, et al. Patients with hypertension-associated thrombotic microangiopathy may present with complement abnormalities. Kidney Int. 2017;91(6):1420–5.

# Acute Kidney Injury in Liver Disease

# 10

Akash Deep and Romit Saxena

**Case Vignette**

An 8-month-old child diagnosed to have biliary atresia in infancy had undergone Kasai porto-enterostomy at 8 weeks of age. Unfortunately, the Kasai operation was unsuccessful and the child progressed gradually to chronic liver disease with rising bilirubin, ascites and portal hypertension. He was eventually listed for liver transplantation and was being followed up on an outpatient basis.

He was admitted to our emergency department with vomiting, loose stools, lethargy, decreased oral acceptance and increased abdominal distention (due to ascites). His investigations revealed transaminitis, hyperbilirubinaemia and hypoalbuminaemia with increased creatinine. The question here was what has caused the kidney injury, i.e. the differential diagnosis of the aetiology of AKI. Was it related to the acute precipitating event—hypovolaemia, sepsis and increased ascites or was it hepatorenal syndrome (HRS) as both liver and kidneys were affected or was it the normal progression of chronic liver disease with its attendant complications including renal dysfunction? The management including candidacy for liver transplantation would vary based on aetiology. The above example illustrates the complex nature of kidney injury in the setting of liver failure as the treatment of each of the aetiologies is

A. Deep (✉)
Paediatric Intensive Care Unit, King's College Hospital, London, UK

Renal/CRRT Section of the European Society of Pediatric and Neonatal Intensive Care (ESPNIC), Geneva, Switzerland
e-mail: akash.deep@nhs.net

R. Saxena
Paediatric Intensive Care Unit, King's College Hospital, London, UK

Paediatric Intensive Care Unit, Great Ormond Street Hospital, London, UK

 
A. Deep, S. L. Goldstein (eds.), *Critical Care Nephrology and Renal Replacement Therapy in Children*, https://doi.org/10.1007/978-3-319-90281-4_10

different. In this chapter we explore the current literature on this fascinating yet less researched topic: Acute kidney injury in liver failure. Unfortunately, most of the data and research in the field of AKI in liver disease is limited to adults and paediatric practice is extrapolated from the adult literature. We shall share our experience of managing patients with AKI in liver disease at King's College Hospital, London, to demonstrate the current practice.

## 10.1 Introduction

The association between liver disease and renal failure has been known for over a century. In 1800s, Flint and co-workers published a case series on this association of kidney involvement in patients with liver disease [1]. Since then, a lot of research has been done on the concept and the importance of acute kidney injury (AKI) in patients with liver disease. AKI in liver failure is a relatively common entity with an incidence that varies depending on the liver disease in question—acute liver failure, chronic liver disease, acute-on-chronic liver failure or post-liver transplantation. AKI is associated with an increased mortality in patients admitted to critical care especially in context of post liver transplant recipients [2, 3]. It has been observed that approximately 20% of patients hospitalized with cirrhosis develop AKI [4]. In this chapter, we shall explore some of these issues and current dilemmas in AKI with liver failure especially in patients with liver disease. We emphasize that there is an extreme paucity of data in paediatric literature, and most of the concepts are an extrapolation from the adult literature.

## 10.2 Acute Kidney Injury in Acute Liver Failure

When we talk about AKI epidemiology in acute liver failure (ALF), most patients have no pre-existing disease and the Kidney Disease Improving Global Outcomes (KDIGO) criteria used to define and stage AKI in non-liver failure patients can be used to define AKI in this group of patients as well.

AKI is common in ALF. A retrospective review of patients enrolled in the Acute Liver Failure Study Group (1998–2010) indicated that 70% of patients with ALF developed AKI and a third received renal replacement therapy (RRT) [5].

The most common causes of AKI in ALF include sepsis, hypovolaemia, direct nephrotoxicity and acute tubular necrosis. Sepsis and the related inflammatory response can contribute to significant vasomotor changes which can affect renal perfusion [6]. Ischaemia secondary to poor perfusion or toxins can cause loss of cellular integrity in proximal tubules and induce apoptosis [7]. Direct nephrotoxicity and acute tubular necrosis can be multifactorial. In cases like acetaminophen overdose, AKI can be due to antioxidant (glutathione) depletion. A retrospective review showed that the median maximum serum creatinine (SCr) level was higher for acetaminophen (APAP) (acetyl-para-aminophenol) related ALF as compared to other aetiologies [5].

Renal injury in association with muscle injury can be associated in patients with shock, drugs or crush injury due to trauma. Shock-related and APAP-related ALF cases had a higher level of creatine kinase as compared with the other aetiologies [5] AKI in association with ALF is known to reduce the overall survival and often delays the spontaneous regeneration of the liver prompting liver transplantation. However, the incidence of chronic kidney disease or dependence on dialysis is minimal. It was observed that only 4% of patients requiring RRT (amongst patients with AKI in ALF) became dependent on dialysis [5].

## 10.3 Acute Kidney Injury in Chronic Liver Failure

Cirrhosis is the end-stage of every chronic liver disease. Its natural history is characterized by an asymptomatic phase, termed 'compensated' cirrhosis followed by a rapidly progressive phase marked by the development of complications of portal hypertension and/or liver dysfunction, termed 'decompensated cirrhosis'. Here we need to differentiate between a cirrhotic patient whose underlying liver disease worsens and complications including portal hypertension and renal dysfunction develop as opposed to a stable cirrhotic with a reasonable liver reserve who is exposed to a precipitating factor such as bleeding, infections, volume loss which leads to multi-organ failure. Both the aetiologies though different in nature, can lead to renal injury. Hence, because of this multifactorial nature, the definitions of AKI employed in studies involving patients with cirrhosis have not been standardized. They often lack sensitivity and are often limited to narrow clinical settings [8].

## 10.4 Problems with Existing Kidney Function Parameters

Urine output and SCr have been the benchmark of defining AKI in patients. However, there is a problem with both these parameters in patients with cirrhosis. SCr is affected by two important factors: muscle mass and liver synthetic function, both of which are impaired in advanced liver disease. Baseline SCr is also significantly lower due to protein malnutrition and muscle wasting. More than 50% of glomerular function can be lost before SCr rises, thus delaying the diagnosis of AKI [9]. In addition, high bilirubin is known to interfere with creatinine assays [10].

Use of oliguria as a diagnostic criterion for AKI in patients with cirrhosis is equally filled with flaws. These patients might have decreased urine output, yet may have relatively normal GFR. Urine output might also be decreased because of intra-abdominal hypertension secondary to massive ascites. On the other hand, urine output may be artificially increased with the use of diuretics. Therefore, decreased or increased urine output in patients with cirrhosis must be interpreted with caution.

## 10.5 New Definitions

Defining AKI in patients with chronic liver disease has been difficult and many groups have tried to attain consensus on the same. Acute Dialysis Quality Initiative (ADQI) in 2010 defined the term 'hepatorenal disorders (HRD)' to describe patients with advanced cirrhosis and concomitant renal dysfunction to include any form of kidney disease occurring in patients with cirrhosis [11]. Table 10.1 illustrates the revised definitions as proposed by International Club of Ascites (ICA).

In 2012, ICA met to define the concept of AKI in patients with liver disease and give objective criterion for the diagnosis. These AKI criteria are different to those with non-liver disorders, in that there is:

1. No urine output criteria: as these patients often have decreased urine output, and retain sodium and may also have normal GFR (contributed to by reduction in fluid and sodium delivery to the distal nephron, increase in proximal sodium reabsorption and loss of tubulo-glomerular feedback) [12].
2. Serum creatinine rise rather than absolute value is taken presuming the rise is within the last 7 days, so the conventional criteria of a rise of creatinine to reach an absolute value of 1.5 mg/dL is removed. There is no absolute value except in stage 3 (ICA-AKI criterion) (Table 10.2). This is different from the existing standards [13, 14]. It was found that though the cut-off of SCr ≥1.5 mg/dL (133 μmol/L), correlated with mortality and progression to higher AKI stages, even small changes in serum creatinine could influence the outcome, thus a more sensitive target was needed. Hence, the lowering of the creatinine threshold was proposed [15–17].
3. Baseline SCr: ICA proposed that serum creatinine in the last 3 months before admission could be used as the baseline reference value. ICA did not include the Cockcroft-Gault or Modification of Diet in Renal Disease (MDRD) formulas as they were felt to be inaccurate in calculation of kidney function in cirrhosis with ascites as they overestimate true GFR, especially in patients younger than 50 years or with ascites [10, 15, 16, 18].

**Table 10.1** Criterion for AKI in liver disease [16]

| |
|---|
| **Baseline SCr**: A value of SCr obtained in the previous 3 months, when available, can be used as baseline SCr. In patients with more than one value within the previous 3 months, the value closest to the admission time to the hospital should be used.<br>In patients without a previous SCr value, the SCr on admission should be used as baseline. |
| **Definition of AKI**<br>• Increase in SCr ≥0.3 mg/dL (≥26.5 μmol/L) within 48 h; or,<br>• A percentage increase SCr ≥50% from baseline which is known, or presumed, to have occurred within the prior 7 days |
| **Definition of response**<br>**No response:** No regression of AKI<br>**Partial response:** Regression of AKI stage with a reduction of SCr to ≥0.3 mg/dL (26.5 μmol/L) above the baseline value<br>**Full response:** Return of SCr to a value within 0.3 mg/dL (26.5 μmol/L) of the baseline value |

*AKI* acute kidney injury, *SCr* serum creatinine

A further classification is described below in Table 10.2 but it is predominantly extrapolated from adult literature, and care should be taken while applying these principles to paediatric practice.

## 10.6 Aetiology of AKI in Chronic Liver Disease

AKI in liver failure can be multifactorial. The predominant causes of AKI in cirrhosis can be either functional or structural as described in Table 10.2. The functional group includes prerenal azotemia due to various causes and hepatorenal syndrome while the structural causes are predominantly due to intrinsic renal disease which may be tubulointerstitial or glomerular in origin [19]. Ascertaining the cause of AKI in these patients is equally important. The importance of ascertaining the exact cause of AKI was demonstrated by Martín-Llahí [20], who found that the most common causes of AKI in cirrhosis were prerenal azotemia, acute tubular necrosis (ATN) and HRS. The 3-month probability of survival was highest with parenchymal nephropathy (73%), followed by hypovolaemia-associated renal failure (46%). About one-third of patients with infection associated renal failure survive to 3 months, yet survival is lower (15%) for patients with HRS [4]. Therefore, knowing the aetiology of AKI in ALF helps not only in precise management of the causative condition but also predicts prognosis.

**Table 10.2** Classification of acute kidney injury in liver failure [4, 11, 16, 19, 20, 22, 46]

| **1. Kidney injury based on acuteness of presentation** [11, 15, 47] | |
|---|---|
| **(a) Acute kidney Injury**<br>* | A rise in SCr ≥ 50% from baseline, or a rise SCr > 0.3 mg/dL<br>Type-1 HRS is a specific form of acute kidney injury |
| **(b) Chronic kidney disease** | GFR < 60 mL/min for >3 month calculated using MDRD-6 formula |
| **(c) Acute-on-chronic kidney disease** | Rise in SCr ≥ 50% from baseline or a rise of SCr > 0.3 mg/dL in a patient with cirrhosis whose GFR is <60 mL/min for >3 month calculated using MDRD-6 formula |
| **2. Kidney injury based on the cause of renal injury** | |
| **Functional Causes:**<br>(a) Prerenal azotemia: volume responsive states<br>(b) HRS type 1 and 2: (volume unresponsive state): now called as HRS-AKI [16]<br>**Structural Causes:**<br>(a) Intrinsic renal disease as acute tubular necrosis (ATN), tubulointerstitial and glomerular diseases [19].<br>(b) Post renal ARF<br>**Post-transplant ARF:** can be a separate entity in itself with multifactorial causation | |
| **3. On basis of severity (ICA-AKI CRITERION)** [16] | |
| **Staging of AKI**<br>• **Stage 1:** increase in SCr ≥0.3 mg/dL (26.5 μmol/L) or increase in SCr ≥1.5 to 2-fold from baseline.<br>• **Stage 2:** increase in SCr >2-fold to 3-fold from baseline<br>• **Stage 3:** increase of SCr >3-fold from baseline or SCr ≥4.0 mg/dL (353.6 μmol/L) with an acute increase ≥0.3 mg/dL (26.5 μmol/L) or initiation of renal replacement therapy. | |

Amongst genetic causes, renal involvement in childhood liver diseases with multi-system involvement is not unusual. These include Alagille syndrome and hepatorenal fibrocystic disorders (ciliopathies) (including autosomal dominant polycystic kidney disease *(ADPKD)* and autosomal recessive polycystic kidney disease *(ARPKD)*, Caroli syndrome and congenital hepatic fibrosis) and rarer conditions such as Bardet Biedl syndrome and Joubert syndrome.

## 10.7 Hepatorenal Syndrome

A common prevalent myth is that every kidney dysfunction in a patient with liver disease is hepatorenal syndrome (HRS). But this is not true and in fact of all cases of acute kidney injury in liver failure patients, only a small proportion of patients have the HRS. In an analysis of 129 cirrhotic patients with ascites and AKI, HRS was responsible for the deterioration of kidney function in only 7.6% [21].

Broadly speaking, HRS is defined as the occurrence of renal failure in a patient with advanced liver disease in the absence of an identifiable cause of renal failure and the diagnosis rests on the exclusion of other causes of AKI with concomitant unresponsiveness to volume expansion and meeting the diagnostic criteria for HRS. The ICA met in 2012 to propose the latest criterion to redefine AKI in patients with liver failure (on the basis of a baseline creatinine). They tried to quantify response to treatment and explored the concept of HRS as HRS-AKI [16, 22, 23], Table 10.3 elaborates the differences between the criteria proposed by ICA 2012 and 2007.

**Table 10.3** Classification of hepatorenal syndrome [16, 22, 23, 26, 48]

| |
|---|
| **HRS-AKI (ICA 2012 criterion)**<br>• Diagnosis of cirrhosis and ascites<br>• Diagnosis of AKI according to ICA-AKI criteria<br>• No response after 2 consecutive days of diuretic withdrawal and plasma volume expansion with albumin 1 g per kg of body weight<br>• Absence of shock<br>• No current or recent use of nephrotoxic drugs (NSAIDs, aminoglycosides, iodinated contrast media, etc.)<br>• No macroscopic signs of structural kidney injury defined as:<br>– absence of proteinuria (>500 mg/day)<br>– absence of microhaematuria (>50 RBCs per high power field)<br>– normal findings on renal ultrasonography |
| **ICA 2012**: Major differences as compared to ICA 2007<br>1. Serum creatinine 0.133 mmol/L (1.5 mg/dL) criterion has been replaced to AKI definition as per ICA-AKI criterion<br>2. More subjective criterion with respect to improvement after 2 days of diuretic withdrawal and plasma expansion with albumin<br>3. Emphasizes the use of urine biomarkers (as NGAL, KIM1, IL 18, F-ABP and albumin) in differentiating HRS and ATN |

*AKI* acute kidney injury, *ICA-AKI* International Club of Ascites—AKI (ICA-AKI), *NSAID* non-steroidal anti-inflammatory drugs, *NGAL* neutrophil gelatinase-associated lipocalin, *KIM* kidney injury molecule, *F-ABP* liver-type fatty acid binding protein, *HRS* hepatorenal syndrome, *ATN* acute tubular necrosis

It might be a real challenge to distinguish between various causes of AKI in these patients and hence it will not be surprising if, in future, we see the inclusion of urinary biomarkers in the differential diagnosis of various causes of AKI in liver disease.

## 10.8 Kidney Injury in Acute-on-Chronic Liver Disease

Acute-on-chronic liver failure (ACLF) is a specific syndrome characterized by acute decompensation (which may be due to development of ascites, encephalopathy, haemorrhage or bacterial infection) in a patient with chronic liver disease. In adults, a majority of patients who develop ACLF will have chronic liver disease (CLD) of varying aetiologies. Whereas in paediatrics, CLD is easily recognized only in a limited number of conditions like biliary atresia, Wilson's disease and autoimmune liver disease. Triggers for precipitation of acute liver insufficiency depend upon geographic location, timing of diagnosis and severity of the presentation amongst others.

The EASL-Chronic Liver Failure (CLIF) Consortium (CANONIC study: EASL-CLIF Acute-on-Chronic Liver Failure Study) (2013), proposed screening all cirrhotic patients at admission for organ dysfunction (CLIF Consortium Organ Failure score) for the diagnosis of ACLF [24]. This scores unlike the previous scores for liver patients has kidney dysfunction at the heart of classifying patients into severity of liver failure and subsequent management and transplantation. Alam demonstrated the application and reliability of the CLIF-SOFA score in a paediatric setting and its preference over other severity scores including model for end-stage liver disease and paediatric end-stage liver disease [25].

## 10.9 Pathogenesis of Hepatorenal Syndrome

Now the question is what causes renal failure and hepatorenal syndrome in patients with cirrhosis? Of vital importance is an understanding of what happens when portal hypertension develops. The mononuclear-phagocyte system of the liver (hepatocytes and Kupffer cells) is important in clearing organisms from the portal circulation. During genesis of cirrhosis, the drained portal blood is obstructed, leading to swollen mucosa and weakened intestinal movements which bring about massive bacterial overgrowth in the lumen of the bowel, particularly Gram-negative enteric organisms and the production of endotoxin. Defects in mucosal barrier function, reduction in healthy normal functioning hepatocytes or Kupffer cells and portal-systemic shunts can cause invasion of enteric organisms/endotoxin into blood resulting in bacterial translocation, bacteraemia and intestinal endotoxaemia. This may elicit an inflammatory response, with increased production of pro-inflammatory cytokines mainly tumour necrosis factor $\alpha$ and interleukin-6. These mediators release vasodilator factors especially nitric oxide in the splanchnic area; this response leads to vasodilatation of the splanchnic arterial vessels. The consequence of this splanchnic vasodilatation is a reduction in systemic vascular resistance and a decrease in the effective circulating blood volume which in turn activates the Renin Angiotensin Aldosterone System (RAAS), unloads the high-pressure baroreceptors in the carotid body and aortic arch with a subsequent activation of the sympathetic nervous system, and induces non-osmotic release of vasopressin. These changes lead to intense renal vasoconstriction and reduced glomerular filtration rate (GFR). With worsening of the liver disease and progression of cirrhosis, further splanchnic vasodilatation occurs, creating a vicious cycle that favours further activation of the RAAS, sympathetic nervous system, and vasopressin release, and subsequent intensification of renal vasoconstriction [16, 26, 27].

In patients with advanced cirrhosis, events that lead to the slightest change in perfusion pressure will translate into a major decrease in renal blood flow that might precipitate intense renal vasoconstriction and HRS. Identifiable precipitating events include intravascular volume depletion from aggressive use of diuretics, gastrointestinal bleeding or following large-volume paracentesis without albumin infusion, also known as post-paracentesis syndrome. Non-steroidal anti-inflammatory drugs may also cause renal failure in patients with cirrhosis, since their kidney function is extremely dependent on renal prostaglandin synthesis.

## 10.10 Kidney Injury Post-liver Transplant

Acute and chronic renal injury in non-renal solid organ transplantation such as liver transplantation is multifactorial as explained in Table 10.4. AKI post-transplantation can increase the duration of hospital stay in the intensive care unit, infectious complications and mortality. Presence of AKI and/or and being on renal replacement therapy prior to transplant are important risk factors for renal dysfunction after transplantation. Early implementation of a renoprotective regimen with identification candidates at risk for renal injury are beneficial in preventing post-operative renal injury [28, 29].

Paracentesis is routinely done in patients with large ascites pre-operatively. It causes a decrease in systemic vascular resistance and RAAS activation [29]. One must be aware of the paracentesis-induced circulatory dysfunction (PICD) which is an entity caused due to excessive paracentesis and can be explained by the marked activation of the RAAS activation [30]. Strategies to prevent this entity include the use of plasma expanders such as albumin [30].

After the patient comes back to the ICU from the operating theatres after liver transplantation, it is important to ensure that the patient is intravascularly euvolaemic and remains haemodynamically stable. We at King's College Hospital aggressively treat hypovolaemia using clinical cues along with non-invasive cardiac output monitoring. We also monitor and replace ongoing drain losses with albumin.

In the pre and post-transplant period, potentially nephrotoxic drugs (NSAIDS, angiotensin converting enzyme (ACE) inhibitors, diuretics, aminoglycosides amongst others) should be avoided or used with caution and their need reviewed on a daily basis [31].

**Table 10.4** Risk factors for acute kidney injury post liver transplantation

| |
|---|
| **Pre-transplant:** [28, 29] |
| 1. Pre-transplant renal dysfunction [49] |
| 2. Hepatorenal syndrome [50] |
| 3. Acute physiology and chronic health evaluation (APACHE) II scores |
| 4. High model for end-stage renal disease (MELD) score [51] |
| 5. Infection |
| 6. Baseline age [50] |
| 7. Dilutional hyponatremia [50] |
| 8. Refractory ascites [50] |
| **Intraoperative risk factors** |
| 1. Hemodynamic instability during intraoperative stage [28, 29, 49] |
| 2. Intraoperative bleeding and volume of transfused blood products, especially packed red cells [49] |
| 3. Intraoperative diuresis [49] |
| **Post-operative risk factors** |
| 1. Early (1st week) prerenal and ischemic acute tubular necrosis are the principal causes of acute renal failure<br>(a) Drug toxicity.<br>(b) Allograft dysfunction esp. grade II–IV dysfunction of the liver graft (odd ratio ¼: 5.6, P¼: 0.002) [52] |
| Late (2–4 weeks) [52]: Multifactorial ARF is the most common aetiology<br>Risk factors include<br>1. Intraoperative and 24-h post-transplant creatinine level > 0.9 mg/dL and high-dose tacrolimus-based immunosuppression [53]<br>2. Drug-induced interstitial nephritis [28]<br>3. Graft dysfunction grades III–IV [28]<br>4. Contrast nephropathy [28] |

Post-operatively, calcineurin-induced nephrotoxicity (CNI) can be acute, associated with high trough levels which may ultimately lead to chronic kidney disease. Hence various strategies are employed including CNI minimization protocols, delayed introduction of CNI or CNI withdrawal and conversion to less nephrotoxic agents [32]. For those with renal impairment, a renal sparing immunosuppressive regimen including the use of IL2 blockers in the peri-operative period and rapid introduction of a calcineurin sparing agent such as mycophenolate mofetil or rapamycin post-operatively could be a possibility. In our practice, routine monitoring of renal function post liver transplantation includes routine renal function tests such as urea and serum creatinine as well as Cystatin C levels together with regular blood pressure monitoring. Table 10.4 summarizes the risk factors for AKI in patients post liver transplantation.

## 10.11 Treatment Options

General principles in treating AKI in patients with liver failure remain the same as for treating critically ill children with AKI without liver disease. Scant paediatric data on HRS partly because of small numbers and partly due to difficulty in diagnosing this condition. We present the treatment protocol based on experience and extrapolated from adult literature.

1. *Prophylactic antibiotics*: Bacterial translocation is a major precipitant of vasodilator release mediated through mediators like TNF-α. Prophylactic antibiotics prevent bacterial translocation and suppress pro-inflammatory cytokine formation implicated in the pathogenesis of HRS [33].
2. *Judicious use of nephrotoxic drugs*: One must avoid use of nephrotoxic drugs and if they are being used, their need should be reviewed periodically and stopped at the first available opportunity.
3. *Maintain intravascular volume and avoid fluid overload*: It is important to ensure that the intravascular status of the patient is maintained and child remains haemodynamically stable. The surviving sepsis guidelines [34] emphasize resuscitation in shock with aggressive management with fluids if mean arterial pressure is low or lactate is high. It is therefore recommended to aggressively treat hypovolaemia and maintain mean arterial pressure using bedside clinical cues alongside use of cardiac output monitors (ultrasound or invasive). It is also important to watch for ongoing losses as drain losses and replace them as required. It is equally important to watch for fluid overload and intervene early as fluid overload has been convincingly shown to be associated with increased morbidity and mortality.
4. *Reduction of intra-abdominal pressure and paracentesis*: As cirrhosis progresses, ascites becomes progressively resistant to diuretics and with increasing ascites there is raised intra-abdominal pressure with antecedent adverse effects on renal and systemic haemodynamics. Therefore ascites should be managed with paracentesis followed by albumin infusion. In cirrhotic patients, RAAS activation causes sodium retention and the use of aldosterone antagonists (such as spironolactone) have been effective in the management of ascites [35].

## 10.12 Pharmacological Treatment

1. *Albumin*: Albumin used in combination with vasoconstrictors represents the therapeutic gold standard for the hepatorenal syndrome (HRS) [36]. Its role in cirrhosis is secondary to its ability to mobilize ascitic fluid due to its plasma volume expander property as well as its efficacy in restoring plasmatic oncotic pressure. But the benefits are more far reaching and include the role of albumin in binding and transportation of substances (exogenous/endogenous), anti-inflammatory, antioxidant, immunomodulatory role and its role in endothelial stabilization [37].
2. *Vasoconstrictors*: Arterial vasodilation is considered an important pathophysiologic mechanism of HRS, hence use of arterial vasoconstrictors can be therapeutic, especially in type 1 HRS. A number of vasoconstrictors including terlipressin, ornipressin, midodrine plus octreotide, and norepinephrine have been used.

Terlipressin is the most widely used vasoconstrictor. It is a prodrug which is converted to its active form lysine vasopressin. The effect half-life of terlipressin is 6 h. Since lysine vasopressin is released over a sustained period, it can be administered by bolus injection rather than by continuous infusion [38]. Terlipressin causes vasoconstriction in the arterioles of the splanchnic circulation, decreasing portal flow, and therefore, redistributing the blood flow to the kidneys [39]. However, one needs to carefully monitor the ischaemic side effects of terlipressin.

*Vaptans*: Vaptans are V2 receptor antagonists. They are aquaretic agents that promote water excretion and diuresis with dilute urine and improve hyponatremia. They also block V2 -mediated vasodilatation. Moreover, V2 receptor antagonism increases plasma vasopressin concentration which may cause unopposed hyperstimulation of the vasoconstrictor V1 receptors leading to free water excretion. This improves hyponatremia and therefore ascites.

## 10.13 Supportive Therapies

Since increased portal pressures are important in pathogenesis of hepatorenal syndrome, surgical modalities to decrease the same such as TIPSS (Trans-jugular Intrahepatic Porto-systemic shunt) might have a role in their management. Other supportive therapies as renal replacement, liver assist devices could be considered. If nothing works, liver or even simultaneous liver–kidney transplant is an option.

*TIPSS (Trans-jugular Intrahepatic Porto-systemic shunt)*: There are multiple retrospective case series showing the use of TIPSS. The main advantage is that there is a good response to ascites. But the incidence of encephalopathy increases as well [40].

*Renal Replacement Therapy (RRT)*: Continuous RRT expedites removal of solutes as ammonia, lactate and helps maintain electrolyte balance which is important in acute liver failure patients. RRT is especially indicated in life-threatening complications as severe hyperkalaemia, severe acidosis and other uremic complications. Anticoagulation is tricky in liver failure due to the risk of haemorrhage secondary to clotting factor deficiencies and thrombocytopenia with possible DIC. CRRT can serve as a bridge to liver transplantation but should be considered at an early stage to help prevent further deterioration and allow potential spontaneous recovery or bridge to liver transplantation [41]. Renal replacement therapy carries with it inherent risks, due to episodes of intradialytic hypotension, which can result in changes in intracranial pressure. This is especially significant in patients of hyper-acute liver failure [42, 43].

## 10.14 Extracorporeal Liver Support Systems (ELS)

Extracorporeal liver support systems (ELS) are being increasingly used in clinical practice. They are temporizing artificial support systems which remove toxins from the circulation. The devices available currently include the following: single-pass albumin dialysis (SPAD), plasma exchange combined with haemodialysis/CRRT,

Prometheus™ dialysis and molecular adsorbent recirculating system (MARS™) [44]. Artificial liver support systems include albumin based systems and bio-artificial liver support systems (LSS) (which use human hepatocytes or porcine liver cells). These are described in the chapter on extracorporeal liver assist devices in liver failure.

In patients who do not respond to any treatment modality, liver transplant is the ultimate option. Focus is gradually shifting from liver transplantation to simultaneous liver–kidney transplants. Recent evidence has established criterion for simultaneous liver and kidney transplant in the liver transplant wait-listed candidates who develop simultaneous liver and kidney dysfunction [45].

Table 10.5 summarizes our recommendations to manage AKI in children with liver disease whereas Table 10.6 has a flow chart which we use as our personal practice at King's College Hospital for children with liver disease and suspected or confirmed HRS.

**Table 10.5** Practical management of AKI in children with liver disease

| |
|---|
| **Treat associated conditions** |
| 1. GI bleeding/hypovolaemia—fluid resuscitation |
| 2. Avoid fluid overload |
| 3. Infections—aggressive antibiotics (as per local policy/antibiogram) |
| 4. Adrenal insufficiency |
| 5. Avoid nephrotoxic drugs |
| 6. Treat raised IAP (drain and replace with albumin) |
| 7. Large volume ascites—TIPSS/paracentesis |
| 8. Differentiate between natural progression of liver disease with its complications versus acute AKI with other organ dysfunction |
| 9. Once in ICU—Cardiac output monitoring, fluids, full organ support, prioritize transplant listing |
| **Pharmacological therapy** |
| 1. Albumin |
| 2. Vasoconstrictors including vasopressin and vasopressin analogues, octreotide, norepinephrine—Started early |
| 3. Vaptans (rarely used) |
| **Assist devices** |
| 1. Continuous renal replacement therapy ± Plasmapheresis |
| 2. MARS |
| 3. SPAD |
| **Surgical Therapy** |
| 1. TIPSS: Trans-jugular intrahepatic Porto-systemic shunt (very rarely done) |
| 2. Liver transplant |

*GI* gastrointestinal, *IAP* intra-abdominal pressure, *TIPSS* trans-jugular intrahepatic porto-systemic shunt, *ICU* intensive care unit, *AKI* acute kidney injury, *MARS* molecular adsorbent recirculating system, *SPAD* single-pass albumin dialysis

**Table 10.6** Personal practice for management of hepatorenal syndrome at King's College Hospital, London

| |
|---|
| Target the precipitating factors and address pre-renal issues avoiding fluid overload |
| ⇓ |
| Start noradrenaline (maximum of 1 mcg/kg/min) |
| ⇓ |
| Add Terlipressin infusion– 10 mcg/kg/day (Closely monitor ischemic side effects) |
| ⇓ |
| Double the dose of Terlipressin if no response in 48 h (decrease in serum creatinine and/or sustained rise in blood pressure |
| ⇓ |
| Stop Terlipressin if no response by 5 days |
| ⇓ |
| Continuous Renal Replacement Therapy, TIPSS, OLT |

*TIPSS* trans-jugular intrahepatic porto-systemic shunt, *OLT* orthotopic liver transplantation

## 10.15 Future Directions

The two questions for the future are:

1. Are there any new pharmacological or non-pharmacological treatments available or being researched for the treatment of HRS?
2. Awaiting the availability and accessibility to new therapies, can we do anything to improve the prognosis of these patients who do not seem to respond to standard therapy?

In the management of AKI in liver disease, it is very important to accurately differentiate HRS from other types of AKI especially acute tubular necrosis. Some of the treatment failures are wrongly attributed to terlipressin inefficacy but in fact, are due to use of this drug in incorrectly diagnosed hepatorenal syndrome. Therefore, the role of urine biomarkers, particularly NGAL and interleukin-18 can potentially help in the differential diagnosis between HRS and acute tubular necrosis. If the role of urinary biomarkers in the differential diagnosis of various aetiologies of AKI in liver disease is confirmed in larger studies, it will not be surprising to see the incorporation of urinary biomarkers in the diagnostic algorithm of type-1 HRS. In addition to accurate diagnosis, some drugs under investigation need a special mention. Serelaxin is a recombinant form of the human peptide relaxin-2 that has been shown to be a renal vasodilator in healthy volunteers. Serelaxin selectively and very effectively increases renal blood flow with no alterations in mean arterial pressure. If researchers could replicate the effect of selective renal vasodilation in patients with renal failure, serelexin could prove an invaluable drug in the treatment of HRS-1 where renal vasoconstriction plays an important role in the pathogenesis.

There is a very important role of inflammation in acute-on-chronic liver failure (ACLF) where HRS occurs as a part of multi-organ failure. Here, failure of one organ system can affect the function of another organ system. Therefore, one needs to target not only the systemic vasodilation which plays an important role in the pathogenesis of HRS but also the systemic inflammation and optimization of function of other organs. Removal of inflammatory and vasoactive mediators by the use of plasmapheresis could be a useful therapeutic adjunct. In a recent study on acute liver failure in adults, total plasma exchange decreased systemic inflammatory response and improved organ failures and survival.

## Conclusion

Acute kidney injury in liver failure is a relatively common entity and incidence varies depending on the liver disease in question—acute liver failure, chronic liver disease, acute decompensation of chronic liver failure or post-liver transplantation. Just like AKI in any critical illness, AKI in liver disease carries an equally poor prognosis with increased morbidity and mortality. Though AKI is common in cirrhotic patients with ascites, not all patients of cirrhosis who develop AKI have HRS. Criteria to diagnose AKI in liver patients are different from AKI in patients with non-liver diagnoses, but unfortunately there are no paediatric specific criteria. Though diagnostic criteria exist to diagnose hepatorenal syndrome, differentiating it from other causes of AKI in cirrhotic patients continues to be a challenging task in some patients. Biomarkers may start to play an important role to differentiate between the various causes of AKI in this patient population which is crucial for diagnostic, therapeutic and prognostic purposes. Therefore, it will not be surprising to see incorporation of biomarkers in the definition of AKI in patients with liver disease soon (instead of creatinine). Vasoconstrictors seem to play an important role in the treatment of HRS if they are started early. The role of prolonged vasoconstrictors to bridge these patients to liver transplant is open to debate and future trials.

### Key Learning Points

- AKI can take place in any liver disease—Acute liver failure, chronic liver failure, acute decompensation of chronic liver disease
- Realizing the limitations of existing diagnostic parameters as creatinine and appreciating the use of biomarkers.
- Use of revised criterion for AKI in liver disease in terms of its diagnosis, staging and response to treatment (ICA-AKI/international club of ascites guidelines)
- Recognizing the causes, especially reversible /functional causes of AKI is important.
- Hepatorenal syndrome is rare in paediatrics, but its unique aetiopathogenesis, treatment, types and outcome make it a distinct entity to understand and treat
- In post liver transplant patients, use of renoprotective strategies and recognition of risk factors leading to AKI is important.

## References


1. Flint A. Clinical report on hydro-peritoneum based on an analysis of forty-six cases. Am J Med Sci. 1863;45:306–39.
2. Kaddourah A, Basu RK, Bagshaw SM, Goldstein SL, Investigators A. Epidemiology of acute kidney injury in children and young adults. N Engl J Med. 2017;376(1):11–20.
3. Wei Y, Zhang L, Lin H, Li J, Li B, Yan L, et al. Factors related to post–liver transplantation acute renal failure. Transplant Proc. 2006;38(9):2982–4.
4. Garcia-Tsao G, Parikh CR, Viola A. Acute kidney injury in cirrhosis. Hepatology. 2008;48(6):2064–77.
5. Tujios SR, Hynan LS, Vazquez MA, Larson AM, Seremba E, Sanders CM, et al. Risk factors and outcomes of acute kidney injury in patients with acute liver failure. Clin Gastroenterol Hepatol. 2015;13(2):352–9.
6. Thabut D, Massard J, Gangloff A, Carbonell N, Francoz C, Nguyen-Khac E, et al. Model for end-stage liver disease score and systemic inflammatory response are major prognostic factors in patients with cirrhosis and acute functional renal failure. Hepatology. 2007;46(6):1872–82.
7. Moore K. Renal failure in acute liver failure. Eur J Gastroenterol Hepatol. 1999;11(9):967–75.
8. Belcher JM, Garcia-Tsao G, Sanyal AJ, Bhogal H, Lim JK, Ansari N, et al. Association of AKI with mortality and complications in hospitalized patients with cirrhosis. Hepatology. 2013;57(2):753–62.
9. Slack A, Yeoman A, Wendon J. Renal dysfunction in chronic liver disease. Crit Care. 2010;14(2):214.
10. Francoz C, Prié D, Abdelrazek W, Moreau R, Mandot A, Belghiti J, et al. Inaccuracies of creatinine and creatinine-based equations in candidates for liver transplantation with low creatinine: impact on the model for end-stage liver disease score. Liver Transpl. 2010;16(10):1169–77.
11. Nadim MK, Kellum JA, Davenport A, Wong F, Davis C, Pannu N, et al. Hepatorenal syndrome: the 8th international consensus conference of the Acute Dialysis Quality Initiative (ADQI) Group. Crit Care. 2012;16(1):1.
12. Angeli P, Gatta A, Caregaro L, Menon F, Sacerdoti D, Merkel C, et al. Tubular site of renal sodium retention in ascitic liver cirrhosis evaluated by lithium clearance. Eur J Clin Investig. 1990;20(1):111–7.
13. Bellomo R, Ronco C, Kellum JA, Mehta RL, Palevsky P. Acute renal failure–definition, outcome measures, animal models, fluid therapy and information technology needs: the Second International Consensus Conference of the Acute Dialysis Quality Initiative (ADQI) Group. Crit Care. 2004;8(4):1.
14. KDIGO AKI Guideline.pdf [Internet]. [cited 2016 Dec 4]. http://www.kdigo.org/clinical_practice_guidelines/pdf/KDIGO%20AKI%20Guideline.pdf
15. Wong F, O'Leary JG, Reddy KR, Patton H, Kamath PS, Fallon MB, et al. New consensus definition of acute kidney injury accurately predicts 30-day mortality in patients with cirrhosis and infection. Gastroenterology. 2013;145(6):1280–1288.e1.
16. Angeli P, Ginès P, Wong F, Bernardi M, Boyer TD, Gerbes A, et al. Diagnosis and management of acute kidney injury in patients with cirrhosis: revised consensus recommendations of the International Club of Ascites. J Hepatol. 2015;62(4):968–74.
17. Mindikoglu AL, Weir MR. Current concepts in the diagnosis and classification of renal dysfunction in cirrhosis. Am J Nephrol. 2013;38(4):345.
18. Agarwal B, Davenport A. Difficulties in diagnosing acute kidney injury post liver transplantation using serum creatinine based diagnostic criteria. World J Hepatol. 2014;6(10):696–703.
19. Nayak SL, Maiwall R, Nandwani A, Ramanarayanan S, Mathur RP, Kumar R, et al. Management of acute kidney injury in cirrhosis. Hepatol Int. 2013;7(3):813–9.
20. Martín-Llahí M, Guevara M, Torre A, Fagundes C, Restuccia T, Gilabert R, et al. Prognostic importance of the cause of renal failure in patients with cirrhosis. Gastroenterology. 2011;140(2):488–496.e4.

21. Montoliu S, Ballesté B, Planas R, Alvarez MA, Rivera M, Miquel M, et al. Incidence and prognosis of different types of functional renal failure in cirrhotic patients with ascites. Clin Gastroenterol Hepatol. 2010;8(7):616–22. quiz e80
22. Salerno F, Gerbes A, Ginès P, Wong F, Arroyo V. Diagnosis, prevention and treatment of hepatorenal syndrome in cirrhosis. Gut. 2007;56(9):1310–8.
23. Arab JP, Claro JC, Arancibia JP, et al. Therapeutic alternatives for the treatment of type 1 hepatorenal syndrome: a Delphi technique-based consensus. World J Hepatol. 2016;8(25):1075–86.
24. Acute-on-chronic liver failure: a new syndrome that will re-classify cirrhosis - 1-s2.0-S0168827814009325-main.pdf [Internet]. [cited 2016 Nov 27]. http://ac.els-cdn.com/S0168827814009325/1-s2.0-S0168827814009325-main.pdf?_tid=45fd39b8-b406-11e6-a541-00000aacb35e&acdnat=1480185151_d564d18bb6df3885942409ff765c0c4f
25. Alam S, Lal BB, Sood V, Rawat D. Pediatric acute-on-chronic liver failure in a specialized liver unit: prevalence, profile, outcome, and predictive factors. J Pediatr Gastroenterol Nutr. 2016;63(4):400–5.
26. Barbano B, Sardo L, Gigante A, Gasperini ML, Liberatori M, Giraldi GDL, et al. Pathophysiology, diagnosis and clinical management of hepatorenal syndrome: from classic to new drugs. Curr Vasc Pharmacol. 2014;12(1):125–35.
27. Arroyo V, Colmenero J. Ascites and hepatorenal syndrome in cirrhosis: pathophysiological basis of therapy and current management. J Hepatol. 2003;38(Suppl 1):S69–89.
28. Pham P-TT, Pham P-CT, Wilkinson AH. Management of renal dysfunction in the liver transplant recipient. Curr Opin Organ Transplant. 2009;14(3):231–9.
29. Guerrero-Domínguez R, López-Herrera Rodríguez D, Acosta-Martínez J, Bueno-Pérez M, Jiménez I. Perioperative renal protection strategies in liver transplantation. Nefrologia. 2014;34(3):276–84.
30. Sola-Vera J, Miñana J, Ricart E, Planella M, González B, Torras X, et al. Randomized trial comparing albumin and saline in the prevention of paracentesis-induced circulatory dysfunction in cirrhotic patients with ascites. Hepatology. 2003;37(5):1147–53.
31. Egerod Israelsen M, Gluud LL, Krag A. Acute kidney injury and hepatorenal syndrome in cirrhosis: acute kidney injury. J Gastroenterol Hepatol. 2015;30(2):236–43.
32. LaRosa C, Baluarte HJ, Meyers KEC. Outcomes in pediatric solid-organ transplantation. Pediatr Transplant. 2011;15(2):128–41.
33. Fernández J, Navasa M, Planas R, Montoliu S, Monfort D, Soriano G, et al. Primary prophylaxis of spontaneous bacterial peritonitis delays hepatorenal syndrome and improves survival in cirrhosis. Gastroenterology. 2007;133(3):818–24.
34. Dellinger RP, Levy MM, Rhodes A, Annane D, Gerlach H, Opal SM, et al. Surviving sepsis campaign: international guidelines for management of severe sepsis and septic shock: 2012. Crit Care Med. 2013;41(2):580–637.
35. Bernardi M, Servadei D, Trevisani F, Rusticali AG, Gasbarrini G. Importance of plasma aldosterone concentration on the natriuretic effect of spironolactone in patients with liver cirrhosis and ascites. Digestion. 1985;31(4):189–93.
36. Facciorusso A, Nacchiero MC, Rosania R, Laonigro G, Longo N, Panella C, et al. The use of human albumin for the treatment of ascites in patients with liver cirrhosis: item of safety, facts, controversies and perspectives. Curr Drug Saf. 2011;6(4):267–74.
37. Garcia-Martinez R, Caraceni P, Bernardi M, Gines P, Arroyo V, Jalan R. Albumin: pathophysiologic basis of its role in the treatment of cirrhosis and its complications. Hepatology. 2013;58(5):1836–46.
38. Delmas A, Leone M, Rousseau S, Albanèse J, Martin C. Clinical review: Vasopressin and terlipressin in septic shock patients. Crit Care. 2004;9(2):212.
39. Fayed N, Refaat EK, Yassein TE, Alwaraqy M. Effect of perioperative terlipressin infusion on systemic, hepatic, and renal hemodynamics during living donor liver transplantation. J Crit Care. 2013;28(5):775–82.
40. Rees CJ, Rose JD, Record CO, Day CP, Bassendine MF, James OF, et al. Transjugular intrahepatic portosystemic shunt: a limited role in refractory ascites. Eur J Gastroenterol Hepatol. 1997;9(10):969–73.

41. Deep A, Stewart CE, Dhawan A, Douiri A. Effect of continuous renal replacement therapy on outcome in pediatric acute liver failure. Crit Care Med. 2016;44:1910.
42. Davenport A, Bouman C, Kirpalani A, Skippen P, Tolwani A, Mehta RL, et al. Delivery of renal replacement therapy in acute kidney injury: what are the key issues? Clin J Am Soc Nephrol. 2008;3(3):869–75.
43. Moore JK, Love E, Craig DG, Hayes PC, Simpson KJ. Acute kidney injury in acute liver failure: a review. Expert Rev Gastroenterol Hepatol. 2013;7(8):701–12.
44. Smith SK, Rosenthal P. Pediatric liver failure: we came, we saw, but have we conquered? F1000Research [Internet]. 2017. [cited 2017 Oct 27];6. https://www.ncbi.nlm.nih.gov/pmc/articles/PMC5580426/
45. Nadim MK, Sung RS, Davis CL, Andreoni KA, Biggins SW, Danovitch GM, et al. Simultaneous liver–kidney transplantation summit: current state and future directions. Am J Transplant. 2012;12(11):2901–8.
46. Urrunaga NH, Mindikoglu AL, Rockey DC. Renal dysfunction in cirrhosis. Curr Opin Gastroenterol. 2015;31(3):215–23.
47. Wong F, Nadim MK, Kellum JA, Salerno F, Bellomo R, Gerbes A, et al. Working Party proposal for a revised classification system of renal dysfunction in patients with cirrhosis. Gut. 2011;60(5):702–9.
48. Rognant N. Acute kidney injury in patients with chronic liver disease. World J Hepatol. 2015;7(7):993–1000.
49. Faenza S, Bernardi E, Cimatti M, Dante A, Mancini E, Miklosova Z, et al. Acute renal failure after liver transplantation in MELD era. Transplant Proc. 2007;39(6):1945–6.
50. Planas R, Montoliu S, Ballesté B, Rivera M, Miquel M, Masnou H, et al. Natural history of patients hospitalized for management of cirrhotic ascites. Clin Gastroenterol Hepatol. 2006;4(11):1385–94.
51. Lee JP, Heo NJ, Joo KW, Yi NJ, Suh K-S, Moon KC, et al. Risk factors for consequent kidney impairment and differential impact of liver transplantation on renal function. Nephrol Dial Transplant. 2010;25(8):2772–85.
52. Cabezuelo JB, Ramirez P, Acosta F, Sanchez Bueno F, Robles R, Pons JA, et al. Prognostic factors of early acute renal failure in liver transplantation. Transplant Proc. 2002;34(1):254–5.
53. Smoter P, Nyckowski P, Grat M, Patkowski W, Zieniewicz K, Wronka K, et al. Risk factors of acute renal failure after orthotopic liver transplantation: single-center experience. Transplant Proc. 2014;46(8):2786–9.

# Renal Emergencies in PICU: Electrolyte, Acid Base and Blood Pressure Issues

# 11

Prabhakar Nayak and Manish D. Sinha

**Case Vignettes**

**Case 1:**

A 3-year-old boy who was previously well presented to the emergency department with a short history of fever, diarrhoea and drowsiness. He was found to be severely tachpnoeic, tachycardic, and hypotensive with poor capillary refill. His blood gas showed severe metabolic acidosis and hyperkalaemia. A clinical diagnosis of septic shock was made, he was aggressively fluid resuscitated and antibiotics administered promptly. He required intubation and ventilation and commencement of inotropes. He was transferred to PICU for further management. His blood results revealed evidence of acute kidney injury (AKI) with elevated urea and creatinine and he became oliguric, despite adequate fluid management. His urine output worsened and he started becoming fluid overloaded and hyperkalaemic. He was fluid restricted, administered 'balanced' intravenous maintenance fluids and commenced on diuretics, with close monitoring of his fluid balance. Acidosis was corrected with bicarbonate infusion and hyperkalaemia improved. His condition stabilised with good intensive care management. His AKI reversed, his renal function tests normalised and his urine output improved without the need for renal replacement therapy.

P. Nayak (✉)
Birmingham Children's Hospital, Birmingham Women's and Children's NHS Foundation Trust, Birmingham, UK
e-mail: prabh.nayak@nhs.net

M. D. Sinha
Department of Paediatric Nephrology, Evelina London Children's Hospital, Guy's and St Thomas' NHS Foundation Trust, London, UK
e-mail: manish.sinha@gstt.nhs.uk



A. Deep, S. L. Goldstein (eds.), *Critical Care Nephrology and Renal Replacement Therapy in Children*, https://doi.org/10.1007/978-3-319-90281-4_11

**Case 2:**
A 10-year-old boy AH was brought to the accident and emergency department via ambulance following one short lasting seizure. His mother informed the paramedics that he had been complaining of double vision prior to this and had complained of headaches over the past few days. His blood pressure at the time of retrieval was 180/110 mmHg and this was confirmed on repeated measurement. Manual BP assessed on arrival at the A&E department was 178/100 mmHg; his 99th percentile for age and height was 116/76 mmHg. He was diagnosed to have a hypertensive emergency with evidence of hypertensive encephalopathy. On clinical evaluation he was drowsy, unresponsive and needed intubation and ventilation to secure his airway following another seizure in the emergency department. AH was euvolaemic and had no neurocutaneous lesions, his 4-limb blood pressure was uniformly elevated, and he had bilateral good volume femoral pulses. Examination of his pupils and fundii were unremarkable. His seizures were controlled with a single dose of lorazepam. Venous access was obtained and blood tests taken including full blood count, urea and electrolytes; plans made for obtaining urine specimen for protein. Chest X-ray showed no evidence of cardiomegaly or fluid overload. 12-lead ECG showed evidence of left ventricular hypertrophy (LVH) with echocardiography confirming concentric LVH and well preserved biventricular systolic and diastolic function. There was no evidence of coarctation of aorta. CT brain was not diagnostic and an MRI brain confirmed evidence of posterior reversible encephalopathy syndrome (PRES) with typical bilateral parieto-occipital distribution. Urinary tract ultrasound study was unremarkable except for the bipolar length of the right kidney, which was significantly smaller than the left kidney at 6 versus 9.8 cm, respectively. Doppler assessment of the right kidney showed typical findings of 'parvus et tardus' of Doppler flows involving the main right renal artery with difficulty in obtaining a reasonable Doppler flow for a short segment of the main artery.

AH was treated with intravenous labetalol and his systolic blood pressure precipitously reduced before further reduction in a controlled meticulous manner targeting systolic BP levels at 150–160 mmHg in the initial 4–6 h, than 130–140 mmHg in the next 24–72 h before targeting 110–120 mmHg over the 3–7 days. Amlodipine was added as an oral antihypertensive therapy on day 3 with additional medications in the form of atenolol and doxazosin to achieve adequate blood pressure control. MRA study of the renal vessels showed evidence of right main renal artery stenosis and this was treated with percutaneous balloon angioplasty 6 weeks following initial presentation, with good angiographic appearance post balloon angioplasty. Six months following this initial procedure AH continues to be on a single antihypertensive agent and blood pressure normal at 104/62 mmHg and repeat echocardiogram study now showing no evidence of LVH and continued good biventricular function.

**Table 11.1** Assessment and management of hydration status

| Hydration status | Clinical features | Initial management |
|---|---|---|
| Dehydrated | Tachycardia, cool peripheries, prolonged capillary refill time, low BP (late sign), dry mucous membranes, sunken eyes | Fluid resuscitation 10–20 mL/kg 0.9% saline, assess urine output and repeat if necessary |
| Euvolaemic | | Fluid challenge 10–20 mL/kg 0.9% saline over 1 h, with furosemide 1–2 mg/kg IV |
| Intravascular fluid overload | Tachycardia, gallop rhythm, raised JVP and BP, palpable liver | Furosemide 2–4 mg/kg IV; haemofiltration/dialysis if no response |

In this chapter, we will discuss the common renal emergencies encountered in paediatric critical care setting with special emphasis on fluids, electrolytes, acid-base and blood pressure. Acute Kidney Injury (AKI) causes potentially reversible inability of the kidneys to maintain fluid balance and adequate acid–base balance. It is usually characterised by 'uraemia', raised serum creatinine, hyperkalaemia, metabolic acidosis, potentially reduced consciousness and oliguria in the acute phase. Oliguria is defined as urine output <1 mL/kg/h in neonates and infants, <0.5 mL/kg/h in children and <400 mL/day in older teenagers and adults. Polyuric renal failure is rarely encountered on the PICU.

Aggressive therapy to correct hypovolaemia, hypotension and hypoxia may lead to spontaneous recovery of renal function including oliguria without the need for renal replacement therapy (RRT). Most oliguria respond to IV fluid challenge and it is important not to use diuretics prior to adequate volume replacement. Give 10–20 mL/kg 0.9% saline and assess response using haemodynamic variables like heart rate, capillary refill time, change in central venous pressure (CVP) and toe-core temperature difference. Repeat fluid challenge if necessary. There is an ongoing debate whether to use crystalloids or colloids in fluid resuscitation with no clear-cut answer. This management is summarised in Table 11.1.

If response to fluid resuscitation if poor, one needs to ascertain whether additional fluids should be administered or not as overzealous fluid therapy might worsen the respiratory and/or cardiovascular status. CVP and invasive blood pressure monitoring should be commenced. Blood or appropriate blood products would be indicated if haemoglobin is low or the patient is coagulopathic or thrombocytopenic. Start inotropes/vasopressors/inodilators as appropriate. Functional (Prerenal) and renal disease must be distinguished using urine Na, fractional excretion of sodium (FeNa), urine osmolality, urine urea and creatinine ratios. Following the fluid challenge and if cardiovascularly stable, furosemide 1–2 mg/kg as a bolus or 0.2–1.0 mg/kg/h infusion can be used. This may not improve renal function but may increase urine output and thus the fluid balance.

## 11.1 Hyperkalaemia in AKI

Serum potassium should be regularly measured and aggressive treatment should be initiated if serum potassium is gap between > and 6.5 mmol/L. Normal levels are 3.5–5.0 mmol/L. Hyperkalaemia in AKI results from a profound reduction in the GFR, decreased distal water and solute delivery limiting Na/K exchange and if there is no sufficient time for adaptive mechanisms to develop. It may also be seen in specific conditions, for example, as a part of tumour lysis syndrome at the initiation of antineoplastic therapy for large tumours. Acid–base balance is assessed preferably using an arterial sample, failing which a central venous or free flowing capillary sample could be used. Ensure that squeezed capillary samples don't give erroneous results. Do not attribute high levels to squeezed samples, instead immediately recheck using an appropriate sample. Ensure no potassium is given either in IV fluids or enterally, including feeds and supplements. Initiate emergency treatment of hyperkalaemia. Monitor for signs of toxicity on ECG (peaked T waves, prolongation of PR interval, flattening of P waves, QRS widening). Realising that ventricular arrhythmias or cardiac arrest may occur at any point during worsening hyperkalaemia and that this progression may occur quickly over a matter of minutes is extremely important. Of the various emergency treatment measures for hyperkalaemia, only ion exchange resins remove potassium from the body. Hence it is important to check the serum potassium for rebound frequently. Emergency measures to treat hyperkalaemia are summarised in Table 11.2.

*Severe hypokalaemia* similarly can have serious consequences if left untreated. Moderate hypokalaemia is defined as a serum potassium level of <3.0 mmol/L and severe hypokalaemia is a serum potassium level of <2.5 mmol/L. Decreased extracellular potassium causes myocardial hyperexcitability with the potential to develop re-entrant arrhythmias. Causes of hypokalaemia include diarrhoea, medications like furosemide, steroids, diabetes insipidus, hypoaldosteronism and hypomagnesaemia.

**Table 11.2** Emergency management of hyperkalaemia

| Mechanism of action | Treatment | Dose | Side effects |
|---|---|---|---|
| Reduces toxic effect of K by stabilising the myocardium | 10% calcium gluconate IV | 0.5–1 mL/kg over 5–10 min | Bradycardia, hypercalcaemia |
| Shifts K into cells | Salbutamol nebuliser | 2.5 mg if <25 kg<br>5 mg if >25 kg | Tachycardia, hypertension |
| | Salbutamol IV | 4 mcg over 10 min | |
| | Sodium bicarbonate 8.4% IV | 1–2 mmol(mL)/kg over 10–30 min | Hypernatraemia, decreases ionised calcium |
| | Glucose and insulin IV | 0.5–1 g/kg/h dextrose (2.5–5 mL/kg/h 10% dextrose) and insulin 0.1–0.2 units/kg as a bolus OR continuous infusion of 10% dextrose at 5 mL/kg/h with insulin 0.1 unit/kg/h | Hypoglycaemia, monitor blood glucose every 15 min during bolus and then at least hourly |
| Removal of K from the body | Calcium resonium orally or rectally with oral lactulose | 1 g/kg every 4 h<br>2.5 mL < 1 year; 5 mL 1–5 years; 10 mL > 5 years | Slow effect. Large doses can cause impaction in the gut |

ECG changes include flattening of the T waves; U waves, prolongation of the QT interval, potential to develop ventricular tachycardia/ventricular fibrillation (VF)/ torsades de pointes (torsades) and clinical signs include muscle weakness, ileus and rhabdomyolysis.

*Management of hypokalaemia*: Continuous ECG monitoring is essential. Blood gas monitoring provides excellent 'point-of-care' testing for electrolytes at the bedside as most blood gas machines also provide electrolyte information. Recheck serum potassium on the blood gas every 30 mins. Correct low Mg; hypokalaemia can be refractory till Mg levels rise to 0.7–1.0 mmol/L. *Central potassium chloride (KCl)* 1 mmol/kg is intravenously infused through a central line over 2 h, diluted in 0.9% saline to 0.5 mmol/mL. Dose is repeated until serum potassium is greater than 3.0 mmol. *Only in arrest scenario*, potassium as KCL is given neat over 3–5 mins, central (IV or intraosseous) or peripherally.

*Hypocalcaemia* is said to be present when ionised calcium (iCa) levels are less than 0.8 mmol/L ± ECG changes. Clinical signs include prolonged QT, pulseless electrical activity (PEA)/VF. Management of hypocalcaemia includes IV calcium gluconate, making sure that serum magnesium levels are corrected and maintained between 0.7 and 1.0 mmol/L and if phosphate is low (<2.0 mmol/L), ensure to give calcium phosphate. In an arrest scenario, give calcium gluconate as bolus till iCa is between 1.0 and 1.4 mmol/L checking iCa levels every 30–60 min. One must be aware that correction of acidosis would further decrease the levels of ionised calcium.

*Hypercalcaemia* is said to be present when the ionised calcium is more than 3.0 mmol/L ± ECG changes. Certain high-risk situations like post-rhabdomyolysis, malignancy, primary hyper-parathyroidism and vitamin D disorders, amongst others, can predispose to hypercalcaemia. Patient might have polyuria, tachyarrhythmias, hypertension or coma. Management includes restoring intravascular fluid volume using fluid bolus followed by forced diuresis using furosemide bolus aiming for a neutral fluid balance. If hypercalcaemia is refractory, continuous renal replacement therapy (CRRT) is preferred to peritoneal dialysis. We need to check ionised calcium levels every 30–60 min.

Although crystalloids remain the first choice for fluid therapy, there may be differences in renal outcomes amongst them. Animal studies suggest that *hyperchloraemia* resulting from 0.9% saline infusion may affect renal haemodynamics causing arteriolar vasoconstriction and decreased glomerular filtration rate. Recent studies have demonstrated decreased renal artery flow and cortical perfusion in subjects who received 0.9% saline compared to a balanced solution (Plasma-Lyte 148). Evidence is emerging that shows lower increases in creatinine, lower incidence of pRIFLE 'injury' and need for RRT in critically ill patients treated with a chloride-restrictive approach as opposed to a chloride-liberal strategy. Based on the available evidence now, it appears that 'balanced' salt solutions may be preferable for managing patients at risk of and with AKI.

Urine output is one of the most important features of end-organ perfusion. It not only reflects poor blood flow to the kidneys, it is incorporated in the definition of AKI as well. One has to ensure that oliguria is not present because of a blocked urinary catheter before deciding on the fluids or diuretics. Flush the urinary catheter with 1 mL/kg normal saline to ensure it is not blocked. Ultrasound of the kidneys and the renal tract is important to exclude hydronephrosis, bladder clots and posterior urethral valves in a male patient.

Fluid overload is associated with impaired oxygenation and morbidity in critically ill children [1]. Daily weight measurements and hourly input/output monitoring are the best indicators of fluid balance. Consider restriction of fluids to insensible losses (400 mL/sq.m/day or 30 mL/kg/day) plus urine output and other measured losses. Early initiation of RRT to treat fluid overload is important. During RRT, fluid intake can be liberalised and the critically ill children be given adequate nutritional calories during their period of critical illness. Children with high fluid overload more than 10% at the time of CRRT initiation have a significant higher mortality and poor outcome [2].

There is no evidence that low dose dopamine prevents renal failure or improves renal function. Dopamine may increase renal blood flow and thus urine output but appears to have no significant advantage over other inotropes in hypotensive patients. Drugs that maintain diuresis have a useful role in avoiding fluid overload.

Therefore a vigilant look for fluid balance, type of resuscitation and maintenance fluids administered, nutrition, acid–base status and regular monitoring of electrolytes using at least daily monitoring of urea and electrolytes (U&Es), creatinine, bicarbonate, calcium, magnesium and phosphate will help maintain appropriate milieu for a critically ill child. More frequent monitoring may be required according to clinical picture and aetiology.

## 11.2 Hypertension in the PICU

Hypertension affects significant number of children admitted to the ICU often with variable clinical presentations and underlying causes. Blood pressure (BP) control is regulated by the vascular endothelial system, the renin–angiotensin system and the sympathetic nervous system. Disruption of these pathways as seen in disease states such as systemic inflammation, renal ischaemia and renal parenchymal disease will result in dysregulation of blood pressure. Additional pathways whose dysregulation may result in hypertension include activation of vasoactive mediators, influencing vascular tone (e.g. endothelin and angiotensin II) and those that regulate the intravascular volume such as atrial natriuretic peptides [3].

The pathophysiology of hypertension in these unwell children is multifactorial and often secondary to one or more processes affecting the cardiac output, large arteries, changes in circulating blood volume or the peripheral vascular bed. For example, hypertension in renal disease may be secondary to one or more of several mechanisms including renal ischaemia in renovascular disease, hyper-reninaemia in reflux nephropathy and sodium and fluid retention in acute nephritic syndromes. The onset of renal dysfunction and its progressive worsening clinically manifests with more severe and difficult to control hypertension often with multiple mechanisms being involved in the same patient [4]. Similarly, the cause of the hypertension in patients with coarctation is complex and the main theories include mechanical obstruction, altered autonomic and baroreceptor function and activation of the renin–angiotensin system [5].

Additional important causes of severe hypertension in children that may need more specific management include those affecting the endocrine system including the adrenal gland function that result in the failure of normal feedback by cortisol and thus in the resultant increase in adrenocorticotrophic hormone, giving rise to congenital adrenal hyperplasia. Cushing's syndrome results from excessive production of adrenocorticotrophic hormone, either pituitary or ectopic. Low-renin hypertensive conditions present with cardinal features of hyperaldosteronism including retention of sodium, hypokalaemia, hypertension, and suppressed activity of renin in the plasma, but these conditions have high levels of aldosterone and others have low levels with several conditions secondary to monogenic causes of hypertension. Central nervous system disorders and drug induced hypertension should always be additionally considered as possible causes of hypertension as these may need more specific treatment [4, 6].

### 11.2.1 Definition of Hypertension

In children hypertension is confirmed following finding of systolic BP (SBP) or diastolic BP (DBP) ≥95th percentile for their gender, age and height using an appropriate-sized BP cuff on repeat measurements. Stage 1 hypertension is defined as systolic and/or diastolic BP level between the 95th and up to 5 mmHg above 99th percentile. Stage 2 hypertension is defined as systolic and/or diastolic BP level > 5 mmHg above the 99th percentile. For adolescents 16 years and older, hypertension is defined as BP ≥140/90 mmHg; Stage 1 hypertension as 140–159/90–99 mmHg and Stage 2 hypertension as 160–179/100–110 mmHg [6].

Expert consensus suggests further categorisation of hypertension as 'severe hypertension' at 20% above the stage 2 hypertension threshold or with systolic BP above 180 mmHg in an adolescent 16 years or older [7]. The clinical evaluation of the child with severe hypertension should determine the presence of any acute organ dysfunction that may be evident on history, physical examination or investigation. Organ dysfunction when present usually involves the cardiac, neurological or renal systems although rarely can cause microangiopathic haemolytic anaemia. A 'hypertensive urgency' is defined as a case with severe hypertension but no target organ dysfunction and 'hypertensive emergency' as life-threatening condition in a child with severe hypertension and associated with evidence of target organ dysfunction. 'Malignant hypertension' is a term used to describe an *acute elevation* of BP from a previously normal or abnormal BP level and associated with at least three different organ systems secondary to hypertension and includes presence of microangiopathic haemolytic anaemia [6].

A detailed clinical history and clinical examination should be performed with important points on history and examination as shown in Tables 11.3 and 11.4 [8].

Cardiac and neurological symptoms and signs are commonly the presenting features in children with severe hypertension although sometimes children will present

**Table 11.3** Important points on history in a child with severe hypertension

| |
|---|
| • Maternal history including antenatal imaging findings of oligohydramnios, maternal health and drugs during pregnancy |
| • Neonatal history including prematurity, birth weight, umbilical vessel cannulation, arterial/venous thrombosis, hypoxia, bronchopulmonary dysplasia and medications |
| • History that may suggest other system involvement including cardiac, renal, endocrine or haemoglobinopathies like sickle cell disease |
| • History of taking any prescribed medications, over the counter medications or recreational drugs in adolescents |
| • History for syndromes such as Neurofibromatosis 1 and Williams syndrome |
| • History suggestive of phaechromocytoma |
| • History of headaches, nausea, vomiting, epistaxis, abdominal pain, increasing tiredness or irritability |

Modified with permission from [8]

**Table 11.4** Important points on examination in a child with severe hypertension

| |
|---|
| • Neonates, infants and young children may present with congestive heart failure, shock or with irritability, failure to thrive, seizures, unexplained tachypnoea, apnoea or lethargy |
| • Absent or difficult to palpate femoral pulses |
| • 4-limb blood pressure with discrepant upper limb >lower limb BP levels by >10 mmHg |
| • Clinical findings in keeping with possible causes of renovascular disease including neurofibromatosis 1, Williams syndrome and Ehler's Danlos syndrome |
| • Evaluation for intracranial pathology such as cerebrovascular stroke, intracranial mass or head trauma |

Modified with permission from [8]

with an incidental finding of severe hypertension [9, 10]. Severe hypertension may lead to congestive cardiac failure and fluid overload. These children have evidence of cardiomegaly on chest X-ray, with echocardiography confirming cardiac dilation and impaired ventricular function with mitral incompetence and pulmonary oedema. This life-threatening combination requires intensive care with positive pressure ventilation, diuretic therapy, inotropic support, and sometimes haemofiltration. Paediatric nephrologists, cardiologists, and intensivists should be involved in the investigation and management of severe life-threatening hypertension [4].

The presence of any 'Red flag' symptoms and signs outlined in Table 11.5 in a child with hypertension should alert the clinician of more severely elevated level of hypertension that needs early/urgent investigation and management [3].

Seizures are common [11] although headaches, vomiting and lethargy may also be seen frequently [9, 10]. Facial palsy is seen infrequently [9, 10].

*Hypertensive retinopathy* has been reported in up to 18% of children with severe hypertension [12]. The development of visual disturbances may be secondary to acute encephalopathy or secondary to ophthalmic involvement (caused by retinal involvement, vitreous haemorrhage, and infarction of the anterior visual pathways) and will only be correctly identified following formal ophthalmic assessment [12, 13]. Rarely permanent visual loss may result [12] although more often cortical

**Table 11.5** Red flags on history and physical examination in a child with severe hypertension

| Red flags | End-organ dysfunction |
|---|---|
| Cardiomegaly<br>Gallop rhythm<br>Breathlessness<br>Pulmonary oedema | Cardiac failure |
| Nausea and vomiting<br>Headaches<br>Upper motor neuron signs<br>Hemiparesis or monoparesis<br>Bell's palsy<br>Loss of vision or blurred vision<br>Seizures<br>Altered sensorium<br>Drowsiness/reduced Glasgow coma scale | Hypertensive encephalopathy |
| Acute and chronic hypertensive changes on fundoscopy | Hypertensive vascular changes, retinal bleeding and cotton wool lesions |
| Papilloedema | Increased intracranial pressure |

Modified with permission from [8]

blindness is temporary associated with cerebral oedema and resolves completely leaving no visual impairment.

*Posterior reversible encephalopathy syndrome (PRES)* is a clinico-radiological entity characterised by a variable combination of impairment of consciousness, seizure activity, headaches, visual abnormalities, nausea/vomiting, and focal neurological signs [14–17]. The neurological involvement is secondary to oedema involving the posterior portion of the cerebral hemispheres, especially bilaterally in the parieto-occipital regions but this may spread to involve the cortical (frontal lobe), subcortical (basal ganglia) regions and unusually also to the brainstem and cerebellum [17]. There is usually no change seen on computerised tomographic scans and magnetic resonance imaging is diagnostic and reveals increased signals predominantly involving the posterior regions of the cerebral hemispheres. Vascular/angiographic imaging is not routinely performed or required in these patients but when performed MR angiography shows vasculopathy with multifocal areas of dilatation and narrowing matching the posterior distribution of the changes [15, 17]. Although uncontrolled severe hypertension is the most common trigger for PRES, other aetiologies are also well described such as elevated calcineurin drug levels (e.g. Tacrolimus). In these patients with associated aetiologies, the level of hypertension may not be severe but still needs to be optimally controlled [17].

In all patients with severe hypertension, it is important to carefully evaluate for any evidence of fluid overload and perform essential investigations including chest X-ray and obtain a detailed echocardiogram study to establish any evidence of hypertensive cardiac involvement including evidence of left ventricular hypertrophy, systolic and diastolic ventricular dysfunction.

### 11.2.2 Cause of Hypertension

Younger children are more likely to have secondary hypertension as opposed to adolescents [10, 18], and those with severe hypertension usually display an underlying cause as opposed to those with lower levels of hypertension [18]. The underlying cause of severe hypertension varies with age. In those with an identifiable underlying cause, renal parenchymal, renovascular and coarctation of aorta are more common in the youngest children whilst renal disease, non-adherence to prescribed antihypertensive medication and drug induced hypertension in the older adolescents. Table 11.6 provides an exhaustive although not complete list of causes of hypertension in children [8]. Drug induced hypertension results due to an adverse effect of another drug or due to the antagonising effect on the antihypertensive medication the child may already be on. It should be considered in all causes of unexplained hypertension that is severe or difficult to control [6].

### 11.2.3 Management of Severe Hypertension

All children with severe hypertension should be referred urgently to paediatric intensivists and/or paediatric nephrologists via the Paediatric Emergency department. Timely management of severe hypertension that has not yet resulted in symptomatic target organ involvement (hypertensive urgency) should be controlled urgently to avoid development of a hypertensive emergency. Symptomatic hypertensive patients should be managed on the intensive care unit or high dependency unit with continuous or frequent monitoring of BP by a clinical team that has expertise in the management of severe hypertension and in the use of appropriate antihypertensive agent/s including intravenous medications.

The aim of the management of severe hypertension is to achieve clinical improvement whilst not compromising blood flow to critical organs. All children with a hypertensive emergency should be treated with an intravenous antihypertensive medication to achieve rapid but controlled lowering of blood pressure. This is essential to avoid unexpected hypotension and possible hypoperfusion that may lead to serious adverse outcomes including acute kidney injury or rarely visual loss and permanent brain injury. Clinical improvement in these patients is often seen with relatively small improvements in BP, typically following 10–15% reduction from presenting systolic BP level usually within the 1st hour, therefore, the immediate aim should never be to reduce BP level rapidly to achieve a numerical 'normal' BP level. Following this early controlled lowering of systolic BP levels, as a guide, the eventual target BP should be defined, and the total reduction in systolic blood pressure calculated with the level reduced by 25–33% in the initial 6–8 h, 2/3rds of the total in the next 24–36 h and the total reduction achieved over the subsequent 48–72 h [4, 6]. If blood pressure drops more rapidly than desired than volume expansion with isotonic saline should be considered in addition to slowing or cessation of intravenous antihypertensive medication.

**Table 11.6** Causes of secondary hypertension during childhood

| | |
|---|---|
| **Parenchymal renal disease** | **Cardiovascular** |
| Glomerulonephritis | Coarctation of aorta |
| Post infection | Takayasu's arteritis |
| IgA nephropathy, HSP nephritis | **Central nervous system** |
| Lupus nephritis | Pain |
| ANCA associated nephritis | Convulsions |
| Anti-GBM nephritis | Increased intracranial pressure |
| Focal and segmental glomerulosclerosis | Guillain-Barré syndrome |
| Pyelonephritis related renal scarring | Dysautonomia |
| Acute kidney injury with salt and water Overload | **Malignancy** |
| Polycystic kidney disease | Wilms' tumour (Nephroblastoma) |
| Chronic kidney disease | Neuroblastoma |
| Obstructive uropathy | Pheochromocytoma |
| **Solid organ transplantation** | **Drugs** |
| **Renovascular** | Amphetamine, cocaine or other sympathomimetics |
| Renal artery stenosis | Antidepressants and antipsychotics |
| Idiopathic | Acute Vitamin D intoxication, hypercalcaemia |
| Fibromuscular dysplasia | Oral contraceptive pills |
| Neurofibromatosis type 1 | Calcineurin inhibitors (cyclosporine/ tacrolimus) |
| Williams syndrome | Decongestants containing phenylephrine and pseudoephedrine |
| Mid-aortic syndrome | Erythropoiesis stimulating agents |
| Thrombosis of renal artery or vein | Glucocorticoids |
| Acute or post haemolytic uraemic syndrome | NSAID's |
| Fistulae | Recent discontinuation of antihypertensive/s |
| External compression | **Others** |
| **Endocrine** | Obstructive sleep apnoea |
| Cortisol/glucocorticoid excess | Bronchopulmonary dysplasia |
| Aldosterone/ mineralocorticoid excess | |
| Catecholamine excess | |
| Congenital adrenal hyperplasia | |
| Thyroid disease | |
| **Monogenic causes of hypertension** | |
| Apparent Mineralocorticoid excess | |
| Liddle syndrome | |
| Glucocorticoid remediable aldosteronism | |
| Congenital adrenal hyperplasia | |
| Gordon syndrome | |

Modified with permission from [8]

Children with a hypertensive emergency are often systemically unwell and additionally need supportive management including critical evaluation and monitoring of airway for possible mechanical ventilation; if there are seizures or these develop during antihypertensive therapy they need specific treatment with anti-epileptic medications. Intracranial pathology as cause of severe hypertension should be considered and excluded as its presence secondary to a stroke, intracranial mass or head injury will influence decisions regarding rate of reduction and targeted BP level to be achieved to avoid compromising cerebral perfusion.

A key factor to assess is the degree of extracellular fluid volume overload. In the presence of fluid overload with elevated jugular venous pressure and/or pulmonary oedema, removal of extra fluid by diuretic (e.g. furosemide) challenge or by dialysis in those with associated renal impairment is required. Acute rise in BP level can sometimes be observed in patients with malignant hypertension because of salt and water depletion and resultant peripheral vasoconstriction and these patients require isotonic saline to control their BP. Close monitoring of fluid balance including urine output in addition to cardiac and BP monitoring is therefore essential in all children with severe hypertension [4].

### 11.2.4 Pharmacotherapy

There are several drugs available for use in hypertensive emergencies and urgencies and achieve BP control using different pathways resulting in vasodilatation within seconds to minutes, including (1) calcium channel blockade (intravenous infusion Nicardipine; oral Nifedipine and Isradipine); (2) stimulation of central alpha-2 adrenergic receptors (intravenous bolus Clonidine); (3) reducing vascular tone via increased nitric oxide (intravenous infusion sodium nitroprusside and nitroglycerine); (4) beta blockade (intravenous infusion Esmolol); (5) alpha and beta blockade (intravenous infusion Labetalol); (6) angiotensin converting enzyme inhibitor (ACEi) which leads to reduction of vascular tone and blood volume (intravenous infusion Enalaprilat; oral Captopril and Lisinopril); (7) diuretics by reduction of blood volume (intravenous or oral Furosemide) and (8) direct vasodilatation (intravenous Hydralazine and oral Minoxidil). These are listed in Table 11.7.

Labetalol is an effective first choice in the majority of cases with severe hypertension that require rapid control of BP. Sometimes use of Labetalol may not be possible as a drug of first choice because of severe hypertensive cardiomyopathy or it may be insufficient to control BP level, at which point sodium nitroprusside (SNP) should be added. SNP is especially useful because of its rapid onset and very short duration of action. Constant monitoring of the rate of infusion and blood pressure is required during its use. Thiocyanate toxicity can occur with long-term therapy or with renal insufficiency. Although nitroprusside has been used without ill effects for up to 10 days [19, 20], levels of thiocyanate should be monitored in the blood after 48 h, and treatment discontinued if the concentration exceeds 100 mcg/mL. The solution must be protected from light by shielding the syringe and infusion lines. Hydralazine is another potent and useful intravenous antihypertensive in controlling hypertension especially when SNP needs to be stopped soon because of concerns regarding thiocyanate toxicity and intravenous medication still required. Other intravenous drugs are now available including Nicardipine, Esmolol and Glyceryl trinitrate but their use in children is limited by their availability, clinical experience and reported use in children and young people. In volume expanded states, loop diuretic furosemide is indicated.

**Table 11.7** Antihypertensive medications for severe hypertension presenting as hypertensive emergency, hypertensive urgency and malignant hypertension

| Drug | Onset of action | Dose and route | Mode of action | Comment |
|---|---|---|---|---|
| Labetalol | 2–5 min | 1–3 mg/kg per hour as intravenous infusion | Vasodilatation | Titrate rate of constant infusion against change in blood pressure |
| Hydralazine | 10–20 min | 1. 0.3–0.5 mg/kg as intravenous slow bolus dose; maximum 4-hourly<br>2. 0.025–0.05 mg/kg per hour intravenously to maximum of 3 mg/kg in 24 h | Direct vasodilator | Titrate rate of constant infusion against change in blood pressure<br>Initial dose may cause marked hypotension<br>Adverse events include flushing and tachycardia |
| Nicardipine | 5–10 min | 1–3 µg/kg per min as an intravenous infusion | Calcium channel blocker | Adverse events include tachycardia, headache and thrombophlebitis |
| Esmolol | 1–2 min | 100–500 µg/kg per min as an intravenous infusion | Beta blocker results in vasodilatation | Contraindicated in patients with asthma<br>Adverse events include bradycardia, bronchospasm and heart failure |
| Glyceryl trinitrate | 2–5 min | 0.1–2 µg/kg per min as an intravenous infusion | Vasodilatation by increasing nitric oxide | Adverse events include methaemoglbinaemia, flushing, headache and reflex tachycardia<br>May be helpful in older adolescents |
| Clonidine | 10 min | 2–6 µg/kg per dose as an intravenous bolus | Central alpha agonist | Adverse events include sedation, dry mouth and may cause bradycardia |
| Enalapril | <15 min | 0.005–0.01 mg/kg per dose as an intravenous bolus | Angiotensin converting enzyme inhibitor (ACEi) | Adverse events include marked fall in BP in high renin states, headache and hyperkalaemia<br>Contraindicated in bilateral renovascular disease |
| Furosemide | 5–10 min | 2–5 mg/kg intravenously as a bolus injection or as an infusion if required | Loop diuretic | For severe intravascular volume expansion states<br>Rapid administration of large doses may be ototoxic<br>Hypokalaemia |

(continued)

**Table 11.7** (continued)

| Drug | Onset of action | Dose and route | Mode of action | Comment |
|---|---|---|---|---|
| Nifedipine (capsules) | 20–30 min | 0.25–0.5 mg/kg orally | Calcium channel blocker | Effect is less controllable than with antihypertensive medications given as intravenous infusion; may cause tachycardia; child must bite and swallow capsule, or liquid contents should be removed via a needle and syringe and then swallowed |
| Isradipine | 60 min | 0.05–1 mg/kg per dose orally | Calcium channel blocker | Effect is less controllable than with antihypertensive medications given as intravenous infusion; can cause marked drop in BP level |
| Captopril | 10–20 min | 0.1–0.2 mg/kg per dose orally | Angiotensin converting enzyme inhibitor (ACEi) | Contraindicated in bilateral renovascular disease |
| Minoxidil | 5–10 min | 0.1–0.2 mg/kg orally | Direct vasodilator | Effect is less controllable than with antihypertensive medications given as intravenous infusion May cause fluid retention |

Modified from [4, 6, 19]

Severe hypertension which is asymptomatic and not associated with target organ dysfunction is often managed successfully with oral nifedipine in rapid-acting capsule and requires the child to bite the capsule, as most absorption occurs after swallowing the contained liquid. For young children, a liquid preparation is available, or the contents of a capsule may be aspirated by syringe and fine needle and then administered orally. Intravenous hydralazine may also be used as a rapid-acting vasodilator. Other oral agents that may be used for a hypertensive urgency are listed in Table 11.7 and their use directed by the clinical situation, availability, physician experience and preference. Oral agents or those administered as an intravenous bolus dose give less precise control over the rate of fall of blood pressure, and intravenous infusion treatment is preferred where there is symptomatic severe hypertension that requires more precise controlled reduction of blood pressure level.

### 11.2.5 Change from Intravenous to Oral Antihypertensive Therapy

Once severe hypertension is controlled using an intravenous antihypertensive medication, oral antihypertensive drugs should be commenced to allow ongoing control of hypertension. The underlying cause of severe hypertension, age and associated comorbidities often dictate the choice of antihypertensive therapy. Long acting oral drug such as Amlodipine is an effective first choice for most cases of severe hypertension. Patients with renovascular disease often require two or more medications to control hypertension optimally whilst more specific interventions are planned. Patients with acute kidney injury (AKI), glomerulonephritis and fluid overload have marked improvement of their severe hypertension following management with dialysis and adequate fluid removal, and often regain normal BP control following complete recovery of renal function.

### 11.2.6 Follow-up

All children and young people treated for severe hypertension should have adequate follow-up with a named physician to specifically manage their hypertension, its underlying cause and any associated comorbidities. In the absence of an underlying cardiac cause for hypertension this will often be a paediatric nephrologist along with colleagues in primary and secondary care. Follow-up of these children will include planning any specific treatment as may be indicated in children with renovascular disease, ongoing monitoring of blood pressure level, adjustment of medications and coordinating of further reviews with paediatric neurology and cardiology as indicated. Failure to achieve normal blood pressure in a child with severe hypertension does not mean the failure of antihypertensive management and is likely to be related to the duration and severity of the underlying cause, fixed lesions of renovascular disease that are not amenable to intervention and permanent renal damage, peripheral vascular remodelling or due to unexplained cause. Finally, all children who developed AKI requiring renal replacement therapy (e.g. continuous veno-venous haemofiltration, dialysis) will need follow-up to confirm their renal related parameters including blood pressure, proteinuria and renal function have returned to their previous normal levels.

**Conclusion**

Fluid, acid–base and electrolyte disturbances are very common in children admitted to paediatric critical care. These include hypo/hyperkalaemia, hypo/hypercalcaemia and hypo/hypermagnesaemia. Hyperchloraemia is an important cause of metabolic acidosis that should be kept in mind while analysing and addressing acid–base issues. Fluid overload contributes directly to increased morbidity and mortality and should be vigilantly looked for and addressed. Frequent monitoring of fluid status (amount and type of fluid administered, fluid balance), acid–base and electrolytes is required in any critically ill child admitted to PICU. Hypertension in children is multifactorial and aetiology varies according to age. Hypertensive emergencies should be managed with multidisciplinary input of paediatric intensivists, nephrologists and where indicated, cardiologists and neurologists. Regular follow-up of children is mandatory following PICU/ HDU discharge after the acute episode of hypertension resolves. Finally, all children who develop AKI during PICU admission with hypertension will need follow-up to confirm their renal related parameters including blood pressure, proteinuria and renal function have returned to their previous normal levels.

## References


1. Arikan AA, Zapitelli M, Goldstein SL, Naipaul A, Jefferson LS, Loftis LL. Fluid overload is associated with impaired oxygenation and morbidity in critically ill children. Pediatr Crit Care Med. 2012;13(3):253–8.
2. Gillespie RS, Seidel K, Symons JM. Effect of fluid overload and dose of replacement fluid on survival in hemofiltration. Pediatr Nephrol. 2004;19(12):1394–9.
3. Levy JH, Faraoni D. Pathophysiology and causes of severe hypertension. In: Webb A, Angus D, Finfer S, Gattinoni L, Singer M, editors. Oxford textbook of critical care. 2nd ed. Oxford: Oxford University Press; 2016. Accessed 15 Nov 2017.
4. Sinha MD, Reid CJD. Ch. 58: Systemic arterial hypertension. In: Anderson RH, Baker EJ, Redington A, Rigby ML, Wernovsky G, editors. Paediatric cardiology. 3rd ed. Philadelphia: Elsevier Ltd; 2009. p. 1191–217.
5. Vigneswaran TV, Sinha MD, Valverde I, Simpson JM, Charakida M. Hypertension in coarctation of the aorta: challenges in diagnosis in children. Pediatr Cardiol. 2018;39(1):1–10.
6. Lurbe E, Agabiti-Rosei E, Cruickshank JK, Dominiczak A, Erdine S, Hirth A, Invitti C, Litwin M, Mancia G, Pall D, Rascher W, Redon J, Schaefer F, Seeman T, Sinha M, Stabouli S, Webb NJ, Wühl E, Zanchetti A. 2016 European Society of Hypertension guidelines for the management of high blood pressure in children and adolescents. J Hypertens. 2016;34(10):1887–920.
7. Wu HP, Yang WC, Wu YK, Zhao LL, Chen CY, Fu YC. Clinical significance of blood pressure ratios in hypertensive crisis in children. Arch Dis Child. 2012;97(3):200–5.
8. Singh C, Jones H, Copeman H, Sinha MD. Fifteen-minute consultation: the child with systemic arterial hypertension. Arch Dis Child Educ Pract Ed. 2017;102(1):2–7.
9. Deal JE, Barratt TM, Dillon MJ. Management of hypertensive emergencies. Arch Dis Child. 1992;67(9):1089–92.
10. Flynn J, Zhang Y, Solar-Yohay S, Shi V. Clinical and demographic characteristics of children with hypertension. Hypertension. 2012;60(4):1047–54.
11. Trompeter RS, Smith RL, Neville BCR, Chantler C. Neurological complications of arterial hypertension in children. Arch Dis Child. 1982;57:913–7.
12. Williams KM, Shah AN, Morrison D, Sinha MD. Hypertensive retinopathy in severely hypertensive children: demographic, clinical, and ophthalmoscopic findings from a 30-year British cohort. J Pediatr Ophthalmol Strabismus. 2013;50(4):222–8.
13. Hulse JA, Taylor DSI, Dillon MJ. Blindness and paraplegia in severe childhood hypertension. Lancet. 1979;ii:553–6.
14. Garg RK. Posterior leukoencephalopathy syndrome. Postgrad Med J. 2001;77:24–8.
15. Bartynski W. Posterior reversible encephalopathy syndrome, part 1: fundamental imaging and clinical feature. Am J Neuroradiol. 2008;29:1036–42.
16. Agarwal A, Kapur G, Altinok D. Childhood posterior reversible encephalopathy syndrome: magnetic resonance imaging findings with emphasis on increased leptomeningeal FLAIR signal. Neuroradiol J. 2015;28:638–43.

17. Singh RR, Ozyilmaz N, Waller S, U-King-Im JM, Lim M, Siddiqui A, Sinha MD. A study on clinical and radiological features and outcome in patients with posterior reversible encephalopathy syndrome (PRES). Eur J Pediatr. 2014;173(9):1225–31.
18. Vogt BA. Hypertension in children and adolescents: definition, pathophysiology, risk-factors and long-term sequelae. Curr Ther Res. 2001;62:283–97.
19. Levy JH. Management of severe hypertension in the ICU. In: Webb A, Angus D, Finfer S, Gattinoni L, Singer M, editors. Oxford textbook of critical care. 2nd ed. Oxford: Oxford University Press; 2016. Accessed 15 Nov 2017.
20. Luderer JR, Hayes AH, Dubysisky O, Berlin CM. Longterm administration of sodium nitroprusside in childhood. J Pediatr. 1977;91:490–1.

# Nutrition in a Child with Acute Kidney Injury and on CRRT

# 12

Michael Zappitelli and Timothy E. Bunchman

**Case Vignette**

A 4-year-old girl with cerebral palsy is admitted to the Pediatric Intensive Care Unit (PICU) with severe pneumonia and potentially bacteremia. She is normally tube-fed at home and on multiple medications including anti-seizure and antispasmodic medications. She requires fluid resuscitation, norepinephrine, and invasive mechanical ventilation at admission. By day 2 of PICU admission, her serum creatinine rises from 40 to 120 μmol/L. She has not tolerated an attempt of gastric enteral feeding and is currently receiving dextrose and saline intravenous fluids. By day 5 of PICU admission, she fulfills criteria for renal replacement therapy requirement and continuous renal replacement therapy (CRRT) is initiated. Enteral feeds which were being administered at half-strength are stopped at CRRT initiation. The dietician became involved in the patient's care on PICU day 3. She is now asking what type of formula to use while the patient is on CRRT and questions your suggestion to provide 3 g/kg/day of protein in this child with severe AKI.

M. Zappitelli (✉)
Department of Pediatrics, Division of Nephrology, Toronto Hospital for Sick Children, Toronto, ON, Canada

T. E. Bunchman
Department of Pediatrics, Pediatric Nephrology, Virginia Commonwealth University, Richmond, VA, USA



A. Deep, S. L. Goldstein (eds.), *Critical Care Nephrology and Renal Replacement Therapy in Children*, https://doi.org/10.1007/978-3-319-90281-4_12

## 12.1 Introduction

Malnutrition and protein-energy wasting (or muscle wasting and loss of fat) are common in children in the intensive care unit (ICU) [1]. This is due to many factors, including, but not limited to, hypercatabolism and substrate requirement in the stress-response state, baseline nutritional status prior to acute illness, and ongoing growth needs (including brain growth in infants) [2, 3]. Young children are at highest risk for protein-energy wasting [4, 5]. Children with acute kidney injury (AKI) tend to be among the most critically ill ICU patients and AKI seems to enhance the risk of protein-energy wasting. The presence of AKI and AKI-associated acidosis/uremia alters lipid, carbohydrate, and protein metabolism, leading to promotion of catabolism [2]. With renal replacement therapy (RRT), catabolism is enabled by the addition of nutritional losses caused by RRT, which may worsen preexisting and acute nutritional deficiencies. Finally, fluid overload often occurs in AKI; this poses challenges to providing nutrition. These nutrition problems overlay the fact that underfeeding is common in children admitted to the ICU and is even more prevalent in children with AKI, especially those receiving RRT [6–8]. In children with AKI, the high baseline risk of protein-energy wasting must be appreciated. The goal should be to *provide* and *enhance* nutrition, rather than restrict.

There are no nutrition trials in pediatric AKI. However, observational data support that malnutrition is more common in AKI and contributes to poor outcome [6, 9, 10]. An ongoing multinational pediatric ICU study showed that ICUs with dedicated programs aimed at enteral nutrition advancement had lower infection rates and that adequate protein intake was inversely related to 60-day mortality [11, 12]. Moreover, attesting to the increasingly perceived importance of adequate evaluation and provision of nutrition in critically ill children, consensus guidelines were published in 2017 by the collaboration of two major collaborative groups (American Society of Parenteral and Enteral Nutrition and the Society of Critical Care Medicine) [3]. Table 12.1 provides the non-exhaustive list of selected recommendations from this guideline. Some of the most important conclusions from this guideline was the need for more nutrition research, a more widely systematic approach to nutrition and the need for patient-individualized approach. In recent years, the importance of adequate nutrition in children with AKI is also increasingly appreciated, and is becoming the basic principle of AKI management and often considered an indication for RRT initiation. Children with AKI are indeed the types of patients that require an individualized and thoughtful approach to nutrition. This chapter is not a detailed review on nutrition in critical illness, however references provided were handpicked to provide a comprehensive reading list on this topic. This chapter provides an overview of issues regarding overall assessment of nutritional status, approach and considerations specific to nutrition in children with AKI and those treated with CRRT.

**Table 12.1** Selected recommendations on nutrition in critically ill children (from the recent Society of Critical Care Medicine (SCCM) and American Society for Parenteral and Enteral Nutrition Guideline) [3]

| Recommendation | Brief rationale and additional notes |
|---|---|
| *Nutrition assessment* | |
| Detailed nutritional assessment should be performed within 48 h of PICU admission.<br>Nutritional status should be re-evaluated at least weekly.<br>A nutrition support team, including a dedicated dietitian, should be available on the PICU team. | Observational studies show that malnutrition is associated with adverse clinical outcomes.<br>Patients are at risk of nutritional deterioration throughout hospitalization. |
| *Nutrition measures* | |
| Weight and height/length should be measured at PICU admission.<br>Z-scores for body mass index-for-age (weight-for-length in children <2 years old), or weight-for-age (if accurate, height is not available), should be used to screen for patients at extremes of these values.<br>In children under 36 months old, head circumference must be documented. | Validated screening methods for the PICU population to identify patients at risk of malnutrition must be developed to direct limited resources to high-risk patients.<br>Despite lack of standardized/validated screening methods, collection of growth/nutrition data is better than no data. |
| *Enteral nutrition* | |
| Enteral nutrition should be the preferred mode of nutrient<br>Delivery in all critically ill children, unless contraindicated.<br>Interruptions to enteral nutrition should be minimized.<br>Enteral nutrition should be started within 24–48 h of PICU admission, in eligible patients.<br>Institutional enteral nutrition guidelines should be used and stepwise algorithms provided, that include criteria for enteral nutrition eligibility, timing of initiation, rate of increase and guide managing enteral nutrition intolerance.<br>In children tolerating enteral nutrition, stepwise advancement<br>Should be used and parenteral nutrition should be delayed.<br>Gastric route should be the preferred site for enteral nutrition. Post-pyloric or small intestinal site may be used in patients unable to tolerate gastric feeding or at high risk for aspiration. | Observational studies support feasibility of enteral nutrition, which can be safely delivered to children with medical and surgical diagnoses, and receiving vasoactive medications.<br>Common barriers to enteral nutrition include delayed initiation, interruptions due to perceived intolerance, and prolonged fasting around procedures.<br>Some nutrients delivered as enteral nutrition are likely to be beneficial for gastrointestinal mucosal integrity and motility.<br>Based on large cohort studies, early initiation of enteral nutrition (within 24–48 h of PICU admission) and achievement of up to two thirds of the nutrient goal in the first week of critical illness have been associated with improved clinical outcomes.<br>Existing data are insufficient to make universal recommendations regarding the optimal site to deliver enteral nutrition or regarding use of continuous vs. intermittent gastric feeding. |

(continued)

**Table 12.1** (continued)

| Recommendation | Brief rationale and additional notes |
|---|---|
| *Parenteral nutrition* | |
| The threshold for and timing of parenteral nutrition initiation should be individualized.<br>Based on a single randomized controlled trial, initiating parenteral nutrition is not recommended in the first 24 hours of PICU admission.<br>Based on a single randomized control trial, supplemental parenteral nutrition should be delayed until 1 week after PICU admission *only in* patients with normal baseline nutritional state and low risk of nutritional deterioration.<br>Based on consensus, parenteral nutrition supplementation may be started in children unable to receive enteral nutrition in the 1st PICU week, who are severely malnourished/ at risk of nutrition deterioration or unable to advance past low enteral nutrition volumes | Based on current evidence, the role of supplemental parenteral nutrition to reach a specific goal for energy delivery is not known. The time when parenteral nutrition should be initiated to supplement insufficient enteral nutrition is also unknown. |
| *Energy* | |
| Energy expenditure should be evaluated by indirect calorimetry (resting energy expenditure should be measured) to determine energy requirements and prescribe energy goals.<br>If indirect calorimetry measurement is not feasible, the Schofield equation or food agriculture organization/World Health Organization/United Nations University equation may be used "without" the addition of stress factors to estimate energy expenditure.<br>The Harris-Benedict equations and the recommended daily allowances, should not be used to determine energy requirements in critically ill children.<br>By the end of the first PICU week, caloric delivery of at least two thirds of the prescribed daily energy requirement should be achieved.<br>Energy requirements should be individualized and timely initiation and attaining targets should be a priority. | Observational cohort studies show problems with accuracy and precision of estimating equations, leading to both underfeeding and overfeeding.<br>Cumulative energy deficits during the first week of critical illness may be associated with poor clinical and nutritional outcomes. |

**Table 12.1** (continued)

| Recommendation | Brief rationale and additional notes |
|---|---|
| *Protein* | |
| A minimum protein intake of 1.5 g/kg/d should be administered, keeping in mind that optimal protein intake may be higher in infants and young children.<br>Protein should be provided early in the course of critical illness to attain protein goals and promote positive nitrogen balance.<br>Recommended daily allowances values should not be used to guide protein prescription in critically ill children. | Based on evidence from randomized controlled trials and supported by observational cohort studies, protein intake higher than 1.5 g/kg/day has been shown to prevent cumulative negative protein balance. Observational data suggest higher protein intake may be associated with lower mortality and positive clinical outcomes.<br>Negative protein balance may result in loss of lean muscle mass, which has been associated with poor outcomes in critically ill patients.<br>Recommended daily allowance values were developed for healthy children and often underestimate the protein needs during critical illness. |
| *Immunonutrition* | |
| Immunonutrition is not recommended based on lack of evidence. | |

## 12.2 Assessment and Monitoring of Nutritional Status

Evaluation of the nutritional status in critically ill children is an evolving field. An international consensus group has been working on defining/evaluating effects of malnutrition in ICU children [13]. It is ideal to assess the nutritional status at admission, to elicit evidence of chronic malnutrition; nutritional issues will worsen with critical illness and may be anticipated. History may reveal past growth problems or nutrition deficits. For example, a patient who has been ill with chronic osteomyelitis with 3 months of unexplained fever should immediately trigger the possibility of chronic nutritional issues. Patients with chronic kidney disease, as another example, must be considered as being at high risk for nutrition issues, and ICU admission should include evaluation for iron deficiency and nutrition status. Physical examination (hair, eyes, skin, mouth, extremities) may reveal specific signs of malnutrition or vitamin/mineral deficiencies [2]. Height and weight (with minimal clothing) should be measured in all patients and head circumference in children <2 years old and especially in young infants. This may be challenging because of difficulties in moving patients (if bed scales are not available). Moreover, the presence of fluid overload at admission must be considered. If the patient is edematous, one must be very weary of using admission weight to identify baseline nutrition status. When admission weight is uncertain, ideal body weight may be used for nutritional calculations. An effort should be made to calculate body mass index at admission, which may reveal nutritional problems. These measures should be expressed as corrected age percentiles and z-scores. The 2006 World Health Organization growth-for-age charts have been recommended in children <2 years old and the Center for Disease Control growth charts have been recommended for older children [13]. Height/weight/body mass index z-score < −2 standard deviations from the mean are reasonable ways to screen for poor baseline nutrition status [13]. Others have suggested height-for-age or weight-for-height < 10th percentile as a proxy for poor baseline nutritional status [2]. Several nutrition scores have been published and may be considered [2, 13]. Measuring triceps skinfold thickness and mid upper arm circumference may be useful (expressed as z-scores) [2, 13]. Weight (or triceps skinfold thickness and mid upper arm circumference) may be followed during admission. However, remember that edema/fluid overload may lead to underestimating weight loss. Some ICUs may use more advanced methods to evaluate body composition, most commonly, bioimpedance analysis. Bioimpedance analysis allows for measurement of lean body mass, which may decrease substantially with illness, even though body mass index may not change [14, 15]. However, it is important to accept that bioimpedance analysis measures will be strongly affected by the presence of edema/fluid overload, and thus should be interpreted with caution.

Biochemical parameters (e.g., albumin, prealbumin, visceral proteins) traditionally used to assess nutrition status will often be altered by fluid shifts and should be cautiously interpreted. If there is suspicion for baseline chronic malnutrition, measuring trace elements or vitamin levels at admission may be helpful to guide initial supplementation plans.

As shown, properly evaluating baseline nutrition status and monitoring nutrition status can be quite tedious and may be time consuming. However, waiting 2 or 3 weeks when the patient begins to improve clinically and noting the presence of hand muscle wasting is not acceptable. Despite the challenges of monitoring nutrition status and weight in critically ill patients, routinely collecting the data is more likely to lead to more tailored nutrition than collecting no data at all. The inclusion of a dedicated critical care dietician as an integral part of the multidisciplinary care team is invaluable.

## 12.3 Nutrition Timing, Approach, and Modality in AKI

The goals of nutrition in AKI are similar to other ICU patients, including preventing protein-energy wasting, avoiding further metabolic derangements and complications, allowing growth, and reducing mortality/morbidity. AKI generally occurs early in pediatric ICU admission [16], thus nutritional problems are triggered early in critical illness. Nutrition planning in AKI should begin immediately and not be delayed while awaiting renal function improvement or global clinical improvement. As described above, it is known that children in the ICU are often underfed [17]; this problem is even more prevalent in patients with AKI, for many reasons (e.g., reduced urine output and fluid restriction; enteral feeding intolerance) [6, 7].

Choice of enteral versus parenteral nutrition should be approached similarly to other ICU patients. Enteral nutrition is preferred when possible (with acknowledged advantages like lower cost, manageability, preservation of gastrointestinal function, and integrity) [18]. AKI itself lends no contraindications to enteral feeding [11, 19, 20].

Several studies demonstrate no survival advantage of early parenteral nutrition [21]. Choice of enteral feeding route (gastric; transpyloric) should also be similar to other ICU children, though transpyloric feeding may increase risk for gastrointestinal complications [2, 22].

With hyperphosphatemia or hyperkalemia, low-potassium/phosphate formulas should be used. With continuous RRT (CRRT) or peritoneal dialysis (peritoneal dialysis), regular enteral formulas may be used once electrolyte homeostasis is achieved. However, it is important to remember that formulas and parenteral nutrition electrolyte contents may need to be changed during non-dialytic periods (e.g., stopping CRRT for a head imaging exam). In AKI, feeding should *not* be avoided as a means to avoid RRT [19].

## 12.4 Energy Provision

Without appropriate energy intake, nutrient utilization is suboptimal; overfeeding is also associated with complications. Although nutrient utilization in AKI is thought to be abnormal, how it impacts on caloric needs is unclear [20]. The gold standard method to estimate energy needs is measuring resting energy expenditure. This is most possible in ventilated children, using a metabolic cart and indirect calorimetry (measures oxygen consumption and carbon dioxide production to estimate resting energy expenditure) [23, 24]. There may be concern for resting energy expenditure measurement validity during RRT, due to bicarbonate fluxes at the hemofilter (may affect expired carbon dioxide measurements which are used for estimating resting energy expenditure), but how much RRT affects resting energy expenditure measurement is unclear. Measuring resting energy expenditure in the ICU is feasible but is not commonly done, requires expertise and equipment, and is associated with limitations [20]. Despite these limitations and challenges, current recommendations are to use indirect calorimetry to prescribe energy intake if at all possible [3]. There is extensive literature on different prediction equations for estimating resting energy expenditure in children [24]. Despite the fact that these equations may often not be accurate or precise, they are commonly used and accepted as a surrogate for measured resting energy expenditure. The Caldwell-Kennedy equation (Table 12.2, recommended by the Kidney Disease: Improving Global Outcomes guidelines) was shown to provide the least biased resting energy expenditure estimation in ICU children [19, 24]. Others have suggested using the Schofield equation [2].

While ideal energy requirements remain controversial, some authors recommend caloric intake 20–30% above requirements estimated using prediction equations. This likely provides adequate calories in most children with AKI without significant overfeeding risk. Energy provision should include lipids, protein, and carbohydrates, using insulin as needed to maintain tight glucose control (Table 12.2) [19, 24]. With peritoneal dialysis, the dietician should consider dialysis fluid glucose load when calculating energy intake [2]. If overfeeding is a concern for a child on CRRT, calories from citrate anticoagulation administered may also be included in carbohydrate energy intake calculation.

**Table 12.2** Proposed suggestions on nutrition in children with acute kidney injury

| | |
|---|---|
| Nutrition assessment/mode | • Admission anthropometric measurements ± triceps skinfold thickness or mid upper arm circumference measures (percentile/z-score for age/gender). Monitor throughout admission.<br>• Calculate basal energy needs (resting energy expenditure) with accepted formulas (e.g., Caldwell-Kennedy equation: Resting energy expenditure (kcal/day) = 22 + 31.05 × weight(kg) + 1.16 × age (years); Schofield equation).<br>• Early enteral feeding.<br>• Renal formulas if high potassium or phosphate.<br>• Regular formulas if on CRRT/peritoneal dialysis and electrolyte homeostasis achieved. Reconsider if RRT stopped. |
| Energy | • ~20–30% above basal metabolic needs as measured on metabolic cart or estimated with eqs.<br>• 20–25% carbohydrates (±insulin); 30–35% lipids (20% lipid emulsions); ~50% protein. |
| Protein intake | • At least ~2 g/kg/day with AKI<br>• Increase intake if on CRRT or peritoneal dialysis (by ~30%, or more if high clearance CRRT) |
| Vitamins | • Daily recommended intake.<br>• Monitor serum folate, water-soluble vitamin levels; consider replacement when using prolonged CRRT<br>• Activated vitamin D may be required with prolonged AKI. |
| Trace elements | • Daily recommended intake.<br>• Consider measurement if chronic malnutrition or prolonged RRT, ±increased supplementation. |

## 12.5 Protein Intake

As in adults, critically ill children with AKI have increased protein catabolism, abnormal protein production, and increased protein turnover (amino acids excessively released from skeletal muscle and extracted by other organs), resulting in a negative nitrogen balance [20, 23]. A recent systematic review of 18 studies reflecting over 2000 critically ill children found that a protein intake >1.1–1.5 g/kg/day was significantly associated with reduced mortality [25]. Measuring amino acid levels as a measure of adequate intake is not useful; serum concentrations do not reflect total body stores or utilization. Nitrogen balance measurement is one way proposed to evaluate protein status [14]. It requires measurement of all nitrogen intake (mainly from nutrition) and all nitrogen output (including urine, stool, skin, other fluid losses, and, of course, RRT losses). A negative nitrogen balance implies catabolism and a positive nitrogen balance implies anabolism; the reason it only *implies* anabolism is because this measure does not reflect amino acid *utilization*. Ensuring adequate total energy (caloric) intake will promote better amino acid utilization/anabolism [14]. It is challenging to decrease protein breakdown, but optimizing protein synthesis to preserve skeletal muscle mass and achieve positive nitrogen balance may be enhanced by increasing protein (amino acid) nutrition [4]. Some guidelines suggest protein intakes for critically ill children: 0–2 years, 2–3 g/kg/day;

2–13 years, 1.5–2 g/kg/day; and 13–18 years, 1.5 g/kg/day [26]. Whether these guidelines are valid in AKI is unknown. Most recent guidelines suggest protein intake in critically ill children of 1.5 g/kg/day (Table 12.1) [3]. Given that negative nitrogen balance often occurs in ICU children, despite protein intake similar to those guidelines [27], these protein requirements may not be sufficient in children with AKI.

The challenge of providing adequate protein intake increases with RRT due to losses of amino acids through the hemofilter. Several studies have evaluated nitrogen balance, amino acid concentrations, and clearance in children treated with CRRT. Overall, they show that nitrogen balance is frequently negative using standard protein prescriptions and that amino acid clearance is substantial (Table 12.3). During CRRT, approximately 10–20% of delivered amino acids are estimated to be lost [28–31]; however, this estimate was based on studies using CRRT clearance of 1.5–2 L/1.73 $m^2$/h. With higher clearance, amino acid losses will be greater. For these reasons, in children with AKI, providing ~2 g/kg/day of protein with close monitoring of acid-base status is advisable. In children treated with CRRT, protein intake should be increased by at least 30% (~3 g/kg/day) and increased more with higher clearance.

Peritoneal dialysis is commonly used to treat severe AKI in children, particularly infants. Peritoneal dialysis is known to cause transperitoneal protein losses in children on chronic dialysis [2, 32]. These losses are proportionally higher in younger infants [32]. Recommendations for protein intake in children treated with chronic peritoneal dialysis (ranging from 1.3 in older children to 1.8 g/kg/day in infants [32]) are based on the needs of non-critically ill children and likely inadequate in the critical illness setting. Thus, similar to children treated with CRRT, protein intake should approach at least 3 g/kg/day in children treated with acute peritoneal dialysis.

## 12.6 Electrolytes, Trace Elements, and Vitamins

AKI may lead to hyperkalemia, hyperphosphatemia, hypocalcemia, hypermagnesemia, and metabolic acidosis. Clearly, these laboratory parameters must be monitored and nutrition adjusted accordingly. In children with nephrotoxic AKI or with some congenital renal malformations, potassium, sodium, or phosphate losses may predominate, as a result of predominant tubular dysfunction. Children treated with CRRT very often become hypokalemic, hypophosphatemic, and hypomagnesemic mainly due to enhanced clearance. These should be expected and treated promptly; if phosphate has dropped below normal levels, increase supplementation immediately, do not wait. With frequent monitoring (at least once daily in AKI and twice daily in CRRT or PD) of these electrolytes, there is little reason that patients should have life-threatening electrolyte complications.

Little data exist on trace element metabolism in AKI. However, an excellent resource on evaluation and measurement of trace elements and vitamins in critically ill children is available [33]. In adults with AKI, plasma concentrations of trace

**Table 12.3** Studies on losses from renal replacement therapy of selected nutrition analytes

| Author, year | Intake composition | RRT type | Amino acid losses | Nitrogen balance | Trace elements/vitamins |
|---|---|---|---|---|---|
| Maxvold 2000 | Prot: 1.5 g/kg/d<br>Cal's: 20–30% above resting energy expenditure | CVVH<br>CVVHD<br>(both 2 L/1.73 $m^2$/h) | 7–75 mL/min/1.73 $m^2$<br>8–53 mL/min/1.73 $m^2$<br>(lowest glutamine; highest cysteine) | −4 g/$N_2$/day/1.73 $m^2$<br>−0.4 g/$N_2$/day/1.73 $m^2$ | N/A |
| Zappitelli, 2009 | Prot: ~2 g/kg/d<br>Cal's: ~30–54 kcal/kg/d | CVVHD<br>~2.1 L/1.73$m^2$/hr | 3–51 ml/min/1.73$m^2$/hr | ~−0.23 g $N_2$/kg/day | Selenium: ~8 mL/min/1.73 $m^2$/h<br>Chromium: ~25 mL/min/1.73 $m^2$/h<br>Copper, Zinc, manganese:<5 mL/min/1.73 $m^2$/h<br>Folate: ~16 mL/min/1.73 $m^2$/h |
| Kuttnig, 1991 | Prot: ~0.3 g/kg/d | CAVH | *Losses:* 0.2 g/kg/d | −0.8 to 0.3 g $N_2$/kg/d | N/A |
| Phan, 2006 | N/A:<br>Leucine only examined | CVVH, CVVHDF<br>1–4.5 L/1.73 $m^2$/h<br>HD | 8 mL/min/1.73 $m^2$<br>89–115 mL/min/1.73 $m^2$ | N/A | N/A |
| Sgambat 2016 | Only carnitine examined.<br>Intake not documented. | CVVHDF<br>2 L/1.73 $m^2$/h | N/A | N/A | Carnitine deficiency prevalence doubled after 1 week of CRRT; ~tripled after 3 weeks. |

Abbreviations: *Yr* year, *RRT* renal replacement therapy, *Prot* protein, *Cals'* calories, *CAVH* continuous arteriovenous hemofiltration, *CVVH* continuous veno-venous hemofiltration, *CVVHD* continuous veno-venous hemodialysis, *CVVHDF* continuous veno-venous hemodiafiltration, $N_2$ nitrogen, *N/A* not applicable/not evaluated, *CRRT* continuous renal replacement therapy elements (e.g., selenium, chromium, manganese, copper, zinc) and water-soluble vitamins (e.g. thiamine, folate) may be reduced [31]. However, the reasons for this are unclear, and may include altered protein-binding with critical illness, fluid loss, poor nutritional intake, and baseline nutritional deficiencies [34]. With prolonged AKI or prolonged CRRT, it may be useful to measure plasma concentrations, to help guide supplementation. Trace elements (especially chromium, selenium) and folate clearance on standard CVVHD prescriptions may be substantial (Table 12.3) [31]. Due to protein binding, trace element clearance may be higher with CVVH and losses may be significant with prolonged CRRT. It is likely that there is clearance of other water-soluble vitamins like thiamine [34]. Thiamine clearance should be considered in certain inborn errors of metabolism. While there is no evidence to support this, in cases where thiamine is especially important for a given inborn error of metabolism or is part of the treatment, we have increased thiamine intake by ~30–50% in children treated with CRRT, with monitoring of serum levels. There is no data available to guide supplementation of water-soluble vitamins and trace metals in acute peritoneal dialysis or HD. However, there are likely losses of some water-soluble vitamins with peritoneal dialysis and trace elements in both modalities. A study recently showed that children treated with CRRT became carnitine deficient, presumably due to clearance (carnitine is a water soluble, small molecule), suggesting the need for research to quantify clearance and evaluate supplementation strategies [35]. Given that the effects of increasing trace elements and/or water-soluble vitamin intake are unclear, it is recommended to provide the recommended daily allowances with the exception of vitamin C (should be lower). However, in children treated with RRT (especially CRRT) for >1 week, monitoring plasma concentrations of these elements may help guide supplementation. Finally, especially in patients with underlying chronic kidney disease, patients with prolonged AKI should be considered for vitamin D and/or activated vitamin D supplementation.

**Conclusion**

Suggested recommendations for feeding children with AKI are shown in Table 12.2. Feeding patients with acute kidney injury (AKI), especially when treated with continuous renal replacement therapy (CRRT), remains a delicate yet challenging task for intensive care unit (ICU) clinicians. Indeed, the AKI process itself is accompanied by inherent metabolic and physiological disturbances necessitating careful implementation of ICU feeding protocols. Nutrition provision for these patients is a crucial part of their care and institutions with standardized nutrition programs and care guidelines are more likely to achieve nutrition provision goals [11]. Healthcare providers should also be prepared to recognize signs and symptoms of nutritional toxicities and deficiencies and monitor mineral, protein, and fluid intake while patients are beginning or weaning from CRRT, as therapy becomes intermittent, and in other therapy changes.

**Key Learning Points**

- Critically ill children with acute kidney injury (AKI) are at high risk for malnutrition and for being underfed.
- Children with AKI treated with continuous renal replacement therapy suffer losses of nutritional elements, which must be considered when prescribing nutrition.
- Detailed assessment of nutritional status and evaluation for attaining nutrition goals must be integral to the care of patients with AKI admitted to critical care units
- Protein intake in patients with AKI should be at least 1.5 g/kg/day and must be increased by at least 30% when continuous renal replacement therapy is initiated.
- The presence of AKI should never lead to significant delays in nutrition administration.

## References

1. Hulst JM, van Goudoever JB, Zimmermann LJ, Hop WC, Albers MJ, Tibboel D, et al. The effect of cumulative energy and protein deficiency on anthropometric parameters in a pediatric ICU population. Clin Nutr. 2004;23(6):1381–9.
2. Sethi SK, Maxvold N, Bunchman T, Jha P, Kher V, Raina R. Nutritional management in the critically ill child with acute kidney injury: a review. Pediatr Nephrol. 2017;32(4):589–601.
3. Mehta NM, Skillman HE, Irving SY, Coss-Bu JA, Vermilyea S, Farrington EA, et al. Guidelines for the provision and assessment of nutrition support therapy in the pediatric critically ill patient: Society of Critical Care Medicine and American Society for Parenteral and Enteral Nutrition. Pediatr Crit Care Med. 2017;18(7):675–715.
4. Coss-Bu JA, Jefferson LS, Walding D, David Y, Smith EO, Klish WJ. Resting energy expenditure in children in a pediatric intensive care unit: comparison of Harris-Benedict and Talbot predictions with indirect calorimetry values. Am J Clin Nutr. 1998;67(1):74–80.
5. Owens JL, Musa N. Nutrition support after neonatal cardiac surgery. Nutr Clin Pract. 2009;24(2):242–9.
6. Castillo A, Santiago MJ, Lopez-Herce J, Montoro S, Lopez J, Bustinza A, et al. Nutritional status and clinical outcome of children on continuous renal replacement therapy: a prospective observational study. BMC Nephrol. 2012;13:125.
7. Kyle UG, Akcan-Arikan A, Orellana RA, Coss-Bu JA. Nutrition support among critically ill children with AKI. Clin J Am Soc Nephrol. 2013;8(4):568–74.
8. Zappitelli M, Goldstein SL, Symons JM, Somers MJ, Baum MA, Brophy PD, et al. Protein and calorie prescription for children and young adults receiving continuous renal replacement therapy: a report from the prospective pediatric continuous renal replacement therapy registry group. Crit Care Med. 2008;36(12):3239–45.
9. Martinez EE, Mehta NM. The science and art of pediatric critical care nutrition. Curr Opin Crit Care. 2016;22(4):316–24.
10. Mitting R, Marino L, Macrae D, Shastri N, Meyer R, Pathan N. Nutritional status and clinical outcome in postterm neonates undergoing surgery for congenital heart disease. Pediatr Crit Care Med. 2015;16(5):448–52.

11. Mehta NM, Bechard LJ, Cahill N, Wang M, Day A, Duggan CP, et al. Nutritional practices and their relationship to clinical outcomes in critically ill children--an international multicenter cohort study*. Crit Care Med. 2012;40(7):2204–11.
12. Mehta NM, Bechard LJ, Zurakowski D, Duggan CP, Heyland DK. Adequate enteral protein intake is inversely associated with 60-d mortality in critically ill children: a multicenter, prospective, cohort study. Am J Clin Nutr. 2015;102(1):199–206.
13. Mehta NM, Corkins MR, Lyman B, Malone A, Goday PS, Carney LN, et al. Defining pediatric malnutrition: a paradigm shift toward etiology-related definitions. JPEN J Parenter Enteral Nutr. 2013;37(4):460–81.
14. Coss-Bu JA, Hamilton-Reeves J, Patel JJ, Morris CR, Hurt RT. Protein requirements of the critically ill pediatric patient. Nutr Clin Pract. 2017;32(1_suppl):128S–41S.
15. Kyle UG, Earthman CP, Pichard C, Coss-Bu JA. Body composition during growth in children: limitations and perspectives of bioelectrical impedance analysis. Eur J Clin Nutr. 2015;69(12):1298–305.
16. Alkandari O, Eddington KA, Hyder A, Gauvin F, Ducruet T, Gottesman R, et al. Acute kidney injury is an independent risk factor for pediatric intensive care unit mortality, longer length of stay and prolonged mechanical ventilation in critically ill children: a two-center retrospective cohort study. Crit Care. 2011;15(3):R146.
17. Leroue MK, Good RJ, Skillman HE, Czaja AS. Enteral nutrition practices in critically ill children requiring noninvasive positive pressure ventilation. Pediatr Crit Care Med. 2017;18:1093.
18. Lee JH, Rogers E, Chor YK, Samransamruajkit R, Koh PL, Miqdady M, et al. Optimal nutrition therapy in paediatric critical care in the Asia-Pacific and Middle East: a consensus. Asia Pac J Clin Nutr. 2016;25(4):676–96.
19. Kidney Disease: Improving Global Outcomes Acute Kidney Injury Work Group. KDIGO Clinical Practice Guideline for acute kidney injury. Kidney Int. 2012;2(Suppl):1–138.
20. Sabatino A, Regolisti G, Maggiore U, Fiaccadori E. Protein/energy debt in critically ill children in the pediatric intensive care unit: acute kidney injury as a major risk factor. J Ren Nutr. 2014;24(4):209–18.
21. Fivez T, Kerklaan D, Mesotten D, Verbruggen S, Wouters PJ, Vanhorebeek I, et al. Early versus late parenteral nutrition in critically ill children. N Engl J Med. 2016;374(12):1111–22.
22. Lopez-Herce J, Sanchez C, Carrillo A, Mencia S, Santiago MJ, Bustinza A, et al. Transpyloric enteral nutrition in the critically ill child with renal failure. Intensive Care Med. 2006;32(10):1599–605.
23. Coss-Bu JA, Jefferson LS, Walding D, David Y, Smith EO, Klish WJ. Resting energy expenditure and nitrogen balance in critically ill pediatric patients on mechanical ventilation. Nutrition. 1998;14(9):649–52.
24. White MS, Shepherd RW, McEniery JA. Energy expenditure in 100 ventilated, critically ill children: improving the accuracy of predictive equations. Crit Care Med. 2000;28(7):2307–12.
25. Hauschild DB, Ventura JC, Mehta NM, Moreno YMF. Impact of the structure and dose of protein intake on clinical and metabolic outcomes in critically ill children: a systematic review. Nutrition. 2017;41:97–106.
26. Mehta NM, Compher C, Directors ASPENBo. A.S.P.E.N. Clinical guidelines: nutrition support of the critically ill child. JPEN J Parenter Enteral Nutr. 2009;33(3):260–76.
27. Coss-Bu JA, Klish WJ, Walding D, Stein F, Smith EO, Jefferson LS. Energy metabolism, nitrogen balance, and substrate utilization in critically ill children. Am J Clin Nutr. 2001;74(5):664–9.
28. Kuttnig M, Zobel G, Ring E, Grubbauer HM, Kurz R. Nitrogen and amino acid balance during total parenteral nutrition and continuous arteriovenous hemofiltration in critically ill anuric children. Child Nephrol Urol. 1991;11(2):74–8.
29. Maxvold NJ, Smoyer WE, Custer JR, Bunchman TE. Amino acid loss and nitrogen balance in critically ill children with acute renal failure: a prospective comparison between classic hemofiltration and hemofiltration with dialysis. Crit Care Med. 2000;28(4):1161–5.

30. Phan V, Clermont MJ, Merouani A, Litalien C, Tucci M, Lambert M, et al. Duration of extracorporeal therapy in acute maple syrup urine disease: a kinetic model. Pediatr Nephrol. 2006;21(5):698–704.
31. Zappitelli M, Juarez M, Castillo L, Coss-Bu J, Goldstein SL. Continuous renal replacement therapy amino acid, trace metal and folate clearance in critically ill children. Intensive Care Med. 2009;35(4):698–706.
32. Quan A, Baum M. Protein losses in children on continuous cycler peritoneal dialysis. Pediatr Nephrol. 1996;10(6):728–31.
33. Dao DT, Anez-Bustillos L, Cho BS, Li Z, Puder M, Gura KM. Assessment of micronutrient status in critically ill children: challenges and opportunities. Nutrients. 2017;9(11):E1185.
34. Fiaccadori E, Regolisti G, Cabassi A. Specific nutritional problems in acute kidney injury, treated with non-dialysis and dialytic modalities. NDT Plus. 2010;3(1):1–7.
35. Sgambat K, Moudgil A. Carnitine deficiency in children receiving continuous renal replacement therapy. Hemodial Int. 2016;20(1):63–7.

# 13 Outcomes Following Acute Kidney Injury in Children

Scott M. Sutherland

**Case Vignette**
A 3-year-old boy undergoing a Fontan requires prolonged cardiopulmonary bypass due to intraoperative complications. His creatinine rises from a baseline of 0.6 to 4.6 mg/dL over 4 days, his urine output dwindles despite aggressive diuretic and vasopressor support, and he appears to need dialysis acutely. During the nephrology consult, the family expresses concern about the acute kidney injury. They are particularly concerned about their son's ability to survive this episode and what the dialysis means for them during the hospitalization. Fortunately, the boy only needs a few days of dialysis therapy and his creatinine quickly falls to a nadir of 0.9 mg/dL. As the family is preparing for discharge, they want to know if their son's kidneys are still functioning normally and what they should expect over the years to come.

## 13.1 Introduction

Acute kidney injury (AKI) is a common complication in hospitalized patients which describes a phenomenon marked by impaired elimination of waste products and dysregulation of electrolytes, acid-base status, and fluid balance [1]. Although AKI has significant clinical consequences, describing its outcomes has been difficult given the historical tendency to apply diverse diagnostic criteria [2]. Fortunately, the previously described transformative advances in AKI epidemiology prompted by the establishment of a consensus definition are now expanding into the area of AKI outcomes research [2–5].

S. M. Sutherland
Division of Nephrology, Department of Pediatrics, Stanford University, Stanford, CA, USA
e-mail: suthersm@stanford.edu



A. Deep, S. L. Goldstein (eds.), *Critical Care Nephrology and Renal Replacement Therapy in Children*, https://doi.org/10.1007/978-3-319-90281-4_13

AKI is now known to be a risk factor for poorer short-term outcomes and patients who develop AKI while hospitalized commonly experience adverse consequences; this is especially true in critical care populations [1, 6–8]. More recently, an association between AKI and long-term sequelae has also been established; though initially thought to be self-limited, AKI events have been linked with long-term renal morbidity and chronic renal dysfunction [9–15]. Now that an established approach to AKI identification exists, one of the more challenging aspects of describing post-AKI outcomes is the contemporary shift in AKI epidemiology. Though formerly thought to be due primarily to intrinsic renal disease, AKI is now recognized as being much more commonly caused by systemic illness, multi-organ injury, and the treatments these conditions demand [6, 7, 16–19]. Since many of these conditions are associated independently with poor outcomes, it can prove challenging to isolate the quantifiable effect of AKI on mortality, length of stay, and chronic kidney disease (CKD). Recognizing this, the goal of this chapter is to comprehensively describe outcomes in children who experience AKI. It will focus on studies which have utilized one of the standard, consensus based definitions (RIFLE, pRIFLE, AKIN, and KDIGO), highlight both short- and long-term sequelae, and attempt to isolate the independent impact that AKI has in pediatric patients.

## 13.2 Short-Term Outcomes Following AKI

While AKI can occur in outpatients, it is far more common in hospitalized children and this is the setting where our knowledge is best established. As a result, outcome research has tended to focus on in-hospital sequelae in the short term. The preponderance of data, especially that which is based upon a consensus definitional approach, has demonstrated that in the pediatric population, AKI is associated with the need for ventilator support, longer hospital stays, and higher mortality rates. Although there is a distinct relationship between medical complexity and AKI, rigorous statistical approaches continue to find that the aforementioned association between AKI and outcomes is independent of disease severity and potential confounders.

### 13.2.1 Mechanical Ventilation

Despite its heterogeneous incidence across various patient populations, AKI has remained consistently associated with both the need for mechanical ventilation and its duration [6, 8, 20–25]. For example, across a large, general critical care population, children who developed any AKI (KDIGO defined) required 2.3 additional days of ventilator support; those with Stage 3 AKI received mechanical ventilation for 4.2 additional days [25]. A similar study which examined noncardiac patients admitted to the ICU found that the development of AKI was associated with twice the length of mechanical ventilation (5.4 vs. 2.2 days) [8]. The multicenter, prospective Assessment of Worldwide AKI, Renal angina, and Epidemiology (AWARE) study, which is the largest prospective study to date, was able to demonstrate a stepwise increase in mechanical ventilation use which correlated with AKI severity; patients with Stage 1, Stage 2, and Stage 3 AKI required mechanical ventilation 38.2%, 40.5%, and 50.2% of the time, respectively (vs. no AKI at 29.5%) [6]. The relationship between AKI and the need for mechanical ventilation holds true in homogenous populations as well. Patients undergoing cardiac surgery, neonates, and children with sepsis all experience longer mechanical ventilation courses if they develop AKI [20, 23, 24, 26]. This association is not particularly surprising given the association between AKI and fluid overload, and the relationship between fluid balance and the need for respiratory support [22, 27–30].

The data regarding AKI and mechanical ventilation underscore several important facets of AKI outcomes research. As an example, a study by MacDonald found that among 66 children undergoing cardiac transplantation, AKI (incidence of 73%) was associated with a mechanical ventilation course that was 2 days longer; however, once they adjusted for covariates, this association disappeared [21]. A larger study examined 311 critically ill children and found that AKI (incidence of 42%) was independently associated with longer duration of mechanical ventilation; even after adjusting for confounders, patients with AKI were three times more likely to need mechanical support of moderate duration [20]. These studies and those like them make three things clear. First, disease severity and intergroup differences can confound AKI outcome effects; it is important to adjust for these factors when possible. Second, larger studies may be needed to see some of the outcome effects associated with AKI; this is especially true when the effect size is more moderate. Third, it may be challenging to identify related outcome associations when the incidence of AKI is exceedingly high; results should be interpreted in the context of the study's underlying epidemiology.

### 13.2.2 Length of Stay

AKI has also been closely linked with longer ICU and hospital lengths of stay (LOS) in children. The first consensus pediatric definition based example of this was the original pRIFLE (Pediatric RIFLE) study published in 2007; pRIFLE was an iteration of the RIFLE criteria which was applicable to children [4]. In this analysis patients who experienced any AKI tended to have longer ICU (18 ± 24.3 days vs. 10.1 ± 6.2 days,) and hospital (36.6 ± 40.1 days vs. 20.5 ± 16.6 days) LOS than those without AKI [4]. This study is relevant since pRIFLE tends to be particularly sensitive and is likely to identify milder AKI events, underscoring the strength of the association [1, 31]. The previously described AWARE study also established this association; patients with AKI (increase of 1.33–1.51 days) and severe AKI (increase of 2.77–3 days) had longer ICU LOS even after adjusting for severity of illness (Fig. 13.1) [6]. One critical care population where the data have been somewhat heterogeneous has been children undergoing cardiac surgery. While some studies have found that mild AKI events (Stage 1) are associated with longer LOS, this is not universal. However, nearly all available data support the association between severe AKI (Stage 2/3) and longer LOS even after controlling for severity of illness, case complexity, and potential confounders [20, 23, 32].

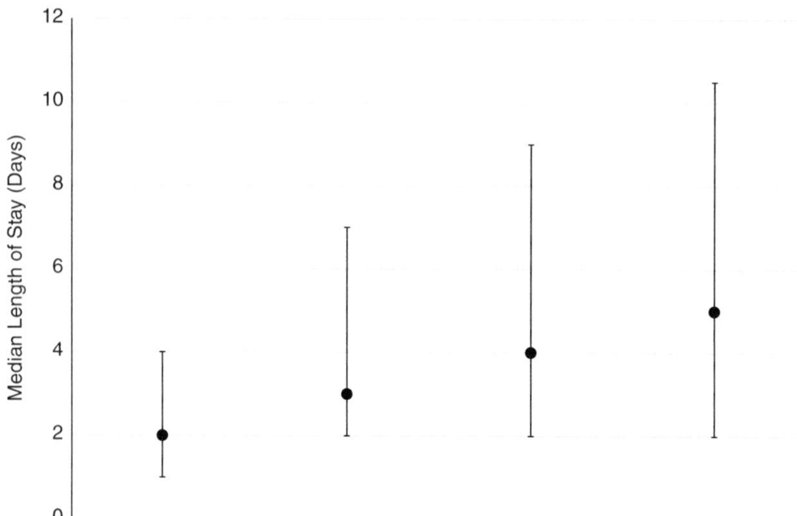


| | No AKI | Stage 1 | Stage 2 | Stage 3 |
|---|---|---|---|---|
| Median LOS | 2 | 3 | 4 | 5 |
| IQR | 1-4 | 2-7 | 2-8 | 2-10.5 |

**Fig. 13.1** Length of ICU stay according to AKI severity stage [6]. In the AWARE study, patients who experienced AKI had prolonged ICU stays. Patients without AKI had a median LOS of 2 days (IQR 1–4). Patients with Stage 1 (Median LOS 3 days, IQR 2–7), Stage 2 (Median LOS 4 days, IQR 2–8), and Stage 3 AKI (Median LOS 5 days, IQR 2–10.5) had longer ICU LOS than children who did not experience AKI ($p < 0.001$)

The association between AKI and LOS is highlighted by the findings of studies performed in non-critically ill children. For example, one study examined 557 children (age 8 ± 5.9 years) on non-critical care wards who received aminoglycoside antibiotics [33]. Even after adjusting for potential confounders, children who developed AKI had prolonged LOS; this effect was more pronounced for children who experienced more severe AKI (Stage 2/3). Interestingly, this study compared the LOS effect of pRIFLE and AKIN defined AKI. Again, the effect was less pronounced when the pRIFLE criteria were used. Application of the pRIFLE criteria enriches the AKI cohort with mild events, whereas AKIN defined AKI tends to be of a more severe phenotype, providing indirect evidence for a dose-dependent effect. Similarly, Rheault *et al.* investigated the impact of AKI among children admitted with nephrotic syndrome [34]. They found that AKI was independently associated with prolonged hospitalization; while they did not examine ICU LOS, they did find that nephrotic syndrome patients who developed AKI were more likely to require ICU care at some point in their hospitalization.

### 13.2.3 Mortality

Among adult patients, AKI has been independently associated with higher mortality rates [35–37]. This effect is distinct and substantial. The multinational, prospective AKI-EPI study demonstrated that KDIGO Stage 2 (adjusted OR 2.95, 95th CI 1.38–6.28) and Stage 3 (adjusted OR 6.88, 95th CI 3.88–12.23) AKI were independently associated with higher mortality among patients admitted to the ICU [37]. Additionally, Chawla found that adults with AKI were two times more likely to die than those who experienced a myocardial infarction [36]. In children, AKI has also been independently associated with death. Alkandari *et al.* examined over 2000 PICU admissions and found that children with AKI were 4–8 times more likely to die than those without [8]. Additionally, those with severe AKI (KDIGO stage 2/3) experienced mortality rates that were 6–10 times higher even after adjusting for severity of illness and intergroup differences. A study of children undergoing corrective cardiac surgery also found an independent effect on survival; children who developed Stage 3 AKI had an adjusted odds ratio for death of nearly 10 [23]. These findings have been corroborated by the aforementioned AWARE study in which KDIGO Stage 2/3 AKI was associated with higher mortality even after adjusting for 16 covariates [6]. Although few studies have been performed, this morality effect seems to be confined to critically ill patients, at least in children. In one representative study, although AKI was associated with higher mortality in the pediatric ICU, this was not the case in patients receiving acute care (Fig. 13.2) [1]. While none of these studies are able to prove true causation, it is clear that the accumulated data available demonstrate that critically ill children who develop AKI experience higher mortality.

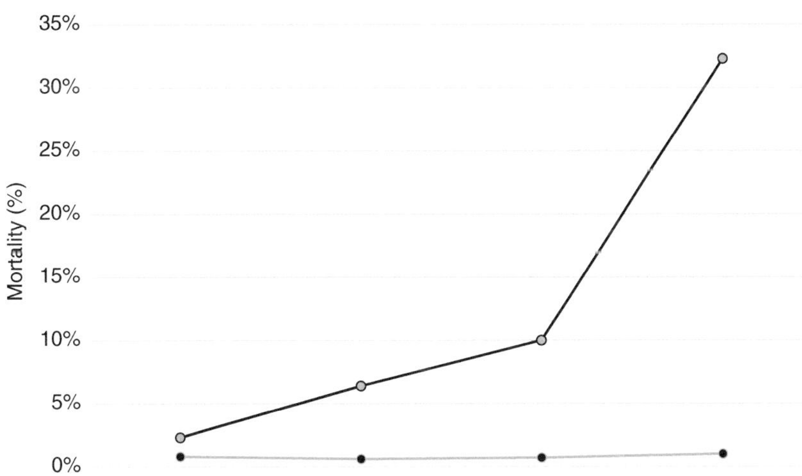


| | No AKI | Stage 1 | Stage 2 | Stage 3 |
|---|---|---|---|---|
| non-ICU | 0.8% | 0.6% | 0.7% | 1.0% |
| ICU | 2.3% | 6.4% | 10.0% | 32.3% |

non-ICU ICU

**Fig. 13.2** AKI mortality in hospitalized children according to severity stage [1]. In non-ICU admissions, mortality among children with and without AKI was similar; this was true regardless of AKI severity stage ($p > 0.05$ for all analyses). In the ICU, mortality was higher among children with AKI than those without. Mortality increased in a stepwise fashion and was higher at each successive severity stage. The increases at Stage 3 and Stage 1 were statistically significant when compared with the prior stage ($p < 0.05$). All stages had significantly higher mortality than patients without AKI ($p < 0.05$)

## 13.3 Longitudinal Outcomes Following AKI

While the short-term, inpatient ramifications of AKI have been studied at length, more recently outcomes research has begun to examine the mid- and long-term impact of AKI among survivors. The data have demonstrated that chronic renal dysfunction is common following AKI and that the prevalence of proteinuria, hypertension, and chronic kidney disease (CKD) are higher than in the general population. Additionally, renal recovery, or the lack thereof, seems to play a significant prognostic role among children who experience AKI while hospitalized.

### 13.3.1 Renal Recovery

Renal recovery is a relatively novel concept which, unfortunately, remains poorly defined [38–40]. Over the past several years, studies have employed various classification schemes for recovery. As a result, renal recovery has been described as a post-AKI serum creatinine <2 mg/dL, a creatinine that is within 1.15×, 1.25×, or 1.5× of baseline, a creatinine that is within 0.3 mg/dL of baseline, no longer requiring RRT, or no longer meeting any AKI criteria [41–47]. While this has created heterogeneity and adds some complexity to the interpretation, the available data demonstrate that it is an important outcome among AKI survivors with prognostic implications.

While the focus of this chapter is on pediatric AKI, the dearth of high-quality data on renal recovery in children necessitates some discussion of the available adult data. A large study of 291 ICUs in France found that among 25,750 adults who required RRT for AKI, renal recovery occurred 86.2% of the time [45]. This is a high rate of recovery relative to other studies, likely reflecting their decision to define recovery as no longer needing RRT. Long *et al.*evaluated 10,419 adults who experienced AKI during their hospitalization; patients were drawn from both ICU and non-critical care wards and were included regardless of receipt of RRT [47]. Overall renal recovery, defined as a serum creatinine <1.5× baseline (no longer meeting Stage 1 AKI criteria), was 67%. Not surprisingly, recovery was less common as AKI severity increased. Renal recovery occurred in 88%, 58%, and 44% of adults with Stage 1, Stage 2, and Stage 3 AKI, respectively; again, there is a clear dose-dependent effect. Renal recovery is also associated with long-term morbidity and mortality. A study of 374 adults undergoing transcatheter aortic valve replacement found that AKI occurred in 98 patients (26%), of which 56% experienced full renal recovery (no longer meeting any Stage 1 AKI criteria at discharge) [48]. While even patients with recovered AKI experienced greater 2-year mortality than adults without AKI (adjusted HR 1.87, 95th CI 1.03–3.23), those with only partial recovery (discharge creatinine >1.5× baseline but not requiring RRT) experienced an even higher 2-year mortality risk of 2.65 (95th CI 1.4–4.7). Notably, those who continued to require RRT at discharge had the highest 2-year mortality risk (HR 10.95, 95th CI 2.59–31.49).

The data on renal recovery in pediatric populations is consistent with the adult findings described above. Basu *et al.* described the post-AKI course of 136 children who developed AKI severe enough to require RRT [44]. In this population, similar to other studies of patients receiving RRT, they defined renal recovery as non-dialysis dependence and of the survivors, 84% had experienced recovery 1 month after the AKI event. At the same time, they did report that only 27% of patients had an eGFR >90 mL/min/1.73 m$^2$ one month later. While a "normal" eGFR is neither a conventional nor precise definition of renal recovery, it does emphasize the point that though many patients may cease needing RRT, a far smaller proportion will experience complete recovery. Additionally, it underscores the need for a standard definitional approach to renal recovery (Fig. 13.3). This concept was also addressed by Hessey *et al.* who examined 2033 pediatric ICU admissions [49].

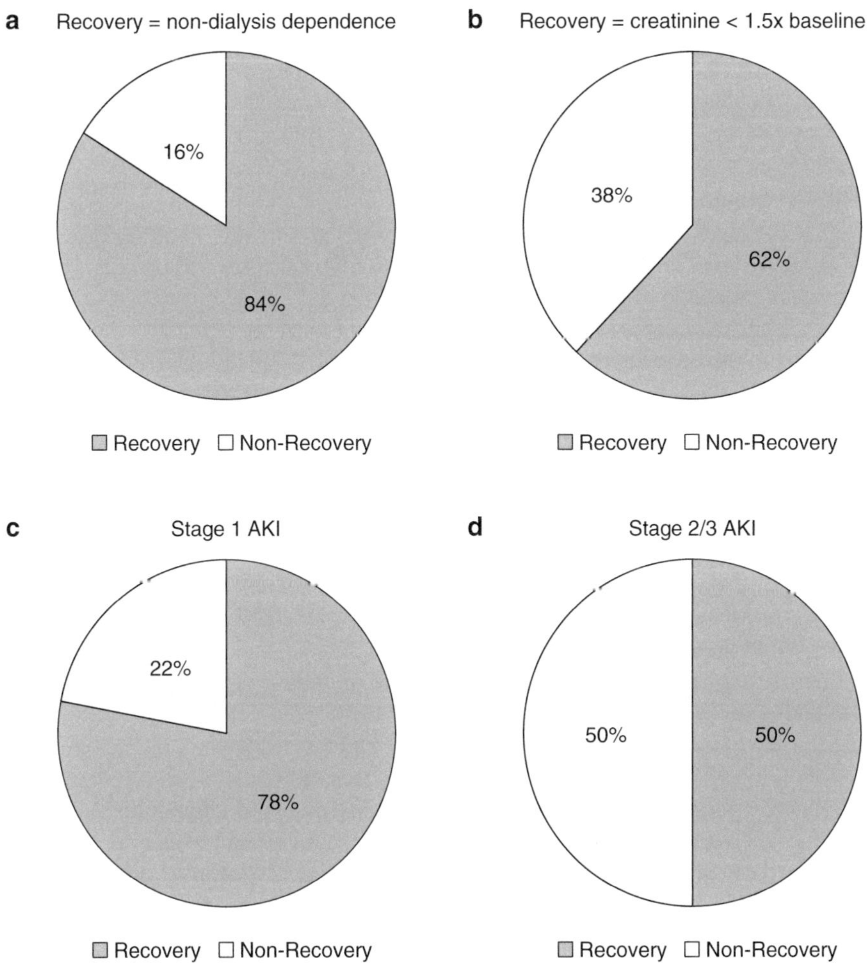


**Fig. 13.3** Renal recovery rates and AKI. While renal recovery rates can vary depending on the definition employed and the population studied, central themes have emerged. In (**a**), renal recovery is defined as non-dialysis dependence; 84% of children with AKI who need dialysis recover enough function to allow cessation of RRT. However, (**b**), where recovery is defined as a creatinine within 1.5× of baseline, demonstrates that only 62% of children with AKI recover enough function to no longer meet AKI definitional criteria. Additionally, recovery is more common in children with mild AKI (78%, **c**) than it is in those with severe AKI (50%, **d**)

They found that the recovery rate differed depending on the defined threshold. 92.5% of patients with AKI recovered function when it was defined as a discharge creatinine <1.5× baseline; however, recovery only occurred in 75.9% of patients when it was defined as discharge creatinine <1.15× baseline. They too found a dose-dependent effect as non-recovery occurred more commonly with more severe AKI. Finally, Hollander *et al.* examined 88 children who underwent cardiac transplantation and found that 62% experienced renal recovery (creatinine <1.5× baseline within 3 months of AKI event) [46]. Notably, recovery was more common in the setting of mild AKI (Stage 1 recovery 78% vs. Stage 2/3 recovery 50%, $p < 0.04$). Perhaps most interestingly, this study found that non-recovery was a risk factor for the subsequent development of CKD. While none of the patients who survived AKI and recovered developed CKD, 18% of those who did not recover from AKI developed CKD (defined as eGFR <60 mL/min/1.73 m$^2$, $p = 0.03$).

### 13.3.2 Chronic Kidney Disease

A number of studies have demonstrated that long-term renal sequelae are highly prevalent following AKI. Askenazi *et al.* examined 29 children with AKI (based upon diagnostic coding) and found that proteinuria and hypertension occurred in more than 20% of survivors; an eGFR <90 mL/min/1.73 m$^2$ (13.8%) was also common [14]. Buysse *et al.* studied 19 children 10 years after they experienced AKI (defined as creatinine 2× normal value) in the setting of septic shock and found nearly identical rates of hypertension and proteinuria [50]. Hingorani *et al.* found that AKI (doubling of serum creatinine) increased the risk for CKD (eGFR <60 mL/min/1.73 m$^2$) by 70% in children undergoing stem cell transplantation [51]. Mammen *et al.* reviewed 126 AKI survivors (AKIN Stage 1 or greater) 1–3 years after ICU discharge. They found only moderate rates of hypertension (3.2%) and proteinuria (9.5%), however, nearly 40% of these children had an eGFR <90 mL/min/1.73 m$^2$ [13]. While these data are compelling, a meta-analysis performed in 2014 underscored some of the issues plaguing the available data [52]. The analysis noted that the studies they reviewed had widely variable follow-up timeframes, identified AKI in a variety of ways, and defined outcomes dissimilarly. The number of patients lost to follow-up was substantial, raising concern for ascertainment bias. Additionally, nearly all of the studies available failed to include a non-AKI comparator group.

Since then, the majority of studies have used, at a minimum, one of the available consensus definitions for AKI. While they have continued to employ disparate definitions for long-term renal sequelae, many of these studies have compared outcomes between AKI and non-AKI cohorts. One such study examined hypertension rates among pediatric stem cell transplant survivors. They found that high blood pressure was common across the entire population, however, AKI (defined as doubling of serum creatinine, equivalent to KDIGO Stage 2 or greater) was associated with a 2.5-fold increased risk for the development of hypertension. Menon *et al.* examined 100 children who developed nephrotoxic medication-associated AKI and found impressively high rates of proteinuria (68.5%), hypertension (37.6%), and an eGFR <90 mL/min/1.73 $m^2$ (23.4%) [15]. When compared with matched non-AKI controls, those who experienced AKI had significantly lower eGFR, more proteinuria, and a higher incidence of hypertension [15].

Two recently published prospective studies deserve special mention. The first is a 5-year follow-up of the Translational Research Investigating Biomarker Endpoints in AKI (TRIBE-AKI) study. This analysis found that hypertension (17%), proteinuria (8%), and an eGFR <90 mL/min/1.73$m^2$ (13%) were common following cardiac surgery, however, these sequelae were not more common among the children who experienced perioperative AKI [53]. The second, entitled, "Follow-up Renal Assessment of Injury Long-term after AKI (FRAIL-AKI)," was able to compare renal findings in 51 children 7 years after they had undergone cardiopulmonary bypass. The 31 AKI and 18 non-AKI patients had similar rates of proteinuria and hypertension as well as comparable eGFRs [54]. However, those with AKI did have higher urinary biomarker levels of interleukin-18 (IL-18) and liver-type fatty acid binding protein (L-FABP) than either the non-AKI patients or healthy controls. This suggests that patients who experience AKI may have subtle evidence of chronic renal injury even in the absence of overt CKD. Interestingly, a subsequently published study did find that cardiac surgery-associated AKI was associated with a greater risk for CKD Stage 2 or greater [55]. The 5-year cumulative incidence of CKD for patients with cardiac surgery-associated AKI was 12% (95th CI 7%–20%), significantly higher than the 3% (95th CI 1%–5%) seen in those without AKI (adjusted HR 3.8, 95th CI 1.4–10.4). While this study was retrospective in nature, it was large, used a consensus definition for AKI, and a rigorous definition of CKD.

## 13.4 Summary

As the clinical emphasis on AKI has grown, we have seen substantial improvement in the scientific rigor of related outcomes research. The development of a consensus definition for AKI has helped eliminate some of the heterogeneity and, as a result, the next decade should provide us with a more detailed and accurate understanding of the manner in which AKI affects short- and long-term outcomes in children. Furthermore, the Acute Dialysis Quality Initiative consortium has developed a series of recommendations and a new definition for the term Acute Kidney Disease, which like the RIFLE criteria will need to be tested by epidemiological study [38]. Currently, we believe that children with AKI will require mechanical ventilation for longer durations, remain in the hospital for greater periods of time, and experience higher mortality. While we cannot yet say that AKI is definitely the *cause* of this, the best available data suggest it. Though AKI was previously thought to be self-limited, we now know that renal recovery is far from universal. Though consensus building around the definition of recovery is necessary, patients with severe AKI are at particularly high risk for non-recovery, portending chronic disease. Additionally, adult and pediatric studies demonstrate that renal sequelae are common following episodes of AKI and suggest that AKI may predispose patients to CKD. After AKI, incident rates of hypertension, proteinuria, and reduced GFR far exceed those in healthy populations. Additionally, many studies have found a dose-dependent association between AKI severity and CKD risk. Thus, there is clearly a strong observational signal and patients who experience AKI should be followed longitudinally, potentially in clinics that are specifically designed to assess outcomes in AKI survivors [56].

**Key Learning Points**

- AKI is associated with longer duration of mechanical ventilation and AKI survivors characteristically experience longer hospital and, if applicable, intensive care unit stays.
- Critically ill children with AKI have higher mortality rates. While an unqualified causal link between AKI and death has not yet been established in children, the fact that the association remains even after adjusting for severity of illness and confounders suggests that AKI is responsible for the increased mortality risk.
- While AKI was traditionally thought to be a self-limited event, a significant proportion of AKI survivors do not experience renal recovery.
- Chronic renal disease is common following AKI and the prevalence of proteinuria, hypertension, and chronic kidney disease (CKD) is significantly higher than the general pediatric population. Patients who do not experience full renal recovery after AKI are at increased risk for development of CKD.
- There is a dose-dependent relationship between AKI and poorer outcomes as higher severity AKI is more strongly associated with morbidity and mortality.

## References

1. Sutherland SM, Byrnes JJ, Kothari M, Longhurst CA, Dutta S, Garcia P, et al. AKI in hospitalized children: comparing the pRIFLE, AKIN, and KDIGO definitions. Clin J Am Soc Nephrol. 2015;10(4):554–61.
2. Bellomo R, Ronco C, Kellum JA, Mehta RL, Palevsky P, Acute Dialysis Quality Initiative w. Acute renal failure – definition, outcome measures, animal models, fluid therapy and information technology needs: the Second International Consensus Conference of the Acute Dialysis Quality Initiative (ADQI) Group. Crit Care. 2004;8(4):R204–12.
3. Kidney Disease: Improving Global Outcomes (KDIGO) Acute Kidney Injury Work Group. KDIGO Clinical Practice Guideline for acute kidney injury. Kidney Int. 2012;2:1–138.
4. Akcan-Arikan A, Zappitelli M, Loftis LL, Washburn KK, Jefferson LS, Goldstein SL. Modified RIFLE criteria in critically ill children with acute kidney injury. Kidney Int. 2007;71(10):1028–35.
5. Mehta RL, Kellum JA, Shah SV, Molitoris BA, Ronco C, Warnock DG, et al. Acute kidney injury network: report of an initiative to improve outcomes in acute kidney injury. Crit Care. 2007;11(2):R31.
6. Kaddourah A, Basu RK, Bagshaw SM, Goldstein SL, Investigators A. Epidemiology of acute kidney injury in critically ill children and young adults. N Engl J Med. 2017;376(1):11–20.

7. Sutherland SM. AKI in hospitalized children: epidemiology and clinical associations in a national cohort. J Pediatr. 2013;8(10):1661–9.
8. Alkandari O, Eddington KA, Hyder A, Gauvin F, Ducruet T, Gottesman R, et al. Acute kidney injury is an independent risk factor for pediatric intensive care unit mortality, longer length of stay and prolonged mechanical ventilation in critically ill children: a two-center retrospective cohort study. Crit Care. 2011;15(3):R146.
9. Chawla LS, Eggers PW, Star RA, Kimmel PL. Acute kidney injury and chronic kidney disease as interconnected syndromes. N Engl J Med. 2014;371(1):58–66.
10. Chawla LS, Amdur RL, Amodeo S, Kimmel PL, Palant CE. The severity of acute kidney injury predicts progression to chronic kidney disease. Kidney Int. 2011;79(12):1361–9.
11. Coca SG, Singanamala S, Parikh CR. Chronic kidney disease after acute kidney injury: a systematic review and meta-analysis. Kidney Int. 2012;81(5):442–8.
12. Hsu CY, Hsu RK, Yang J, Ordonez JD, Zheng S, Go AS. Elevated BP after AKI. J Am Soc Nephrol. 2016;27(3):914–23.
13. Mammen C, Al Abbas A, Skippen P, Nadel H, Levine D, Collet JP, et al. Long-term risk of CKD in children surviving episodes of acute kidney injury in the intensive care unit: a prospective cohort study. Am J Kidney Dis. 2012;59(4):523–30.
14. Askenazi DJ, Feig DI, Graham NM, Hui-Stickle S, Goldstein SL. 3–5 year longitudinal follow-up of pediatric patients after acute renal failure. Kidney Int. 2006;69(1):184–9.
15. Menon S, Kirkendall ES, Nguyen H, Goldstein SL. Acute kidney injury associated with high nephrotoxic medication exposure leads to chronic kidney disease after 6 months. J Pediatr. 2014;165(3):522–7. e2
16. Hui-Stickle S, Brewer ED, Goldstein SL. Pediatric ARF epidemiology at a tertiary care center from 1999 to 2001. Am J Kidney Dis. 2005;45(1):96–101.
17. Goldstein SL. Acute kidney injury in children: prevention, treatment and rehabilitation. Contrib Nephrol. 2011;174:163–72.
18. Williams DM, Sreedhar SS, Mickell JJ, Chan JC. Acute kidney failure: a pediatric experience over 20 years. Arch Pediatr Adolesc Med. 2002;156(9):893–900.
19. Goldstein SL, Kirkendall E, Nguyen H, Schaffzin JK, Bucuvalas J, Bracke T, et al. Electronic health record identification of nephrotoxin exposure and associated acute kidney injury. Pediatrics. 2013;132(3):e756–67.
20. Li S, Krawczeski CD, Zappitelli M, Devarajan P, Thiessen-Philbrook H, Coca SG, et al. Incidence, risk factors, and outcomes of acute kidney injury after pediatric cardiac surgery: a prospective multicenter study. Crit Care Med. 2011;39(6):1493–9.
21. MacDonald C, Norris C, Alton GY, Urschel S, Joffe AR, Morgan CJ, et al. Acute kidney injury after heart transplant in young children: risk factors and outcomes. Pediatr Nephrol. 2016;31(4):671–8.
22. Sutherland SM, Zappitelli M, Alexander SR, Chua AN, Brophy PD, Bunchman TE, et al. Fluid overload and mortality in children receiving continuous renal replacement therapy: the prospective pediatric continuous renal replacement therapy registry. Am J Kidney Dis. 2010;55(2):316–25.
23. Blinder JJ, Goldstein SL, Lee VV, Baycroft A, Fraser CD, Nelson D, et al. Congenital heart surgery in infants: effects of acute kidney injury on outcomes. J Thorac Cardiovasc Surg. 2012;143(2):368–74.
24. Fitzgerald JC, Basu RK, Akcan-Arikan A, Izquierdo LM, Pineres Olave BE, Hassinger AB, et al. Acute kidney injury in pediatric severe sepsis: an independent risk factor for death and new disability. Crit Care Med. 2016;44(12):2241–50.
25. Selewski DT, Cornell TT, Heung M, Troost JP, Ehrmann BJ, Lombel RM, et al. Validation of the KDIGO acute kidney injury criteria in a pediatric critical care population. Intensive Care Med. 2014;40(10):1481–8.
26. Selewski DT, Jordan BK, Askenazi DJ, Dechert RE, Sarkar S. Acute kidney injury in asphyxiated newborns treated with therapeutic hypothermia. J Pediatr. 2013;162(4):725–9.e1.
27. Arikan AA, Zappitelli M, Goldstein SL, Naipaul A, Jefferson LS, Loftis LL. Fluid overload is associated with impaired oxygenation and morbidity in critically ill children*. Pediatr Crit Care Med. 2012;13(3):253–8.

28. Hassinger AB, Wald EL, Goodman DM. Early postoperative fluid overload precedes acute kidney injury and is associated with higher morbidity in pediatric cardiac surgery patients. Pediatr Crit Care Med. 2014;15(2):131–8.
29. Hazle MA, Gajarski RJ, Yu S, Donohue J, Blatt NB. Fluid overload in infants following congenital heart surgery. Pediatr Crit Care Med. 2013;14(1):44.
30. Selewski DT, Cornell TT, Blatt NB, Han YY, Mottes T, Kommareddi M, et al. Fluid overload and fluid removal in pediatric patients on extracorporeal membrane oxygenation requiring continuous renal replacement therapy. Crit Care Med. 2012;40(9):2694–9.
31. Lex DJ, Tóth R, Cserép Z, Alexander SI, Breuer T, Sápi E, et al. A comparison of the systems for the identification of postoperative acute kidney injury in pediatric cardiac patients. Ann Thorac Surg. 2014;97(1):202–10.
32. Taylor ML, Carmona F, Thiagarajan RR, Westgate L, Ferguson MA, del Nido PJ, et al. Mild postoperative acute kidney injury and outcomes after surgery for congenital heart disease. J Thorac Cardiovasc Surg. 2013;146(1):146–52.
33. Zappitelli M, Moffett BS, Hyder A, Goldstein SL. Acute kidney injury in non-critically ill children treated with aminoglycoside antibiotics in a tertiary healthcare centre: a retrospective cohort study. Nephrol Dial Transplant. 2011;26(1):144–50.
34. Rheault MN, Zhang L, Selewski DT, Kallash M, Tran CL, Seamon M, et al. AKI in children hospitalized with nephrotic syndrome. Clin J Am Soc Nephrol. 2015;10(12):2110–8.
35. Bastin AJ, Ostermann M, Slack AJ, Diller GP, Finney SJ, Evans TW. Acute kidney injury after cardiac surgery according to risk/injury/failure/loss/end-stage, acute kidney injury network, and kidney disease: improving global outcomes classifications. J Crit Care. 2013;28(4):389–96.
36. Chawla LS, Amdur RL, Shaw AD, Faselis C, Palant CE, Kimmel PL. Association between AKI and long-term renal and cardiovascular outcomes in United States veterans. Clin J Am Soc Nephrol. 2014;9(3):448–56.
37. Hoste EA, Bagshaw SM, Bellomo R, Cely CM, Colman R, Cruz DN, et al. Epidemiology of acute kidney injury in critically ill patients: the multinational AKI-EPI study. Intensive Care Med. 2015;41(8):1411–23.
38. Chawla LS, Bellomo R, Bihorac A, Goldstein SL, Siew ED, Bagshaw SM, et al. Acute kidney disease and renal recovery: consensus report of the acute disease quality initiative (ADQI) 16 workgroup. Nat Rev Nephrol. 2017;13(4):241–57.
39. Goldstein SL. Renal recovery at different ages. Nephron Clin Pract. 2014;127(1–4):21–4.
40. Goldstein SL, Chawla L, Ronco C, Kellum JA. Renal recovery. Crit Care. 2014;18(1):301.
41. Helgadottir S, Sigurdsson MI, Palsson R, Helgason D, Sigurdsson GH, Gudbjartsson T. Renal recovery and long-term survival following acute kidney injury after coronary artery surgery: a nationwide study. Acta Anaesthesiol Scand. 2016;60(9):1230–40.
42. Heung M, Steffick DE, Zivin K, Gillespie BW, Banerjee T, Hsu CY, et al. Acute kidney injury recovery pattern and subsequent risk of CKD: an analysis of veterans health administration data. Am J Kidney Dis. 2016;67(5):742–52.
43. Laskey HL, Schomaker N, Hung KW, Asrani SK, Jennings L, Nydam TL, et al. Predicting renal recovery after liver transplant with severe pretransplant subacute kidney injury: the impact of warm ischemia time. Liver Transpl. 2016;22(8):1085–91.
44. Basu B, Mahapatra TK, Roy B, Schaefer F. Efficacy and outcomes of continuous peritoneal dialysis versus daily intermittent hemodialysis in pediatric acute kidney injury. Pediatr Nephrol. 2016;31(10):1681–9.
45. Bonnassieux M, Duclos A, Schneider AG, Schmidt A, Benard S, Cancalon C, et al. Renal replacement therapy modality in the ICU and renal recovery at hospital discharge. Crit Care Med. 2018;46(2):e102–10.
46. Hollander SA, Montez-Rath ME, Axelrod DM, Krawczeski CD, May LJ, Maeda K, et al. Recovery from acute kidney injury and CKD following heart transplantation in children, adolescents, and young adults: a retrospective cohort study. Am J Kidney Dis. 2016;68(2):212–8.
47. Long TE, Sigurdsson MI, Sigurdsson GH, Indridason OS. Improved long-term survival and renal recovery after acute kidney injury in hospitalized patients: a 20 year experience. Nephrology. 2016;21(12):1027–33.

48. Thongprayoon C, Cheungpasitporn W, Srivali N, Kittanamongkolchai W, Sakhuja A, Greason KL, et al. The association between renal recovery after acute kidney injury and long-term mortality after transcatheter aortic valve replacement. PLoS One. 2017;12(8):e0183350.
49. Hessey E, Ali R, Dorais M, Morissette G, Pizzi M, Rink N, et al. Renal function follow-up and renal recovery after acute kidney injury in critically ill children. Pediatr Crit Care Med. 2017;18(8):733–40.
50. Buysse CM, Raat H, Hazelzet JA, Hulst JM, Cransberg K, Hop WC, et al. Long-term health status in childhood survivors of meningococcal septic shock. Arch Pediatr Adolesc Med. 2008;162(11):1036–41.
51. Hingorani S, Guthrie KA, Schoch G, Weiss NS, McDonald GB. Chronic kidney disease in long-term survivors of hematopoietic cell transplant. Bone Marrow Transplant. 2007;39(4):223–9.
52. Greenberg JH, Coca S, Parikh CR. Long-term risk of chronic kidney disease and mortality in children after acute kidney injury: a systematic review. BMC Nephrol. 2014;15:184.
53. Greenberg JH, Zappitelli M, Devarajan P, Thiessen-Philbrook HR, Krawczeski C, Li S, et al. Kidney outcomes 5 years after pediatric cardiac surgery: the TRIBE-AKI study. JAMA Pediatr. 2016;170(11):1071–8.
54. Cooper DS, Claes D, Goldstein SL, Bennett MR, Ma Q, Devarajan P, et al. Follow-up renal assessment of injury long-term after acute kidney injury (FRAIL-AKI). Clin J Am Soc Nephrol. 2016;11(1):21–9.
55. Madsen NL, Goldstein SL, Froslev T, Christiansen CF, Olsen M. Cardiac surgery in patients with congenital heart disease is associated with acute kidney injury and the risk of chronic kidney disease. Kidney Int. 2017;92(3):751–6.
56. Silver SA, Goldstein SL, Harel Z, Harvey A, Rompies EJ, Adhikari NK, et al. Ambulatory care after acute kidney injury: an opportunity to improve patient outcomes. Can J Kidney Health Dis. 2015;2:36.

# Part II

# Renal Replacement Therapy

# 14 CRRT: Technology and Basic Concepts

Shina Menon and Jordan M. Symons

## 14.1 Introduction

Continuous renal replacement therapy (CRRT) has become the preferred modality to manage acute kidney injury (AKI) and fluid overload in critically ill children [1, 2]. Advances in technology allowing precise control of ultrafiltration, more accurate fluid balance, and better control of blood flow have made CRRT more reliable and easier to operate. CRRT allows molecular clearance and ultrafiltration to occur gradually and continuously over an extended period. Hemodynamically unstable patients who may not tolerate the rapid volume and solute concentration changes seen with standard hemodialysis (HD) can be managed safely and effectively with CRRT. While peritoneal dialysis (PD) also provides gradual clearance and ultrafiltration, CRRT provides more accurate control of fluid removal, along with the ability to independently adjust composition of the extracellular fluid [3]. This chapter aims to describe the principles of pediatric CRRT and review mechanisms of clearance in CRRT, thus providing background for optimal use of the therapy.

Pediatric CRRT has evolved over the last 40 years since Kramer et al. first described free-flow, non-pumped arteriovenous hemofiltration in the late 1970s, followed by the successful adaptation of the technique for use in an infant in 1981 [4, 5]. For pediatric use, membranes and filters were specifically designed to obtain low-resistance extracorporeal circuits and low ultrafiltration rates (1–3 mL/min) [6]. The arteriovenous pressure gradient provided the force to move blood through the circuit, which was challenging in small children due to lower systemic pressures. The technique became more popular in pediatric AKI after the advent of pumped venovenous machines, which mitigated the problem of low driving pressures in pediatric patients.

S. Menon · J. M. Symons (✉)
Division of Nephrology, Department of Pediatrics, University of Washington School of Medicine, Seattle Children's Hospital, Seattle, WA, USA
e-mail: Shina.Menon@seattlechildrens.org; jordan.symons@seattlechildrens.org



A. Deep, S. L. Goldstein (eds.), *Critical Care Nephrology and Renal Replacement Therapy in Children*, https://doi.org/10.1007/978-3-319-90281-4_14

While CRRT technology has advanced significantly over the years including development of pediatric-specific devices, the majority of pediatric patients still receive CRRT using equipment designed for and prescriptions extrapolated from adult patient experience.

## 14.2 Mechanisms of Solute Removal

All modalities of renal replacement therapy, be it PD, HD, or CRRT, involve transfer of solutes and fluid across a semipermeable membrane. Solute removal is governed by the physical principles of molecular movement (Fig. 14.1). In CRRT, this may occur

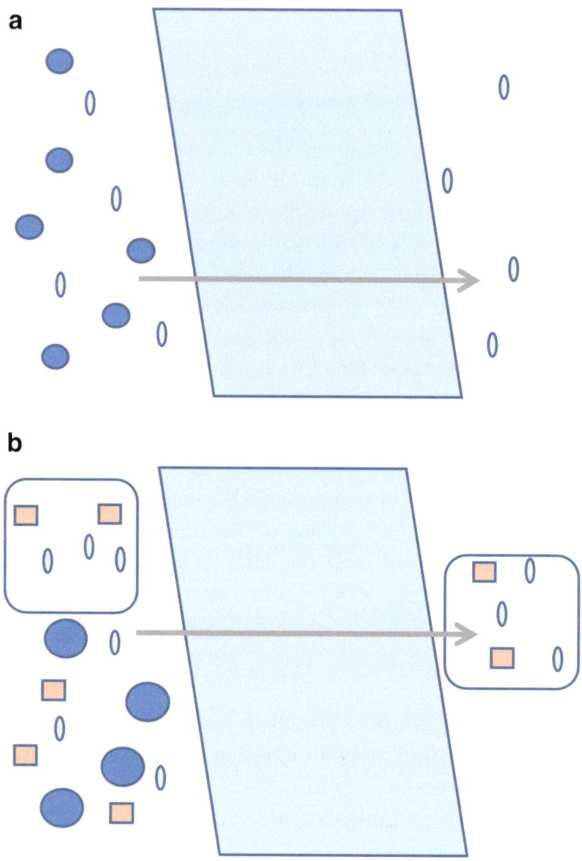


**Fig. 14.1** Schematic representations of diffusion and convection. (**a**) In diffusion, a substance flows down its concentration gradient across a semipermeable membrane. This movement of molecules down their concentration gradient from one solution to another continues until equilibrium is achieved on both sides. Diffusion is more efficient in the clearance of small molecular weight solutes. (**b**) In convection, solutes move across a membrane with solvent drag. The concentration of a solute is similar on either side of the membrane. Convection is more efficient at the clearance of larger molecular weight solutes

via diffusion, convection, adsorption, or a combination of these methods [7]. Fluid removal (ultrafiltration) is driven by hydrostatic pressure across the membrane.

Diffusion is the movement of dissolved particles across a semipermeable membrane from an area of high concentration to an area of low concentration. Any modality that uses dialysate relies on the process of diffusion for removal of solutes. The concentration gradient is maximized and maintained throughout the length of the membrane by running the dialysate countercurrent to the blood flow. The amount of solute removed (clearance) depends on the magnitude of the concentration gradient, the size of the molecule, and the surface area across which diffusion takes place. Diffusion is more efficient in clearing low molecular weight solutes like urea and creatinine, than those of higher molecular weight like beta 2 microglobulin and cytokines.

Convection describes the flow of dissolved particles across a semipermeable membrane from solvent flux due to the effects of a pressure gradient. Because the solute and solvent are moving together, the removed solute appears in the effluent at the same concentration as in the origin solution. The movement of a specific solute across the membrane is dependent not only on the charge and size of the solute but also on the size of the pores in the membrane. The ability of the solute to cross the membrane by convection is expressed as the sieving coefficient, and is calculated as the ratio of the solute concentration in the effluent and blood. The sieving coefficient for a particular solute may decline over the duration of treatment as plasma proteins that are too large to cross the membrane accumulate along the membrane surface. This phenomenon of protein concentration polarization can potentially change the charge of the pores and restrict access to them.

Adsorption is the adherence of solutes (particularly peptides and proteins) to surfaces within the extracorporeal circuit. Adsorption of solutes occurs to varying degrees in all CRRT circuits and can contribute to large-molecule removal, particularly with the polyacrylonitrile membrane. Adsorption may vary with the size, charge, and structure of the molecule and the characteristics of the membrane (porosity, composition) [8]. The contribution of adsorption to solute removal decreases over time as the membrane becomes saturated with the substance [7].

Ultrafiltration is the movement of water across the semipermeable membrane secondary to a transmembrane pressure (TMP) gradient. The ultrafiltration rate is determined by the hydraulic permeability of the membrane, the membrane surface area, and the TMP. Convection occurs with ultrafiltration, and high rates of ultrafiltration will remove both small and larger particles by convection, up to the limits of the membrane.

## 14.3 Modalities of Continuous Renal Replacement Therapy

The various subcategories of CRRT are named based on the primary method of solute clearance (Fig. 14.2). Slow continuous ultrafiltration (SCUF) uses ultrafiltration exclusively without fluid replacement. This is primarily used to treat fluid overload. Solute removal is minimal due to the slow rate of ultrafiltration (low convection)

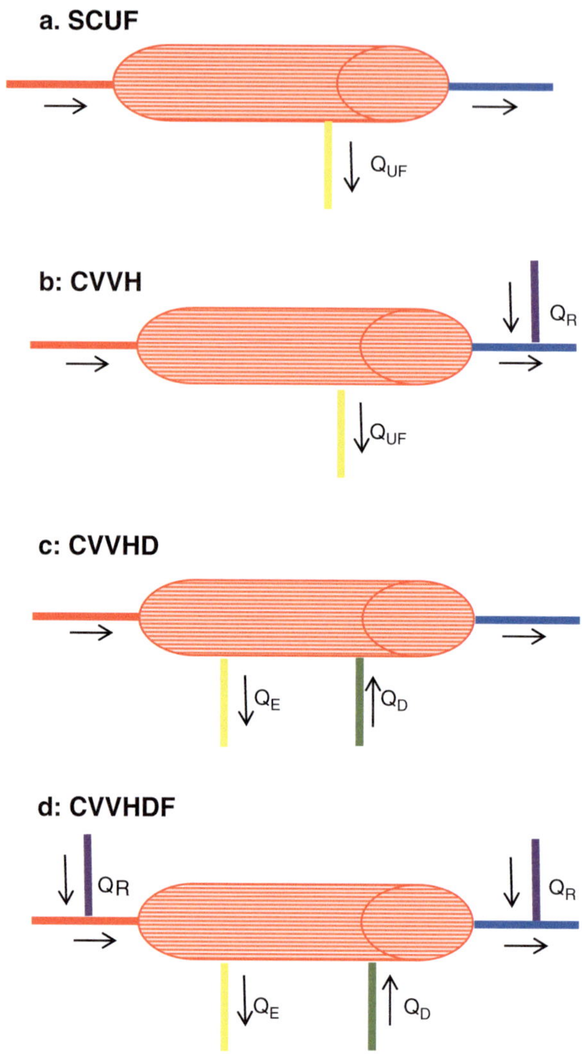


**Fig. 14.2** Schematic representation of common modalities of continuous renal replacement therapy. (**a**) SCUF, (**b**) CVVH, (**c**) CVVHD, (**d**) CVVHDF. Abbreviations: $Q_B$ blood flow rate, $Q_{UF}$ ultrafiltration flow rate, $Q_D$ dialysate flow rate, $Q_R$ total replacement flow rate, $Q_E$ effluent flow rate, *SCUF* slow continuous ultrafiltration, *CVVH* continuous venovenous hemofiltration, *CVVHD* continuous venovenous hemodialysis, *CVVHDF* continuous venovenous hemodiafiltration

and lack of dialysis. Continuous venovenous hemofiltration (CVVH) relies on higher rates of convection and requires a substitution fluid to replace part or all of the ultrafiltrate. The composition of this replacement fluid can be varied based on the patient's requirements and it can be infused pre- or postfilter. Continuous venovenous hemodialysis (CVVHD) uses dialysate to generate diffusive clearance.

Finally, continuous venovenous hemodiafiltration (CVVHDF) uses both dialysate and replacement fluids for combined diffusion and high-grade convection.

## 14.4 Calculation of Solute Clearance

Solute clearance can be calculated based on either the disappearance of solute from the blood or its appearance in the effluent fluids. During CVVH, the solute concentration of ultrafiltrate is similar to that of plasma and the variation in plasma solute concentration over the length of the hemofilters tends to be small. Additionally, during CVVHD, the dialysate flow is significantly less than the blood flow. As a result, the appearance of the solute in the effluent is more commonly used to estimate clearance.

Using the solute appearance in the effluent, clearance ($K$) during CRRT can be expressed as:

$$K = \left[\left(Q_E C_E\right) - \left(Q_D C_D\right)\right] / C_B,$$

where $Q_D$ and $Q_E$ are the dialysate inflow and effluent outflow rates, respectively, and $C_B$, $C_D$, and $C_E$ are the concentrations of solute in the blood, dialysate, and effluent, respectively. Given that the ultrafiltration rate ($Q_{UF}$) is equal to the difference between the effluent outflow and dialysate inflow rates, ($Q_{UF} = Q_E - Q_D$), clearance ($K$) may be rewritten as:

$$K = \left(Q_{UF} C_E\right) / C_B + \left[Q_D \left(C_E - C_D\right)\right] / C_B.$$

The first part of the equation [$(Q_{UF}C_E)/C_B$] represents clearance that occurs in the absence of dialysate flow and approximates the convective clearance. The convective clearance ($K_C$) can also be written as $Q_{UF}S$, where $S$ is the sieving coefficient ($S = C_E/C_B$).

The second half of the equation, [$Q_D(C_E - C_D)]/C_B$, estimates clearance in the absence of ultrafiltration and is a measure of the diffusive component of clearance. For solutes that are not present in the dialysate, the equation can be simplified to $Q_D C_E/C_B$.

Solute clearance is also affected by the site of infusion of replacement fluid in the circuit, prefilter (predilution) or postfilter (postdilution). For low molecular weight solutes with sieving coefficients close to unity, the solute clearance during postdilution CVVH is approximately equal to the ultrafiltration rate [9]. Clearance can be increased with higher ultrafiltration rates to an extent. However, this may also result in an increase in the filtration fraction (FF), which is the ratio of ultrafiltration rate ($Q_{UF}$) to plasma flow rate, and is determined as follows:

$$\text{FF} = Q_{UF} / Q_B \left(1 - \text{hematocrit}\right)$$

A filtration fraction greater than 20–30% can result in hemoconcentration and increased risk of clotting. Higher ultrafiltration rates require larger blood flows to avoid elevated FF and filter clotting.

Administration of the replacement fluid prefilter reduces the solute concentration in the blood entering the filter, and is useful in preventing clotting of the circuit. However, this dilution of blood entering the filter also reduces the clearance in predilution CVVH. Clearance is calculated by the effluent rate corrected for the dilution factor.

In CVVHD, due to relatively lower dialysate flow rates compared with intermittent HD, near complete equilibration can occur between blood and dialysate for low molecular weight solutes. This results in a nearly linear relationship between dialysate flow and small solute clearance. The clearance of higher molecular weight solutes is limited by their slower rates of diffusion and not dependent on dialysate flow.

In general, for most small molecules solute removal is approximated by the effluent rate in milliliters/kilogram/hour. This may however overestimate the true clearance, because it does not account for filter clotting and circuit down time due to other reasons. Measuring solute removal in the effluent and calculating clearance based on the mass extracted is considered the gold-standard method to assess delivered dose.

## 14.5 Technical Aspects of Continuous Renal Replacement Therapy

*CRRT Devices*: Across the globe, various CRRT devices are available from different manufacturers, each with its own distinctive features. The choice of CRRT device for pediatric patients depends on cost, availability, and local expertise. CRRT for children incurs added risks secondary to higher circuit extracorporeal volumes relative to patient blood volume, higher relative blood flows, and alternative indications/diseases. Most of the current devices were designed for adults and have been adapted for use in pediatrics with smaller circuits and lines. In recent years there has been significant progress in the creation of pediatric-specific devices that may revolutionize the practice of pediatric CRRT. These newer devices are discussed in more detail in Chap. 17.

Despite the differences in the CRRT machines and devices, the key technical aspects of pediatric CRRT can be generalized.

*Vascular Access*: The success of CRRT treatment depends on the quality of vascular access. Adequate blood flow ($Q_B$) is required to generate appropriate access and return pressures to prevent related complications. As defined by Poiseuille's law, resistance is directly proportional to length and inversely proportional to radius to the fourth power. Based on this, the shortest and widest catheter will provide maximum blood flow. The Prospective Pediatric Continuous Renal Replacement Therapy (ppCRRT) Registry evaluated the effect of vascular access size and location on circuit survival [10]. They noted that the survival of the CRRT circuit was significantly higher when larger catheters were used. The 48-hour survival with 8-French catheters was 76%, compared to 26% with 7-French catheters. In this study, the standard single lumen 5-French catheter used in small infants fared poorly with low circuit survival. El Masri and colleagues recently published their experience in infants who received CRRT via two hemostasis valve sheaths (3, 4, and 5-French) placed into separate veins for dialysis access and return [11]. These sheaths are different in that their internal diameter is significantly larger than conventional catheters with similar external diameter. Consequently, they had low resistance and provided excellent blood flow but their thin walls were prone to kinking.

Temporary or tunneled cuffed hemodialysis catheters are currently used as vascular access for CRRT. The Kidney Disease: Improving Global Outcomes (KDIGO) guideline recommends ultrasound guidance for catheter placement to reduce the failure and complication rates of central venous catheter insertion [12]. For patients requiring more than a week of acute dialysis therapy, tunneled, cuffed, double-lumen catheters are better [7].

The optimal site for catheter placement is dependent on various factors including the risks of the procedure, possibility of thrombosis, stenosis, and infection. The internal jugular vein is preferred (particularly right over the left) because of its large caliber, more direct route to the superior vena cava, and lower recirculation rate [12]. Femoral veins, while not ideal, are often considered as the second choice due to their accessibility. However, they are associated with higher recirculation rates and potential for flow interference secondary to patient movement or increased intraabdominal pressure. Subclavian vein cannulation is usually avoided due to the risk of stenosis, which may interfere with arteriovenous graft or fistula creation in the future should the patient develop chronic kidney disease. Table 14.1 shows suggested weight and size based temporary catheters for CRRT access.

## 14.6 Blood Flow Rates

The presence of a good-sized catheter in the right location allows adjustment of the blood flow ($Q_B$) according to the size of the patient. The recommended blood flow rates in pediatrics have been extrapolated from adults and are typically in the range of 3–10 mL/kg/min. Higher blood flow (10–12 mL/kg/min) is usually necessary in neonates and small infants when using adult sized CRRT devices. While a higher $Q_B$

**Table 14.1** Suggested weight/size-based temporary catheters for acute continuous renal replacement therapy access

| Patient size | Catheter size |
|---|---|
| Neonates | Double lumen 7 French |
| 3–6 kg | Double lumen 7 French |
| 6–12 kg | Double lumen 8 French |
| 12–20 kg | Double lumen 9 French |
| 20–30 kg | Double lumen 10 French |
| 30+ kg | Double lumen 10 or 11 French<br>Triple lumen 11.5 French |

may reduce the risk for intrafiber clotting and prolong circuit life span, it is unlikely to increase small solute clearance (as seen in hemodialysis). In patients with predilution CVVH or CVVHDF, it mitigates the reduced efficiency resulting from predilution. Smaller patients, particularly those with disproportionately larger CRRT circuits, may not tolerate maximal blood flow at the initiation of CRRT and the $Q_B$ should be gradually advanced to the targeted rate as tolerated.

## 14.7 Membrane and CRRT Filters

A number of hemofilters and membranes have been developed for use with CRRT, and the choice of hemofilter usually depends on the CRRT machine being used. Membrane characteristics like thickness, pore size, charge, and adsorptive properties determine the solute removal capacity during CRRT.

While none of the membranes has been shown to be superior, one highly biocompatible membrane, the AN-69 polyacrylonitrile membrane has been associated with the bradykinin release syndrome particularly when used in conjunction with a blood prime [13]. The syndrome is characterized by a precipitous drop in blood pressure 5–10 min after initiation of CRRT. It occurs secondary to the exposure of the blood to the negatively charged AN-69 membrane, which activates pre-kallikrein and Hageman factor resulting in the release of bradykinin, a powerful vasodilator. Several strategies have been proposed to prevent this syndrome, including buffering the blood to physiological pH before priming the circuit, infusing the blood post filter at the same rate as a blood transfusion, or completely avoiding the AN-69 membrane [13–15]. A variant, the AN-69ST membrane, where the electronegativity of polyacrylonitrile is neutralized by treating the surface with polyethyleneimine, has the potential to mitigate blood–membrane contact reactions and release of bradykinin [16]. However, these filters may not be available everywhere, and there is limited pediatric safety and efficacy data [17].

Polyacrylonitrile membrane is sometimes recommended for patients with sepsis due to greater cytokine sieving coefficients when compared to other membranes. While inflammatory mediators (interleukin 6 [IL-6], IL-8, IL-1, and tumor necrosis factor) can be removed by convection according to the molecular weight and degree of plasma protein binding, studies have not shown that cytokine removal improves the survival of septic patients receiving CRRT [18–20].

Polysulfone derivative membranes [polyarylethersulfone (PAES) or polyethersulfone] are alternatives to the AN-69 membrane that have not been shown to cause bradykinin release [21]. However, they may not be available in pediatric-specific sizes.

*Anticoagulation*: The contact of circulating blood with the extracorporeal circuit, tubing, and membrane activates platelets and inflammatory and prothrombotic mediators. In pediatric patients, the risk of clotting is exacerbated by lower blood flow rates, turbulent flow, small catheters, and high hematocrits. The resultant fibrin deposition reduces the surface of the membrane available for diffusion or convection and consequently the efficiency of solute clearance. To prevent clotting and prolong CRRT circuit life span, anticoagulation is commonly employed. Several methods of anticoagulation are now available, with unfractionated heparin and sodium citrate being the most common. These will be discussed in more detail in a separate chapter.

*Solutions for dialysate and replacement fluids*: For CRRT, solutions can either be compounded in the institutional pharmacy or purchased commercially. While the former method may be less expensive, it increases the risk of contamination and error [22]. Preprepared solutions are usually more expensive but have long shelf lives and high reliability. The varieties of solutions available commercially are too extensive to list here, and the choice of fluids available in a certain institution is dependent on the local anticoagulation practices, solute composition, and regulatory body approval status among other factors.

The composition of solutions used in CRRT has changed significantly in recent times, with the use of lactate-based fluids gradually decreasing. In the past when lactate was used as the buffer, lactic acidosis and subsequent cardiac dysfunction was commonly seen [23]. KDIGO recommends using bicarbonate based fluids for CRRT, particularly in patients with AKI and circulatory shock, or AKI and liver failure [12]. Many of the commercially available preparations still contain a small, clinically insignificant amount of lactate to improve stability.

In addition to a buffer, CRRT solutions also contain varying amounts of sodium, potassium, chloride, glucose, calcium, and magnesium; the composition varies according to the manufacturers. The goal for fluid composition during CRRT is precise management of the solute composition of the plasma. The fluid composition may change over the course of CRRT therapy. While treatment is often started with a fluid that is low in potassium and phosphorous, most patients develop hypokalemia and hypophosphatemia shortly thereafter, especially with higher doses of CRRT. Hypophosphatemia, which is particularly common due to larger filter pore size and ongoing intercompartmental mass transfer, can lead to respiratory and cardiac depression, and immune dysfunction [7]. Supplementation of the replacement solutions with the requisite electrolytes by the pharmacy results in a more physiologic fluid for the patient. There is however the potential for pharmacy errors with this approach. Phosphate-containing CRRT replacement fluids are now commercially available [24].

It is practical to have the same composition for the replacement and dialysate fluids when using CVVHDF. This reduces the risk of error.

## Conclusion

CRRT is becoming a common modality to manage critically ill children with AKI. While there are no data to suggest its superiority over hemodialysis or peritoneal dialysis, it may be well tolerated by children with hemodynamic instability. Significant research is still needed in several aspects, including timing of initiation and optimal dose. Newer advances like smaller miniaturized circuits and membranes, and more accurate devices are promising.

**Key Learning Points**

- Renal replacement therapy may be required in patients with severe acute kidney injury. Several RRT modalities, including peritoneal dialysis, intermittent hemodialysis, and continuous RRT, are available to manage pediatric patients with AKI.
- The selection of modality is based on patient factors (size, underlying illness, hemodynamic stability, ability to obtain access), the local expertise and experience, and available resources.
- CRRT involves either diffusion-based solute removal (dialysis) or convection-based solute and water removal or a combination of both.
- Due to the slower rate of solute or fluid removal, CRRT is generally better tolerated than intermittent RRT.
- Multiple different CRRT devices are available worldwide but all operate under the same physical principles.
- Most CRRT devices were designed for adults and adapted to pediatric care; newer pediatric-specific devices are now becoming available.

## References


1. Goldstein SL, et al. Pediatric patients with multi-organ dysfunction syndrome receiving continuous renal replacement therapy. Kidney Int. 2005;67(2):653–8.
2. Ricci Z, Goldstein SL. Pediatric continuous renal replacement therapy. Contrib Nephrol. 2016;187:121–30.
3. Maxvold NJ, Bunchman TE. Renal failure and renal replacement therapy. Crit Care Clin. 2003;19(3):563–75.
4. Kramer P, et al. Continuous arteriovenous haemofiltration. A new kidney replacement therapy. Proc Eur Dial Transplant Assoc. 1981;18:743–9.
5. Ronco C, et al. Treatment of acute renal failure in the newborn by continuous arteriovenous hemofiltration. Trans Am Soc Artif Intern Organs. 1985;31:634–8.
6. Garzotto F, Zanella M, Ronco C. The evolution of pediatric continuous renal replacement therapy. Nephron Clin Pract. 2014;127(1–4):172–5.
7. Macedo E, Mehta RL. Continuous dialysis therapies: core curriculum 2016. Am J Kidney Dis. 2016;68(4):645–57.
8. Neri M, et al. Nomenclature for renal replacement therapy in acute kidney injury: basic principles. Crit Care. 2016;20(1):318.
9. Troyanov S, et al. Solute clearances during continuous venovenous haemofiltration at various ultrafiltration flow rates using Multiflow-100 and HF1000 filters. Nephrol Dial Transplant. 2003;18(5):961–6.
10. Hackbarth R, et al. The effect of vascular access location and size on circuit survival in pediatric continuous renal replacement therapy: a report from the PPCRRT registry. Int J Artif Organs. 2007;30(12):1116–21.
11. El Masri K, et al. Successful continuous renal replacement therapy using two single-lumen catheters in neonates and infants with cardiac disease. Pediatr Nephrol. 2013;28(12):2383–7.
12. Kidney Disease: Improving Global Outcomes (KDIGO) Acute Kidney Injury Work Group. KDIGO clinical practice guideline for acute kidney injury. Kidney Int. 2012;2:1–138.
13. Bunchman TE, Brophy PD, Goldstein SL. Technical considerations for renal replacement therapy in children. Semin Nephrol. 2008;28(5):488–92.

14. Brophy PD, et al. AN-69 membrane reactions are pH-dependent and preventable. Am J Kidney Dis. 2001;38(1):173–8.
15. Pasko DA, Mottes TA, Mueller BA. Pre dialysis of blood prime in continuous hemodialysis normalizes pH and electrolytes. Pediatr Nephrol. 2003;18(11):1177–83.
16. Desormeaux A, et al. The effect of electronegativity and angiotensin-converting enzyme inhibition on the kinin-forming capacity of polyacrylonitrile dialysis membranes. Biomaterials. 2008;29(9):1139–46.
17. Hothi DK, et al. Continuous renal replacement therapy (CRRT) in children using the AQUARIUS. Nephrol Dial Transplant. 2006;21(8):2296–300.
18. Bellomo R, Tipping P, Boyce N. Continuous veno-venous hemofiltration with dialysis removes cytokines from the circulation of septic patients. Crit Care Med. 1993;21(4):522–6.
19. Cole L, et al. Cytokine removal during continuous renal replacement therapy: an ex vivo comparison of convection and diffusion. Int J Artif Organs. 2004;27(5):388–97.
20. Bellomo R, et al. Intensity of continuous renal-replacement therapy in critically ill patients. N Engl J Med. 2009;361(17):1627–38.
21. Sutherland SM, Alexander SR. Continuous renal replacement therapy in children. Pediatr Nephrol. 2012;27(11):2007–16.
22. Barletta JF, et al. Medication errors and patient complications with continuous renal replacement therapy. Pediatr Nephrol. 2006;21(6):842–5.
23. Davenport A, Will EJ, Davison AM. Hyperlactataemia and metabolic acidosis during haemofiltration using lactate-buffered fluids. Nephron. 1991;59(3):461–5.
24. Ronco C, et al. Renal replacement therapy in acute kidney injury: controversy and consensus. Crit Care. 2015;19:146.

# Critical Care Nephrology and Renal Replacement Therapy in Children: Timing of Initiation of CRRT

**15**

David M. Kwiatkowski, Catherine D. Krawczeski, and David T. Selewski

**Case Vignette**

You are caring for a 3 kg 2-week-old infant who is recovering 6 days after a complex palliative cardiac surgery. She had evidence of early acute kidney injury that seemed to improve, but she is not making much urine and continues to have a positive fluid balance each day. She has increasing ascites and requires significant mechanical ventilation due to impaired respiratory mechanics. You advocate for consideration of peritoneal dialysis, but the rest of your team prefers limiting nutrition, increasing inotropic medications and diuretics, contending that all babies just have to get through this period of fluid overload and that the risks of renal replacement therapy outweigh the benefits.

The indications for the initiation of renal replacement therapy (RRT) in pediatric patients are well established in critical care nephrology, including the need for ultrafiltration for fluid removal and solute removal of a dialyzable agent, electrolyte or for uremia. The development of acute kidney injury (AKI) and the need for RRT are recognized risk factors for worse outcomes in many critical illnesses in pediatrics;

D. M. Kwiatkowski · C. D. Krawczeski (✉)
Division of Pediatric Cardiology, Department of Pediatrics, Stanford University School of Medicine, Palo Alto, CA, USA
e-mail: ckraw@stanford.edu

D. T. Selewski
Division of Pediatric Nephrology, Department of Pediatrics, University of Michigan School of Medicine, Ann Arbor, MI, USA



A. Deep, S. L. Goldstein (eds.), *Critical Care Nephrology and Renal Replacement Therapy in Children*, https://doi.org/10.1007/978-3-319-90281-4_15

thus focus has turned to modifiable variables in the care of patients with renal injury, including the timing of RRT. Whereas the classic RRT indications for solute removal remain relatively unchanged, the specific indications and timing for RRT initiation for fluid removal has become an area of academic interest.

Earlier initiation of RRT for prevention and treatment of fluid overload has been advocated, as evidence supports worse outcomes with greater degrees of fluid overload [1–3]. Furthermore, early and aggressive fluid removal may permit better nutritional support and allow necessary blood products and medications. However, it must be remembered that RRT, in every modality, is an invasive procedure with its own inherent risks, which are often greater in smaller patients. Since the indications for RRT to remove solutes are less contentious, the goal of this chapter is to review outcomes associated with fluid overload, and to discuss considerations of timing of initiation of the various forms of RRT in various patient populations to guide more judicious use of this intervention.

## 15.1 The Problem of Fluid Overload in Pediatric Patients

Impaired urine output and the subsequent development of fluid overload is a devastating consequence of acute kidney injury, likely accounting for much of its associated morbidity. Renal tubular injury and hypoperfusion lead to a decrease in glomerular filtration and subsequent retention of fluid. The presence of inflammation and the subsequent capillary leak associated with critical illness, such as sepsis or with cardiopulmonary bypass, contributes further to tissue and organ edema which is then exacerbated by fluid resuscitation. Low cardiac output may also activate neurohormonal pathways, including the renin-angiotensin system, adding to fluid and salt retention. The combination of these factors culminates in fluid accumulation in each organ system leading to organ dysfunction.

Perhaps the most visible consequence of fluid overload is the development of skin edema, or in severe cases, anasarca. While also "cosmetic," altered tissue integrity can lead to important morbidities such as skin ulceration, poor wound healing, and infection. In the lungs, fluid overload is manifest as pulmonary edema and pleural effusions, which contribute to impaired gas exchange and altered lung compliance. In the abdomen, the development of gut edema and ascites causes feeding intolerance and poor gut motility, while the associated increased abdominal pressure decreases cardiac preload, worsens respiratory dynamics, and further impairs kidney perfusion [4]. Edema in the myocardium is manifest as diastolic dysfunction and decreased contractility. These, along with diminished preload and elevated venous pressures, contribute to further renal dysfunction. These effects are progressive and additive, and can quickly lead to major morbidity and mortality.

While previously thought to be insignificant or transient, it is now well recognized that even lesser amounts of fluid overload are associated with worse outcomes. In a large study from the prospective pediatric CRRT registry, a greater percentage of fluid overload at the time of CRRT initiation independently predicted mortality, with each additional 1% of fluid overload present at the time of CRRT institution conferring a 3% increase in mortality [1, 5]. Of note, those with >20%

fluid overload had an over 8 times higher risk of mortality. Conversely, early renal replacement therapy prior to the onset of fluid overload has been associated with a higher incidence of renal recovery at 1 year [6]. In the pediatric population, early postoperative fluid overload is directly associated with worse outcomes, including duration of intensive care, inotropic medication use, length of mechanical ventilation, oxygenation index, rate of mechanical circulatory support, and mortality [7–11]. Further, the risk of poor outcome increases with longer time to fluid removal in the postoperative period [2]. It is important to note that the presence of fluid overload may precede and be associated with the subsequent development of AKI [7, 12] but worse outcomes have been noted with fluid overload even in the absence of AKI, confirming its independent effects [13]. Similar poor outcomes with fluid overload have been demonstrated in other critically ill populations with a linear relationship between increasing fluid overload and declining oxygen index, longer length of mechanical ventilation, and higher mortality [14, 15].

Accurate assessment of volume status may be difficult in the pediatric patient, but is vital to aid in management decisions. Fluid overload is most typically denoted as a percentage and is calculated as [16]:

$$\%\mathrm{FO} = \left[\left(\text{Fluid In}(\mathrm{L}) - \text{Fluid Out}(\mathrm{L})\right) / \text{Admit Weight}(\mathrm{kg})\right] \times 100$$

While this calculation does not take into account insensible losses, which may vary among patients, percentage fluid overload using this formula has been shown to correlate with outcomes in multiple populations in both adults and pediatrics [7, 9, 11, 17]. Alternatively, the weight-based calculation uses change in weight rather than fluid intake and output to determine percent fluid overload. While daily weights may be impractical in some populations, such as early postoperative cardiac patients, due to instability, it may be more accurate in others, such as neonates, where insensible losses may impact fluid status to a larger degree [18]. It may be calculated as:

$$\%\mathrm{FO} = \left[\left(\text{Daily Weight}(\mathrm{Kg}) - \text{ICU Admit Weight}(\mathrm{Kg})\right) / \text{ICU Admit Weight}\right] \times 100$$

Fluid overload calculated by weight changes has also been shown to correlate with adverse outcomes in several populations [2, 3, 19, 20].

In addition to its negative effects on organ function, fluid overload may also mask the recognition of AKI if the excess intravascular volume dilutes the measured serum creatinine concentration. Thus, the use of "corrected" serum creatinine has been suggested to be a more accurate assessment of true changes in its concentration and may be calculated as:

$$\text{Corrected SCr} = \text{Measured SCr} \times \left[1 + \left(\text{cumulative net fluid balance} / \text{total body water}\right)\right]$$

where total body water = 0.6 × weight (kg).

The use of the corrected serum creatinine concentration may reclassify patients with fluid overload and previously unrecognized AKI or those with volume depletion who were incorrectly diagnosed with AKI, improving the prediction of poor outcome and aiding in management decision [21–23]. Elevation in the corrected serum creatinine has been shown to improve the predictive value and be associated with worse outcomes in postoperative cardiac patients [21]. The impact of intravascular volume (both by dilution or concentration) on diagnostic accuracy might be decreased or eliminated in the future by the use of more specific and accurate biomarkers.

Despite multiple studies of pharmacologic treatments, no medication has been shown to treat or prevent AKI in humans [24]. There are a number of reasons that likely underlie this lack of success, including the multifactorial cause of AKI (such that one single intervention may not be successful for all forms of AKI), the delayed recognition of AKI in most patients which prevents treatment within a very narrow therapeutic window of opportunity, and the inability to remove the inciting cause of injury in many patients (e.g., low cardiac output). Given this, the focus of management remains the treatment or prevention of fluid overload. The simplest strategy, at first glance, is typically restriction of fluid input. While this strategy conceptually should be easy and successful, the practicality of it is unfortunately limited, since patients with AKI tend to be critically ill and the necessary medications (such as vasoactive infusions, continuous sedation medications, diuretics, antibiotics, electrolyte replacements, and line flushes) often exceed the desired restriction alone, even if adequate nutrition is withheld. This is particularly problematic in neonates and infants, who have smaller fluid requirements. Furthermore, additional fluid administration may be necessary to maintain adequate preload and cardiac output in critically ill patients with impaired ventricular function or with sepsis.

With this in mind, attention typically turns to augmentation of urine output. Pharmacologic therapies intended to improve urine output include diuretics, renal vasodilators, and medications to improve cardiac output. While there are some exceptions, most diuretics exert their action by decreasing reabsorption of sodium, thereby increasing fluid loss.

The use of diuretics in critically ill patients with AKI is ubiquitous, however they are often ineffective, and at worse may even be detrimental, associated in some studies with a higher risk of mortality [25–27]. Importantly, almost all diuretics must reach the tubular lumen by glomerular filtration or proximal tubular secretion to exert their action [28]. Thus, if AKI causes a decrease in glomerular filtration, diuretic delivery and subsequent efficacy is impeded. Newer diuretics such as vasopressor receptor antagonists are being used more frequently in pediatric patients and early studies have demonstrated improved urine output [29] but results from a multicenter study are pending (ClinicalTrials.gov NCT02012959).

Renal vasodilators and medications to improve cardiac output are theorized to increase glomerular perfusion, therefore improving urine output. Dopamine has been used for decades in "renal doses," intended to increase renal blood flow and urine production [30]. In healthy adults, it has been shown to improve GFR and renal blood flow [30] but studies in critically ill populations have failed to consistently demonstrate an improvement in urine output with no difference in incidence of AKI or need for renal replacement therapy [31, 32]. Retrospective studies of fenoldopam and aminophylline have suggested an improvement in urine output in neonates after cardiac surgery [33, 34]. However, study results have been conflicting and in pediatric randomized controlled trials none of the investigated renal vasodilators have consistently been shown to decrease the incidence of AKI or augment urine output [35–39].

As medical interventions are often ineffective at preventing and treating fluid overload, early renal replacement therapy is becoming increasingly used in pediatric patients, in many cases to avoid the onset fluid overload.

## 15.2 Initiation of Continuous Renal Replacement Therapy

In pediatric critical care there has been a transition in the choice of modality for providing renal replacement therapy. This first became evident from survey data in 2000 describing the increasing use of CRRT as the modality of choice for renal replacement therapy in critically ill children [40]. CRRT has several advantages over other modalities in critically ill children. The major advantage to CRRT in critically ill children is its ability to provide renal replacement therapy with good hemodynamic tolerance. Furthermore, the continuous nature of this modality allows for slower fluid removal without large fluid shifts that may occur with intermittent hemodialysis. At the same time, the amount of fluid removed can be precisely set, which is advantageous when compared to a modality such as peritoneal dialysis. CRRT provides cumulative solute clearance similar to intermittent hemodialysis but with better hemodynamic tolerance. As a result of the combination of precise volume control and clearance characteristics, CRRT allows for the provision of volume to a patient that is sufficient for adequate nutrition, medications, and blood products [41, 42]. CRRT also provides the theoretical benefit of immunomodulation, a detailed discussion of which is outside of the scope of this chapter.

The indications for CRRT are fundamentally similar to other renal replacement modalities including refractory acidosis, electrolyte abnormalities, uremia, fluid overload, inability to provide adequate nutrition, and certain intoxications. In 2005, the prospective pediatric CRRT Registry (ppCRRT) provided an evaluation of CRRT indications from a registry of 370 children receiving CRRT at 13 centers. This study showed that fluid management and fluid overload were the indication for CRRT in 78% of the cohort (46% combined fluid/electrolyte, 29% fluid overload, 3% prevention of fluid overload) [43]. Single-center studies have confirmed these findings repeatedly reporting fluid overload as the most common indication for CRRT [3, 44]. Pediatricians have been at the forefront of recognizing the deleterious impact of the degree of fluid overload at CRRT initiation. This is exemplified by the seminal publication in 2010 from the ppCRRT registry that evaluated the impact of fluid overload in 297 patients from the registry. This study described increasing mortality with higher degrees of fluid overload at time of CRRT initiation (29.6% mortality in <10% fluid overload, 43.1% mortality in 10–20% fluid overload, and 65.6% mortality in >20% fluid overload). Furthermore, on multivariable analysis accounting for severity of illness, this study showed that children who had >20% FO at CRRT initiation had increased mortality (OR 8.5) [1]. Several single-center studies have produced similar findings [3, 20, 44, 45]. The cumulative data from a multitude of observational studies show that mortality increases significantly when CRRT is initiated at 10–20%. As a result, expert consensus has suggested that fluid overload 10–20% represents a critical value to consider definitive intervention dependent on disease course [46, 47].

While the observational data to date have suggested that earlier intervention with CRRT prior to the development of significant fluid overload would improve outcomes, there has not been a confirmatory prospective study or clinical trial in children. To date there have been few studies evaluating the impact of timing of CRRT in general pediatric populations. Modem evaluated the impact of the timing of CRRT initiation in a single-center study of 190 children on CRRT for AKI and or fluid overload. In this study, patients who had later initiation (>5 days) after ICU admission had increased mortality by adjusted analysis (HR 1.56, 95%CI 1.56) [48]. In a small study of 27 children aged <16 with severe sepsis with multi-organ dysfunction syndrome who required CRRT, Gulla found that survival was significantly higher in those that received CRRT within 48 h of admission (61.1 vs. 33.3%, $p < 0.001$) [49]. Further work is warranted to better delineate the impact of the timing of initiation of CRRT on outcomes in critically ill children.

## 15.3 Initiation of Peritoneal Dialysis

Management of acute kidney injury and fluid overload is particularly challenging among infants and small children as this population is often more sensitive to acute volume shifts, has more challenges with the achievement of optimal anticoagulation, and has smaller blood vessels through which to perform hemodialysis. For these reasons and others, the use of peritoneal dialysis (PD) is a common modality of RRT in smaller patients, especially in infants and small children after heart surgery with cardiopulmonary bypass. However, even within this population, its use is rare, at only 2% of the population [50]. The use of PD for RRT in this cohort has been endorsed by The Kidney Disease: Improving Global Outcomes (KDIGO) Clinical Practice Guideline for Acute Kidney Injury and the International Consensus Conference of the Acute Dialysis Quality Initiative (ADQI) Group [51, 52]. However, incomplete data about the risks and benefits of this intervention create tremendous institutional variation in practice. The mechanisms by which PD provides beneficial effect are multifactorial although poorly understood. While much of the effect of PD is due to the direct effects of interstitial fluid removal, some believe removal of pro-inflammatory cytokines prevent maladaptive inflammatory processes which limit negative sequelae of AKI [53]. Some also hypothesize that prevention of ascites collection may prevent or lessen the compression of the inferior vena cava and resulting elevated renal venous pressures, which when uncontrolled will decrease renal perfusion pressure and further propagate development of AKI [4].

The majority of literature on the initiation of PD in pediatric populations has focused on infants and children after cardiac surgery. Although there are some studies that find association between the use of PD and worse outcomes including mortality [50, 54], it has been suggested that these poor outcomes are not related to the use of PD, but rather the *need* for PD and may have been mitigated by earlier use of RRT [54]. In an effort to prevent the onset of fluid overload in infants at high risk for AKI after cardiac surgery, some centers have advocated for the early institution of peritoneal dialysis at the time of oliguria [55], while others support the practice of prophylactic peritoneal dialysis [56] in at-risk populations, such as neonates undergoing cardiopulmonary bypass. The decision to proceed with PD requires a thoughtful comparison of the benefits of PD to the potential risks of peritonitis, bowel injury, bleeding, and hemodynamic instability. However, PD is generally considered a safe intervention, and multiple studies have demonstrated that PD is associated with a very rare incidence of adverse events, particularly when the catheter is placed in the operating room [55, 57–61].

Association of earlier PD initiation and better survival in children after cardiac surgery was demonstrated by Bojan in a propensity score-matched study of 146 infants who utilized postoperative PD [60]. Controlling for illness severity and other risk factors, dialysis initiation within the first postoperative day was associated with a 40% decrease in 30- and 90-day mortality compared to PD initiated later. A similar single-center retrospective study that included all forms of RRT (78% PD) after pediatric cardiac surgery also found that earlier initiation of therapy was associated with lower incidence of mortality when controlled for illness severity score [62].

There are several centers that place PD catheters at the time of cardiac surgery in patients at high risk for AKI and fluid overload for planned dialysis initiation at the time of oliguria [59, 63]. A retrospective matched-cohort study compared infants with the placement of catheters to those without [59]. This study found that patients with catheters were more likely to have a negative fluid balance and had shorter durations of mechanical ventilation, even when including patients who did not develop oliguria and only had the catheter open to drain. Cost analysis showed that additional costs associated in the delivery of PD were offset by savings from improved resource utilization elsewhere in care. Similar association of isolated peritoneal drainage with improved fluid balance was seen in a single-center retrospective study of infants after cardiac surgery [64]. The benefits of postoperative PD use were best validated in a prospective trial of 73 infants with PD catheters placed at the time of surgery that randomized patients with postoperative oliguria to receive either standard diuretics or PD initiation [55]. Infants randomized to diuretics were three times more likely to develop fluid overload, were more likely to have prolonged ventilation, and had a longer duration of inotropic use. The incidence of adverse events related to the PD catheter placement and use was very low.

The use of prophylactic peritoneal dialysis (pPD) has been proposed in high-risk cohorts, including neonates with major cardiac surgery [56–58, 65]. Single-center retrospective studies have found an association of pPD with improved fluid balance, greater urine output, and decreased need for inotropes [57, 58]. In this population, the patient cohort does not yet have fluid overload or even oliguria, so some have hypothesized the effects may be due to removal of pro-inflammatory cytokines, which has been supported in several studies [53, 57]. This has been hypothesized to prevent renal tubule injury, capillary leak, and vasomotor instability, each contributing to the development of fluid overload. However, pPD remains controversial as studies have mixed results, including one small randomized study on neonates after the Norwood palliation surgery which found an increased incidence of adverse events without an improvement of fluid balance [56]. It should be noted that this study had significant flaws in its balance of baseline characteristics, design, and delivery of intended randomized arms.

The core conundrum with initiation of PD, or any modality of RRT, is the identification of a patient in need. Although there is acceptance that RRT is beneficial in a patient with fluid overload, the question of how soon to initiate PD remains unclear. Universal PD catheter placement introduces undue risk to some patients who may not need intervention. The ultimate goal would be the identification of early biomarkers or genetic polymorphisms that would help identify patients at highest risk for AKI and fluid overload such that they could undergo catheter placement in the operating room and undergo earlier intervention.

Literature on the use of peritoneal dialysis in other pediatric patient populations is limited. Continuous renal replacement therapy (CRRT) has largely replaced PD as the most common RRT modality in North America as the technology for CRRT has improved, allowing smaller access, smaller prime volumes, and more reliable filtration rates [66, 67]. One particular exception continues to be small patients including infants who have inadequate access for CRRT. However, there are currently no major studies that investigate the timing of initiation or PD on patients with AKI outside of the cardiac population. Therefore, the decision for initiation of PD in these populations must rely upon literature on other forms of CRRT, modified for differences in risk profile.

## 15.4 Renal Replacement Therapy During Extracorporeal Membrane Oxygenation

The timing of renal replacement in children treated with extracorporeal membrane oxygenation (ECMO) warrants special discussion as this represents a unique patient population particularly prone to the development of AKI and FO. In a 6-center 5-year retrospective cohort study of 832 children treated with ECMO the Kidney Interventions During Extracorporeal Membrane Oxygenation (KIDMO) study group recently reported 72% incidence of AKI and a clear association with increased mortality and length of stay [68], which is consistent with single-center studies [69–71]. The KIDMO study group then went on to evaluate the incidence and impact of fluid overload in a cohort of 656 children. This study showed that fluid overload occurs commonly (median peak fluid overload on ECMO 30.9%, IQR 15.4–54.8%) and is associated with increased mortality. Furthermore, when considering patient peak fluid overload during ECMO, 84.8% had a peak fluid overload ≥10%; 67.2% peak fluid overload ≥20%; and 29% peak fluid overload ≥50% [72]. This study showed that mortality increased significantly when peak fluid overload on ECMO was ≥30% and proposed this as a point to consider intervention. This data clearly shows that AKI and FO occur commonly in children on ECMO and are associated with adverse outcomes.

While it is clear that fluid overload occurs commonly in children treated with ECMO, the role and optimal timing for the initiation of CRRT is less clear. The KIDMO study group performed a survey of Extracorporeal Life Support Organization (ELSO) centers evaluating renal replacement practices and demonstrated that the most common indications were fluid overload (43%), AKI (35%), and the prevention of fluid overload (16%) [73]. Studies evaluating the impact of CRRT in children on ECMO have shown improved fluid management and fluid balance, suggesting a role for CRRT in fluid management on ECMO [74–76]. In 2015 Blijdorp published an evaluation of the impact of hemofiltration on fluid management in a cohort of neonates on ECMO, demonstrating that those treated with CRRT had shorter median duration of ECMO (98 h (IQR48,178) vs. 126 h (IQR 24,403)) with no increased mortality [76]. Two recent studies in neonatal ECMO have evaluated the impact of earlier initiation of CRRT. In the first study evaluating 42 neonates, those who received early CRRT initiation (within 48 h of ECMO cannulation) were able to receive higher volumes of parenteral nutrition and protein without increased mortality [77]. This same group recently published their experience describing the impact of standardized institution of early CRRT (within 48 h of ECMO cannulation), which showed there was improved fluid management and more rapid return to baseline weight without increased mortality with early CRRT initiation [78]. To date there has been a single study evaluating the impact of the timing of CRRT initiation on outcomes in older children on ECMO [79]. In a retrospective study of 153 cardiac patients treated with ECMO Wolf et al. reported an increased mortality (adjusted OR 3.02; 95% CI 1.32–6.9, $p = 0.009$) with early CRRT initiation (within 48 h of ECMO cannulation) [79]. Following that publication, Lou evaluated the impact of CRRT on outcomes in a retrospective propensity-matched cohort study of 86 children and showed no increased mortality associated with CRRT [75]. There has been a small single-center evaluation of the association of FO with outcomes at CRRT initiation children on ECMO ($N = 53$ treated with CRRT, which showed that the median FO at CRRT initiation was lower in survivors (24.5 vs. 38%) [20]. Early in the history of ECMO and CRRT there was concern that the utilization of CRRT led to poor renal outcomes. Paden et al. challenged this belief in a study evaluating the renal outcomes in 154 children treated concurrently with CRRT while on ECMO, which showed renal recovery (dialysis free) in all patients that did not have primary renal disease [80]. In summary, the literature shows that fluid overload occurs commonly and impacts outcomes on ECMO, CRRT can assist with fluid management on ECMO, and CRRT is not associated with deleterious renal outcomes. Further study on the optimal timing for intervention and the impact of CRRT on outcomes is necessary.

## 15.5 Modified Ultrafiltration During Cardiopulmonary Bypass

It is well established that cardiopulmonary bypass during cardiac surgery is a major risk factor for the development of AKI and fluid overload in infants and children due to multiple mechanisms, including ischemic-reperfusion injury and the upregulation of pro-inflammatory pathways [7, 81]. For this reason and others, attempts to limit or modify this necessary intervention have been explored. The use of conventional ultrafiltration (CUF) during cardiopulmonary bypass is a widely utilized mechanism employed to minimize fluid overload during cardiac surgery. There are centers that believe continuation of ultrafiltration after completion of bypass through a process called modified ultrafiltration (MUF) may provide additional benefit. It is hypothesized that this prolonged filtration of blood may allow greater free water elimination and potentially removal of pro-inflammatory cytokines and thereby may prevent or limit negative sequelae of bypass. Some also hypothesize that hemoconcentration with MUF minimizes the need for blood transfusions, which is an established risk factor for AKI [82]. Data supporting this practice are limited, and therefore there is tremendous practice variation among different surgical centers.

Retrospective studies and small-randomized trials in adults and children have demonstrated potential benefit to the use of MUF after cardiac surgery, showing MUF to be associated with lower inflammatory cytokine levels [83–85], improved cardiovascular performance [85–87], improved pulmonary mechanics [88, 89], fewer blood product replacements [85, 86], and potentially lower mortality [87, 90] in infants undergoing heart surgery.

Despite these encouraging data, a majority of larger pediatric and adult studies have shown no benefit associated with the additional use of MUF to standard CUF. Studies have demonstrated no difference in duration of mechanical ventilation or ICU stays time, blood product administration, or inflammatory profiles [91–95], and therefore the practice is not uniformly practiced. Many of the studies that demonstrate improvement in outcomes only show differences for the first several post-operative hours [85, 88, 91]. Although better understanding of this modifiable outcome would certainly be useful to perioperative care, adequate studies are difficult due to a heterogeneous population, with small sample sizes, and innumerable confounders. Furthermore each center has different practices with respect to blood and fluid administration during perfusion and degrees of fluid removal via CUF and MUF. While adequately powered randomized trials have not been performed among pediatric patients, at current time there does not appear adequate evidence to recommend routine use of MUF.

## 15.6 Conclusions and Future Considerations

In summary, there is no debate that RRT should be used in patients with fluid overload, however it is less clear what degree of fluid overload justifies the risks of intervention. A recent meta-analysis of 44 pediatric studies (most of which have been discussed above) comprised of 7407 children supports the strong association between fluid overload and poor outcomes across the entire spectrum of pediatric critical illness [96]. The prediction of AKI and need for RRT is hampered by dependence on the flawed and delayed biomarker of creatinine [97]. It is possible that risk stratification for the need for RRT will improve with the advent of novel biomarkers. In addition, the utility of novel biomarkers may aid in the evaluation of these modalities to limit invasive procedures to only those at highest risk. Additionally, miniaturization of RRT devices may decrease the risk profile for fluid removal and thereby change decision factors [98, 99]. Although the masses of recent research have not defined the exact indications for initiation for RRT, they have created greater awareness of the perils of fluid overload and potential benefits of timely intervention.

**Key Learning Points**

- Fluid overload is associated with significant morbidity and mortality in critically ill pediatric patients.
- Delayed initiation of CRRT in patients with fluid overload is associated with increased mortality.
- Peritoneal dialysis is associated with improved fluid balances after cardiac surgery in infants and delayed initiation is associated with worse outcomes.
- Ultrafiltration in patients with fluid overload during ECMO is associated with improved outcomes.
- Institutional variation in the use of Modified Ultrafiltration during cardiopulmonary bypass has led to mixed findings about the associated benefits.

## References


1. Sutherland SM, Zappitelli M, Alexander SR, Chua AN, Brophy PD, Bunchman TE, et al. Fluid overload and mortality in children receiving continuous renal replacement therapy: the prospective pediatric continuous renal replacement therapy registry. Am J Kidney Dis. 2010;55(2):316–25.
2. Hazle MA, Gajarski RJ, Yu S, Donohue J, Blatt NB. Fluid overload in infants following congenital heart surgery. Pediatr Crit Care Med. 2013;14(1):44.
3. Selewski DT, Cornell TT, Lombel RM, Blatt NB, Han YY, Mottes T, et al. Weight-based determination of fluid overload status and mortality in pediatric intensive care unit patients requiring continuous renal replacement therapy. Intensive Care Med. 2011;37(7):1166–73.
4. Kirkpatrick AW, Roberts DJ, De Waele J, Jaeschke R, Malbrain ML, De Keulenaer B, et al. Intra-abdominal hypertension and the abdominal compartment syndrome: updated consensus definitions and clinical practice guidelines from the World Society of the Abdominal Compartment Syndrome. Intensive Care Med. 2013;39(7):1190–206.
5. Sutherland SM, Goldstein SL, Alexander SR. The prospective pediatric continuous renal replacement therapy (ppCRRT) registry: a critical appraisal. Pediatr Nephrol. 2014;29(11):2069–76.
6. Heung M, Wolfgram DF, Kommareddi M, Hu Y, Song PX, Ojo AO. Fluid overload at initiation of renal replacement therapy is associated with lack of renal recovery in patients with acute kidney injury. Nephrol Dial Transplant. 2012;27(3):956–61.
7. Hassinger AB, Wald EL, Goodman DM. Early postoperative fluid overload precedes acute kidney injury and is associated with higher morbidity in pediatric cardiac surgery patients. Pediatr Crit Care Med. 2014;15(2):131–8.
8. Wilder NS, Yu S, Donohue JE, Goldberg CS, Blatt NB. Fluid overload is associated with late poor outcomes in neonates following cardiac surgery. Pediatr Crit Care Med. 2016;17(5):420–7.

9. Seguin J, Albright B, Vertullo L, Lai P, Dancea A, Bernier P-L, et al. Extent, risk factors, and outcome of fluid overload after pediatric heart surgery*. Crit Care Med. 2014;42(12):2591–9.
10. Valentine S, Sapru A, Higgerson R, Spinella P, Flori H, Graham D, et al. Pediatric acute lung injury and Sepsis Investigator's (PALISI) network; acute respiratory distress syndrome clinical research network (ARDSNet). Fluid balance in critically ill children with acute lung injury. Crit Care Med. 2012;40(10):2883–9.
11. Arikan AA, Zappitelli M, Goldstein SL, Naipaul A, Jefferson LS, Loftis LL. Fluid overload is associated with impaired oxygenation and morbidity in critically ill children*. Pediatr Crit Care Med. 2012;13(3):253–8.
12. Bouchard J, Soroko SB, Chertow GM, Himmelfarb J, Ikizler TA, Paganini EP, et al. Fluid accumulation, survival and recovery of kidney function in critically ill patients with acute kidney injury. Kidney Int. 2009;76(4):422–7.
13. Mah KE, Hao S, Sutherland SM, Kwiatkowski DM, Axelrod DM, Almond CS, et al. Fluid overload independent of acute kidney injury predicts poor outcomes in neonates following congenital heart surgery. Pediatr Nephrol. 2018;33(3):511–20.
14. Akcan-Arikan A, Gebhard DJ, Arnold MA, Loftis LL, Kennedy CE. Fluid overload and kidney injury score: a multidimensional real-time assessment of renal disease burden in the critically ill patient. Pediatr Crit Care Med. 2017;18(6):524–30.
15. Alobaidi R, Morgan C, Basu RK, Stenson E, Featherstone R, Majumdar SR, et al. Associations between fluid balance and outcomes in critically ill children: a protocol for a systematic review and meta-analysis. Can J Kidney Health Dis. 2017;4:2054358117692560.
16. Goldstein SL, Currier H, Graf JM, Cosio CC, Brewer ED, Sachdeva R. Outcome in children receiving continuous venovenous hemofiltration. Pediatrics. 2001;107(6):1309–12.
17. Sinitsky L, Walls D, Nadel S, Inwald DP. Fluid overload at 48 hours is associated with respiratory morbidity but not mortality in a general PICU: retrospective cohort study. Pediatr Crit Care Med. 2015;16(3):205–9.
18. van Asperen Y, Brand PL, Bekhof J. Reliability of the fluid balance in neonates. Acta Paediatr. 2012;101(5):479–83.
19. Askenazi DJ, Koralkar R, Hundley HE, Montesanti A, Patil N, Ambalavanan N. Fluid overload and mortality are associated with acute kidney injury in sick near-term/term neonate. Pediatr Nephrol. 2013;28(4):661–6.
20. Selewski DT, Cornell TT, Blatt NB, Han YY, Mottes T, Kommareddi M, et al. Fluid overload and fluid removal in pediatric patients on extracorporeal membrane oxygenation requiring continuous renal replacement therapy. Crit Care Med. 2012;40(9):2694.
21. Basu RK, Andrews A, Krawczeski C, Manning P, Wheeler DS, Goldstein SL. Acute kidney injury based on corrected serum creatinine is associated with increased morbidity in children following the arterial switch operation. Pediatr Crit Care Med. 2013;14(5):e218–e24.
22. Liu KD, Thompson BT, Ancukiewicz M, Steingrub JS, Douglas IS, Matthay MA, et al. Acute kidney injury in patients with acute lung injury: impact of fluid accumulation on classification of acute kidney injury and associated outcomes. Crit Care Med. 2011;39(12):2665.
23. Macedo E, Bouchard J, Soroko SH, Chertow GM, Himmelfarb J, Ikizler TA, et al. Crit Care. 2010;14(3):R82.
24. Kellum JA, Leblanc M, Gibney RTN, Tumlin J, Lieberthal W, Ronco C. Primary prevention of acute renal failure in the critically ill. Curr Opin Crit Care. 2005;11(6):537–41.
25. Sampath S, Moran JL, Graham PL, Rockliff S, Bersten AD, Abrams KR. The efficacy of loop diuretics in acute renal failure: assessment using Bayesian evidence synthesis techniques. Crit Care Med. 2007;35(11):2516–24.
26. Mehta RL, Pascual MT, Soroko S, Chertow GM, Group P.S. Diuretics, mortality, and nonrecovery of renal function in acute renal failure. JAMA. 2002;288(20):2547–53.
27. Bagshaw SM, Bellomo R, Kellum JA. Oliguria, volume overload, and loop diuretics. Crit Care Med. 2008;36(4):S172–S8.
28. van der Vorst MM, Kist JE, van der Heijden AJ, Burggraaf J. Diuretics in pediatrics. Pediatr Drugs. 2006;8(4):245–64.

29. Regen RB, Gonzalez A, Zawodniak K, Leonard D, Quigley R, Barnes AP, et al. Tolvaptan increases serum sodium in pediatric patients with heart failure. Pediatr Cardiol. 2013;34(6):1463–8.
30. McDonald RH Jr, Goldberg LI, McNay JL, Tuttle EP Jr. Effects of dopamine in man: augmentation of sodium excretion, glomerular filtration rate, and renal plasma flow. J Clin Invest. 1964;43(6):1116.
31. Prins I, Plötz FB, Uiterwaal CS, van Vught HJ. Low-dose dopamine in neonatal and pediatric intensive care: a systematic review. Intensive Care Med. 2001;27(1):206–10.
32. Bellomo R, Chapman M, Finfer S, Hickling K, Myburgh J. Low-dose dopamine in patients with early renal dysfunction: a placebo-controlled randomised trial. Australian and New Zealand Intensive Care Society (ANZICS) Clinical Trials Group. Lancet. 2000;356(9248):2139–43.
33. Axelrod DM, Anglemyer AT, Sherman-Levine SF, Zhu A, Grimm PC, Roth SJ, et al. Initial experience using aminophylline to improve renal dysfunction in the pediatric cardiovascular ICU. Pediatr Crit Care Med. 2014;15(1):21–7.
34. Costello JM, Thiagarajan RR, Dionne RE, Allan CK, Booth KL, Burmester M, et al. Initial experience with fenoldopam after cardiac surgery in neonates with an insufficient response to conventional diuretics. Pediatr Crit Care Med. 2006;7(1):28–33.
35. Ricci Z, Luciano R, Favia I, Garisto C, Muraca M, Morelli S, et al. High-dose fenoldopam reduces postoperative neutrophil gelatinase-associated lipocaline and cystatin C levels in pediatric cardiac surgery. Crit Care. 2011;15(3):R160.
36. Ricci Z, Stazi GV, Di Chiara L, Morelli S, Vitale V, Giorni C, et al. Fenoldopam in newborn patients undergoing cardiopulmonary bypass: controlled clinical trial. Interact Cardiovasc Thorac Surg. 2008;7(6):1049–53.
37. Axelrod DM, Sutherland SM, Anglemyer A, Grimm PC, Roth SJ. A double blinded, randomized, placebo-controlled clinical trial of aminophylline to prevent acute kidney injury in children following congenital heart surgery with cardiopulmonary bypass. Pediatr Crit Care Med. 2016;17(2):135.
38. Yoder SE, Yoder BA. An evaluation of off-label fenoldopam use in the neonatal intensive care unit. Am J Perinatol. 2009;26(10):745–50.
39. Tamburro RF, Thomas NJ, Ceneviva GD, Dettorre MD, Brummel GL, Lucking SE. A prospective assessment of the effect of aminophylline therapy on urine output and inflammation in critically ill children. Front Pediatr. 2014;2:59.
40. Warady BA, Bunchman T. Dialysis therapy for children with acute renal failure: survey results. Pediatr Nephrol. 2000;15(1–2):11–3.
41. Walters S, Porter C, Brophy PD. Dialysis and pediatric acute kidney injury: choice of renal support modality. Pediatr Nephrol. 2009;24(1):37–48.
42. Sutherland SM, Alexander SR. Continuous renal replacement therapy in children. Pediatr Nephrol. 2012;27(11):2007–16.
43. Symons JM, Chua AN, Somers MJ, Baum MA, Bunchman TE, Benfield MR, et al. Demographic characteristics of pediatric continuous renal replacement therapy: a report of the prospective pediatric continuous renal replacement therapy registry. Clin J Am Soc Nephrol. 2007;2(4):732–8.
44. Foland JA, Fortenberry JD, Warshaw BL, Pettignano R, Merritt RK, Heard ML, et al. Fluid overload before continuous hemofiltration and survival in critically ill children: a retrospective analysis. Crit Care Med. 2004;32(8):1771–6.
45. Hayes LW, Oster RA, Tofil NM, Tolwani AJ. Outcomes of critically ill children requiring continuous renal replacement therapy. J Crit Care. 2009;24(3):394–400.
46. Goldstein SL. Continuous renal replacement therapy: mechanism of clearance, fluid removal, indications and outcomes. Curr Opin Pediatr. 2011;23(2):181–5.
47. Selewski DT, Goldstein SL. The role of fluid overload in the prediction of outcome in acute kidney injury. Pediatr Nephrol. 2018;33(1):13–24.
48. Modem V, Thompson M, Gollhofer D, Dhar AV, Quigley R. Timing of continuous renal replacement therapy and mortality in critically ill children*. Crit Care Med. 2014;42(4):943–53.

49. Gulla KM, Sachdev A, Gupta D, Gupta N, Anand K, Pruthi PK. Continuous renal replacement therapy in children with severe sepsis and multiorgan dysfunction – a pilot study on timing of initiation. Indian J Crit Care Med. 2015;19(10):613–7.
50. Madenci AL, Thiagarajan RR, Stoffan AP, Emani SM, Rajagopal SK, Weldon CB. Characterizing peritoneal dialysis catheter use in pediatric patients after cardiac surgery. J Thorac Cardiovasc Surg. 2013;146(2):334–8.
51. Kellum JA, Lameire N. Diagnosis, evaluation, and management of acute kidney injury: a KDIGO summary (part 1). Crit Care. 2013;17(1):204.
52. Bellomo R, Ronco C, Kellum JA, Mehta RL, Palevsky P. Acute renal failure–definition, outcome measures, animal models, fluid therapy and information technology needs: the second international consensus conference of the acute Dialysis quality initiative (ADQI) group. Crit Care. 2004;8(4):R204.
53. Dittrich S, Aktuerk D, Seitz S, Mehwald P, Schulte-Mönting J, Schlensak C, et al. Effects of ultrafiltration and peritoneal dialysis on proinflammatory cytokines during cardiopulmonary bypass surgery in newborns and infants. Eur J Cardiothorac Surg. 2004;25(6):935–40.
54. Madenci AL, Stoffan AP, Rajagopal SK, Blinder JJ, Emani SM, Thiagarajan RR, et al. Factors associated with survival in patients who undergo peritoneal dialysis catheter placement following cardiac surgery. J Pediatr Surg. 2013;48(6):1269–76.
55. Kwiatkowski DM, Goldstein SL, Cooper DS, Nelson DP, Morales DS, Krawczeski CD. Peritoneal dialysis vs furosemide for prevention of fluid overload in infants after cardiac surgery: a randomized clinical trial. JAMA Pediatr. 2017;171:357.
56. Ryerson LM, Mackie AS, Atallah J, Joffe AR, Rebeyka IM, Ross DB, et al. Prophylactic peritoneal dialysis catheter does not decrease time to achieve a negative fluid balance after the Norwood procedure: a randomized controlled trial. J Thorac Cardiovasc Surg. 2015;149(1):222–8.
57. Sasser WC, Dabal RJ, Askenazi DJ, Borasino S, Moellinger AB, Kirklin JK, et al. Prophylactic peritoneal dialysis following cardiopulmonary bypass in children is associated with decreased inflammation and improved clinical outcomes. Congenit Heart Dis. 2014;9(2):106–15.
58. Alkan T, Akçevin A, Türkoglu H, Paker T, Sasmazel A, Bayer V, et al. Postoperative prophylactic peritoneal dialysis in neonates and infants after complex congenital cardiac surgery. ASAIO J. 2006;52(6):693–7.
59. Kwiatkowski DM, Menon S, Krawczeski CD, Goldstein SL, Morales DL, Phillips A, et al. Improved outcomes with peritoneal dialysis catheter placement after cardiopulmonary bypass in infants. J Thorac Cardiovasc Surg. 2015;149(1):230–6.
60. Bojan M, Gioanni S, Vouhé PR, Journois D, Pouard P. Early initiation of peritoneal dialysis in neonates and infants with acute kidney injury following cardiac surgery is associated with a significant decrease in mortality. Kidney Int. 2012;82(4):474–81.
61. Murala JSK, Singappuli K, Provenzano SC, Nunn G. Techniques of inserting peritoneal dialysis catheters in neonates and infants undergoing open heart surgery. J Thorac Cardiovasc Surg. 2010;139(2):503–5.
62. Sanchez-de-Toledo J, Perez-Ortiz A, Gil L, Baust T, Linés-Palazón M, Perez-Hoyos S, et al. Early initiation of renal replacement therapy in pediatric heart surgery is associated with lower mortality. Pediatr Cardiol. 2016;37(4):623–8.
63. Sorof JM, Stromberg D, Brewer ED, Feltes TF, Fraser CD Jr. Early initiation of peritoneal dialysis after surgical repair of congenital heart disease. Pediatr Nephrol. 1999;13(8):641–5.
64. Saini A, Delius RE, Seshadri S, Walters H III, Mastropietro CW. Passive peritoneal drainage improves fluid balance after surgery for congenital heart disease. Eur J Cardiothorac Surg. 2012;41(2):256–60.
65. Dittrich S, Dähnert I, Vogel M, Stiller B, Haas NA, Alexi-Meskishvili V, et al. Peritoneal dialysis after infant open heart surgery: observations in 27 patients. Ann Thorac Surg. 1999;68(1):160–3.
66. Weaver DJ, Somers MJ, Martz K, Mitsnefes MM. Clinical outcomes and survival in pediatric patients initiating chronic dialysis: a report of the NAPRTCS registry. Pediatr Nephrol. 2017;32(12):2319–30.

67. Zaritsky J, Warady BA. Peritoneal dialysis in infants and young children. Semin Nephrol. 2011;31(2):213–24. Elsevier
68. Fleming GM, Sahay R, Zappitelli M, King E, Askenazi DJ, Bridges BC, et al. The incidence of acute kidney injury and its effect on neonatal and pediatric extracorporeal membrane oxygenation outcomes: a multicenter report from the kidney intervention during extracorporeal membrane oxygenation study group. Pediatr Crit Care Med. 2016;17(12):1157–69.
69. Zwiers AJ, de Wildt SN, Hop WC, Dorresteijn EM, Gischler SJ, Tibboel D, et al. Acute kidney injury is a frequent complication in critically ill neonates receiving extracorporeal membrane oxygenation: a 14-year cohort study. Crit Care. 2013;17(4):R151.
70. Gadepalli SK, Selewski DT, Drongowski RA, Mychaliska GB. Acute kidney injury in congenital diaphragmatic hernia requiring extracorporeal life support: an insidious problem. J Pediatr Surg. 2011;46(4):630–5.
71. Smith AH, Hardison DC, Worden CR, Fleming GM, Taylor MB. Acute renal failure during extracorporeal support in the pediatric cardiac patient. ASAIO J. 2009;55(4):412–6.
72. Selewski DT, Askenazi DJ, Bridges BC, Cooper DS, Fleming GM, Paden ML, et al. The impact of fluid overload on outcomes in children treated with extracorporeal membrane oxygenation: a multicenter retrospective cohort study. Pediatr Crit Care Med. 2017;18(12):1126–35.
73. Fleming GM, Askenazi DJ, Bridges BC, Cooper DS, Paden ML, Selewski DT, et al. A multicenter international survey of renal supportive therapy during ECMO: the kidney intervention during extracorporeal membrane oxygenation (KIDMO) group. ASAIO J. 2012;58(4):407–14.
74. Hoover NG, Heard M, Reid C, Wagoner S, Rogers K, Foland J, et al. Enhanced fluid management with continuous venovenous hemofiltration in pediatric respiratory failure patients receiving extracorporeal membrane oxygenation support. Intensive Care Med. 2008;34(12):2241–7.
75. Lou S, MacLaren G, Paul E, Best D, Delzoppo C, Butt W. Hemofiltration is not associated with increased mortality in children receiving extracorporeal membrane oxygenation. Pediatr Crit Care Med. 2015;16(2):161–6.
76. Blijdorp K, Cransberg K, Wildschut ED, Gischler SJ, Jan Houmes R, Wolff ED, et al. Haemofiltration in newborns treated with extracorporeal membrane oxygenation: a case-comparison study. Crit Care. 2009;13(2):R48.
77. Murphy HJ, Cahill JB, Twombley KE, Kiger JR. Early continuous renal replacement therapy improves nutrition delivery in neonates during extracorporeal life support. J Ren Nutr. 2018;28(1):64–70.
78. Murphy HJ, Cahill JB, Twombley KE, Annibale DJ, Kiger JR. Implementing a practice change: early initiation of continuous renal replacement therapy during neonatal extracorporeal life support standardizes care and improves short-term outcomes. J Artif Organs. 2018;21(1):76–85.
79. Wolf MJ, Chanani NK, Heard ML, Kanter KR, Mahle WT. Early renal replacement therapy during pediatric cardiac extracorporeal support increases mortality. Ann Thorac Surg. 2013;96(3):917–22.
80. Paden ML, Warshaw BL, Heard ML, Fortenberry JD. Recovery of renal function and survival after continuous renal replacement therapy during extracorporeal membrane oxygenation. Pediatr Crit Care Med. 2011;12(2):153–8.
81. Li S, Krawczeski CD, Zappitelli M, Devarajan P, Thiessen-Philbrook H, Coca SG, et al. Incidence, risk factors, and outcomes of acute kidney injury after pediatric cardiac surgery–a prospective multicenter study. Crit Care Med. 2011;39(6):1493.
82. Haase M, Bellomo R, Story D, Letis A, Klemz K, Matalanis G, et al. Effect of mean arterial pressure, haemoglobin and blood transfusion during cardiopulmonary bypass on postoperative acute kidney injury. Nephrol Dial Transplant. 2011;27(1):153–60.
83. Wang W, Huang HM, Zhu DM, Chen H, Su ZK, Ding WX. Modified ultrafiltration in paediatric cardiopulmonary bypass. Perfusion. 1998;13(5):304–10.
84. Portela F, Español R, Quintáns J, Pensado A, Vazquez A, Sánchez A, et al. Combined perioperative ultrafiltration in pediatric cardiac surgery. The preliminary results. Rev Esp Cardiol. 1999;52(12):1075–82.

85. Zhou G, Feng Z, Xiong H, Duan W, Jin Z. A combined ultrafiltration strategy during pediatric cardiac surgery: a prospective, randomized, controlled study with clinical outcomes. J Cardiothorac Vasc Anesth. 2013;27(5):897–902.
86. Koutlas TC, Gaynor JW, Nicolson SC, Steven JM, Wernovsky G, Spray TL. Modified ultrafiltration reduces postoperative morbidity after cavopulmonary connection. Ann Thorac Surg. 1997;64(1):37–43.
87. Naik SK, Knight A, Elliott M. A prospective randomized study of a modified technique of ultrafiltration during pediatric open-heart surgery. Circulation. 1991;84(5 Suppl):III422–31.
88. Keenan HT, Thiagarajan R, Stephens KE, Williams G, Ramamoorthy C, Lupinetti FM. Pulmonary function after modified venovenous ultrafiltration in infants: a prospective, randomized trial. J Thorac Cardiovasc Surg. 2000;119(3):501–7.
89. Liu J, Long C, Feng Z, Ji B, Li C. Comparative study of pulmonary function after conventional ultrafiltration or modified ultrafiltration during cardiac surgery of infants. Zhongguo Yi Xue Ke Xue Yuan Xue Bao. 2002;24(4):364–6.
90. Tweddell JS, Hoffman GM, Mussatto KA, Fedderly RT, Berger S, Jaquiss RD, et al. Improved survival of patients undergoing palliation of hypoplastic left heart syndrome: lessons learned from 115 consecutive patients. Circulation. 2002;106(12 Suppl 1):I82–9.
91. Pearl JM, Manning PB, McNamara JL, Saucier MM, Thomas DW. Effect of modified ultrafiltration on plasma thromboxane B2, leukotriene B4, and endothelin-1 in infants undergoing cardiopulmonary bypass. Ann Thorac Surg. 1999;68(4):1369–75.
92. McRobb CM, Ing RJ, Lawson DS, Jaggers J, Twite M. Retrospective analysis of eliminating modified ultrafiltration after pediatric cardiopulmonary bypass. Perfusion. 2017;32(2):97–109.
93. Chew MS, Brix-Christensen V, Ravn HB, Brandslund I, Ditlevsen E, Pedersen J, et al. Effect of modified ultrafiltration on the inflammatory response in paediatric open-heart surgery: a prospective, randomized study. Perfusion. 2002;17(5):327–33.
94. Kuratani N, Bunsangjaroen P, Srimueang T, Masaki E, Suzuki T, Katogi T. Modified versus conventional ultrafiltration in pediatric cardiac surgery: a meta-analysis of randomized controlled trials comparing clinical outcome parameters. J Thorac Cardiovasc Surg. 2011;142(4):861–7.
95. Mahmoud A-BS, Burhani MS, Hannef AA, Jamjoom AA, Al-Githmi IS, Baslaim GM. Effect of modified ultrafiltration on pulmonary function after cardiopulmonary bypass. Chest J. 2005;128(5):3447–53.
96. Alobaidi R, Morgan C, Basu RK, Stenson E, Featherstone R, Majumdar SR, et al. Association between fluid balance and outcomes in critically ill children: a systematic review and meta-analysis. JAMA Pediatr. 2018;172(3):257–68.
97. Murray PT, Mehta RL, Shaw A, Ronco C, Endre Z, Kellum JA, et al. Potential use of biomarkers in acute kidney injury: report and summary of recommendations from the 10th acute Dialysis quality initiative consensus conference. Kidney Int. 2014;85(3):513–21.
98. Askenazi D, Ingram D, White S, Cramer M, Borasino S, Coghill C, et al. Smaller circuits for smaller patients: improving renal support therapy with Aquadex™. Pediatr Nephrol. 2016;31(5):853–60.
99. Ronco C, Garzotto F, Brendolan A, Zanella M, Bellettato M, Vedovato S, et al. Continuous renal replacement therapy in neonates and small infants: development and first-in-human use of a miniaturised machine (CARPEDIEM). Lancet. 2014;383(9931):1807–13.

# Management Considerations for the Delivery of CRRT in Children

**16**

Francisco X. Flores

**Case Vignette**

A 7-month-old male, status post bone marrow transplantation with veno-occlusive disease is receiving cefepime, vancomycin, and acyclovir for a recent fever and presumed infection. His weight today is 9 kg (from 8 kg, yesterday), length of 68 cm, and his body surface area is 0.38 $m^2$. His urine output in the last 12 h was <0.3 mL/kg/h and today's laboratory studies reported sodium of 138 mmoL/L, potassium 6 mmoL/L, carbon dioxide 13 mmoL/L, calcium 8 mg/dL, phosphorus 10 mg/dL, BUN 100 mg/dL, creatinine of 2 mg/dL (3 days ago creatinine was 0.4 mg/dL), elevated LFTs, INR of 2.6, bilirubin of 15 mg/dL, and a serum albumin of 2 g/dL. Due to deterioration of his clinical status, the patient was transferred to the pediatric intensive care and you are consulted to assist in the management of AKI.

## 16.1 Introduction

In clinical practice, the provision of continuous renal replacement therapy (CRRT) requires a careful consideration of the technical aspects of the therapy and the elements that should be included in the CRRT prescription. These technical aspects include vascular access, anticoagulation, thermal regulation and CRRT replacement and dialysis fluid solutions. The CRRT prescription in pediatric patients should include the blood flow rate, the size/type of the hemofilter, the CRRT modality, the

F. X. Flores
Division of Nephrology and Hypertension, Cincinnati Children's Hospital Medical Center, Cincinnati, OH, USA
e-mail: Francisco.flores@cchmc.org



A. Deep, S. L. Goldstein (eds.), *Critical Care Nephrology and Renal Replacement Therapy in Children*, https://doi.org/10.1007/978-3-319-90281-4_16

CRRT dose, and ultrafiltration rate. An important aspect of pediatric CRRT provision is the spectrum of the patient's age and size from neonates to young adults. Therefore, a one-size-fits-all approach is not appropriate for pediatric CRRT, and the prescription will vary based on the patient size and underlying disease state. This chapter will focus on all the aspects of pediatric CRRT prescription, with the exception of anticoagulation which is covered in a Chap. 17.

## 16.2 Technical Aspects of CRRT

### 16.2.1 Vascular Access

A properly functioning and reliable vascular access is one of the most important determinants for the delivery of pediatric CRRT. The flows obtained from the catheter will impact the adequacy of the therapy, the CRRT circuit life, and staff satisfaction. Of the catheter-related characteristics, the diameter is critical in determining the resistance to flow, more than the length of the catheter [1]. However, in some circumstances, longer catheters are needed to allow access to a larger blood vessel to be able to obtain higher blood flow rates. Suggested catheter sizes based on a patient's weight in Table 16.1.

Although the use of two 5-French single lumen catheters was previously reported as a viable alternative for neonates, Hackbarth reported a circuit survival of less than 20 h when using two single-lumen 5-French catheters [2]. Therefore, due to poor circuit survival, which will preclude the delivery of adequate CRRT, the use of this particular size catheter is not generally recommended.

The catheter's anatomical location also has a significant impact on circuit survival. Factors influencing the decision regarding the location of the vascular access include: clinical expertise, patient's body habitus, the presence of other catheters and coagulopathy or abdominal distention. The femoral location, compared to internal jugular (IJ) and subclavian, is more often preferred due to easy placement (69% vs. 16% vs. 8%) [2], but femoral catheters often require the patient to be sedated or paralyzed to avoid intermittent interruption of the blood flow due to kinking of the vascular access. In addition, femoral catheters have an increased risk of recirculation and they tend to perform poorly in the presence of high pressure ascites or intraabdominal compartment syndrome.

**Table 16.1** Recommended weight-based temporary catheters for acute CRRT access

| Patient weight | Catheter size |
|---|---|
| Neonate | Dual-lumen 7 French |
| 3–6 kg | Dual-lumen 7 French |
| 6–12 kg | Dual-lumen 8 French |
| 12–20 kg | Dual-lumen 9 French |
| 20–30 kg | Dual-lumen 10 French |
| >30 kg | Dual or triple-lumen 10–12.5 French |

*Adapted from Cincinnati Children's Hospital Medical Center for Acute Care Nephrology Access Guideline

**Table 16.2** A 60-h circuit survival rates [2]

| Catheter size (French) | Number of patients | % Survival at 60 h |
|---|---|---|
| 5 | 6 | 0 ($p < 0.0001$) |
| 7 | 57 | 43 ($p < 0.002$) |
| 8 | 65 | 55 (NS) |
| 9 | 35 | 51 ($p < 0.002$) |
| 10 | 46 | 53 (NS) |
| 11.5 | 71 | 57 (NS) |
| 12.5 | 64 | 60 (NS) |
| *Insertion site* | | |
| Internal jugular | 58 | 60 ($p < 0.05$) |
| Subclavian | 31 | 51 (NS) |
| Femoral | 260 | 52 (NS) |

The availability of bedside ultrasound devices has made the IJ vein insertion easy and safe. More often, the tip of the catheter lays in the right atrium, which reduces the risk of recirculation and the chances of the catheter getting stuck against the blood vessel's wall. IJ catheters are also associated with a significantly higher circuit survival when compared to femoral or subclavian catheters (60% vs. 52% vs. 51% at 60 h) (Table 16.2) [2].

Unless there is no other available vascular access, the placement of subclavian catheters is not recommended due to the high risk of stenosis of the subclavian vein, therefore preventing its use for long-term vascular access creation if the acute kidney injury patient does not recover renal function [3].

### 16.2.2 Anticoagulation

Anticoagulation is another important component of CRRT provision since it will affect the dose delivered, staff satisfaction, and cost of the therapy. Most pediatric centers choose either systemic anticoagulation with heparin or regional anticoagulation with citrate to prevent clotting of the CRRT circuit. Citrate anticoagulation allows a longer life span of the circuits when compared to systemic anticoagulation [4], and in 2012, the Kidney Disease Improving Global Outcome (KDIGO) guideline suggested the use of citrate anticoagulation in CRRT for patients with or without risk of bleeding [5]. However, in cases where either the patient's condition prevented the use of systemic anticoagulation or citrate was not available for regional anticoagulation, critically ill patients have received CRRT without any form of anticoagulation. Based on the pediatric prospective CRRT Registry's (ppCRRT) experience, it is not recommended to provide CRRT without any form of anticoagulation. In this report, the comparison of CRRT provided with no anticoagulation vs. heparin or citrate anticoagulation, showed a reduction in the duration of therapy in terms of hours and in the % of circuits working at 60 h [5]. As noted above, this important technical aspect will be reviewed in depth in Chap. 17.

### 16.2.3 Thermal Regulation

It is common for small patients to develop hypothermia while receiving CRRT due to the large extracorporeal blood volume. Interventions such as placing infants in radiant warmers and using heating blankets can be performed to either prevent or manage hypothermia. Some CRRT machines provide blood warmers that prevent heat loss and allow patients to be comfortable during the therapy. One of these blood warming devices uses an electric heating sleeve that is placed at the venous return to the patient and the temperature of the blood can be adjusted between 33 and 43 °C.

### 16.2.4 CRRT Solutions

The purpose of the CRRT solution is to provide a safe and consistent metabolic control and to be adaptive to the choice of therapy; continuous venovenous hemofiltration (CVVH) vs. continuous venovenous hemodialysis (CVVHD) vs. continuous venovenous hemodiafiltration (CVVHDF). The ideal solution needs to be physiologic, reliable, inexpensive, easy to prepare, simple to store, available, and fully compatible. The CRRT solutions contain various concentrations of sodium, potassium, chloride, glucose, phosphate, calcium, and magnesium, and in general, the electrolyte concentration should be equal in the dialysate and in the replacement solutions. In circumstances where the electrolyte abnormality requires a slow correction such as in hypo- or hypernatremia, the sodium composition of the CRRT solutions can be modified to provide a slow and stepwise correction [6]. The use of lactate as the solution buffer, resulted in the development of lactic acidosis, cardiac dysfunction, and hypotension [7]. Currently, industry made, pharmaceutical grade bicarbonate-based dialysis/replacement solutions are the standard of care in adults and children receiving CRRT, since they have demonstrated superiority to the lactate-based solutions [8, 9]. Despite of the bicarbonate concentration (22–32 mEq/L), many of the solutions contain 3 mEq/L of lactate to provide stability and physiological pH in the solution. When providing systemic anticoagulation with heparin or regional anticoagulation with citrate it is important to consider the calcium concentration (0–3.5 mEq/L) when choosing the CRRT solution. Patients receiving regional citrate anticoagulation should receive calcium-free solutions to avoid the development of hypercalcemia, since these patients are already receiving intravenous calcium supplementation.

## 16.3 CRRT Prescription

### 16.3.1 Blood Flow Rates

The blood flow rate (Qb; milliliters per minute) is generally dependent on the vascular access, the CRRT machine and the hemodynamic stability of the patient. The recommended blood flow rates based on patient weight (kg) are 3–10 mL/kg/min, however higher rates of 10–12 mL/kg/min are usually necessary in neonates and small infants to be able to generate adequate access and return pressures to prevent clotting of the circuit or setting off alarms from the CRRT machine. Data from the ppCRRT Registry reported a mean blood flow rate of 97.9 mL/min (range 10–350 mL/min; median 100 mL/min), with a mean blood flow rate scaled to body weight of 5 mL/kg/min (range 0.6–53.6 mL/kg/min; median 4.1 mL/kg/min) [10].

Higher blood flow rates can extend the circuit life span by reducing the risk of intrafiber clotting, especially when no anticoagulation is used. But in comparison to intermittent hemodialysis, a higher blood flow rate will not necessarily increase small molecule clearance in CRRT, given the relatively low effluent rate (Qeff; replacement fluid rate + dialysis fluid rate + ultrafiltration rate in mL/h) compared to the Qb (mL/min). A Qeff/Qb ratio of >1.5 is needed to give Qb precedence for clearance, which is generally not achievable on CRRT.

### 16.3.2 Hemofilter

When selecting the CRRT hemofilter, it is important to consider the size and the characteristics of the membrane. In general terms, the size of the hemofilter should be comparable to the patient's body surface area. In addition, one needs to consider the priming volume of the hemofilter, since it will determine the need of blood priming and the potential blood loss volume to the patient. The AN-69 is a polyacrylonitrile membrane with a higher sieving coefficient, a greater ability to remove cytokines and/or inflammatory mediators and the one associated with the development of bradykinin release syndrome [11–13]. Polyarylethersulphone membranes (PAES) are not associated with bradykinin release syndrome, but they are not available in pediatric sizes. The exception is the HF-20 filter (Baxter Healthcare Corporation, Deerfield, IL), which has a 0.2 $m^2$ surface area and a priming volume of 60 mL. It is currently available in Europe and undergoing clinical trial in the United States [14].

When the extracorporeal circuit priming volume for the hemofilter exceeds 10–15% of the patient's total blood volume, physicians prescribing the therapy need to consider priming solution for the circuit. In clinical practice, priming with packed red blood cells (PRBC) (Hct 60%) or a mix of 1:1 PRBC: albumin (estimated Hct 35%) can prevent hypotension and hemodilution at CRRT initiation. However, this practice can be associated with electrolyte abnormalities such as hyperkalemia, hypocalcemia, and the delivery of an acid load. The development of bradykinin release syndrome is characterized by the sudden onset of mucosal congestion, bronchospasm, and hypotension at the time of CRRT initiation. This phenomenon seems to be pH sensitive and related to the release of bradykinin when the patient's blood comes in contact with the AN-69 membrane [15]. Techniques attempting to prevent bradykinin release syndrome include the bypass system [15], recirculation system [16], changing the circuit's pH with bicarbonate infusion during the priming process or by completely avoiding the use of AN-69 membranes.

**Table 16.3** Convection vs. diffusion [17]

| Solute (MW) | Sieving coefficient | Diffusion coefficient |
|---|---|---|
| Urea (60) | 1.01 ± 0.05 | 1.01 ± 0.07 |
| Creatinine (113) | 1.00 ± 0.09 | 1.01 ± 0.06 |
| Uric acid (168) | 1.01 ± 0.04 | 0.97 ± 0.04* |
| Vancomycin (1148) | 0.84 ± 0.10 | 0.74 ± 0.04** |

*$p < 0.05$ vs. sieving coefficient
**$p < 0.01$ sieving coefficient

### 16.3.3 Modality

The CRRT modalities are defined by the main solute clearance mechanism, where convection is the mechanism used to provide continuous venovenous hemofiltration (CVVH), diffusion is used to provide continuous venovenous hemodialysis and the combination of diffusion and convection is used for continuous venovenous hemodiafiltration (CVVHDF). Slow continuous ultrafiltration (SCUF) is a CRRT modality that provides minimal clearance and it is used mainly for volume removal. CVVH provides convective therapy by infusing replacement solutions pre-filter or post-filter. CVVHD provides diffusive therapy by infusing a dialysis solution in a countercurrent fashion. In terms of which modality provides better clearance, CVVH and CVVHD provide an equivalent small solute clearance, but middle and large solute removal, theoretically is enhanced by CVVH (Table 16.3) [18].

### 16.3.4 Dose

The conceptual definition of CRRT dose is the amount of CRRT delivered to control uremic toxins. In clinical practice, the delivered dose is considered to be the equivalent of the total effluent volume expressed in mL/kg/h and estimates the clearance of small solutes such as urea nitrogen. This concept of CRRT dose was first introduced in 2000, when Ronco and colleagues reported their randomized controlled study evaluating the impact of CRRT dose on outcome [19]. 425 patients were randomized to receive 20 mL/kg/h (conventional-dose group), 35 mL/kg/h (moderate-dose group), or 45 mL/kg/h (high-dose group) and the primary end point of the study was to determine the survival rate at 15 days after the last CRRT treatment. Patients in the intermediate and high-dose group had a significantly higher survival rate than those patients in the conventional-dose group.

The VA/NIH Acute Renal Failure Network study (ATN) and the Randomized Evaluation of Normal versus Augmented Level (RENAL) Replacement Therapy studies are the two most recent studies looking into the impact of CRRT dose and outcomes. The ATN study in 2008 randomized 1124 patients to receive more intensive therapy or less intensive therapy based on their hemodynamic stability. In patients who were hemodynamically stable, the more intensive group received intermittent hemodialysis six times per week with a minimum KT/V of 1.2 per session or intermittent hemodialysis three times per week with a minimum KT/V of 1.2

per session in the less intensive group. Unstable patients were randomized to the more intensive CRRT group (35 mL/kg/h) or to the less intensive CRRT group (20 mL/kg/h) [20]. This study did not find any difference in the 60-day survival rates between two groups. The RENAL study in 2009 randomized 1508 patients to receive intensive CRRT (40 mL/kg/h) or conventional CRRT (25 mL/kg/h). This study also did not show any survival difference at 90 days between the intensive CRRT group and the conventional CRRT group. Based on the results of these two studies, it appears that there is no difference in terms of survival or recovery of the kidney function, by trying to deliver a dose greater than 20–25 mL/kg/h [21].

But the prescribed dose is often not the delivered dose. There are multiple factors that can affect the ability to deliver the prescribed dose; they include scheduled filter change, circuit clotting, vascular access problems, therapy interruption due to patient's issues, and the dilutional effect when using pre-filter replacement solutions. To compensate for the difference between the prescribed and delivered dose, KDIGO recommends to prescribe 25–30 mL/kg/h in order to achieve a delivered dose of 20–25 mL/kg/h, and to minimize therapy interruptions [3].

In pediatric practice, this adult CRRT dosing extrapolates to a dose of 2000–3000 mL/1.73m$^2$/h but potentially different rates might be needed if increased citrate clearance is required during episodes of citrate intoxication or in neonates with hyperammonemia. In this particular situation, when CRRT is used as the first line of renal replacement therapy, a dose of 8000 mL/1.73m$^2$/h has been reported to provide adequate clearance with an expected ammonia reduction rate of 70% at 2 h of therapy [22]. It is important to keep in mind that delivering this high clearance rate is associated with significant depletion of electrolytes such as potassium, phosphorus, and magnesium; therefore it is important to add them to the dialysate/replacement solutions and follow the blood levels of these electrolytes, closely.

### 16.3.5 Ultrafiltration

During CRRT, prescribing ultrafiltration allows for the balance of the fluid input and the removal of excessive fluid over time, which serves to make room to maximize nutrition and provide solute clearance by a convective mechanism.

At the time of prescribing CRRT, it is important to determine the desired targeted fluid status for the patient. In patients requiring CRRT mainly for solute removal, the goal would be to achieve an even net fluid balance; that means that the CRRT machine will be programed to remove all fluids that the patient receives, minus the patient's output. On the other hand, in patients with fluid overload who require extra fluid removal, the machine will be programed to remove all fluids that the patient receives, minus the patient's output, plus an additional volume or net ultrafiltration volume. This net ultrafiltration volume can be estimated by calculating an extra removal rate of 0.5–2 mL/kg/h or 1–3% of the patient's blood volume per hour. The targeted 24 h net ultrafiltration volume will be determined based on the percentage of fluid overload, cardiovascular stability, and patient's ability to tolerate fluid removal. A safety feature that some CRRT machines provide is an alarm when a 3 h fluid balance limit is achieved. This feature aims to prevent less than 5% of blood volume error over 3 h in small children and less than 10% over 3 h for larger patients. This 3 h fluid limit should be set at the time of programing the CRRT machine with the prescription. In our institution, we have chosen to set this 3 h fluid limit alarm at 150 mL for patients who are less than 30 kg, 200 mL for patients weighing 30–50 kg, and 300 mL for patients weighing more than 50 kg.

## 16.4 Practical Consideration in Pediatric CRRT

### 16.4.1 Electrolyte and Glucose Balance

The development of hyponatremia while delivering CRRT should raise the concerns of mixing errors in the preparation of the dialysate/replacement solutions in institutions that are not using commercially available solutions. On the other hand, hypernatremia during CRRT is usually related to the sodium ($Na^+$) concentration in the intravenous fluids or in the total parenteral nutrition (TPN), the $Na^+$ bicarbonate in the dialysate/replacement solution (22–32 mEq/L) and the use of anticoagulant citrate dextrose solution- A (ACD-A solution, CitraLabs, LLC, Braintree, MA (ACD-A)) for regional anticoagulation (220 mEq/L of $Na^+$). In 2006, Barletta and colleagues reported a survey of three pediatric list serves, where 16 out of 31 programs reported errors in the preparation of dialysate or replacement solutions, which resulted in six episodes of seizures due to hypo or hypernatremia [23]. The management of hyponatremia in patients receiving CRRT requires a slow correction of the serum $Na^+$, no faster that 8–10 mEq/day, and this correction can be provided in a stepwise fashion by using successively higher $Na^+$ concentration in the dialysate/replacement solutions. The management of hypernatremia, on the other hand, includes a slow reduction of the $Na^+$ content in the TPN, increasing the free water delivery or by changing the $Na^+$ concentration in the dialysate/replacement solutions [6].

Hypokalemia is a common electrolyte abnormality in patients receiving CRRT. It is mainly related to the potassium restriction prior to CRRT initiation, insufficient supplementation in the intravenous fluids or in the TPN or due to clearance provided by the therapy. The management of hypokalemia includes increasing potassium supplementation in the TPN, changing CRRT solutions to ones with higher potassium concentration or the addition of potassium chloride or potassium phosphate to the dialysate/replacement solutions.

Citrate toxicity results from the liver's inability to metabolize the delivered citrate and can be observed in infants and patients with liver disease or severe hypoperfusion states. During citrate toxicity, the total calcium levels rise, the ionized calcium levels decline, and the total calcium/ionized calcium ratio is >2.5 [24]. In patients at risk of developing citrate toxicity, it is recommended to initiate the citrate infusion rate at approximately 50% of the standard infusion rate, while maintaining the standard calcium infusion rate. Patients who develop citrate toxicity can be managed by reducing the citrate infusion rate, increasing the citrate clearance rate or stopping the citrate infusion rate for 1–4 h, while following the patient's ionized calcium concentration. Once the patient's ionized calcium is higher than 0.9 mmoL/L, the citrate infusion is restarted at 70% the previous infusion rate.

Metabolic alkalosis occurs frequently after initiation of CRRT. Factors contributing to the development of this electrolyte abnormality include the increased concentration of bicarbonate/acetate in the intravenous fluids and in the TPN that was delivered in an attempt to control metabolic acidosis prior to CRRT initiation, the bicarbonate concentration in the dialysate/replacement solutions (22–32 mEq/L), the use of citrate for regional anticoagulation (a healthy liver will metabolize citrate to bicarbonate in a 3:1 ratio) and chloride losses due to nasogastric tube suctioning or emesis. Interventions to prevent and manage this electrolyte abnormality include discontinuation of the bicarbonate/acetate in the intravenous fluids and in the TPN at the time of CRRT initiation, changing the dialysate/replacement solutions to one with lower bicarbonate concentrations, changing the dialysis/replacement solution to 0.9% normal saline solution (pH 5.4) at a rate to provide 30% of the CRRT dose, reducing the citrate infusion rate or increasing the citrate clearance, if alkalosis is believed to be related to citrate toxicity.

Santiago and colleagues reported hypophosphatemia in 68% and severe hypophosphatemia in 39% of pediatric patients receiving CRRT. They observed that the phosphate levels decreased in the first 24 h of CRRT initiation and the incidence of hypophosphatemia was as high as 85% in the patients who did not receive any phosphate supplementation in the dialysate or replacement solution. Patients who were not receiving phosphate supplementation, those who were receiving high CRRT dose and whose age was less than 6 years, were at a higher risk of developing hypophosphatemia [25]. Hypophosphatemia can be managed by the addition of phosphate to the TPN, or by the addition of 2–4 mEq/L of potassium phosphate, 0.8 mL (1 mmoL/1 mL) monosodium phosphate to the dialysate/replacement solutions or by using phosphate containing dialysate/replacement solutions (Phoxilium® 1.1 mmoL/L. Baxter Healthcare Corporation. Deerfield, IL) [26]. The use of Phoxillium® has also reduced the need of magnesium supplementation in patients receiving CRRT. Many factors can contribute to the development of hypomagnesemia in critically ill patients receiving CRRT, including malnutrition, inadequate supplementation and chelation by the citrate used for regional anticoagulation. The management of hypomagnesemia includes increasing the magnesium supplementation in the TPN or adding magnesium sulfate to the dialysate/replacement solutions.

The development of hyperglycemia while delivering CRRT in pediatric patients is more common when the therapy is provided to infants and they are receiving citrate regional anticoagulation. The most common citrate solution used for regional anticoagulation is ACD-A and provides 2.45 g/dL of dextrose. Other potential contributors to the development of hyperglycemia include the dextrose concentration in the dialysate/replacement solutions (100–110 mg/dL) and the dextrose concentration in the TPN. If the patient develops hyperglycemia while on CRRT, the dextrose concentration in the patient's TPN needs to be adjusted without compromising nutritional support and/or the initiation of an insulin infusion needs to be discussed with the ICU team.

### 16.4.2 Nutrition

This important aspect in the care of children while receiving CRRT will be reviewed extensively in Chap. 12. But in general, in an attempt to maximize nutritional support while the patient is receiving therapy, we need to assure a delivery of 2.5–3 grams/kg/day of total protein and the caloric intake should be 20–30% above the resting energy expenditure [27].

### 16.4.3 Drug Dosing

Little clinical data exist surrounding the effect of acute kidney injury (AKI) and modern continuous renal replacement therapy (CRRT) methods on drug disposition (pharmacokinetics, PK) and response for adults or children receiving CRRT [28]. Data are often extrapolated from the adult or pediatric end-stage renal disease literature, which may not be appropriate given the different fluid overload status, increased metabolic rates, increased non-renal clearance and changing kidney function in patients with AKI. Recent in silico modeling of meropenem pharmacokinetics using the demographic and CRRT prescription data have shown that the predicted PK differed based on patient age and size [29], with children less than 5 years of age requiring three times daily dosing compared to twice daily dosing to achieve target concentrations. These predictions were subsequently validated in vivo in seven children who received CRRT and meropenem [30].

Given that few serum medication concentrations are readily measurable by most clinical labs, the critical care nephrology community has highlighted this gap in clinical care as a public health priority [31]. In 2016, the Kidney Health Initiative, which is supported by the American Society of Nephrology and the United States Food and Drug Administration and nephrology stakeholder, published a white paper outlining the parameters and need to fill this gap, and provided recommendations for the systematic assessment of all relevant medications provided to critically ill patients who receive CRRT [32]. The physiochemical properties of a drug are important to determine the likelihood of increased clearance by CRRT and these include: small molecular weight (<5000 Daltons), low plasma protein binding (<80%), low volume of distribution (<1 L/kg of body weight), and limited extrarenal clearance [33]. In the absence of published PK and PD data in patients receiving CRRT, integrating rounding pharmacist recommendation for drug dosing has been associated with lower adverse drug events and improved ICU costs [34, 35].

## References

1. Depner TA. Catheter performance. Semin Dial. 2001;14(6):425–31.
2. Hackbarth R, Bunchman TE, Chua AN, Somers MJ, Baum M, Symons JM, et al. The effect of vascular access location and size on circuit survival in pediatric continuous renal replacement therapy: a report from the PPCRRT registry. Int J Artif Organs. 2007;30(12):1116–21.

3. Khwaja A. KDIGO clinical practice guidelines for acute kidney injury. Nephron Clin Pract. 2012;120(4):c179–84.
4. Raymakers-Janssen P, Lilien M, van Kessel IA, Veldhoen ES, Wosten-van Asperen RM, van Gestel JPJ. Citrate versus heparin anticoagulation in continuous renal replacement therapy in small children. Pediatr Nephrol. 2017;32(10):1971–8.
5. Brophy PD, Somers MJ, Baum MA, Symons JM, McAfee N, Fortenberry JD, et al. Multi-Centre evaluation of anticoagulation in patients receiving continuous renal replacement therapy (CRRT). Nephrol Dial Transplant. 2005;20(7):1416–21.
6. Ostermann M, Dickie H, Tovey L, Treacher D. Management of sodium disorders during continuous haemofiltration. Crit Care. 2010;14(3):418.
7. Davenport A, Will EJ, Davison AM. Hyperlactataemia and metabolic acidosis during haemofiltration using lactate-buffered fluids. Nephron. 1991;59(3):461–5.
8. Zimmerman D, Cotman P, Ting R, Karanicolas S, Tobe SW. Continuous veno-venous haemodialysis with a novel bicarbonate dialysis solution: prospective cross-over comparison with a lactate buffered solution. Nephrol Dial Transplant. 1999;14(10):2387–91.
9. Barenbrock M, Hausberg M, Matzkies F, de la Motte S, Schaefer RM. Effects of bicarbonate- and lactate-buffered replacement fluids on cardiovascular outcome in CVVH patients. Kidney Int. 2000;58(4):1751–7.
10. Symons JM, Chua AN, Somers MJ, Baum MA, Bunchman TE, Benfield MR, et al. Demographic characteristics of pediatric continuous renal replacement therapy: a report of the prospective pediatric continuous renal replacement therapy registry. Clin J Am Soc Nephrol. 2007;2(4):732–8.
11. Peng Y, Yuan Z, Li H. Removal of inflammatory cytokines and endotoxin by veno-venous continuous renal replacement therapy for burned patients with sepsis. Burns. 2005;31(5):623–8.
12. Bellomo R, Tipping P, Boyce N. Continuous veno-venous hemofiltration with dialysis removes cytokines from the circulation of septic patients. Crit Care Med. 1993;21(4):522–6.
13. Stoves J, Goode NP, Visvanathan R, Jones CH, Shires M, Will EJ, et al. The bradykinin response and early hypotension at the introduction of continuous renal replacement therapy in the intensive care unit. Artif Organs. 2001;25(12):1009–13.
14. Liu ID, Ng KH, Lau PY, Yeo WS, Koh PL, Yap HK. Use of HF20 membrane in critically ill unstable low-body-weight infants on inotropic support. Pediatr Nephrol. 2013;28(5):819–22.
15. Brophy PD, Mottes TA, Kudelka TL, McBryde KD, Gardner JJ, Maxvold NJ, et al. AN-69 membrane reactions are pH-dependent and preventable. Am J Kidney Dis. 2001;38(1):173–8.
16. Pasko DA, Mottes TA, Mueller BA. Pre dialysis of blood prime in continuous hemodialysis normalizes pH and electrolytes. Pediatr Nephrol. 2003;18(11):1177–83.
17. Bunchman TE, Brophy PD, Goldstein SL. Technical considerations for renal replacement therapy in children. Semin Nephrol. 2008;28(5):488–92.
18. Jeffrey RF, Khan AA, Prabhu P, Todd N, Goutcher E, Will EJ, et al. A comparison of molecular clearance rates during continuous hemofiltration and hemodialysis with a novel volumetric continuous renal replacement system. Artif Organs. 1994;18(6):425–8.
19. Ronco C, Bellomo R, Homel P, Brendolan A, Dan M, Piccinni P, et al. Effects of different doses in continuous veno-venous haemofiltration on outcomes of acute renal failure: a prospective randomised trial. Lancet. 2000;356(9223):26–30.
20. Network VNARFT, Palevsky PM, Zhang JH, O'Connor TZ, Chertow GM, Crowley ST, et al. Intensity of renal support in critically ill patients with acute kidney injury. N Engl J Med. 2008;359(1):7–20.
21. Investigators RRTS, Bellomo R, Cass A, Cole L, Finfer S, Gallagher M, et al. Intensity of continuous renal-replacement therapy in critically ill patients. N Engl J Med. 2009;361(17):1627–38.
22. Spinale JM, Laskin BL, Sondheimer N, Swartz SJ, Goldstein SL. High-dose continuous renal replacement therapy for neonatal hyperammonemia. Pediatr Nephrol. 2013;28(6):983–6.
23. Barletta JF, Barletta GM, Brophy PD, Maxvold NJ, Hackbarth RM, Bunchman TE. Medication errors and patient complications with continuous renal replacement therapy. Pediatr Nephrol. 2006;21(6):842–5.

24. Meier-Kriesche HU, Gitomer J, Finkel K, DuBose T. Increased total to ionized calcium ratio during continuous venovenous hemodialysis with regional citrate anticoagulation. Crit Care Med. 2001;29(4):748–52.
25. Santiago MJ, Lopez-Herce J, Urbano J, Bellon JM, del Castillo J, Carrillo A. Hypophosphatemia and phosphate supplementation during continuous renal replacement therapy in children. Kidney Int. 2009;75(3):312–6.
26. Godaly G, Carlsson O, Broman M. Phoxilium((R)) reduces hypophosphataemia and magnesium supplementation during continuous renal replacement therapy. Clin Kidney J. 2016;9(2):205–10.
27. Zappitelli M, Goldstein SL, Symons JM, Somers MJ, Baum MA, Brophy PD, et al. Protein and calorie prescription for children and young adults receiving continuous renal replacement therapy: a report from the prospective pediatric continuous renal replacement therapy registry group. Crit Care Med. 2008;36(12):3239–45.
28. Mueller BA, Smoyer WE. Challenges in developing evidence-based drug dosing guidelines for adults and children receiving renal replacement therapy. Clin Pharmacol Ther. 2009;86(5):479–82.
29. Nehus EJ, Mouksassi S, Vinks AA, Goldstein S. Meropenem in children receiving continuous renal replacement therapy: clinical trial simulations using realistic covariates. J Clin Pharmacol. 2014;54(12):1421–8.
30. Nehus EJ, Mizuno T, Cox S, Goldstein SL, Vinks AA. Pharmacokinetics of meropenem in children receiving continuous renal replacement therapy: validation of clinical trial simulations. J Clin Pharmacol. 2016;56(3):291–7.
31. Goldstein SL, Nolin TD. Lack of drug dosing guidelines for critically ill patients receiving continuous renal replacement therapy. Clin Pharmacol Ther. 2014;96(2):159–61.
32. Nolin TD, Aronoff GR, Fissell WH, Jain L, Madabushi R, Reynolds K, et al. Pharmacokinetic assessment in patients receiving continuous RRT: perspectives from the kidney health initiative. Clin J Am Soc Nephrol. 2015;10(1):159–64.
33. Schetz M. Drug dosing in continuous renal replacement therapy: general rules. Curr Opin Crit Care. 2007;13(6):645–51.
34. Jiang SP, Zhu ZY, Wu XL, Lu XY, Zhang XG, Wu BH. Effectiveness of pharmacist dosing adjustment for critically ill patients receiving continuous renal replacement therapy: a comparative study. Ther Clin Risk Manag. 2014;10:405–12.
35. Jiang SP, Zhu ZY, Ma KF, Zheng X, Lu XY. Impact of pharmacist antimicrobial dosing adjustments in septic patients on continuous renal replacement therapy in an intensive care unit. Scand J Infect Dis. 2013;45(12):891–9.

# 17 Anticoagulation in CRRT

Patrick Brophy, Irfan Khan, and Akash Deep

**Case Vignette**

A 3-year-old male child with acute liver failure (ALF) gets admitted to the Pediatric Intensive Care Unit (PICU) in hepatic encephalopathy grade 3. He is intubated and ventilated and in view of high ammonia (324 μmol/L) and oliguria is commenced on CRRT (continuous renal replacement therapy). Since CRRT in this patient is started for high ammonia, it was imperative that downtimes for the circuit were minimized. Patient's INR was 7.2 IU, platelets were 67, and lactate was 5.4. To achieve acceptable filter life, the options we had were no anticoagulation, only saline flushes (high INR, low platelets), low-dose heparin (risk of bleeding), citrate (risk of citrate toxicity due to liver failure), or antiplatelet agent like prostacyclin. The decision to start anticoagulation is always complicated as we need to balance the safety, efficacy, and risk profiles of the agent we choose. The agent chosen should be effective in maintaining the desired half-life of at least 48–72 h while minimizing the side effects. Taking the full patient profile into account, we started this patient on 4 ng/kg/min of prostacyclin closely watching for bleeding episodes and hypotension. The circuit life was approximately 72 h, ammonia levels decreased

---

P. Brophy
Department of Pediatrics, University of Rochester School of Medicine and Dentistry, Rochester, NY, USA

Golisano Children's Hospital, University of Rochester Medical Center, Rochester, NY, USA

I. Khan
Presbyterian Hospital, Albuquerque, NM, USA

A. Deep (✉)
Paediatric Intensive Care Unit, King's College Hospital, London, UK

Renal/CRRT Section of the European Society of Pediatric and Neonatal Intensive Care (ESPNIC), Geneva, Switzerland
e-mail: akash.deep@nhs.net



A. Deep, S. L. Goldstein (eds.), *Critical Care Nephrology and Renal Replacement Therapy in Children*, https://doi.org/10.1007/978-3-319-90281-4_17

from 324 to 112 in 48 h, and liver transplant was performed after 72 h of admission. There was no bleeding episodes or hypotension encountered. We continued CRRT post liver transplant and the child regained renal function and was discharged from PICU on Day 6 posttransplant with intact neurology.

## 17.1 Introduction

Acute kidney injury in critically ill children and young adults is an independent risk factor for a prolonged ICU stay and death [1]. Hemodynamically unstable patients with multi-organ dysfunction fail to tolerate intermittent HD, and hence are candidates for continuous renal replacement therapy (CRRT). The delivered dialysis dose for CRRT often varies from the prescribed dose depending on the longevity of the filter and performance of the CRRT circuit which are key elements that determine the successful running of the CRRT circuit. To achieve this besides optimizing non-circuit factors, one of the key things to do is to use an anticoagulant which maintains the fluidity of blood in the circuit and yet have minimal effects on systemic circulation.

A variety of anticoagulants have been used in CRRT (Table 17.1). Each one has its advantages, disadvantages, ease of use and cost implications and complications. An ideal anticoagulant strategy should be readily available, selectively active, and durable (in terms of filter life span) in the extracorporeal circuit, with minimal effects on patient hemostasis. The monitoring should be rapid, simple, and in the case of complications, anticoagulation should be rapidly reversible. All staff involved should be well trained in the use and recognition of side effects of the used anticoagulant.

Unfractionated heparin provides systemic anticoagulation and is cheap and easy to use by physicians and nurses who feel comfortable with its protocol. There is no special preparation needed and it requires an uncomplicated monitoring method (see Table 17.2). However, recent advances in the use of commercially prepared standardized citrate solutions, the use of mathematical algorithms and simplified protocols for the use of citrate in a variety of populations have contributed for its expanded use in multiple centers across the world [6–18].

**Table 17.1** List of various anticoagulants used in CRRT

| |
|---|
| • Saline flushes |
| • Heparin (unfractionated) |
| • Low molecular weight heparin |
| • Citrate regional anticoagulation |
| • Prostacyclin |
| • Nafamostat mesilate |
| • Danaparoid |
| • Hirudin/Lepirudin |
| • Argatroban (thrombin inhibitor) |

**Table 17.2** Select Randomized clinical studies comparing citrate with heparin anticoagulation for continuous renal replacement therapy (CRRT)

| | | Circuit life (hours) | | Bleeding | | Transfusion (RBC/day) | | Survival | |
|---|---|---|---|---|---|---|---|---|---|
| Reference | Design | Citrate | Heparin | Citrate | Heparin | Citrate | Heparin | Citrate | Heparin |
| Monchi and colleagues [2] | RCOT, $n = 20$ | 70 (44–140), $p < 0.001$ | 40 (17–48) | $n = 0$ | $n = 1$ | 0.2 (0–0.4), $p < 0.001$ | 1.0 (0–2.0) | | |
| Kutsogiannis and colleagues [3] | RCT, $n = 30$ | 125 (95–157), $p < 0.001$ | 38 (25–62) | RR 0.17 (0.03–1.04), $p = 0.06$ | | 0.53 (0.24–1.20), $p = 0.13$ | | | |
| Betjes and colleagues [4] | RCT, $n = 48$ | | | 0% $p < 0.01$ | 33% | 0.43, $p = 0.01$ | 0.88 | | |
| Hetzel and colleagues [5] | RCT, $n = 170$ | 37.5 + 23, $p < 0.001$ | 26.1 + 19.2 | 14.5%, $p = 0.06$ | 5.7% | | | +30%, NS | +43% |

### 17.1.1 Unfractionated Heparin for Anticoagulation

Unfractionated heparin has traditionally been the most popular anticoagulant for use in patients undergoing CRRT [19]. Its main advantages are its ease of use, simple monitoring, reversal with protamine, and low cost.

It is a relatively large molecule with a molecular weight of 12–15 kDa. Its half-life is approximately 30 min in healthy patients and about 90 min in patients with renal failure. Heparin binds to the enzyme inhibitor antithrombin (AT) activating it, which in turn inactivates thrombin, factor Xa, and other proteases. The formation of the quaternary bond between heparin, AT, and thrombin results in the inactivation of thrombin. Heparin also has anti-Xa activity in its unfractionated form [20]. Both high AT consumption and increased AT degradation contribute to heparin resistance during critical illness.

The effect of heparin can be measured using the activated partial thromboplastin time (aPTT) and the activated clotting time (ACT).

### 17.1.2 Heparin Protocol

A variety of heparin protocols exist (see Fig. 17.1). In general, heparin is infused pre-filter for patients on CRRT unless the patient is on heparin infusion for other reasons. The heparinized filtered blood is then returned to the patient, who is now systemically anticoagulated. There are no defined standard rates of heparin infusion in use with CRRT. In most cases, patients are started with a baseline measurement of baseline aPTT and administering a 25–50 units/kg bolus of heparin (if aPTT is <35 s) into the circuit priming solution before the blood comes in contact with the circuit surfaces. This is followed by an infusion rate of 10–20 units/kg/h titrated by nurses to keep the aPTT of patient's blood in the 45–65 s range. Repeat aPTT testing is performed at least every 4 h according to a standardized dosing nomogram [3, 21]. The heparin infusion is adjusted up or down on 10% titrations for therapeutic aPTT out of the desired range, small boluses of heparin can be administered intermittently if necessary. Alternately, ACT measurements can be used to titrate heparin dosing at the bedside when that option is available aiming for ACT between 180–220 s. This is a bedside test and can be easily performed by the nursing team. However, there is always a debate whether ACT levels correlate with efficacy of unfractionated heparin.

### 17.1.3 Side Effects of Unfractionated Heparin

Children are relatively more prone to low AT levels, especially during sepsis, and if higher than normal heparin infusion rates (possibly indicative of heparin resistance) are required, an antithrombin level should be checked and AT replaced with a full vial for levels less than 70% [22].

Full blood count is closely monitored for any evidence of a significant drop in platelet count and/or clotting. If the platelet levels fall rapidly, then heparin is eliminated and a screen for heparin-induced thrombocytopenia sent [23]. In about 1–5%

**PATIENT COAGULATION/ANTICOAGULANT THERAPY:**
**(before initiating therapy)**

1. Obtain PT/PTT, Platelet count, *ACT baseline (by dialysis nurse).
2. In the absence of coagulopathy (patient's ACT <150 secs), give bolus of ____ units heparin (25 units/kg) to patient and recheck ACT. Repe at heparin bolus and ACT check until ACT >180 secs (maximum:repeat x 2)

**(during hemofiltration)**

1. Heparin infusion: When ACT > 180 secs, start heparin drip 10 units/ml in CRRT circuit at 10 units/kg/hr = ____ units/hr or ____ ml/hr. Check system ACT.
2. Titrate heparin drip to keep post-filter ACT between 180-220 seconds
   - If ACT is <180 secs, increase heparin drip by 1 unit/k g/hr.
   - If ACT is >220 secs, decrease the heparin drip by 1 unit/kg/hr

Anticoagulation monitoring: **With each circuit change and when platelets or blood are administered to the patient**, obtain postfilter (blue port) ACT q 20 minutes until stable.

Monitor ACT q 20-30 min. for an hour after any heparin

changes. Monitor ACTs every four hours once stable

Adapted from: http://www.pcrrt.com/ProtocolsAccess.html

**Fig. 17.1** Heparin protocol

of the patients receiving heparin, heparin-induced thrombocytopenia (HIT) develops [24, 25]. It is related to the binding of heparin to platelet factor 4 released from activated platelets. Some patients develop antibodies against these heparin-platelet factor 4 complexes. The antibody-platelet factor 4-heparin complex subsequently binds to platelets, inducing platelet activation, aggregation and activation of the coagulation pathways. This sequence results in a loss of circulating platelets and a prothrombotic state [26].

Despite the vast experience in the use of unfractionated heparin, it has several side effects which are clinically significant. The main one being the patient's risk of bleeding. Severe bleeding events are reported in 10–50% of cases, depending on the population and the degree of anticoagulation.

Another issue is the unpredictable pharmacokinetics of heparin—the pharmacokinetics of heparin are not only time- and dose-dependent but also unpredictable due to inter- and intra-patient variability, which is related to an interaction with a variety of proteins and cells and can thereby interfere with the inflammatory cascade and, altogether, confer unpredictable consequences for critically ill patients.

### 17.1.4 Regional Citrate Anticoagulation

Citrate has been recognized as an anticoagulant for over 100 years [27]. Indeed it was first used as a regional approach in hemodialysis (HD) [28–31], especially in HD patients at risk for bleeding [29].

The initial use of regional citrate anticoagulation (RCA) for CRRT involved 18 adult patients with AKI in an ICU setting whereby trisodium citrate vs. heparin vs. saline flushes were employed as anticoagulation strategies. Since then, multiple studies have described various citrate protocols that have been progressively simplified with the use of standardized commercially available citrate solutions and development of mathematical algorithms to titrate citrate and calcium infusion rates.

### 17.1.5 The Main Components of the Citrate Protocol Include

**Prefilter anticoagulation solution:** The goal of the prefilter solution is to administer enough citrate to quickly chelate and reduce the filter ionized calcium levels to around 0.25–0.35 mmol/L. Low ionized calcium levels inhibit the generation of thrombin by suppressing the coagulation cascade, as ionized calcium is a cofactor for the final common pathway and activation of factors II, X, XIII and fibrin formation. Trisodium citrate [sodium content (220 mmol/L)] solutions were initially prepared in house by pharmacies but were costly and at risk for error. The advent of commercially prepared solutions like the ACD-A solution (acid citrate dextrose) has led to much wider use of the RCA protocol in various studies and centers.

**Post-filter solution**: The unused citrate which is returned to the patient can have metabolic consequences like systemic hypocalcemia from continued chelation of the calcium in patient's blood and is metabolized by the liver into bicarbonate occasionally resulting in metabolic alkalosis. In order to neutralize the citrate, a calcium gluconate or chloride containing solution is infused via the hemocatheter or a central line into the patient's blood and the rate of infusion is titrated to maintain the iCa in the patient's blood around 1.1–1.3 mmol/L.

**Citrate protocols:** Mehta et al. [32] described the procedural details of using citrate anticoagulation with trisodium citrate. The importance of prefilter citrate rates, prefilter replacement solution to maintain convective clearance, and post-filter calcium infusion rates were introduced for the first time. A variety of studies have modified this protocol and simplified its application [3, 7, 9, 12, 18, 21, 33, 34] (see Fig. 17.2).

## 17.2 RCA Side Effects

A phenomenon called citrate toxicity or citrate lock may occur if the total serum calcium as compared to an ionised calcium (iCa) rises disproportionately. This is directly proportional to the concentration of **citrate** in the blood. An elevated total to iCa ratio of greater than 2.5 is indicative of citrate toxicity. Given that the total citrate concentration in this case can exceed the body's ability to metabolize it, a variety of

1. Prime in CVVHDF Mode using ordered dialysate and replacement solutions.

    Dialysate: HCO3-based without Ca
    Replacement: normal saline or bicarb-based industry made solution

2. Place a 3 way stop cock to both the "arterial" and venous ports of the dialysis access. Attach the Citrate ACD(A) Solution 1000 cc to a regular IV pump and then attach it to the "arterial" stop cock.

3. When ready to start, the citrate rate in ccs/hr will be 1.5 x the blood flow rate of the PRISMA machine at ccs/min. (eg Start Citrate at 150 mls/hr if the BFR is 100mls/min)

4. Set up the Ca++ infusion (ie. 8gms Calcium Chloride in 1L NS or 23.5 gms of Calcium Gluconate in 1L of NS) as ordered via central line other than the dialysis access. This will run at 40% of the citrate flow rate. (eg if citrate rate = 150 mls/hr then CaCl rate = 60 mls/hr)

5. Set the flow rates in Hemofiltration machine as ordered.

6. Patient Fluid Removal Rate is calculated by:
   Net Ultrafiltration rate + Citrate rate + Calcium infusion rate = Pt. Fluid Removal Rate.

7. Connect the Hemofiltration machine circuit to the dialysis catheter as per procedure and press start.

8. 2 hour after initiation of therapy and every 6 hours thereafter, send the following blood work:

    Post-filter ionized Ca++ (drawn fromthe return line, blue sample port) Systemic ionized Ca++ (drawn from patient (true) arterial line or peripheral draw)
    Bloods for biochemistry (eg Lytes, Bun, Cr, Ca, Phos, Albumin) (see # 14 for citrate and calcium adjustment)

9. Metabolic alkalosis occurs due to citrate metabolism to bicarbonate and due to bicarbonate in the Dialysate. Call Pediatric Nephrologist if the Serum Bicarb is > 35 meq/l. In that case the Pediatric Nephrologist will add in NS as a replacement solution by 200-400 cc/hr and decrease the dialysate rate by the same amount. This will give an acid load from the NS and diminish the HCO3 from the bath at the same time.

10. Notify MD for the following:
    a. Systemic Ionized Ca++ < 0.75 mmol/L. (Consider holding citrate for 1 hour and resuming infusion at 30% of the citrate flow rate and bolus with 10 mg/kg of CaCl and increase Ca infusion by 10%)
    b. Na+ > 150 mmol/L. Consider changing replacement solution to 0.45% NaCl.

**Fig. 17.2** Citrate protocols

11. If the filter clots, stop the citrate and Ca++ infusions and discontinue the filter.

12. **In children less then 10kg who require a blood transfusion when going on CRRT, avoid the use of citrate for the first 15 minutes for it may exacerbate the Bradykinin release syndrome seen in some children.**

13. Citrate Lock occurs when the total calcium rises with a dropping ionized calcium. This is due to the fact of the citrate infusion exceeds the clearance on dialysis and from hepatic metabolism. When this is seen, stop the citrate for 2-4 hours then restart at 70% of the previous dose. Watch the ionized calcium during this time to avoid inadequate anticoagulation of the circuit (i.e.the ionized calcium of the system rising causing system clotting).

14. Titrate the Citrate infusion according to the citrate sliding scale below:

| Prisma ionized Ca++ (mmol/L) | **Citrate Infusion Adjustment** | |
|---|---|---|
| | > 20 kg | < 20 kg |
| < 0.35 | ↓ rate by 10 ml/hr | ↓ rate by 5 ml/hr |
| 0.35 –0.5 (Optimum Range) | No adjustment | |
| 0.5 – 0.6 | ↑ rate by 10 ml/hr | ↑ rate by 5 ml/hr |
| > 0.6 | ↑ rate by 20 ml/hr | ↑ rate by 10 ml/hr |
| NOTIFY MD IF CITRATE INFUSION RATE > 200 ml/hr | | |

Titrate the Calciumin fusion according to the calcium sliding scale below:

| Patient ionized Ca++ (mmol/L) | **Calcium Infusion Adjustment** | |
|---|---|---|
| | > 20 kg | < 20 kg |
| > 1.3 | ↓ rate by 10 ml/hr | ↓ rate by 5 ml/hr |
| 1.1-1.3 (Optimum Range) | No adjustment | |
| 0.9-1.1 | ↑ rate by 10 ml/hr | ↑ rate by 5 ml/hr |
| < 0.9 | ↑ rate by 20 ml/hr | ↑ rate by 10 ml/hr |
| NOTIFY MD IF Calcium INFUSION RATE > 200 ml/hr | | |

**Fig. 17.2** (continued)

options exist to improve clearance including withholding the citrate infusion and/or increasing the ultrafiltration rate. If continued issues exist, it is reasonable to evaluate the patient for possible hepatic dysfunction. Initial and continued analysis of electrolytes is warranted in order to evaluate for evolving sodium, potassium, magnesium, phosphorus, and acid–base status.

In summary, RCA protocols for CRRT vary depending on the citrate concentration used, the choice and position of the replacement/dialysate fluid, and the rate of blood flow.

### 17.2.1 Comparison of Heparin vs. Citrate for Anticoagulation

To compare the two methods of anticoagulation, we need to review the literature supporting their efficacies in terms of circuit survival, effect on cost, requirement for special personnel training and complications or side effect profiles [35, 36].

### 17.2.2 Randomized Control Trials (Table 17.2)

**Monchi et al.** [2]: Forty-nine circuits were analyzed in ICU patients at a single center: 23 with heparin and 26 with citrate. The median lifetime of hemofilters was longer with citrate anticoagulation ($p = 0.0007$). One major bleeding event occurred during heparin anticoagulation and one episode of metabolic alkalosis ($pH = 7.60$) was noted with citrate after a protocol violation. Transfusion rates (units of red blood cells (RBC) per day of CVVH) were higher in the heparin group ($p = 0.0008$).

**Kutsogiannis et al.** [3]: In 30 patients requiring CRRT and randomly assigned to receive RCA vs. heparin, median hemofilter survival time was 124.5 h (95% CI 95.3–157.4) in the citrate group, which was significantly longer than the 38.3 h (95% CI 24.8–61.9) in the heparin group ($p < 0.001$). The relative risk of hemorrhage with citrate anticoagulation was significantly lower than that with heparin ($p = 0.05$).

**Betjes et al.** [4]: 48 patients (21 for RCA and 27 for heparin) were randomized and circuit survival was similar in both groups. Major bleeding risk was higher in the heparin group ($p < 0.01$) and so was the RBC transfusion need (0.88 vs. 0.43, $p = 0.01$) and drop in hemoglobin. No adverse metabolic events reported in the RCA group.

**Hetzel et al.** [5]: In a prospective randomized multicenter trial, 174 mechanically ventilated adult patients at nine different centers receiving CRRT were studied. Patient mortality was similar ($p = 0.67$); however, the use of citrate resulted in less systemic anticoagulation, a lower risk of bleeding ($p = 0.06$), and a longer hemofilter patency ($p < 0.001$). Metabolic acidosis requiring bicarbonate infusion ($p = 0.07$), hypocalcemia ($p < 0.001$), and hypercalcemia ($p < 0.001$) occurred more frequently in the RCA group.

**Schilder et al.** [37]: In this multicenter non-blinded, prospective randomized clinical trial performed in 10 ICUs in the Netherlands, 139 patients were enrolled, 66 were randomized to citrate and 73 to heparin. Mortality rates at 28–90 days were similar in both groups ($p = 1.00$ for both). Renal outcome, measured as dependence on RRT at 28 days from initiation, did not differ between groups ($p = 0.82$). Filter survival rates were superior for citrate (median 46 vs. 32 h, $p = 0.02$), as were the number of filters used ($p = 0.002$) and time off filter within 72 h ($p = 0.002$). The costs during the first 72 h of prescribed CVVH were lower in citrate-based CVVH. Citrate accumulation was proved in 6% of the patients assigned to RCA. Clinically suspected HIT was reported in 8% of patients on heparin. There was a trend for fewer bleeding episodes in the citrate group ($p = 0.08$), however, this did not result in significant PRBC transfusions difference between the 2 groups. ($p = 0.68$). Fewer filters were used in the citrate group ($p = 0.04$), as well as time on CVVH was higher for the citrate group ($p = 0.04$). Circuit clotting resulting in filter change was higher in the heparin group ($p = 0.001$). There was a statistically significant decrease in cost for CVVH in the citrate group ($p < 0.001$).

**Brian MJ et al.** [38]: In this Australian study, 30 patients were randomly assigned by a computer to undergo RCA vs. heparin anticoagulation for CRRT. Significant crossover occurred from citrate to heparin group hampering conclusions. However, median filter survival, by intention to treat, was not significantly different ($p = 0.58$) between the two groups. Per-protocol filter survival was higher for citrate ($p = 0.004$).

**Stucker et al.** [39]: 103 patients were randomized to either CRRT with RCA or heparin anticoagulation. Median CRRT duration was 3.0 (2–6) days. Effective delivered daily RRT doses and filter life spans was higher in the RCA group ($p = 0.005$ and $p = 0.004$). Survival rates were similar in the two groups. Patients treated with RCA didn't have any significant electrolyte and acid–base abnormalities.

### 17.2.3 Meta-analysis of the RCTs

Bai M et al. [40], in 2015, evaluated 11 RCTs on 992 patients and determined that citrate for CRRT significantly reduced the risk of circuit loss compared to systemic heparin ($p = 0.04$). Filter failure was much lower in the citrate group ($p = 0.04$). There was a lower bleeding risk in the citrate group ($p < 0.001$).The incidences of heparin-induced thrombocytopenia (HIT) and hypocalcemia were increased in the heparin and citrate groups, respectively. There was no difference in survival between the groups.

### 17.2.4 Prospective Studies

**Brophy et al.** [16]: In this largest pediatric study, 138 patients from 1 day to 25 years old from seven US centers receiving RCA vs. heparin vs. no anticoagulation were prospectively studied. Mean circuit survival was similar between the two groups. Nine patients in the heparin group developed systemic bleeding, including intracranial, epistaxis, pulmonary, gastrointestinal, bladder, and vaginal bleeding, resulting in termination of heparin. One patient developed HIT and was switched to no heparin.

One patient in the RCA group developed metabolic alkalosis managed by titration of normocarb. Two patients with hepatic failure developed citrate lock managed by titration of the ACD-A solution.

**Raymakers-Janssen et al.** [21]: In this prospective study in small children undergoing CRRT with the smallest filters, heparin (6 patients) was compared with citrate (14 patients). Median circuit survival time with heparin was 21 h compared to 45.2 h with citrate ($p < 0.001$). Actual administered effluent dose compared to prescribed dose was 85% with heparin compared to 92% with citrate ($p = 0.31$). No patient treated with citrate developed citrate toxicity. No other differences in electrolytes were found between the two CRRT regimes. In the heparin group, a median of 6.5 units of red blood cells (IQR 1.5–23.8) were given during CRRT, compared to three in the citrate group (IQR 2.0–5.0, $p = 0.12$).

Just as heparin can be a concern in those with bleeding abnormalities, citrate metabolism can be a concern in those with liver dysfunction. Use of citrate is not universal and requires very close monitoring of ionized calcium and acid base balance.

#### 17.2.4.1 Other Anticoagulants

Neither heparin nor citrate anticoagulation provides a perfect solution for prolonging circuit longevity, and so the possibility of an alternative, safe, and efficacious CRRT anticoagulation agent remains an attractive prospect. An important alternative is prostacyclin which is an effective anticoagulant which can be used in situations where heparin or citrate cannot be used or may be ineffective, particularly in patients with coagulopathy as in liver failure.

### 17.2.5 Prostacyclin

Prostacyclin (also called Prostaglandin I2 or PGI2) is a member of the family of lipid molecules called eicosanoids, synthesized from the arachidonic acid pathway by cyclooxygenase enzymes. It is produced by endothelial cells of blood vessels. It is both a potent vasodilator and inhibitor of platelet aggregation. Epoprostenol, the synthetic equivalent of prostacyclin, is the drug currently used as an anticoagulant for pediatric CRRT

#### 17.2.5.1 Pharmacological Properties

Prostacyclin is metabolized rapidly and has a very short half-life (42 s) [41]. Furthermore, its low molecular weight of 374.45 Daltons and its low protein-binding fraction preclude significant elimination by ultra-filtrate and dialysate fluids. Prostacyclin acts as a potent vasodilator and is a major inhibitor of platelet aggregation. In addition to beneficial effects of prostacyclin as an anticoagulant, it can potentially help to optimize oxygen delivery and uptake in critically ill patients. This property of PGI2 can be of advantage in critically ill children with multi-organ failure who are hemodynamically stable.

#### 17.2.5.2 Mechanism of Action

The anticoagulant effects of prostacyclin are mainly mediated through its antiplatelet effect. Prostacyclin reversibly inhibits platelet function and reduces heterotypic platelet leukocyte aggregation during clinical hemofiltration in critically ill patients [42].

Prostacyclin activates adenylate cyclase, leading to an increase in cyclic AMP levels. Cyclic AMP mediates phosphorylation of VASP (Vasodilator stimulated phosphoprotein) to VASP-P (phosphorylated form), which inhibits glycoprotein IIb-IIIa receptor activation, thereby inhibiting platelet aggregation and finally the process of thrombus formation.

It also has a heparin sparing effect, which can be crucial to prevent the side effects of higher doses of heparin. Prostacyclin can significantly reduce the amount of heparin needed for effective anticoagulation—probably because of the reduced inhibition of unfractionated heparin by platelet factor 4. It has been shown that prostacyclin can inhibit the release of platelet factor-4 by 85–95% [43].

Therefore, the same amount of anticoagulation can be achieved by using lower doses of heparin when prostacyclin is added to heparin. Turney et al. have shown that prostacyclin can also prolong the half-life of heparin by up to 40% [44].

#### 17.2.5.3 Side Effects

Due to its short half-life, complications of prostacyclin are minimal. The main side effect described is hypotension due to vasodilatation. This complication usually responds to intravascular volume expansion with fluids, addition or increase in the dose of vasopressors, or decrease in the dosage of prostacyclin. There might be an increased incidence of bleeding in patients with esophageal varices due to inhibition of platelets and increased blood flow in the portal venous system. Systemic side effects (hypotension, and an increase of intracranial pressure) can be further prevented or limited by infusion into the extracorporeal circuit, reducing the systemic levels due to extracorporeal elimination [45].

Prostacyclin can also cause ventilation perfusion mismatch with an increase in alveolar-arterial oxygen tension gradient. This might be clinically significant in those with reflex hypoxic pulmonary vasoconstriction [46].

Safety of intravenous prostacyclin has also been demonstrated in neonates receiving this drug for severe pulmonary hypertension [47]. Prostacyclin is therefore a safe drug when used regionally as an anticoagulant in the CRRT circuit.

### 17.2.6 Marketing

Epoprostenol is marketed as Flolan® (GlaxoSmithKline plc, London, UK) and is also available as a generic drug (Teva Pharmaceutical Industries Ltd., Petah Tikva, Israel). Since 2008, a room-temperature stable (RTS) formulation of epoprostenol (Veletri®, Action Pharmaceuticals Ltd., Allschwil, Switzerland) has also been available.

## 17.3 Guidelines for the Use of Prostacyclin (Epoprostenol) in Children on CRRT

We propose the following protocol for the use of prostacyclin as an anticoagulant in CRRT (Fig. 17.3) This protocol is being used in the PICU of King's College Hospital, London.

### 17.3.1 Method of Administration

Due to its short-half life, epoprostenol is used as a continuous infusion into the extracorporeal circuit. The infusion should be stopped when CRRT is discontinued. Epoprostenol has a vasodilatory effect at 20 ng/kg/min and an antiplatelet effect at 2–8 ng/kg/min.

### 17.3.2 Monitoring

Prostacyclin use for pediatric CRRT does not need complex monitoring. Side effects can be monitored clinically—bleeding and systemic hemodynamics. Further monitoring with platelet function tests can be done but will incur costs and results are not

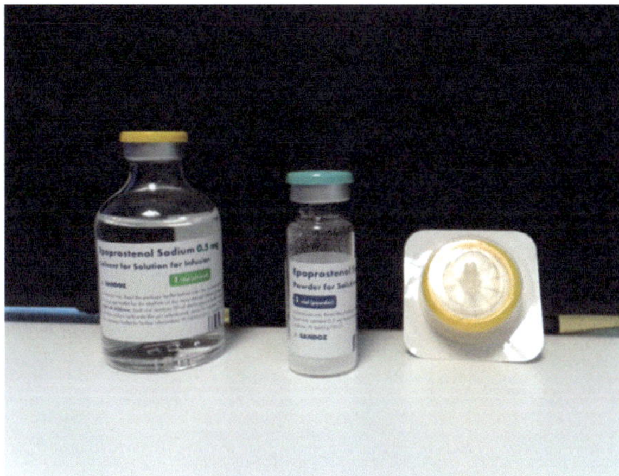

**Fig. 17.3** Prostacyclin protocol for CRRT

readily available. These tests are not routinely employed in clinical practice. Thromboelastography (TEG) or ROTEM (Rotational Thromboelastometry) may be useful.

### 17.3.3 Cost-Effectiveness

Cost can be an important factor while using prostacyclin as an anticoagulant. However, when one considers the cost of changing clotted filters and circuits, including the costs of monitoring tests with other anticoagulants, the overall cost of using prostacyclin might be less.

As discussed before, heparin-sparing effect can be effectively used in patients requiring escalating doses of heparin to achieve the desired ACT, and in those where filters/circuits clot frequently. For example, in patients who are extremely sick and septic with low AT-III, using heparin alone in these patients may require increasing doses to achieve the same anticoagulation effect. Therefore, we use the combination of low-dose heparin and prostacyclin quite commonly in our institute. Prostacyclin, by its antiplatelet and heparin-sparing effects, increases ACT and helps maintain longer filter life. We attach a 3-way tap and combine the two anticoagulants for the desired effect (Fig. 17.4).

## 17.4 Evidence for the Use of Prostacyclin as an Anticoagulant

Prostacyclin has been commonly used for treating pulmonary hypertension in children, but its use in pediatric CRRT has been limited. The literature search on prostacyclin in pediatric CRRT is rather frustrating with mainly case series and observational studies. Use of prostacyclin as an anticoagulant is described in adults with acute kidney injury. Most of the studies were conducted where heparin was contraindicated or caused side effects.

We have used prostacyclin safely and effectively in critically ill patients with both liver and non-liver problems. Use of an anticoagulant in patients with liver

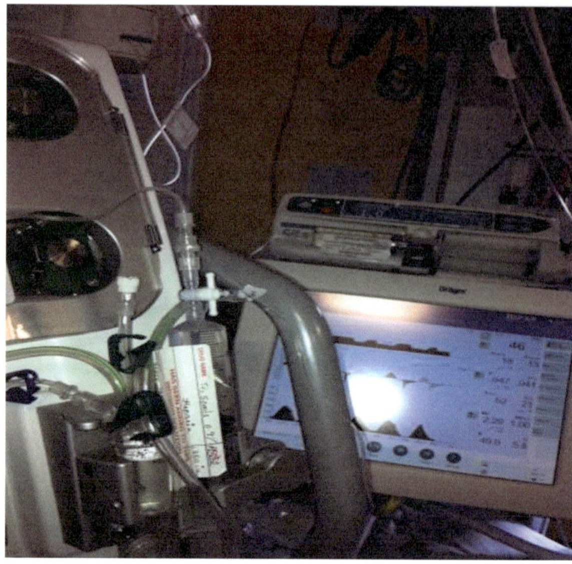

**Fig. 17.4** Combined use of heparin and prostacyclin as anticoagulants in CRRT

failure is always a topic of debate. Clinicians are hesitant to use any anticoagulation due to abnormal clotting tests and perceived risk of bleeding. In fact, most of these patients are pro-coagulant and require anticoagulation [48].

Zobel G et al. had earlier reported to have used prostacyclin either alone or with heparin in six children with preexisting coagulopathy and high risk of bleeding. There was an approximately 20% increase in filter life in the heparin/prostacyclin combined group compared to heparin alone. No adverse events were reported [49].

Zobel G et al. have also reported the use of prostacyclin for continuous arterio-venous hemofiltration (CAVH) in five critically ill premature infants with a mean gestational age of 31.8 +/− 3.8 weeks. Prostacyclin was the sole anticoagulant [dose of 5–10 ng/kg/min] in four, with heparin in one. The filter life was 14 h, with no reported side effects due to prostacyclin. This is the earliest report of the use of prostacyclin in premature infants [49].

Although these studies were mainly conducted in adult patients, children with a similar pathophysiology could have similar results. However, further studies in children are necessary. Some of the relevant studies are summarized in Table 17.3 [52, 54, 57–59].

Prostacyclin (epoprostenol) can be an effective alternate anticoagulant either alone or in conjunction with heparin for pediatric CRRT. It can be safely used in patients with thrombocytopenia and/or increased risk of bleeding both in patients with liver and non-liver disorders. Although heparin and citrate are the most commonly used anticoagulants, prostacyclin is an attractive alternative, with a favorable safety and efficacy profile. While the protocol and the safety profile have been promising, more research, particularly in children, is necessary for it to be accepted as a universal add-on or sole anticoagulant.

**Table 17.3** Summary of relevant studies using prostacyclin as an anticoagulant for CRRT

| Reference | Age group | Patient/circuits characteristics | Dosage | Results | Comments |
|---|---|---|---|---|---|
| Goonasekera et al. [50] | 0–18 years | 62 filtration episodes.<br>Liver dysfunction | Prostacyclin-4 ng/kg/min | Mean duration of circuit use −53 h | No reported complications |
| Zobel et al. [51] | 6 children [10 days to 12 years] | Preexisting coagulopathy/thrombocytopenia | Prostacyclin as sole or with heparin. | 20% increase in filter life when prostacyclin was added. | No adverse events reported. |
| Zobel et al. [49] | 5 preterm infants<br>31.8 +/−3.8 weeks | Mean duration of CAVH 53.6+/−14 h | Prostacyclin:<br>5-10 ng/kg/min | Mean circuit use—14 h | No side effects observed |
| Langenecker et al. [52] | Adults | 3 groups<br>Gr 1: UFH ($n = 13$)<br>Gr 2: PGI2 ($n = 14$)<br>Gr3: UFH+ PGI2($n = 19$)<br>Critically ill on CVVH | Prostacyclin alone: 7.7 +/−0.7 ng/kg/min.<br>With heparin 6.4 +/−0.3 ng | Circuit life longest when prostacyclin + heparin (22 h) | Better hemodynamic profiles.<br>No bleeding complications |
| Gainza et al. [53] | Adult | 38 patients | Prostacyclin-5 ng/kg/min | Circuit life increased by 50% | Bleeding (18%) fall in BP [18%]<br>Recovered in 24 hours |
| Fabbri et al. [54] | Adult<br>Prospective RCT. | 90 patients<br>Critically ill patients with ARF<br>UFH + PGI2($n = 46$) vs. UFH($n = 44$) | Prostacyclin-<br>4 ng/kg/min | Circuit life-<br>68 h vs. 19 h | Platelets reduced progressively while on heparin alone |
| Balik et al. [55] | Adult<br>Compared with citrate as an alternative coagulant. | 32 patients<br>UFH + PGI2($n = 17$)<br>vs.<br>Citrate ($n = 15$) | Prostacyclin-<br>4-10 ng/kg/mt | Circuit life<br>26 h vs. 36.5 h | Hypotension 23% in 1st gp.<br>Increased dose of PGI2 doesn't increase hemodynamic side effects. |
| Herrera-Gutiérrez et al. [56] | Adult | 389 patients.<br>Prostacyclin used in those with risk of bleeding.<br>Combined with UFH—When issues with early clotting of filters. | Prostacyclin<br>4–5 ng/kg/mt either when isolated or when combined with UFH | Circuit life almost doubled when combined with UFH [27 h] | Mild bleeding in 3% patients. |
| Fiaccadori et al. [57] | Adult [SLED]] | 35 patients.<br>Prostacyclin given directly to patient-1/2 dose. | Prostacyclin 6 ng/kg/mt | 90% sessions completed as prescribed | No increase in risk of bleeding |

Therefore, to choose between three of these discussed anticoagulants is not an easy decision—while heparin and citrate are the most commonly used anticoagulants, they have well recognized side effects especially bleeding in heparin and metabolic complications in citrate. Though citrate use has revolutionized anticoagulation options, it is still not universally used. Prostacyclin is a useful option in patients with bleeding diathesis but the cost is always an issue.

Thus, to conclude, there exists no perfect anticoagulant in literature, it is very important to have a complete picture in mind including patient's basic disease process, vascular access issues, and blood product usage. Depending upon the local usage and patient population, one needs to choose an anticoagulant, make easy to follow protocols and train its staff who run the shop floor.

## References


1. Kaddourah A, Basu RK, Bagshaw SM, Goldstein SL, for the AWARE Investigators. Epidemiology of acute kidney injury in critically ill children and young adults. N Engl J Med. 2017;376:11–20.
2. Monchi M, Berghmans D, Ledoux D, Canivet JL, Dubois B, Damas P. Citrate vs. heparin for anticoagulation in continuous venovenous hemofiltration: a prospective randomized study. Intensive Care Med. 2004;30(2):260–5. Epub 2003 Nov 5.
3. Kutsogiannis DJ, Gibney RT, Stollery D, Gao J. Regional citrate versus systemic heparin anticoagulation for continuous renal replacement in critically ill patients. Kidney Int. 2005;67(6):2361–7.
4. Betjes MG, van Oosterom D, van Agteren M, van de Wetering J. Regional citrate versus heparin anticoagulation during venovenous hemofiltration in patients at low risk for bleeding: similar hemofilter survival but significantly less bleeding. J Nephrol. 2007;20(5):602–8.
5. Hetzel GR, Schmitz M, Wissing H, Ries W, Schott G, Heering PJ, Isgro F, Kribben A, Himmele R, Grabensee B, Rump LC. See comment in PubMed commons belowRegional citrate versus systemic heparin for anticoagulation in critically ill patients on continuous venovenous haemofiltration: a prospective randomized multicentre trial. Nephrol Dial Transplant. 2011;26(1):232–9.
6. Davies H, Morgan D, Leslie G. A regional citrate anticoagulation protocol for pre-dilutional CVVHDf: the 'modified Alabama protocol'. Aust Crit Care. 2008;21(3):154–65. https://doi.org/10.1016/j.aucc.2008.04.002. Epub 2008 Jul 16.
7. Tobe SW, Aujla P, Walele AA, Oliver MJ, Naimark DM, Perkins NJ, Beardsall M. A novel regional citrate anticoagulation protocol for CRRT using only commercially available solutions. J Crit Care. 2003;18(2):121–9.
8. Tolwani AJ, Prendergast MB, Speer RR, Stofan BS, Wille KM. A practical citrate anticoagulation continuous venovenous hemodiafiltration protocol for metabolic control and high solute clearance. Clin J Am Soc Nephrol. 2006;1(1):79–87. Epub 2005 Nov 23.
9. Bunchman TE, Maxvold NJ, Barnett J, Hutchings A, Benfield MR. Pediatric hemofiltration: normocarb dialysate solution with citrate anticoagulation. Pediatr Nephrol. 2002;17(3):150–4.
10. Chadha V, Garg U, Warady BA, Alon US. Citrate clearance in children receiving continuous venovenous renal replacement therapy. Pediatr Nephrol. 2002;17(10):819–24. Epub 2002 Sep 7.
11. Symons JM, Brophy PD, Gregory MJ, McAfee N, Somers MJ, Bunchman TE, Goldstein SL. Continuous renal replacement therapy in children up to 10 kg. Am J Kidney Dis. 2003;41(5):984–9.

12. Elhanan N, Skippen P, Nuthall G, Krahn G, Seear M. Citrate anticoagulation in pediatric continuous venovenous hemofiltration. Pediatr Nephrol. 2004;19(2):208–12. Epub 2003 Dec 11.
13. Hothi DK, St George-Hyslop C, Geary D, Bohn D, Harvey E. Continuous renal replacement therapy (CRRT) in children using the AQUARIUS. Nephrol Dial Transplant. 2006;21(8):2296–300.
14. Rajasekaran S, Jones DP, Avent Y, Shaffer ML, Elbahlawan L, Henderson N, Barfield RC, Morrison RR, Tamburro RF. Outcomes of hematopoietic stem cell transplant patients who received continuous renal replacement therapy in a pediatric oncology intensive care unit. Pediatr Crit Care Med. 2010;11(6):699–706.
15. Symons JM, Chua AN, Somers MJ, Baum MA, Bunchman TE, Benfield MR, Brophy PD, Blowey D, Fortenberry JD, Chand D, Flores FX, Hackbarth R, Alexander SR, Mahan J, McBryde KD, Goldstein SL. Demographic characteristics of pediatric continuous renal replacement therapy: a report of the prospective pediatric continuous renal replacement therapy registry. Clin J Am Soc Nephrol. 2007;2(4):732–8. Epub 2007 May 18.
16. Brophy PD, Somers MJ, Baum MA, Symons JM, McAfee N, Fortenberry JD, Rogers K, Barnett J, Blowey D, Baker C, Bunchman TE, Goldstein SL. Multi-Centre evaluation of anticoagulation in patients receiving continuous renal replacement therapy (CRRT). Nephrol Dial Transplant. 2005;20(7):1416–21. Epub 2005 Apr 26.
17. Askenazi DJ, Goldstein SL, Koralkar R, Fortenberry J, Baum M, Hackbarth R, Blowey D, Bunchman TE, Brophy PD, Symons J, Chua A, Flores F, Somers MJ. Continuous renal replacement therapy for children ≤10 kg: a report from the prospective pediatric continuous renal replacement therapy registry. J Pediatr. 2013;162(3):587–592.e3. https://doi.org/10.1016/j.jpeds.2012.08.044. Epub 2012 Oct 24.
18. Musielak A, Warzywoda A, Wojtalik M, Kociński B, Kroll P, Ostalska-Nowicka D, Zachwieja J. Outcomes of continuous renal replacement therapy with regional citrate anticoagulation in small children after cardiac surgery: experience and protocol from a single center. Ther Apher Dial. 2016;20(6):639–44.
19. Uchino S, Bellomo R, Morimatsu H, Morgera S, Schetz M, Tan I, Bouman C, Macedo E, Gibney N, Tolwani A, Oudemans-van Straaten H, Ronco C, Kellum JA. Continuous renal replacement therapy: a worldwide practice survey. The beginning and ending supportive therapy for the kidney (B.E.S.T. Kidney) investigators. Intensive Care Med. 2007;33(9):1563–70. Epub 2007 Jun 27.
20. Hirsh J, Warkentin TE, Shaughnessy SG, Anand SS, Halperin JL, Raschke R, Granger C, Ohman EM, Dalen JE. Heparin and low-molecular-weight heparin: mechanisms of action, pharmacokinetics, dosing, monitoring, efficacy, and safety. Chest. 2001;119(1 Suppl):64S–94S.
21. Raymakers-Janssen PAMA, Lilien M, van Kessel IA, Veldhoen ES, Wösten-van Asperen RM, van Gestel JPJ. Citrate versus heparin anticoagulation in continuous renal replacement therapy in small children. Pediatr Nephrol. 2017;32(10):1971–8.
22. Stockton WM, Padilla-Tolentino E, Ragsdale CE. Antithrombin III doses rounded to available vial sizes in critically ill pediatric patients. J Pediatr Pharmacol Ther. 2017;22(1):15–21.
23. Ferreira JA, Johnson DW. The incidence of thrombocytopenia associated with continuous renal replacement therapy in critically ill patients. Ren Fail. 2015;37(7):1232–6.
24. Verma AK, Levine M, Shalansky SJ, Carter CJ, Kelton JG. Frequency of heparin-induced thrombocytopenia in critical care patients. Pharmacotherapy. 2003;23(6):745–53.
25. Selleng S, Selleng K, Wollert HG, Muellejans B, Lietz T, Warkentin TE, Greinacher A. Heparin-induced thrombocytopenia in patients requiring prolonged intensive care unit treatment after cardiopulmonary bypass. J Thromb Haemost. 2008;6(3):428–35.
26. Warkentin TE. Heparin-induced thrombocytopenia: diagnosis and management. Circulation. 2004;110(18):454–8.
27. Weil R. Sodium citrate in transfusion of blood. JAMA. 1915;64:425.
28. Morita Y, Johnson RW, Dorn RE, Hall DS. Regional anticoagulation during hemodialysis using citrate. Am J Med Sci. 1961;242:32–43.

29. Pinnick RV, Wiegmann TB, Diederich DA. Regional citrate anticoagulation for hemodialysis in the patient at high risk for bleeding. N Engl J Med. 1983;308(5):258–61.
30. Golper TA, Ronco C, Kaplan AA. Continuous arteriovenous hemofiltration: improvements, modifications, and future directions. Semin Dialysis. 1988;1:50–4.
31. von Brecht JH, Flanigan MJ, Freeman RM, Lim VS. Regional anticoagulation: hemodialysis with hypertonic trisodium citrate. Am J Kidney Dis. 1986;8(3):196–201.
32. Mehta RL, McDonald BR, Aguilar MM, Ward DM. Regional citrate anticoagulation for continuous arteriovenous hemodialysis in critically ill patients. Kidney Int. 1990;38(5):976–81.
33. Tolwani AJ, Campbell RC, Schenk MB, Allon M, Warnock DG. Simplified citrate anticoagulation for continuous renal replacement therapy. Kidney Int. 2001;60(1):370–4.
34. Rodriguez K, Srivaths PR, Tal L, Watson MN, Riley AA, Himes RW, Desai MS, Braun MC, Akcan Arikan A. Regional citrate anticoagulation for continuous renal replacement therapy in pediatric patients with liver failure. PLoS One. 2017;12(8):e0182134. Published online 2017 Aug 8. https://doi.org/10.1371/journal.pone.0182134.
35. Soltysiak J, Warzywoda A, Kociński B, Ostalska-Nowicka D, Benedyk A, Silska-Dittmar M, Zachwieja J. Citrate anticoagulation for continuous renal replacement therapy in small children. Pediatr Nephrol. 2014;29(3):469–75.
36. Fernández SN, Santiago MJ, López-Herce J, García M, Del Castillo J, Alcaraz AJ, Bellón JM. Citrate anticoagulation for CRRT in children: comparison with heparin. Biomed Res Int. 2014;2014:786301.
37. Schilder L, Nurmohamed SA, Bosch FH, Purmer IM, den Boer SS, Kleppe CG, Vervloet MG, Beishuizen A, Girbes AR, Ter Wee PM, Groeneveld AB, CASH study group. Citrate anticoagulation versus systemic heparinisation in continuous venovenous hemofiltration in critically ill patients with acute kidney injury: a multi-center randomized clinical trial. Crit Care. 2014;18(4):472.
38. Brain MJ, Roodenburg OS, Adams N, McCracken P, Hockings L, Musgrave S, Butt W, Scheinkestel C. Randomised trial of software algorithm driven regional citrate anticoagulation versus heparin in continuous renal replacement therapy: the filter life in renal replacement therapy pilot trial. Crit Care Resusc. 2014;16(2):131–7.
39. Stucker F, Ponte B, Tataw J, Martin PY, Wozniak H, Pugin J, Saudan P. Efficacy and safety of citrate-based anticoagulation compared to heparin in patients with acute kidney injury requiring continuous renal replacement therapy: a randomized controlled trial. Crit Care. 2015;19:91.
40. Bai M, Zhou M, He L, Ma F, Li Y, Yu Y, Wang P, Li L, Jing R, Zhao L, Sun S. Citrate versus heparin anticoagulation for continuous renal replacement therapy: an updated meta-analysis of RCTs. Intensive Care Med. 2015;41(12):2098–110.
41. Cawello W, Schweer H, Müller R, Bonn R, Seyberth HW. Metabolism and pharmacokinetics of prostaglandin E1 administered by intravenous infusion in human subjects. Eur J Clin Pharmacol. 1994;46(3):275–7.
42. Kozek-Langenecker SA, Spiss CK, Michalek-Sauberer A, Felfernig M, Zimpfer M. Effect of prostacyclin on platelets, polymorphonuclear cells, and heterotypic cell aggregation during hemofiltration. Crit Care Med. 2003;31:864–8.
43. Shuman MA, Levine SP. Relationship between secretion of platelet factor 4 and thrombin generation during in vitro blood clotting. J Clin Invest. 1980;65(2):307–13.
44. Turney JH, Williams LC, Fewell MR, Parsons V, Weston MJ. Use of prostacyclin in regular dialysis therapy. Proc EDTA. 1980;17:318–22.
45. Davenport A, Will EJ, Davison AM. Comparison of the use of standard heparin and prostacyclin anticoagulation in spontaneous and pump-driven extracorporeal circuits in patients with combined acute renal and hepatic failure. Nephron. 1994;66(4):431–7.
46. Max M, Rossaint R. Inhaled prostacyclin in the treatment of pulmonary hypertension. Eur J Pediatr. 1999;158(Suppl 1):S23–6.
47. McIntyre CM, Hanna BD, Rintoul N, Ramsey EZ. Safety of epoprostenol and treprostinil in children less than 12 months of age. Pulm Circ. 2013;3(4):862–9.

48. Habib M, Roberts LN, Patel RK, Wendon J, Bernal W, Arya R. Evidence of rebalanced coagulation in acute liver injury and acute liver failure as measured by thrombin generation. Liver Int. 2014;34(5):672–8.
49. Zobel G, Ring E, Müller W. Continuous arteriovenous hemofiltration in premature infants. Crit Care Med. 1989;17(6):534–6.
50. Goonasekera CD Wang J, Bunchman TE, Deep A. Factors affecting circuit life during continuous renal replacement therapy in children with liver failure. Ther Apher Dial. 2015;19(1):16–22. https://doi.org/10.1111/1744-9987.12224. PMID: 25195689.
51. Zobel G, Trop M, Muntean W, Ring E, Gleispach H. Anticoagulation for continuous arteriovenous hemofiltration in children. Blood Purif. 1988;6(2):90–5.
52. Langenecker SA, Felfernig M, Werba A, Mueller CM, Chiari A, Zimpfer M. Anticoagulation with prostacyclin and heparin during continuous venovenous hemofiltration. Crit Care Med. 1994;22(11):1774–81.
53. Gainza F, Quintanilla N, Pijoan JI, Delgado S, Urbizu JM, Lampreabe I. Role of prostacyclin (epoprostenol) as anticoagulant in continuous renal replacement therapies: efficacy, security and cost analysis. J Nephrol. 2006;19(5):648–55. PMID: 17136695.
54. Fabbri LP, Nucera M, Al Malyan M, Becchi C. Regional anticoagulation and anti-aggregation for CVVH in critically ill patients: a prospective, randomized, controlled pilot study. Acta Anaesthesiol Scand. 2010;54(1):92–7.
55. Balik M, Waldauf P, Plásil P, Pachl J. Prostacyclin versus citrate in continuous haemodiafiltration: an observational study in patients with high risk of bleeding. Blood Purif. 2005;23(4):325–9. Epub 2005 Aug 23. PMID:16118487.
56. Herrera-Gutiérrez ME, Seller-Pérez G, Lebrón-Gallardo M, De La Cruz-Cortés JP, González-Correa JA. Use of isolated epoprostenol or associated to heparin for the maintenance of the patency of the continuous renal replacement technical circuits. Med Intensiva. 2006;30(7):314–21. Spanish. PMID: 17067504.
57. Fiaccadori E, Maggiore U, Parenti E, Giacosa R, Picetti E, Rotelli C, Tagliavini D, Cabassi A. Sustained low-efficiency dialysis (SLED) with prostacyclin in critically ill patients with acute renal failure. Nephrol Dial Transplant. 2007;22:529–37.
58. Schultheiß C, Saugel B, Phillip V, Thies P, Noe S, Mayr U, Haller B, Einwächter H, Schmid RM, Huber W. Continuous venovenous hemodialysis with regional citrate anticoagulation in patients with liver failure: a prospective observational study. Crit Care. 2012;16(4):1–10.
59. Kozek-Langenecker SA, Kettner SC, Oismueller C, Gonano C, Speiser W, Zimpfer M. Anticoagulation with prostaglandin E1 and unfractionated heparin during continuous venovenous hemofiltration. Crit Care Med. 1998;26:1208–12.
60. http://www.pcrrt.com/ProtocolsAccess.html.

# Haemodialysis

# 18

Evgenia Preka and Rukshana Shroff

## 18.1 Introduction

Paediatric intensive care units (PICU) have to deal with fluid, electrolyte and pH homeostasis abnormalities in critically ill children with acute kidney injury (AKI) and/or end-stage kidney disease (ESKD). The application of the paediatric RIFLE criteria (pRIFLE) have confirmed that AKI is an independent risk factor for death in PICU patients [1]. AKI in the severely ill child has been significantly associated with longer hospital stay, increased morbidity and mortality after application of the pRIFLE, AKIN (Acute Kidney Injury Network) or KDIGO (Kidney Disease: Improving Global Outcomes) definitions [2].

In PICU, the available modalities of acute renal replacement therapy (RRT) include intermittent haemodialysis (iHD), peritoneal dialysis (PD) and continuous renal replacement therapies (CRRT). CRRT is the most widely used modality of RRT in PICU due to its better haemodynamic stability and control of uremic solute clearances. In younger children weighing less than 8–10 kg, PD was historically used and still remains the treatment of choice in most of the neonatal and paediatric units. However, advances in technology and the availability of new dialysis machines that allow exquisite control of ultrafiltration (UF) volume have allowed intermittent haemodialysis, haemodiafiltration (iHDF) or their combination to be safely applied in critically ill children. Most of the times intermittent HD is performed in the PICU when plasmapheresis or plasma exchange has to be performed simultaneously. Small randomized clinical trials and subsequent meta-analyses comparing iHD and CRRT have shown no difference in patient survival [3]. However, the final decision about dialysis modality should be based on local expertise, available resources and the child's clinical status [4].

E. Preka · R. Shroff (✉)
Great Ormond Street Hospital, London, UK
e-mail: Rukshana.Shroff@gosh.nhs.uk



A. Deep, S. L. Goldstein (eds.), *Critical Care Nephrology and Renal Replacement Therapy in Children*, https://doi.org/10.1007/978-3-319-90281-4_18

In this chapter, we discuss the principles and practice of haemodialysis, writing a standard HD prescription, common complications and the management of HD in special situations.

## 18.2 Principles of Haemodialysis

The purpose of haemodialysis is to mimic the role of the kidney, removing waste products and prescribed quantities of solutes and fluids that have accumulated between dialysis sessions. The three main principles used in haemodialysis are diffusion, convection and ultrafiltration. All of the above use a semipermeable membrane, which allows the passage of water and small-to-medium molecular weight molecules (by diffusion and convection), inhibits the movement of large molecules and allows the water removal by ultrafiltration depending on the process.

A schematic review of the three principles and their details are shown in Fig. 18.1. In conventional dialysis, the use of high-flux membranes has been associated with a better survival especially in high risk adult patients [5] and should be preferred even in children [6].

**Haemodialysis** provides diffusive small-solute transport that involves the movement of molecules from an area of high concentration to an area of low concentration across a semipermeable membrane. Diffusion principally depends on the dialysis fluid flow and the dialyzer surface area (which determines the mass transfer area coefficient ($K_oA$) and consequently, the solute permeability of the membrane) (Table 18.1).

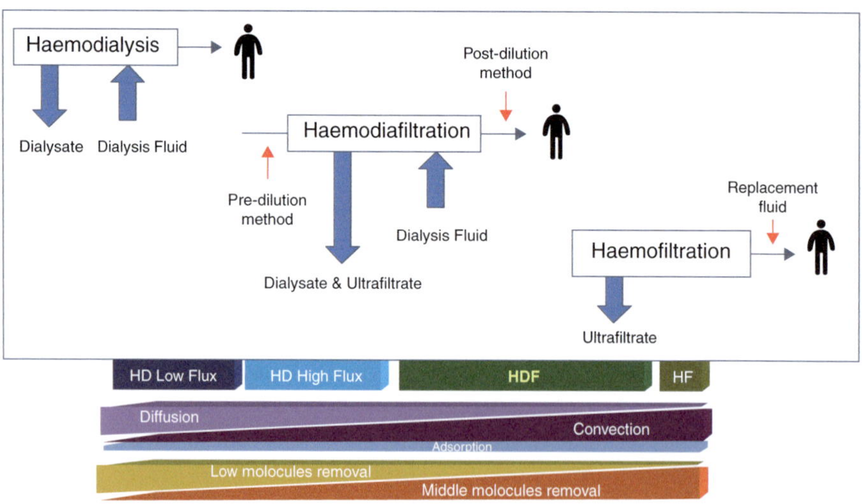


**Fig. 18.1** Conventional haemodialysis and haemodiafiltration types and the different adsorption principles used

**Table 18.1** Dialytic solute removal depending on each dialysis modality

| Dialytic solute removal | Haemodialysis | Haemofiltration | Haemodiafiltration |
|---|---|---|---|
| Type of process involved | Diffusion | Convection | Diffusion and convection |
| Description of the process | Movement down a concentration gradient | Passive movement of solute through the semipermeable membrane influenced by the osmotic/pressure gradient | Dialysis derived both by the concentration gradient across the membrane and the osmotic/pressure gradient. |
| Highly effective clearance for | Small molecules (e.g. urea, creatinine) | Fluid removal medium-sized molecules (<60KDa) (e.g. b2-microglobulin, vitamin B12, kappa light chains, sepsis mediators*) and large-sized proteins (e.g. Albumin) | Small and medium-sized molecules and ultrafiltration |
| Determinants of the process | 1. Characteristics of the solute (size, charge, protein binding)<br>2. Dialysis membrane (type, porosity, thickness, surface area)<br>3. Rate of the delivery (blood flow rate, dialysate rate)<br>4. Dialysate's temperature | 1. Ultrafiltration rate<br>2. Dialyzer<br>3. Porosity of the membrane | 1. Solute molecular size<br>2. Protein-binding molecules<br>3. Filter porosity |
| Formulas calculating clearance | $K_{HD} = Q_B \times (c_i\text{-}c_0)/c_i$ | $K_{HF} = Q_{UF} \times S$/post-dilution<br>$K_{HF} = Q_B \times Q_{UF} \times S$/pre-dilution | $K_{HDF} = K_{HD} \times S/Q_B) + K_{HF}$ |

Mediators in sepsis (IL-8, TNF, IL-10, IL-6, complement, eicosanoids, platelet activating factor, myocardial depressants)
$K_{HD}$ = Haemodialysis clearance, $K_{HF}$ = Haemofiltration clearance, $Q_{UF}$ = Ultrafiltration flow $C_{UF}$ = Ultrafiltrate solute concentration, $S$ = Sieving coefficient [$S = 2\ C_{UF}/(c_1 + c_0)$], $C_i$ = in solute concentration, $C_o$ = out solute concentration

**Haemofiltration** provides convective transport of small and medium-sized molecules that can be similarly quantified by the filtrate saturation of the urea. In haemofiltration, the ultrafiltration flow is mainly dependent on the transmembrane pressure gradient (TMP) applied to the hydraulic permeability of the membranes. In practice, membranes with a sieving curve similar to that of the glomerular basement membrane even allows the removal of large-sized molecules, but prevent the passage of albumin (molecular weight 68KDa) [7]. In haemofiltration, clearance is determined by the site of fluid replacement, which can be infused either into the arterial blood line leading to the haemofilter (pre-dilution) or into the venous blood line leaving the haemofilter (post-dilution) (Fig. 18.1). To optimize clearance, post-dilution HF is more often used, as with pre-dilution the filtrate is generated from blood diluted with replacement fluid and therefore contains a lower concentration of uremic toxins. Using this technique, small-solute clearance is reduced by 15% at low ultrafiltration rate (UFR), while this figure increases to 40% with a higher UFR [8]. However, UFR should not exceed 30% of the plasma water flow rate (filtration fraction less than 0.30) so as to prevent haemofilter haemoconcentration and therefore filter clotting. In children where usually we have low blood flows, or in all patients with high haematocrit and/or elevated plasma protein (conditions that limit the filtration capacity), pre-dilution has been proven to be of significant clinical benefit, with considerably less risk of membrane clotting [7].

**Haemodiafiltration** optimizes the removal of middle (up to 300-500KDa molecular weight [MW]) and larger molecules (>15–60 kDa MW), by combining the two principles of diffusion and convection. However, if the clearance of low molecular weight solutes such as urea have reached maximal clearance by HD, then the addition of HDF will not improve clearance further (Table 18.1). With HDF there is no osmotic disequilibrium while arriving at a maximum of the urea clearance as the continuous iso-osmotic HF substitution fluid inflow allows keeping an osmotic stability throughout the whole dialysis session. The effectiveness of a membrane to ultrafiltrate fluid is described by the UF coefficient ($K_{UF}$), which is $Q_{UF}$/deltaP (volume of UF per unit time, divided by the pressure gradient across the membrane; TMP). Filtration fraction (FF) is the fraction of plasma that is removed from the blood during haemofiltration, and the relationship between TMP and oncotic pressure determines the FF. In HDF, a high sieving coefficient is required for middle molecule removal.

## 18.3 Advantages of Haemodiafiltration (HDF) over Conventional Haemodialysis (HD) in the Paediatric Population [7]

1. Increased clearance of middle-molecules, e.g. β2-microglobulin.
2. Increased clearance of plasma phosphate compared with HD.
3. Reduced resistance to erythropoietin possibly related to reduced inflammation and removal of erythropoiesis-inhibiting factors.
4. Improved haemodynamic stability, leading to less intra-dialytic hypotension and faster recovery time after dialysis.
5. Decreased inflammation related to better biocompatibility and the use of ultrapure dialysate.
6. Improved growth, possible anabolic effect of HDF.
7. Overall, improved survival and reduced cardiovascular complications, when higher convection volumes (>17.4 L and 20 L) are used.

## 18.4 Choice of the Vascular Access

Independent of the acute renal replacement therapy HD choice, a reliable vascular catheter is essential as it determines the quality of dialysis. The type and size of catheter, the catheter site, and the technique for insertion need to be considered in order to choose the right catheter for each patient. In the acute setting, an uncuffed non-tunnelled (temporary) double lumen catheter in the internal jugular, subclavian or femoral vein is the preferred access type. Femoral catheters, although easiest to insert, should be used only for "rescue and transient" access if intensive care is needed: they carry a higher risk of infection and thrombosis [6]. Although subclavian catheters are associated with less infectious complications [9], they are clearly associated with more procedural complications and post-operative stenosis [10] which consequently doesn't allow an adequate dialysis. A study of 100 patients dialysed either by a subclavian or internal jugular catheter (50 in each group) showed that 42% of the subclavian group had a stenosis of the subclavian/brachiocephalic vein, compared to 10% of the internal jugular group [11]. In order to increase the success rate of insertion while decreasing the mechanical complications rate the ultrasound-guided technique should be applied. If the clinician feels that the catheter might be needed for more than 10–14 days, a tunnelled catheter should be considered. Left-sided internal jugular and subclavian catheters provide flows that are more erratic and up to 100 mL/min lower than elsewhere, because their tips abut the vein walls. As a consequence, right-sided internal jugular catheters are the gold standard of practice as they can provide the best blood flow rates necessary for a sufficient solute clearance with the less complications.

In order to achieve satisfactory blood speeds, the larger the gauge of the access, the better, but the size of the catheter must depend on the size of the child and their vessel (Table 18.2). The rate of blood flow is proportional to the fourth power of the radius of the catheter. Most lines are dual lumen, allowing a continuous flow of blood around the circuit. However, HD can also be achieved using single lumen access. In very small children single lumen access may be more appropriate as the

**Table 18.2** An example of catheter sizes commonly used based on the weight of the child

| Non-tunnelled haemodialysis central venous catheter (temporary CVC) | | | | |
|---|---|---|---|---|
| Approx child weight | Type[a] | A | V | Vessel |
| < 5 kg | 6.5 FG 10 cm | 0.75 | 0.78 | IJV and femoral |
| 10–20 kg | 8.0 FG 10 cm | 0.8 | 0.82 | IJV |
| 10–20 kg | 8.0 FG 12.5 cm | 0.84 | 0.86 | Femoral |
| 20–30 kg | 11 FG 12.5 cm | 0.96 | 1.02 | IJV and femoral |
| >30 kg | 11 FG 15 cm | 1.04 | 1.10 | IJV and femoral |

*A* arterial lumen
*V* venous lumen
*IJV* internal jugular vein
[a]All of these catheters are examples of catheter size (lumen) and length from the tip to the internal cuff and based on Gambro products. Several other makes and sizes of catheters are available

lumen of the catheter will be larger and therefore the flow that can be obtained through it is relatively greater. In order to obtain two directional blood flows with a single lumen line, the dialysis circuit has to be modified. This can be achieved by the double-pump method, using two blood pumps which pump alternately, or by using a single pump which pumps intermittently, using gravity to let blood flow back in to the child. Disadvantages of the single lumen catheter are that an expansion chamber is necessary in the circuit to allow for the pressure changes and this increases the volume of the blood circuit; also blood flow rates are compromised by a greater degree of recirculation.

The Centers for Disease Control and Prevention recommend that temporary catheters in the ICU setting should be changed when it is clinically indicated rather than routinely because the risks of the catheterization outweigh the supposed benefit of reduced infection risk [12]. KDOQI recommend that subclavian and internal jugular catheters should be changed after 3 weeks and femoral after 5 days in the non-ICU setting due to the increased risk of infections [13].

Other types of vascular access include arterio-venous fistulae or arterio-venous grafts, but these are seldom used in the ICU setting, unless a child with pre-existing ESKD who already has this access needs ICU treatment. It may need the involvement of the nephrology specialist's nursing team during the venipuncture procedure [14].

## 18.5 Choice of the Dialyzer

The haemodialyzer is composed of two compartments, one for blood and one for dialysate, which are separated by the semipermeable membrane. A capillary (hollow fibre) configuration achieves the maximal membrane surface area over which blood and dialysate make contact in a relatively low fill volume with low compliance. The membrane can be composed of modified cellulose or a synthetic material. Unmodified cellulose membranes (e.g. cuprophan) are the least biocompatible, and may cause activation of complement and leucocytes and a severe allergic reaction within minutes of starting dialysis. Synthetic membranes (e.g. Polysulfone, polycarbonate, polyamide or polyacryl-polyamide acrylate) are relatively more biocompatible, but can rarely cause hypotension, inflammatory hyperaemia, oedema, and pain (bradykinin-mediated reaction). Synthetic membranes have high adsorption properties, and are therefore the haemofilter of choice for albumin dialysis or acute toxicities where the undesired plasma toxin is highly protein bound.

Dialyzers are described based on their solute transport properties expressed as the mass transfer-area coefficient (KoA) and ultrafiltration coefficient (KUf). Dialyzers of usual efficiency (for removal of small solutes) have a KoA of 300–500; high-efficiency dialyzers may have a KoA of more than 700. Precise clearance values for creatinine, urea, vitamin $B_{12}$ and phosphate are given for all dialyzers in the manufacturer's specification sheet. Clearance of a solute is inversely proportional to the molecular size; most dialyzers allow the passage of solutes of up to 5–10,000 Daltons. The ultrafiltration coefficient (KUf) describes its ability to remove water. For example, a KUf of 2.0 means that 2 mL/h of UF will occur for each mmHg of TMP at a blood flow rate of 200 mL/min. KUf depends on the surface area of the dialyzer as well as its membrane characteristics. Dialyzers with KUfs of less than 10 are referred to a low-flux and those with a rate of 15–60 mL/h/mmHg are called high-flux. Synthetic membranes tend to be high-flux.

Dialyzers may be sterilized with irradiation, steam or ethylene oxide. Steam sterilization or gamma irradiation reduces the allergic reactions (compared to ethylene oxide). Priming the circuit with one to two litres of saline to expel air and prepare the capillaries for use will also help flush out remaining ethylene oxide and other soluble compounds in the circuit, which may be toxic or cause allergic reactions at the commencement of dialysis.

The choice of the haemodialyzer for any patient must take into consideration the membrane characteristics and size. Synthetic high-flux membranes are generally preferred. The surface area of the dialyzer must equal, but not exceed, the surface area of the child.

## 18.6 Choice of the Dialysate

Dialysate is prepared during the dialysis session. Sodium, potassium, magnesium, calcium, chloride, dextrose and bicarbonate are added to the purified water by the machine and their concentrations can be varied within prescribed limits, and adjusted depending on the patient's needs They are mixed and proportionated by the dialysis machine. Standard settings are 138-140 mmol/L for sodium, 2 mmol/L for potassium, 1.25–1.75 mmol/L for calcium, 0.5-1 mmol/L for magnesium and 1 g/L for glucose. The dialysis machine monitors the electrical conductivity of the dialysis solution to ensure the correct proportion of water to concentrate is occurring before it is delivered to the haemodialyzer.

**(a) Sodium:** Isonatric dialysis should be targeted whenever UF is not needed. When hyponatric dialysis is done, there is an osmotic fluid shift from the extracellular to the intracellular compartment, contributing to dialysis disequilibrium disorder and intradialytic hypotension while hypernatric dialysis may cause interstitial oedema, increased intradialytic thirst and weight gain, as well as worsening hypertension.

A recent meta-analysis showed that Na profiling (step, linear or exponential) might be useful [15] in which the dialysate Na concentration is changed during the dialysis section to meet the individual's needs. Na profiling has been shown to increase stability of intradialytic cramps and interdialytic fatigue in children and adults [16, 17]. Step profiles are most effective at attenuating postdialytic hypotension and early intradialytic hypotension, whereas linear profiles best reduce cramps and late intradialytic hypotension [18] Na profile is also indicated in the prevention of dialysis disequilibrium syndrome.

**(b) Potassium:** Adjustments are done based on the pre-dialysis K levels. Remember that the rate of K removal is highest at the start of dialysis when the diffusion gradient is high.

- Typically: 1–2 mmol/L
- Severe hyperkalaemia: 0-1 mmol/L
- Normokalaemia: 3–4 mmol/L

Of note, using 0 or 1 mmol potassium tanks can induce rapid clearance of K+ by diffusion and precipitate arrhythmias.

**(c) Bicarbonate:** Bicarbonate is used as a buffer. The bicarbonate preparation has a separate acidic component to prevent precipitation of calcium and magnesium carbonate and is added by a second proportionating pump. Inevitably with time there will be deposition of calcium and magnesium salts, so the dialysate system needs daily decalcification.

In general, plasma bicarbonate levels rise by 4–5 mmol/L and then fall to pre-dialysis levels by 48 h [19]. The adjusted survival of HD patients decreases with pre-dialysis acidosis (<18 mmol/L) and with post-dialysis alkalosis (>24 mmol/L) [19, 20] suggesting a U-shaped correlation with mortality. The severity of metabolic acidosis/alkalosis in HD patients also correlates with a higher risk of fractures [21]. Special consideration should be given to possible sudden drops in plasma potassium and calcium due to the transient alkalosis that might lead to intradialytic vascular and cardiac instability.

**(d) Calcium:** typically used at a concentration of 1.25 mmol/L, allows higher doses of vitamin D and calcium-based phosphate binders. Remember that in case the patient develops hypocalcaemia, this might worsen the hyperparathyroidism, apart from decreasing myocardial contractility, reduced vascular reactivity and thus increase the risk of intradialytic hypotension.

**(e) Phosphate:** mainly intracellular anion which decreases at the start of dialysis but increases post-dialysis with a rebound effect for up to 4 h. Phosphate purification gets improved with higher bicarbonate baths and by quotidian dialysis.

**(f) Magnesium:** typically 0.5–1 mmol/L. Low magnesium levels can result in cramps and arrhythmias. Higher magnesium baths help improve cardiovascular stability and intradialytic symptoms.

**(g) Glucose:** normally 100–200 mg/dL (6–11 mmol/L). Caution with higher glucose concentration in baths, as hypertriglyceridemia and less effective K purification can happen.

**Dialysate temperature:** the dialysate is warmed to 35.5–37.5° C depending on the patient's pre-dialysis temperature, in order to compensate for losses of heat in the extracorporeal circuit and to keep the physiologic normal values. Lower temperatures are associated with less hypotensive events, but diffusion is increased at higher temperatures. Standard dialysate flow is 500mL/min (range 300–800 mL/min).

**Table 18.3** European Pharmacopoeia definitions for the upper limit of water quality

| | Bacterial growth (cfu/mL) | Endotoxin (EU/mL) | Cytokine induction |
|---|---|---|---|
| Mains water | 200 | 5 | + |
| Regular water | 100 | 0.25 | + |
| Ultrapure | 0.01 | 0.03 | – |
| Sterile | $10^{-6}$ | 0.03 | – |

*CFU* colony forming units
*EU* Endotoxin units

## 18.7 Dialysate Quality

Even though national quality standards may be slightly different among different countries, it is imperative that disinfection practices and regular surveillance are applied so as to ensure a secure dialysis session [22]. Dialysate quality has been shown to have a positive impact on inflammation, oxidative stress biomarkers, as well as on oxidative parameters [23]. Water quality is defined as "pure" or "ultrapure". Pure water is adequate for conventional dialysis, but ultrapure water is preferable, and is essential for high-flux dialyzers (when backfiltration can occur) and particularly in HDF, when large volumes of replacement fluids are used. Even very low levels of endotoxin in the water can cause cytokine-mediated inflammation. The degree of cytokine stimulation is related to the concentration of endotoxin and other "cytokine-induced substances" in the dialysate compartment and to the permeability of the dialysis membranes to these substances. The superiority of ultrapure dialysate has been shown when using highly permeable membranes as inflammatory markers as CRP and IL-6 have been shown to be decreased when comparing contaminated dialysate samples [24].

The European Pharmacopoeia definitions for the upper limit of water quality are described in Table 18.3.

## 18.8 Choice of the Anticoagulation

The risk of circuit clotting with consequent blood loss and reduced dialysis efficacy clearly indicates the need for a systemic anticoagulation in HD patients. In paediatrics, unfractionated heparin (UFH) is primarily used, with some units preferring low-molecular-weight heparin (LMWH) (Table 18.4). In patients with bleeding risk, citrate is gaining popularity but can be more technically demanding to use [25]. Comparing the safety and efficacy of LMWH with UFH, different meta-analysis have revealed that LMWH seem to be as safe as UFH in terms of bleeding complications and as effective as UFH in preventing extracorporeal circuit thrombosis [26, 27]. However, based on the fact that LMWH has unpredictable kinetics in ESRD patients and prolonged T ½ without any antidote, we cannot advise routine use of LMWH in children until an evidence of an anticoagulation advantage over UFH.

**Table 18.4** Anticoagulation choices in HD patients

| | Dose schedule | Control | Tips |
|---|---|---|---|
| Unfractionated heparin (UFH) | Bolus dose:<br>15–20 units/kg<br>Continuous infusion:<br>20–30 units/kg/h | APTT, ACT<br>PLT periodically (heparin-toxicity) | • Level of anticoagulation can vary depending on the risk of bleeding versus risk of clotting<br>• Risk of clotting is inversely related to the dialysis blood flow rate and is higher in less biocompatible dialyzers (e.g. Cuprophane)<br>• A 50% above baseline ACT is proposed to achieve adequate anticoagulation. |
| Low-molecular-weight-heparin (LMWH) | Charge dose:<br>0.5-1 mg/kg<br>During HD: May need to repeat the dose in the middle if duration of HD >4 h | Anti-Xa levels | • LMWH is principally by the kidney → in ESRD kinetics are unpredictable (prolonged T ½)<br>• LMWH has negative charge → impermeable across dialysis membranes (insignificant clearance by HD/HDF)<br>• Disadvantage: Lack of antidote<br>• Advantage of a single bolus dose at the start of dialysis |

*APTT* activated partial thromboplastin time; *ACT* activated clotting time

Further details on anticoagulation in dialysis circuits are provided in Chap. 17, though in patients with continuous RRT.

## 18.9 Writing a Standard HD or HDF Prescription

A stepwise approach and key points to keep in mind when writing a dialysis prescription are:

1. *The extracorporeal blood volume (ECV) is 8–10% of the total blood volume (TBV).* The lines and the haemodialyzer are selected on the basis that the child can tolerate 8–10% of their total blood volume (TBV, 80 mL/kg estimated dry weight) in the extracorporeal circuit. For example, a child weighing 10 kg has a TBV of 800mL (10 × 80 mL), therefore the extracorporeal circuit can be 64–80mL. The total volume of the lines and haemodialyzer therefore must not exceed 64–80mL. There are lines that are made in a variety of sizes by different companies. Some examples are shown in Table 18.5.
2. *Total circuit volume (TCV) = priming volume of the lines + dialyzer. The TCV should never exceed the ECV calculated above.*
   Lines are primed with saline. However, in the very young, even the smallest circuit may exceed the safe extracorporeal volume. In this situation, the circuit must be primed with blood. The blood is not washed back into the child at the completion of dialysis to prevent haemoconcentration. Obviously this is not ideal

**Table 18.5** Volumes of lines available for dialysis according to the size of the patient

| | Venous (mL) | Arterial (mL) | Total (mL) |
|---|---|---|---|
| Mini-neonatal (<6 kg) | 21 | 8 | 29 |
| Neonatal (6–12 kg) | 22 | 18 | 40 |
| Paediatric | 42 | 30 | 72 |
| Adult | 70 | 62 | 132 |

**Table 18.6** Useful formulas for an HD/HF/HDF prescription

| | |
|---|---|
| Total blood volume (TBV) | BW × 80mL |
| Extracorporeal volume (ECV) | 8–10% of the TBV [(BW × 80 × 8)/100–(BW × 80 × 8)/100] |
| Heparin (UFH) | 0–30 units/kg/h depending on clotting. Start at 10 units/kg/h |
| Low molecular weight heparin (e.g. Dalteparin) | 50 units/kg as a single dose pre-dialysis |
| Mannitol | 0.5–1 g/kg infused into the venous bubble trap, during HD only, over 1–2 h (helps especially in the prevention) |
| Dialysate sodium | Within 4 mmols of serum Na levels |
| Blood transfusion | Body weight × 3 × number of grams required to raise Hb |
| Fluid loss | 10 mL/kg/h or 1–2% of the BW/h; maximum of 5% of body weight |

*BW* Body weight
*TBC* total body volume
*ECV* extracorporeal volume
*UFH* unfractioned heparin

because the repeated prescription of blood increases the risks of HLA sensitisation, with its consequent difficulties for transplantation.

3. *The surface area of the dialyzer should be less or equal to child's surface area, especially if it is the first session.*
4. *Blood flow rate*
   The speed at which the blood is pumped out of the child and around the circuit is calculated as the equivalent of their extracorporeal volume total, i.e. up to body wt (kg) × 8 mL/min. Thus, the 10 kg child, with an extracorporeal circuit of 64–80 mL, can have blood speeds of up to 80 mL/min. The blood pump flow rate is a very important determinant of solute clearance, allowing maximum diffusion and convection.

Some useful formulae are given in Table 18.6 and an example of an HD/HDF prescription sheet is presented in Fig. 18.2.

### 18.9.1 Special Circumstances to Consider Are

1. In the 1st session: the blood flow rate should be no more than 3 mL/kg (or 90 mL/BSA) in order to avoid disequilibrium syndrome. The duration should be short (no more than 3 h)
2. If Urea >40 mmol/L pre-dialysis, consider use of mannitol; limit time to 1–2 h, consider low blood flow rate, down-size dialyzer surface area; decrease dialysate flow.

Name:
Hospital Number:
Date of Birth:

**HDx Single Needle Treatment Chart**

Date

| | | | | | | | |
|---|---|---|---|---|---|---|---|
| Weight Pre Dialysis: | | Pre BP: | | HD/SN: | | Plan of Care: | Machine No: |
| Weight Last dialysis/aim: | | Pre HR: | | Vol/Press Control: | | | Bed No: Saline ☐ |
| Weight Gain: | | Temp: | | Pre/Post Dilution: | | | Dialyser size: |
| Infusions: | | Bloods Taken: | | Sys Press setting: | | | Heparin: iu/hr \| Stop limit: |
| Drinks: | | | | Dialysate Flow: | | | O2 & Suction check ☐ |
| Extra Fluid Loss: | | | | Sodium: | | | ID Band on patient ☐ or PPID used<br>Check Prescription ☐ |
| Washback: | | | | Bicarb: | | Machine Double Checked ☐ | Signature: |
| Total Planned UF: | | | | Select Bag: | | | Print Name: |

| Model | Time | BP | HR | Art Flow | Mean BFR | Low Pv | High Pv | V Time | A Time | SV | TMP | UFR | UF Vol | Lines | Comments | Initial |
|---|---|---|---|---|---|---|---|---|---|---|---|---|---|---|---|---|
| | | | | | | | | | | | | | | | | |
| | | | | | | | | | | | | | | | | |
| | | | | | | | | | | | | | | | | |
| | | | | | | | | | | | | | | | | |
| | | | | | | | | | | | | | | | | |
| | | | | | | | | | | | | | | | | |
| | | | | | | | | | | | | | | | | |

Evaluation:

| | | | | |
|---|---|---|---|---|
| Post Weight: | | | | |
| Post BP: | | | | |
| Weight Gain: | | | | |
| UF (Pre-Post): | | | | |
| Final BVS (%): | | | | |
| Litres Processed: | | | | |
| Vol Infused: | | | | |
| Time Dialysed: | | Total heparin infused recorded? ☐ Risk Assessment completed? ☐ Recorded Weight on chart? ☐ CVAD chart completed? ☐ | | |
| Dressing: | | Date: | Signature: | Print & Designation: |

**Fig. 18.2** Example of an HD/HDF prescription sheet

### 18.9.2 Estimation of the Optimal Weight

Optimal (or 'dry') weight is the post-dialysis weight at which the patient is euvolaemic, and below which the patient will become hypotensive. It needs regular assessment, especially in a growing child and there is no single optimal method of assessment. The common techniques for the estimation of the dry weight are:

- **Clinical assessment**: orthostatic vital signs, jugular venous distention (the most accurate marker, especially in children where heart failure is absent) [28].
- **Biochemical markers**: Atrial natriuretic peptide (ANP) correlates with increased plasma volume in renal failure, but can remain elevated in volume-contracted status [29]. Cyclic GMP has no specificity in patients with cardiac/valvular dysfunction. Brain natriuretic peptide (BNP) is usually elevated in patients with overload and is superior to ANP in predicting left ventricular hypertrophy and dysfunction [30].
- **Inferior Vena Cava Diameter (IVCD):** An accurate non-invasive tool of dry weight estimation, guided by ultrasound. An IVCD between 8.0 and 11.5 mm/m$^2$ and a collapse index between 40 and 75% is considered as normovolaemia. It cannot be used as a stand-alone measure, and needs to be correlated with clinical judgement [6].
- **Bioelectric Impedance Study (BIS)**: Measures ECFV and ICFV, and thus estimates fluid shifts from various compartments; strongly correlates with ultrafiltration volume in HD, with biomarkers like N-terminal pro-brain natriuretic peptide (NT-proBNP) and CV measures like left ventricular end-diastolic diameter (LVEDd) which have been shown to predict all cause mortality in chronic HD [31].
- **Non-invasive Blood Volume Monitors**: 'Crash" Hct is the level of Hct at which the patient has lost more than 10% of his blood volume in 3 h time. It's easy to use and is validated in children [28] but it has to be used as a real-time monitoring in order to avoid hypovolaemia during HD, rather than a pre-session estimation of dry weight.

### 18.9.3 Special Considerations

#### 18.9.3.1 Intradialytic Nutrition

In patients with intradialytic hypotension, the intradialytic nutrition should be limited as it inverses the attended vasoconstriction of the splanchnic bed and consequently the blood that returns to heart and maintains the cardiac refilling. Intradialytic total parenteral nutrition (TPN) is an alternative method of providing calories and protein during HD; it can be used for short-term nutritional support in severely malnourished children.

#### 18.9.3.2 HD in Young Children <10 kg

Children weighing less than 10 kg usually need at least 4–5 sessions per week, so as to enable adequate nutrition in terms of volume. Special attention should be paid to the volume and type of fluid used for extracorporeal blood replacement at the end of the session; blood products, albumin or normal saline have been used [6].

Recently, a group in Newcastle presented the NIDUS programme, which can provide HD in the PICU and outpatient intermittent HD without blood priming for babies less than 8 kg. They have shown that this technique improves urea, creatinine and phosphate clearances compared to PD, and delivers more precise ultrafiltration control than either PD or conventional HD [32].

#### 18.9.3.3 Metabolic Diseases

Intermittent haemodialysis provides higher clearances in patients with an inborn error of metabolism disease (e.g. maple syrup urine disease, urea cycle disorders like ornithine transcarbamylase deficiency, propionic acidaemia) and requires shorter sessions when comparing with CRRT [33–35]. A close collaboration between the intensive care, metabolic and nephrology team is required. Further details are provided in Chap. 27.

#### 18.9.3.4 Drug Intoxications

Depending on the physicochemical properties of the substance (molecular weight, degree of protein binding, solubility and volume of distribution), the clinician should decide the appropriate modality of RRT [36] (Fig. 18.3). Further details are provided in Chap. 28.

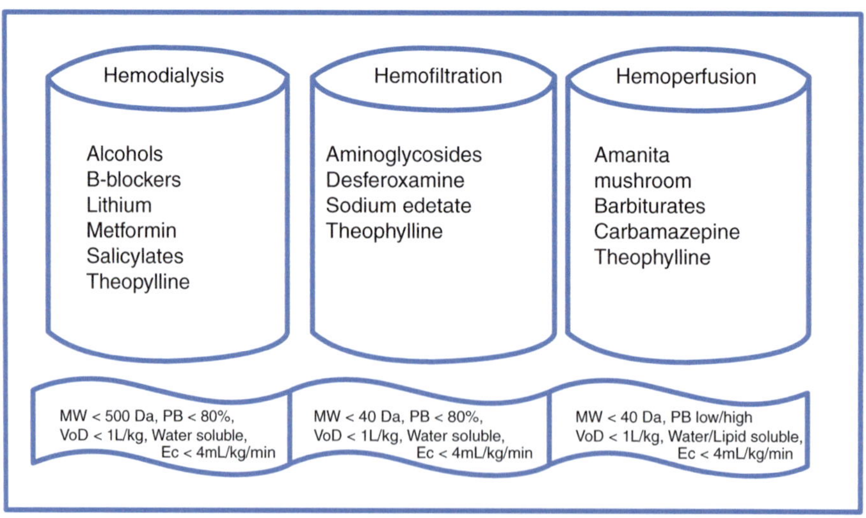


**Fig. 18.3** Specific toxic substances, physicochemical characteristics and the optimal extracorporeal removal modality. *MW* Molecular weight; *PB* Protein binding; *VoD* Volume of distribution; *EC* Endogenous clearance

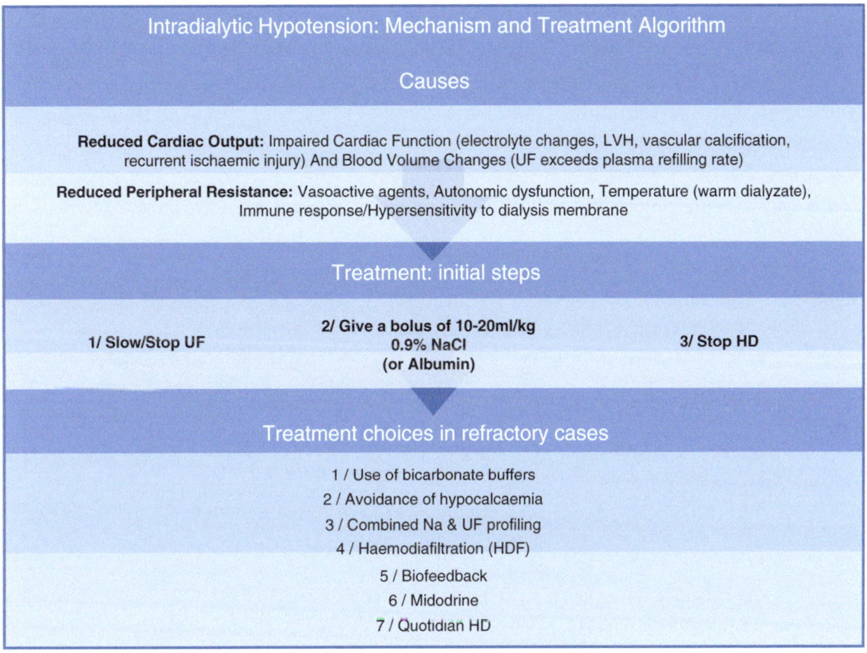


**Fig. 18.4** Intradialytic hypotension: mechanisms and treatment options

### 18.9.4 Complications of Conventional Dialysis

Intradialytic symptoms and especially intradialytic hypotension can result and lead to premature discontinuation of treatment and suboptimal dialysis. Repeated episodes of intradialytic hypotension are associated with increased risk of mortality.

Emerging data support a multifactorial aetiology and different strategies have been proposed [37] (Fig. 18.4).

### 18.9.5 Treatment Options in Refractory Cases

1. Use of bicarbonate buffers: improvement in the haemodynamic stability.
2. Avoidance of hypocalcaemia: avoidance of the acute disturbances in the cardiac function.
3. Combined sodium and UF profiling (theoretically superior to using either in isolation): Better vascular stability, reduced intra- and inter-dialytic symptoms and a post-dialysis weight closer to the dry weight of the patient [38].
4. Haemodiafiltration: In children HDF has been associated with improved haemodynamic stability, reduced left ventricular hypertrophy and a decreased requirement for antihypertensives in a pilot study with daily on-line pre-dilutional haemodiafiltration (3 h, six times/week) [39]. An international study across Europe is ongoing.

5. Biofeedback: more often blood volume controlled feedback systems which respond to relative blood volume (RBV) changes and adjust the UF rate and dialyzate conductivity to maintain RBV along pre-set targets.
6. Midodrine: Recommended only for acute and refractory cases, as there is known tachyphylaxis to the drug and the data in paediatric population is limited [40].

**Table 18.7** Complications in haemodialysis: aetiology and immediate treatment in the acute setting

| Complications of dialysis | | Aetiology/risk factors | Treatment |
|---|---|---|---|
| Common | Dialysis-related Hypertension | Sodium/water overload<br>Inappropriate excretion of renin | • Increase fluid removal (if overload)—more frequent dialysis is preferred to increasing the % body weight ultrafiltration >4% per session<br>• ACE inhibiters (in renin-dependant HTN) |
| | Cramps | Excessive or rapid ultrafiltration<br>Underestimation of dry weight<br>Hypomagnesaemia | • Stop UF ± bolus of NaCl<br>• Warm compresses, massage<br>• Correct any Ca, Mg, Ph abnormalities |
| | Headaches | Moderate DDS<br>Hypocalcaemia<br>Hypotension or HTN | • Paracetamol<br>• Stop UF ± bolus of NaCl<br>• Mannitol |
| | Nausea | Hypotension<br>At the start of DDS | • Slow/Stop UF ± bolus of NaCl<br>• Mannitol? |
| Serious | Dialysis disequilibrium syndrome (DDS) | 1st sessions<br>High urea levels at the start of the dialysis | • Perfusion of NaCl (reconstitution of plasma osmolality)<br>• Mannitol IV<br>• Avoid dropping urea >50% in the 1st session |
| | Air embolism (AE) | Aspiration in the circuit/in a cannula<br>Problem with the air detector | • Trendelenburg manoeuvre<br>• Oxygen 100%<br>• Hyperbaric $O_2$ in cases of massive AE |
| | Haemolysis | Technical machine problems<br>Inadequate water treatment | • STOP dialysis immediately<br>• DO NOT reconstitute the blood back to the patient<br>• Check potassium—Treat hypokalaemia if needed<br>• Change the dialysis circuit and machine before the next session<br>• Check the dialysis water for excess of trace elements (e.g. cu) and antimicrobial quality |
| | Bacteraemia/ septicaemia | Presence of endotoxins in the water<br>Viral contaminants (HepB, HepC, HIV)<br>Nosocomial infection/ contamination | • Stop dialysis<br>• Treat by broad-spectrum antibiotics (until finding the cause/negative cultures) |

*HTN* Hypertension; *Ca* Calcium; *Mg* Magnesium; *Ph* Phosphate

7. Quotidian haemodialysis: Improvement in the interdialytic haemodynamic stability, decrease in the LVH rate and the use of antihypertensives is reported. Short daily (2–3 h treatment, 5–6×/week) or nocturnal HD (8 h treatment on alternate days) has been used.

Apart from intradialytic hypotension, other complications may occur as in every dialysis modality. Table 18.7 summarizes the most common and the most serious complications, their main risk factors and the immediate treatment in the acute setting.

**Conclusion**

In conclusion, we present the technical details of dialysis therapy, details of vascular access, dialysis adequacy, fluid removal, and the common infectious and non-infectious complications of dialysis. Optimal vascular access is crucial to achieve optimal clearances and fluid control, and this is often better achieved via an arteriovenous fistula rather than a central venous line. Haemodiafiltration has shown promising results in adults, and needs further studies in children.

## References


1. Akcan-Arikan A, Zappitelli M, Loftis LL, Washburn KK, Jefferson LS, Goldstein SL. Modified RIFLE criteria in critically ill children with acute kidney injury. Kidney Int. 2007;71:1028–35.
2. Sytherland SM, Byrnes JJ, Kothari M, Longhurst CA, Dutta S, Garcia P, Goldstein SL. AKI in hospitalized children: comparing the pRIFLE, AKIN, and KDIGO definitions. Clin J Am Soc Nephrol. 2015;10:554–61. https://doi.org/10.2215/CJN.01900214.
3. Pannu N, Klarenbach S, Wiebe N, et al. Renal Remplacement therapy in patients with acute renal failure: a systematic review. JAMA. 2008;299:793–805.
4. Gaillot T, Ozanne B, Betremieux P, Tirel O, Ecoffey C. Acute renal replacement therapy in pediatrics. Ann Fr Anesth Reanim. 2013;32(12):e231–6.
5. Tattersall J, Canaud B, Heimburger O, Pedrini L, Schneditz D, Biesen WV, European Renal Best Practice advisory Board. High-flux or low-flux dialysis: a position statement following publication of the membrane permeability outcome study. Nephrol Dial Transplant. 2010;25(4):1230–2.
6. Fischbach M, Edefonti A, Schroöder C, Watson A, The European Pediatric Dialysis Working Group. Hemodialysis in children: general practical guidelines. Pediatr Nephrol. 2005;20:1054–66.
7. Fischbach M, Zaloszyc A, Shroff R. Hemodiafiltration in children: an ultrapure complete blood purification. In: Handbook of dialysis therapy E-book (Chapter 75).
8. Troyanov S, Cardinal J, Geadah D, et al. Solute clearances during continuous venovenous haemofiltration at various ultrafiltration flow rates using Multiflow-100 and HF1000 filters. Nephrol Dial Transplant. 2003;18:961–6.
9. Akaraborworn O. A review in emergency central venous catheterization. Chin J Traumatol. 2017;20(3):137–40.
10. Schwab SJ, Quarles LD, Middleton JP, et al. Hemodialysis-associated subclavian vein stenosis. Kidney Int. 1988;33:1156–9.
11. Schillinger F, Schillinger D, Montagnac R, et al. Post catheterisation vein stenosis in haemodialysis: comparative angiographic study of 50 subclavian and 50 internal jugular accesses. Nephrol Dial Transplant. 1991;6:722–4.

12. Centers for Disease Control and Prevention. Guidelines for the prevention of intravascular catheter-related infections. MMWR. 2002;51(RR-10):1–26.
13. National Kidney Foundation. K/DOQI clinical practice guidelines for vascular access, 2000. Am J Kidney Dis. 2001;37(Suppl 1):S137–81.
14. Calder F, Gogalniceanu P, Shroff R. Paediatric vascular access for haemodialysis – a rough guide. London, UK: Guy's and St.Thomas NHS Trust & Great Ormond Street Hospitals.
15. Dunne N. A meta-analysis of sodium profiling techniques and the impact on intradialytic hypotension. Hemodial Int. 2017;21(3):312–22. https://doi.org/10.1111/hdi.12488.
16. Zhou YL, Liu HL, Duan XF, Sun Y, Liu Q. Impact of sodium and ultrafiltration profiling on haemodialysis-related hypotension. Nephrol Dial Transplant. 2006;21(11):3231–7.
17. Hothi DK, Harvey E, Goia CM, Geary DF. Evaluating methods for improving ultrafiltration in pediatric hemodialysis. Pediatr Nephrol. 2008;23(4):631–8. https://doi.org/10.1007/s00467-007-0716.
18. Hothi DK, Geary DF. Pediatric hemodialysis prescription, Efficacy, and outcome. In: Comprehensive pediatric nephrology (Chapter 57).
19. Viegas M, Candido C, Felqueiras J, Clemente J, Barros S, Farbota R, Vera F, Matos A, Sousa F. Dialysate bicarbonate variation in maintenance hemodiafiltration patients: impact on serum bicarbonate, intradialytic hypotension and interdialytic weight gain. Hemodial Int. 2017;21(3):385–92.
20. Yamamoto T, Shojl S, Yamakawa T, Wada A, Suzuki K, Iseki K, Tsubakihara Y. Predialysis and postdialysis pH and bicarbonate and risk of all-cause and cardiovascular mortality in long-term hemodialysis patients. Am J Kidney Dis. 2015;66(3):469–78.
21. Kato A, Kido R, Onishi Y, Kurita N, Fukagawa M, Akizawa T, Fukuhara S. Association of serum bicarbonate with bone fractures in hemodialysis patients: the mineral and bone disorder outcomes study for Japanese CKD stage 5D patients (MBD-5D). Nephron Clin Pract. 2014;128(1–2):79–87.
22. Penne EL, Visser L, van den Dorpel MA, van der Weerd NC, Mazairac AH, van Jaarsveld BC, Koopman MG, Vos P, Feith GW, Kremer Hovinga TK, van Hamersvelt HW, Wauters IM, Bots ML, Nube MJ, Ter Wee PM, Blankestijn PJ, Grooteman MP. Microbiological quality and quality control of purified water and ultrapure dialysis fluids for online hemodiafiltration in routine clinical practice. Kidney Int. 2009;76(6):665–72.
23. Gonzalez-Diez B, Cavia M, Torres G, Abalgar P, Camarero V, Muniz P. The effects of 1-year treatment with a haemodiafiltration with on-ine regeneration of ultrafiltrate (HFR) dialysis on biomarkers of oxidative stress in patients with chronic renal failure. Mol Biol Rep. 2012;39(1):629–34.
24. Praditpornsilpa K, Tiranathanagul K, Susantitaphong P, Katavetin P, Trakarnvanich T, Townamchai N, Kanjanabuch T, Avihingsanon Y, Tungsanga K, Elam-Ong S. Effects of different levels of endotoxin contamination on inflammatory cytokine production by peripheral blood mononuclear cells after high-flux hemodialysis. Blood Purif. 2011;32(2):112–6.
25. Davenport A. Alternatives to standard unfractionated heparin for pediatric hemodialysis treatments. Pediatr Nephrol. 2012;27(10):1869–79.
26. Lim W, Cook DJ, Crowther MA. Safety and efficacy of low molecular weight heparins for hemodialysis in patients with end-stage renal failure: a meta-analysis of randomized trials. J Am Soc Nephrol. 2004;15(12):3192–206.
27. Lazrak HH, Rene E, Elftouh N, Leblanc M, Lafrance JP. Safety of low-molecular-weight heparin compared to unfractionated heparin in hemodialysis: a systematic review and meta-analysis. BMC Nephrol. 2017;18(1):187.
28. Ishibe S, Peixoto AJ. Methods of assessment of volume status and intercompartmental fluid shifts in hemodialysis patients: implications in clinical practice. Semin Dial. 2004;17(1):37–43.
29. Kouw PM, Kooman JP, Cheriex EC, Olthof CG, de Vries PM, Leunissen KM. Assessment of postdialysis dry weight: a comparison of techniques. J Am Soc Nephrol. 1993;4:98–104.
30. Nishikimi T, Futoo Y, Tamano K, Takahashi M, Suzuki T, Minami J, et al. Plasma brain natriuretic peptide levels in chronic hemodialysis patients: influence of coronary artery disease. Am J Kidney Dis. 2001;37:1201–8.

31. Eng CSY, Bhowruth D, Mayes M, Stronach L, Blaauw M, Barber A, Rees L, Shroff RC. Assessing the hydration status of children with chronic kidney disease and on dialysis: a comparison of techniques. Nephrol Dial Transplant. 2017:1–9. https://doi.org/10.1093/ndt/gfx287.
32. Coulthard MG, Crosier J, Griffiths C, Smith J, Drinnan M, Whitaker M, Beckwith R, Matthews JN, Flecknell P, Lambert HJ. Haemodialysing babies weighing <8kg with Newcastle infant dialysis and ultrafiltration system (Nidus): a comparison with peritoneal and conventional haemodialysis. Pediatr Nephrol. 2014;29(10):1873–81.
33. Phan V, Clermont MJ, Merouani A, Litalien C, Tucci M, Lambert M, Mitchell G, Jouvet P. Duration of extracorporeal therapy in acute marple syrup urine disease: a kinetic model. Pediatr Nephrol. 2006;21(5):698–704.
34. Rafique M. Emerging trends in management of propionic acidemia. Arg Bras Endocrinol Metabol. 2014;58(3):237–42.
35. Picca S, Bartuli A, Dionisi-Vici C. Medical management and dialysis therapy for the infant with an inborn error of metabolism. Semin Nephrol. 2008;28(5):477–80.
36. Mirrakhimov AE, Barbaryan A, Gray A, Ayach T. The role of renal replacement therapy in the management of pharmacologic poisings. Int J Nephrol. 2016;2016:3047329. https://doi.org/10.1155/2016/3047329.
37. Hayes W, Hothi DK. Intradialytic hypotension. Pediatr Nephrol. 2011;26:867–79.
38. Song JH, Park GH, Lee SY, Lee SW, Kim MJ. Effect of sodium balance and the combination of ultrafiltration profile during sodium profiling hemodialysis on the maintenance of the quality of dialysis and sodium and fluid balances. J Am Soc Nephrol. 2005;16:237–46.
39. Fischbach M, Terzie J, Laugel V, Dheu C, Menouer S, Helms P, Livolsi A. Daily on-line haemofiltration; a pilot trial in children. Nephrol Dial Transplant. 2004;19:2360–7
40. Hothi DK, Harvey E, Goia C, Geary D. The value of sequential dialysis, mannitol and midodrine in children prone to dialysis failure. Pediatr Nephrol. 2009;24:1587–91.

# 19 Sustained Low-Efficiency Dialysis (SLED) and Hybrid Therapies in Children

Valentine Lobo

## 19.1 Definition and History of Prolonged Intermittent Renal Replacement Therapy

In 1946, Wilhem Kolff first carried out a successful 690 min dialysis session on a patient of acute kidney injury and severe hyperkalemia. Blood flow was 116 mL/min, urea clearance 87 mL/min, and Kt/V of 1.4 [1]. This prolonged session with low blood flow and clearances could be described as the first prolonged intermittent renal replacement therapy (PIRRT), a term employed by Fealy, Baldwin, and Bellomo in 2004 [2]. Although continuous renal replacement therapy (CRRT) was first used by Kramer in 1979, the large majority of adult patients with acute kidney injury continued to be treated with intermittent hemodialysis similar to those with chronic kidney disease. In the late 1980s and 1990s Schlaper et al. extended the length of intermittent hemodialysis sessions and by 2000 the terms extended dialysis(ED), extended daily dialysis(EDD), slow low efficiency daily dialysis(SLEDD), sustained low efficiency dialysis(SLED) had been coined. Early sessions varied from 8 to 12 h on single pass machines, to 18 h on the Genius machine. The continuous mode with sessions lasting 24 h was described by Salahudeen [3] in 2009, and the criteria became more variable with some workers using sessions as short as 6 h.

The technical difficulties of performing intermittent hemodialysis in small children and infants have meant that peritoneal dialysis and CRRT have been the mainstay of renal replacement therapy in developed and developing countries, respectively. A recent survey including 60 centers from the USA and 48 from the Indian subcontinent and Latin America revealed a marked geographical variation in RRT practices. Limited availability, expertise, and high costs limit CRRT in developing countries. SLEDD however was used in 25% of centers in developing countries as compared to 20% in developed countries [4].

V. Lobo
Department of Nephrology, King Edward Memorial Hospital, Pune, India



A. Deep, S. L. Goldstein (eds.), *Critical Care Nephrology and Renal Replacement Therapy in Children*, https://doi.org/10.1007/978-3-319-90281-4_19

**Sustained low efficiency dialysis is a conceptual and technical hybrid of continuous renal replacement therapy (CRRT) and intermittent hemodialysis (IHD), combining the desirable properties of each modality** [5]:

1. A reduced rate of ultrafiltration for optimized hemodynamic stability.
2. Low-efficiency solute removal to minimize solute disequilibrium.
3. Sustained treatment duration to maximize dialysis dose.
4. Intermittent nature for convenient access to patients for out-of-unit diagnostic and therapeutic procedures during scheduled downtime.

**Case Vignette**

An 8-year-old child, weighing 19 kg, admitted in the Pediatric Intensive Care Unit, following a blunt trauma, had a distended, tender abdomen with guarding, and anuria for 8 h after the event. He had received around 1000 mL of crystalloid at the time of surgical evacuation. At ICU admission his blood pressure (BP) was 90/40 mm of Hg, RR 26/min, heart rate 170/min, and CVP 4 cm $H_2O$. As further fluid resuscitation and dopamine infusion did not improve urine output, a CT scan of the abdomen was done. This revealed a solitary left kidney, a non-visualized renal artery, splenic hematoma, multiple lacerations in the body and tail of pancreas, and numerous large and small intraperitoneal collections. Exploratory laparotomy showed hemoperitoneum with anterior abdominal wall necrosis, widespread intra- and retroperitoneal fat necrosis, liquefaction of the jejunal wall, edematous pancreas with slough collection, and omentum covered with slough, a thrombosed left renal artery with cyanotic kidney and splenic hematoma. Left nephrectomy with de-sloughing, drain insertion, splenectomy, and feeding jejunostomy was done. Postoperatively, he received antibiotics, noradrenaline, intravenous fluids, elective ventilation, and hemodialysis. On the third postoperative day, he developed sudden bleeding from the peritoneal drain and his hemoglobin dropped to 2.6 g%, platelet count to 47,000/$mm^3$, prothrombin and activated thromboplastin time were prolonged. Despite transfusions he developed shock with a systolic BP of 60 mm of Hg, hypoxia, bradycardia, and a cardiac arrest requiring CPR. The following day his circulation was stabilized with noradrenaline and vasopressin. His blood reports showed pH of 7.00, bicarbonate of 7.3 mmol/L, blood urea of 167 mg/dL, creatinine of 7.3 mg/dL, and serum potassium of 6.5 mmol/L. He received 41 h of continuous veno-venous hemofiltration with a blood flow of 100 mL/min, replacement fluid (Prismasol) at 600 mL/h, and ultrafiltration of 50 mL/h. Regional heparinization was used with monitoring of the patient's and extracorporeal circuit aPTT individually. The procedure was stopped when the filter clotted, by which time the noradrenaline dose had decreased to 0.12 mcg/kg/min.

He required amphotericin B for candidemia. His coagulopathy continued to require blood products. He was taken for sustained low efficiency daily dialysis for 10 h daily using the ArrT plus machine at a blood flow of 135 mL/min, citrate bicarbonate dialysate at 200 mL/min with 800 mL of ultrafiltration per session and no anticoagulant. After three sessions he was extubated, and noradrenaline discontinued after the seventh session. He was discharged from the ICU on the 29th postoperative day, a cuffed tunneled catheter was inserted in the left internal jugular vein and he was placed on a maintenance hemodialysis program.

## 19.2 Introduction

The case described above highlights the indications, and the problems with providing renal replacement therapy to the critically ill child. What is unique about these patients is that multiple indications for renal replacement therapy may exist simultaneously and a balance may have to be created between providing biochemical correction of hyperkalemia, acidosis and uremia, fluid removal for pulmonary edema, and maintenance of blood pressure in a patient with increased extravascular volume, inotrope need and increased permeability of capillaries and veins.

**Box1: Indications for SLED**

- Clinically significant fluid overload of more than 10% above baseline in AKI not responding to high dose diuretics.
- Severe metabolic acidosis with other signs of decreased end-organ perfusion.
- Hyperkalemia (plasma $K^+ > 6.5$ meq/L or rapidly rising).
- Azotemia (BUN >100 mg/dL).
- Uremic organ involvement (pericarditis, encephalopathy, neuropathy, myopathy).
- Progressive severe dysnatremia ($Na^+ > 160$ or < 115 meq/L).
- Nonobstructive oliguria (<0.5 mL/kg/h for more than 6 h).
- Malignant hyperthermia.
- Overdose with a dialysable drug.
- Neonatal hyperammonemia and other inborn errors of metabolism.
- Coagulopathy requiring large amounts of blood products in patients at risk of pulmonary edema or ARDS.

## 19.3 Procedure of Sustained Low Efficiency Dialysis

SLED is typically carried out using equipment used for conventional hemodialysis, easily available in dialysis units and familiar to dialysis nurses. While many centers rely on dialysis nurses or technicians to initiate the procedure with troubleshooting from ICU personnel, Marshall reported a study in which the entire procedure of

SLEDD-f was carried out by ICU nurses trained for this purpose [5]. In our own unit the process has evolved from a largely nocturnal procedure where machines shifted from the dialysis unit were operated by dialysis personnel after the daily maintenance dialysis was over, to stationing of machines permanently in the ICU and operated by ICU nurses and technicians. The responsibility and treatment objectives, goals, and plan are shared jointly by nephrologists and intensivists. An overview of machines available for SLEDD with their specifications is shown in Table 19.1. Dialyzers can be low flux for SLEDD, but either high flux dialyzers or hemofilters are required if online hemodiafiltration (SLEDD-f) is prescribed. The dialyzer needs to be appropriately chosen for the patient's size, a slightly smaller dialyzer with lower clearance and KoA is appropriate as it reduces the risk of disequilibrium and hypotension further, while dose delivery is compensated for, by the increased session length. Similarly blood tubings for pediatric treatments may require adjustment of the blood pump occlusion diameter if the same machine is used with standard 6.4 mm sets.

The vascular access should be chosen according to the size of the child and the blood flow requirement [6]. Care should be taken while siting the vascular access for dialysis and central venous access for giving inotropes, antibiotics, etc. as the proximity of these two accesses can cause siphoning of drugs given through the central access by the negative pressure applied to the dialysis catheter. A brief overview of dialyzers for SLEDD is given in Table 19.2. Although the hemofilters from the AV series have been used in SLEDD-f in adults, they appear to be too large for use in children and an equally efficient treatment can be carried out using high flux dialyzers.

## 19.4 Fluid Removal

Large volumes of fluid for maintaining adequate nutrition and hydration, blood products to combat DIC and coagulopathy, antibiotic infusions, inotropes and pressors all increase the total daily administered fluid. In an anuric patient, this mandates fluid removal to prevent pulmonary edema. An increasing body of evidence indicates that volume overload which is invariably an unavoidable consequence of resuscitation is associated with increased mortality, morbidity, and hospital stay [7, 8]. In fact, in children an increase in body weight of 10%, and definitely of 20%, is associated with increased mortality and considered an indication for dialysis [6, 8]. In a study from India, an even lower degree of fluid overload increased mortality [9].

Continuous therapies achieve a better reduction in fluid accumulation compared to intermittent ones, underscoring the importance of extending the time available for ultrafiltration to maintain hemodynamic stability [7, 10]. Many patients with AKI diagnosed as having acute respiratory distress syndrome (ARDS) actually have pulmonary edema, as cardiac function can also be profoundly impaired by fluid overload. Such patients achieve normal lung compliance and improved oxygenation with fluid removal by dialysis. Systemic hemodynamics remain stable as long as the rate of fluid removal does not exceed the rate of mobilization of interstitial fluid into

**Table 19.1** Machines for SLEDD

| Parameter | Fresenius 4008 NG | Fresenius 5008 | DBB-07 Nikissho | Artis (Gambro) | Diamax (Nipro) |
|---|---|---|---|---|---|
| Water requirement | 1.5–3 bar | 1.5–6 bar | 1– 7 bar | 1– 6 bar | 1– 4 bar |
| Electricity requirements | 100– 240 V AC, 47–63 Hz | 100– 240 V AC, 47–63 Hz | 220–240 V AC, 50/60 Hz | 220–240 V AC, 50/60 Hz | 220–240 V AC, 50/60 Hz |
| Blood flow | 5–500 mL/min | 30–600 mL/ | 40–600 mL/min | 0–580 mL/min | 15–600 mL/min |
| Dialysate flow | 300, 500, and 800 mL/min | 0–1000 mL/min in increments of 100 | 300–700 mL/min in increments of 100 | 300–800 mL/min in increments of 100 | 300–700 mL/min in increments of 100 |
| Heparin pump | Syringe 0.5–10 mL/h | Syringe 0.5–10 mL/h | Syringe 0–9.9 mL/h | Syringe | Syringe |
| Ultrafiltration | 1 mL/h to maximum of 9990 mL | 0–4000 mL/h (in steps of 10 mL) | 0.1–4000 mL/h | 0–4000 mL/h | 100–5000 mL/h |
| Maximum treatment time | 10 h | 24 h | 12 h | 24 h | 6 h |
| Compatibility with multiple dialyzer and tubing sets | Yes | Dedicated tubing sets | Yes | Yes | Yes |
| Sodium and ultrafiltration profiling | Custom | Custom | Also bicarbonate profiling. | Also bicarbonate | Flexible |
| Dialysate sodium/conductivity range | 128–148 meq/L | 125–151 mmol/L, (12.8–15.7 mS/cm) | 12.5–15.5 mS/cm | 130–160 mmol/L | 10–17 mS/cm |
| Dialysate temperature range | 35–39 °C | 34–39 °C | 34–40 °C | 30–39 °C | 30–40 °C |
| Dry powder concentrate use* | Bibag | Bibag (650 or 900 g) | No | Yes (Bicart) acetate free citrate bicarb sterile concentrate available | No |
| Online replacement fluid preparation | No | Yes 25–600 mL/min | 0.1–30 L/h online. Also external scale for fluid bags | Yes (U 9000 disposable filter required) auto TMP monitored and manual options available | No |

(continued)

**Table 19.1** (continued)

| Parameter | Fresenius 4008 NG | Fresenius 5008 | DBB-07 Nikissho | Artis (Gambro) | Diamax (Nipro) |
|---|---|---|---|---|---|
| Disinfection options | | | | | |
| Heated citrate | (85 °C) | 85 °C | 85 °C | 85 °C | (65 °C) |
| Peracetic acid/sodium hypochlorite | 37 °C | 37 °C | 37 °C | 37 °C | Not specified |
| System self test | Yes | Yes | Yes | Yes | Yes |
| Additional features | OCM, | OCM, BTM, and BPM | DDM, BVM, and BPM | Diascan and Hemoscan monitors | Not specified |

**Table 19.2** Dialyzers/Hemofilters for SLEDD

| Parameter | Dialyzer | | | | |
|---|---|---|---|---|---|
| | Sureflux 5 N (Nipro) | F3 (Fresenius) | FX40 (Fresenius) | FX ped (Fresenius) | Polyflux 6H (Gambro) |
| Surface area ($m^2$) | 0.5 | 0.4 | 0.6 | 0.2 | 0.6 |
| Priming volume (mL) | 34 | 28 | 53 | 18 | 52 |
| Ultrafiltration coefficient | 2.7 | 1.7 | 20 | 7 | 33 |
| Urea clearance | 130[a] | 125[b] | 170[b] | 76[c] | 50[d] |
| Creatinine clearance | 109[a] | 95[b] | 144[b] | 64[c] | 50[d] |
| Phosphate clearance | 62[a] | 50[b] | 138[b] | 57[c] | 49[d] |
| Material | Cellulose triacetate | Polysulfone | Helixone | Helixone | Polyflux[e] |
| Fiber inner diameter (micron) | 200 | 200 | 185 | 220 | 215 |
| Thickness | 15 | 40 | 35 | 35 | 50 |
| Blood flow (mL/min) | | 50–200 | 50–200 | 30–100 | 50–200 |
| Sterilization | Gamma ray | ETO | Inline steam | Inline steam | Inline steam |

[a]At Qb = 200 mL/min
[b]At Qb = 200 mL/min
[c]At Qb = 100 mL/min
[d]At Qb = 50 mL/min
[e]Polyflux is a blend of Polyarylethersulfone, Polyvinylpyrrolidone, Polyamide

the vascular compartment. Kumar et al. [11] achieved a median UF of 3000 mL/day with both 7.5 h EDD sessions and 19.5 h CRRT sessions in adults, with excellent maintenance of MAP and similar hypotensive episodes in the two therapies. This permitted obligatory fluid administration, even in anuric patients, though the patients did not necessarily achieve overall negative fluid balance. While patients with chronic kidney disease (CKD) with hypertension were shown in the HEMO study [12] to tolerate ultrafiltration of 10–12 mL/kg/h, the patient with high pressor support, increased capillary permeability and hypoalbuminemia would simply not tolerate such rates. Most studies on SLED in adults report total ultrafiltration achieved but not the hourly rate. In a multicenter study in children from India [9], the reported rate was 9.28 ± 6.67 mL/kg/h. However in 30% of these sessions performed in patients who were not on inotropes, intradialytic hypotension was seen in 31 of 211 sessions with termination in 20. It may be prudent to restrict ultrafiltration rates to a lower level in the interest of hemodynamic stability, probably around 4–5 mL/kg/h. This entails increasing the duration of the session and thus the desired ultrafiltration will drive the session length. The dialysate flow rate is reduced both to decrease the consumption of dialysate and the biochemical clearance. Lonemann et al. [13] using the Genius machine with blood and dialysate flow both set at 70 mL/min carried out 18 h sessions in adult patients with 4000 mL of ultrafiltration and an increase in mean arterial pressure from 69 to 81 mm of Hg. A longer and slower dialysis reduces the rate of change of the plasma osmolality, which also enhances hemodynamic stability and reduces the incidence of disequilibrium. Additionally, use of sodium profiling, cooled dialysate and increased dialysate calcium or potassium can also be used although their role in the critically ill patient is less clear. In the recently conducted RESCUE study [14], the mean duration of daily SLEDD session was 14.9 h and CRRT session was 15.9 h daily, while 24 h SLEDD sessions have also been conducted [3]. Once the duration and dialysate flow have been chosen, blood flow can be adjusted according to the desired clearance and the dialyzer specifications. The flexibility of varying the dialysate flow rate, composition, ultrafiltration rate, blood flow and dialyzer to adapt a treatment on a standard dialysis machine for this patient subset are some of the unique features of SLEDD.

## 19.5 Anticoagulation

While SLEDD can be performed using standard unfractionated heparin as with intermittent hemodialysis, a single dose of Enoxaparin 1 mg/kg or regional citrate can also provide adequate and safe anticoagulation for a 8 h session. Perhaps the greatest advantage of SLEDD over CRRT is the ability to conduct a complete session without the need for any anticoagulation. Kumar et al. [11] found that patients on EDD required significantly less heparin than those treated with CVVH. 117 EDD treatment days (31.9%) were done without heparin compared to only three CVVH treatment days (2.7%). Of over 3000 sessions of SLEDD in our unit, almost half were performed without anticoagulation. We generally increase the blood flow rate by 20–25% for anticoagulant free sessions. Since 2014 we have successfully used dry citrate bicarbonate dialysate concentrate for all SLEDD sessions, as described by Suhail Ahmed [15], which produces a dialysate citrate concentration of 3–4 mmol/L, protecting the dialyzer from clotting without producing systemic anticoagulation. It is important to confirm that the machine proportioning system is configured for the compatible citrate concentrate, that the contribution of the acid concentrate to the final conductivity is at least 9.4 mS/cm and that the dialysate flow is switched on during the priming procedure.

**Table 19.3** Prescription for SLEDD

| |
|---|
| Patient described in the case vignette has undergone nephrectomy and is now anuric. |
| The volume of blood products, antibiotic and pressor infusions, amphotericin B and intravenous fluids amount to 54 mL/h. Within 36 h he will gain 10% of his dry weight. |
| He also has pulmonary edema and is on noradrenaline and vasopressin infusions. |
| *Vascular Access*: We will use 8F double lumen cannula. While the right internal jugular vein is preferred, this is being used for multiple infusions already, hence I would choose the left femoral. |
| *Dialyzer*: his body surface area is $0.8m^2$, so we choose a dialyzer of $0.6–0.8m^2$. FX40, F4HPS, or Polyflux 6 L; all these are appropriate and will give adequate small solute clearance. FX40, F40S or Polyflux 6H have ultrafiltration coefficients capable of being used for HDF. |
| *Blood Flow*: at 5 mL/kg/min this is 95 mL/min, so we will start with 100 mL/min. If HDF is being used, blood flow is increased to 120 mL/min, easily achievable with a 8F cannula. |
| *Dialysate Composition and Flow*: ideally 100 mL/min or the lowest possible on the machine(see Table 19.2).Ensuring dialysate sodium of 140 mmol/L or higher for the first session. As there is severe acidosis and hyperkalemia, bicarbonate of ≥32 mmol/L and potassium of 2.1 mmol/L(default) are used. |
| *Ultrafiltration rate and duration*: patient has a daily input of 1300 mL/day. In addition to treating pulmonary edema and decreasing ventilator settings, we need to remove additional fluid. Adding an additional 500 mL gives us a target UF of 1800 mL. If we target 100 mL/h (5 mL/kg/h), this gives us an 18 h session, which would be well tolerated. This can be modified during the session depending on MAP, fluid intake and $PaO_2/FiO_2$ ratio. |
| *Anticoagulation*: none as the patient is coagulopathic and is actively bleeding, in addition, he has had major surgery recently.<br>*Convection (Optional)*: we can add replacement fluid prefilter. The smallest permissible amount (25 mL/min) is around 75 mL/kg/h for this child and would give a filtration fraction of 25% at 100 mL/min of blood flow and 20% at 120 mL/min. |

A sample algorithm, taking into account the need for ultrafiltration, fluid intake, anticoagulation, correction of metabolic parameters, and patient size for the patient described, is provided in Table 19.3 and also in a recent review [16].

## 19.6 Solute Clearance and Control

The solute clearances in SLED are low compared to conventional hemodialysis because of the low blood flow and dialysate flow. This decreases the rapid osmolar shifts induced by hemodialysis, the risk of disequilibrium, fluid shifts from intravascular to interstitial and intracellular space and maintains blood pressure, permitting ultrafiltration (Fig. 19.1). As the session length is greater, the net solute removal is enhanced despite the lower clearance and the equivalent solute clearance may be expected to be higher than for intermittent hemodialysis (Fig. 19.2). This has actually been shown by Marshall et al. [5] who obtained an equivalent renal urea clearance of 35.7 mL/min with 8 h SLEDD-f sessions and a single pool Kt/V of 1.43 for urea and 1.02 for vitamin B12. In fact various SLEDD regimens have shown EKR levels of 25.1–36.8 mL/min, and with daily 8 h sessions, the overall efficacy may be equivalent to or slightly higher than CRRT prescribed at 30–35 mL/kg/h [5].

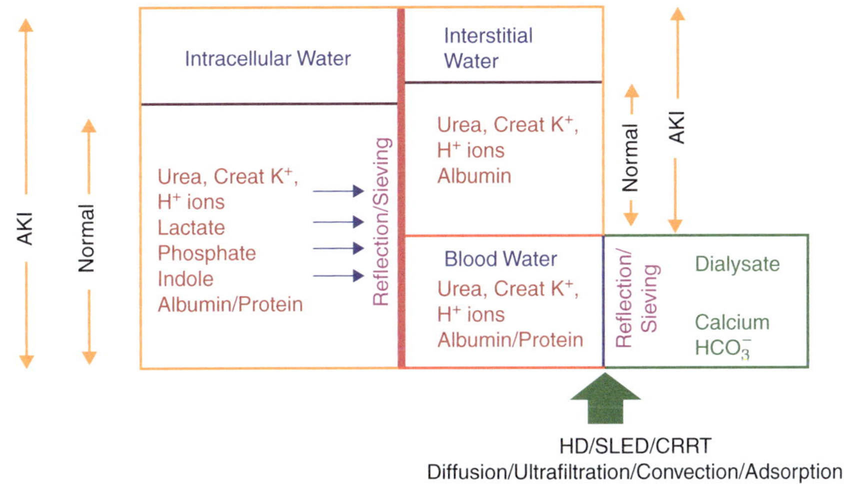


**Fig. 19.1** SLED: Only blood water is cleared directly by the dialyzer. The equivalent solute and water clearances are dependent on equilibration between the various body water compartments

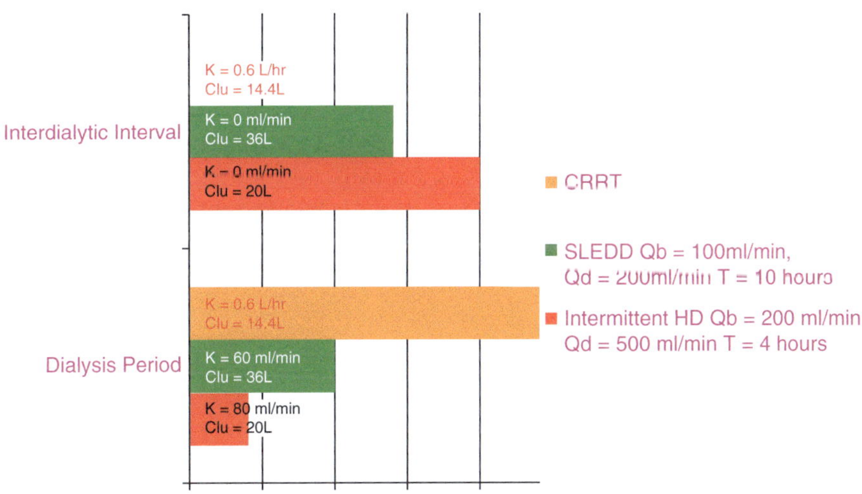


**Fig. 19.2** SLEDD: In an anuric patient weighing 20 kg, urea clearances and rebound with SLEDD are intermediate between intermittent HD and CRRT

Wu et al. also found a higher dialysis dose in SLED than CVVH after 8-h dialysis (equivalent urea clearance, 62.7 ± 4.4 vs. 50.2 ± 3.9 mL/min, $p = 0.002$) [15].

The extended sessions allow solute equilibration between intracellular and extra-cellular fluid with more efficient removal of phosphates, which may have to be replaced to prevent deficiency. The serum ET-1 level increased after CVVH (p = 0.019) but not after SLED treatment in a study by Wu which also found equivalent effects on intracranial pressure by both modalities [17].

While no renal replacement therapy has been shown to clear lactate, SLEDD provides an almost unlimited source of bicarbonate buffer which corrects metabolic acidosis and may improve mean arterial pressure, tissue perfusion and decrease pressor requirement. This is our own observation, and is also described in the retrospective pediatric study from India [16] and in C-SLEDD [3], where pH normalized at 12 h and was sustained up to 48 h.

## 19.7 Complications

Both technical and medical complications occur in SLEDD. Studies investigating complications have largely focused on hypotension, an inevitable occurrence in this population of already hemodynamically unstable patients, and the frequency has been estimated at around 50% [18]. However in a recent randomized study comparing two different session lengths of SLEDD, the incidence of hypotension was 82.6%, with no significant difference between 6 and 10 h sessions [19]. An attempt to decrease hypotension by increasing the session length is balanced by an increased risk of circuit clotting and filter loss which was encountered in 25.3% of sessions.

We counter hypokalemia by using a dialysate potassium of 4 mmol/L in patients at risk, and monitor phosphate levels every 3 days, after starting SLEDD. Hypophosphatemia and hypomagnesemia may be minimized by intravenous or oral supplementation, or by increasing the dialysate content, a flexibility which is unique to SLEDD.

Concerns have also been raised about the microbiological purity of the dialysate. With the use of the Genius machine and the online replacement fluid in SLEDD-f (see below), these have been addressed in studies by Dhondt and Lonnemann [13, 20].

## 19.8 Outcomes with SLEDD

Controversy continues to surround the utility of SLEDD and its advantages/disadvantages compared to CRRT. Till date only two observational studies on SLEDD in children have been published, a single center study from Taiwan [21] and a multicenter study from India [9]. The mortality was 28.6 and 42.6%, respectively, however these studies appear to have included a heterogeneous population and in the Taiwanese study the sickest patients were not considered for SLEDD, but taken for CRRT.

An increasing number of studies in adults have compared CRRT and SLEDD in recent years. In a non-randomized study Kitchlu [22] compared 158 patients undergoing CRRT with 74 patients undergoing SLEDD for an average duration of 7.11 h.

All-cause mortality at 30 days was 54% and 61% among SLED and CRRT-treated patients respectively (adjusted OR 1.07, 95% CI 0.56–2.03). Secondary outcomes including fluid removal after 7 days, was also similar between the two therapies.

In a longitudinal study between 1995 and 2005, involving 1347 patients from ICUs of three different hospitals, Marshall et al. observed that the switch from CRRT to PIRRT use was not associated with any increase in mortality rate, with an adjusted IRR of 1.02 (0.61–1.71). The IRR was virtually identical in the three ICUs (P-value = 0.63 for the difference in the IRR between ICUs) [23]. In the largest RCT comprising 232 patients, the RESCUE study [14], the duration of CRRT and SLEDD barely differed by 1 hour (14.9 vs. 15.9 h, despite the SLED prescription being 12 h), and the 90-day mortality was also similar (49.6 vs. 55.6%, $p = 0.43$). Systolic blood pressure improved after SLED, but not CRRT without increase in the vasopressor doses and with similar ultrafiltration. There was also a significantly lower ICU stay, duration of mechanical ventilation, and RRT requirement with SLED compared with CRRT. This underscores the point that CRRT for technical and logistic reasons is almost never continuous and that SLEDD needs to be more than 12 h long to allow optimum ultrafiltration without compromising hemodynamics and yet maintain the flexibility of allowing out of ICU procedures.

In a recent meta analysis, involving 18 studies, only four were of high quality. In the primary outcome analysis of renal recovery no difference was found between CRRT and SLEDD (OR = 0.87, 95% CI = 0.63–1.20), but a small mortality benefit was actually found with SLEDD (OR for mortality with CRRT = 1.21, 95% CI = 1.02–1.43) [24] The analysis included both randomized controlled and observational studies and the difference was not present in a sensitivity analyses for only RCTs. A similar finding was noted in an earlier analysis of 17 studies, indicating that a marked selection bias may exist in observational studies [25]. In conclusion, SLEDD appears to offer similar survival benefits as CRRT, lower anticoagulation requirements, technical ease and lower costs. Future trials, designed like the RESCUE study and importantly more studies in children are needed to address these issues.

## 19.9 Adaptations of SLEDD

*Drug dose modifications*—The increased solute removal with SLEDD over the longer duration means greater drug removal. This is particularly critical for the septic shock patient receiving antibiotics which are cleared to a level intermediate between intermittent hemodialysis and CRRT. Extensive studies are still lacking except for a few drugs like Meropenem [26], which should be dosed either side of an extended dialysis session. In a review by Sinha et al. [16] recommendations are provided for drug dosing based on adult studies as no specific data is available in children.

### 19.9.1 Adding a Convective Component (SLEDD-f)

Sustained low efficiency daily diafiltration (SLEDD-f) is possible with the new generation of machines (Table 19.1). They possess the feature of cold sterilization or ultrafiltration of the dialysate through ultrafilters having a pore size of 0.05μm, which results in a 4-log reduction of bacteria and a 2-log reduction in endotoxin, producing almost unlimited quantities of a sterile, pyrogen-free fluid suitable for intravenous infusion. The process of cold sterilization by ultrafiltration was validated by Lebedo [27], for the Gambro system and Vasalaki [28], for the Fresenius system. One dry powder bicarbonate cartridge generally allows around 160–200 L of dialysate generation. With a dialysate flow of 100 mL/min and a replacement of 30 mL/kg/h for a 20-kg child, a treatment could actually be run for 24 h. A complete description of the process of obtaining and ensuring ultrapure water is beyond the scope of this chapter, but should confirm to the EU standards for generation and monitoring.

SLEDD-f enables adding a convective component to the predominant diffusion clearance of the standard HD machines. Ultrapure water and sterile dry powder concentrates usually dedicated for individual machines are required for the dialysate preparation. High flux dialyzers or hemofilters having UF coefficients >20 mL/mmHg/h, are mandatory. At least a part of the replacement fluid should be delivered prefilter to reduce the viscosity of the blood caused by the high ultrafiltration rates and the blood flow has to be proportionally higher than usual in order to avoid a filtration fraction >25%, which predisposes to circuit clotting and filter loss. The ultrafiltration actually carried out is the sum of the replacement fluid rate and the desired ultrafiltration and is calculated by the machine software.

Several small series have demonstrated encouraging results with Marshall et al. using the technique in 24 critically ill patients, while Holt and White noted a 30-day survival of 100% in the SLEDD-f group, despite higher APACHE II scores, against 38% in the SLEDD group. Furthermore, all patients in the SLEDD-f group recovered significant renal function to allow discontinuation of RRT [29]. In another small study from Eucador, Dario et al. showed a small non-significant survival benefit from online hemodiafiltration, and a significantly shorter pressor requirement time and ICU stay [30].

Coupling SLEDD with hemoperfusion and plasma exchange has been successfully carried out (Figs. 19.3 and 19.4) using both the charcoal hemoperfusion device and cytokine removal cartridges. In a case of fulminant drug overdose with liver and kidney injury, we have used an external roller pump at a speed of 50 mL/min to perform coupled plasma filtration adsorption with SLEDD. The blood pump of the dialysis machine drives blood from the access to a plasma filter with an external pump to control plasma removal rate and perfuse the charcoal hemoperfusion cartridge before it is reinfused into the venous bubble chamber, while the blood exiting the plasma filter is dialyzed using a low flux or high flux dialyzer. When using cytokine removal devices, we connect them in series with the dialyzer using the blood

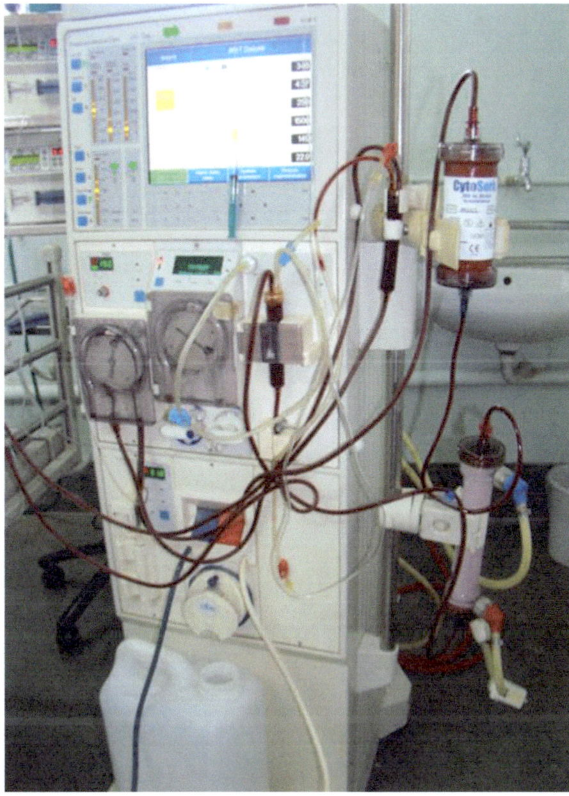


**Fig. 19.3** The cytokine adsorption cartridge Cytosorb connected in series with a hemodialyzer during SLEDD. The total volume of the circuit will be increased by 300 mL making this problematic in very small children

pump to drive the circuit, this may not be feasible in very small children as the extracorporeal volume is increased, in older children, priming the circuit with blood should sort out this issue.

### 19.9.2 SLED in ECMO

The use of extracorporeal membrane oxygenation in ARDS delivers one cardiac output to an external oxygenator via a centrifugal pump, operating with a veno-venous access. In the case of low cardiac output, a veno-arterial access is used. In patients with concomitant AKI requiring SLEDD and ECMO, a portion of the blood (usually between 100 and 200 mL/min) being delivered to the oxygenator is shunted through a parallel circuit to the dialysis machine (Fig. 19.5). The return of blood is always pre-oxygenator and it should be noted that the pre-pump arterial pressure in such a SLEDD circuit is positive rather than negative and the machine software may not be able to calculate the actual blood flow.

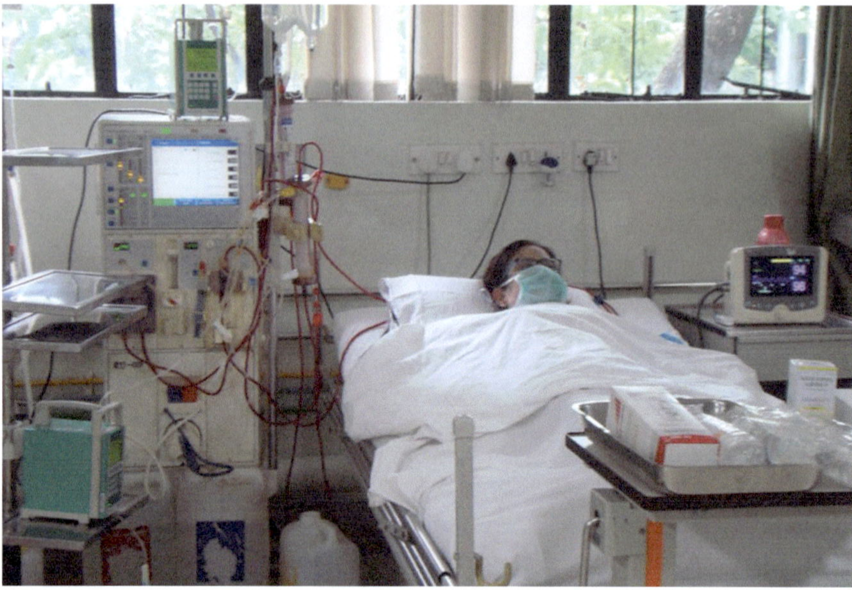

**Fig. 19.4** Plasma exchange coupled with SLEDD. The plasma filter and hemodialyzer are connected in series and the removal and replacement of plasma is controlled by two matched infusion pumps

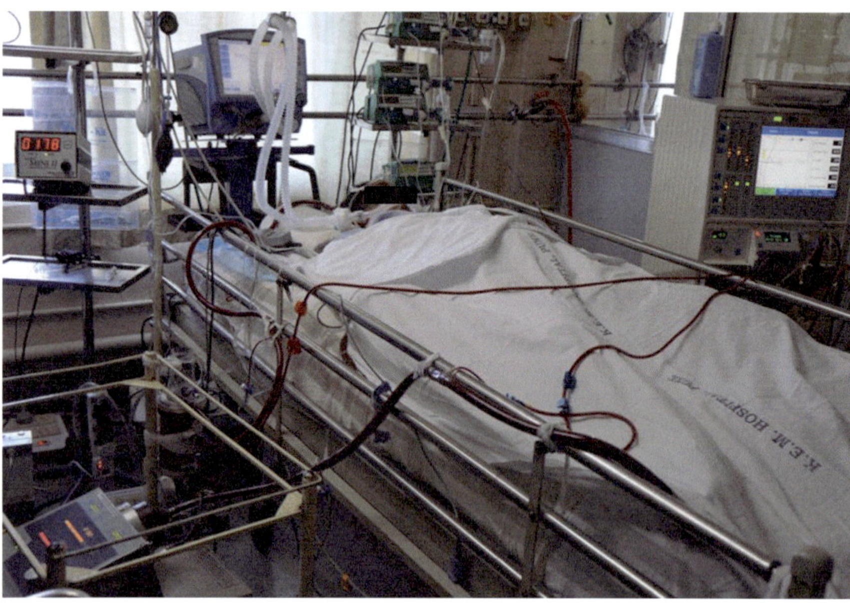

**Fig. 19.5** A patient of H1N1 ARDS and multi-organ failure receiving SLEDD and ECMO. The two circuits are connected in parallel

**Key Learning Points**

- SLEDD is a hybrid therapy with remarkable flexibility and has been adapted by nephrologists and intensivists to suit the needs of individual patients.
- It provides adequate small solute clearance, correction of acidosis and fluid removal while maintaining hemodynamic stability.
- Convective clearance can be added with the use of a sterile online substitution fluid prepared by the machine from ultrapure water and dry powder concentrates.
- Survival, renal recovery, ICU stay and hemodynamic stability are similar to that of CRRT.
- Future developments will include exact determination of drug dosing especially antibiotics during this therapy, and further adaptations for special situations like septic shock and ARDS requiring other extracorporeal therapies.

## References


1. Fliser D, Kielstein JT. Technology insight: treatment of renal failure in the intensive care unit with extended dialysis. Nat Clin Pract Nephrol. 2006;2:32–9.
2. Bellomo R, Baldwin I, Fealy N. Prolonged intermittent renal replacement therapy in the intensive care unit. Crit Care Resusc. 2002;4:281–90.
3. Salahudeen AK, Kumar V, Madan N, Xiao L, Lahoti A, Samuels J, et al. Sustained low efficiency dialysis in the continuous mode (C-SLED): dialysis efficacy, clinical outcomes, and survival predictors in critically ill cancer patients. Clin J Am Soc Nephrol. 2009;4:1338–46.
4. Raina R, Chauvin A, Bunchman T, Askenazi D, Deep A, Ensley M, Krishnappa V, Sethi S. Treatment of AKI in developing and developed countries: an international survey of pediatric dialysis modalities. Plos One. 2017:1–9.
5. Marshall M, Ma T, Galler D, Patrick A, Rankin N, Williams A. Sustained low-efficiency daily diafiltration (SLEDD-f) for critically ill patients requiring renal replacement therapy: towards an adequate therapy. Nephrol Dial Transplant. 2004;19:877–84.
6. Vinsonneau C, Allain-Launay E, Blayau C, et al. Renal replacement therapy in adult and pediatric intensive care - recommendations by an expert panel from the French Intensive Care Society (SRLF) with the French Society of Anesthesia Intensive Care (SFAR) French Group for Pediatric Intensive Care Emergencies (GFRUP) the French dialysis society (SFD). Ann Intensive Care. 2015;5:58–76.
7. Ostermann M, Oudemans-van Straaten HM, Forni L. Fluid overload and acute kidney injury cause or consequence? Crit Care. 2015;19:443–5.
8. Schrier R. AKI: fluid overload and mortality. Nat Rev Nephrol. 2009;5:485.
9. Sethi S, Sinha R, Jha P, Wadhwani N, Ragunathan V, Dhaliwal M, Shyam B, Bansal S, Kher V, Lobo V, Sharma J, Raina R. Feasibility of sustained low efficiency dialysis in critically sick pediatric patients: A multicentric retrospective study. Hemodial Int. 2017;22:228–34.
10. Augustine JJ, Sandy D, Seifert TH, Paganini EP. A randomized controlled trial comparing intermittent with continuous dialysis in patients with ARF. Am J Kidney Dis. 2004;44(6):1000–7.
11. Kumar VA, Craig M, Depner T, Jane Y, Yeun J. Extended daily dialysis: a new approach to renal replacement for acute renal failure in the intensive care unit. Am J Kidney Dis. 2000;36(2):294–300.

12. Eknoyan G, Beck G, Cheung A, et al. Effect of dialysis dose and membrane flux in maintenance hemodialysis. N Engl J Med. 2002;347:2010–9.
13. Lonnemann G, Jurgen Floege J, Kliem V, Brunkhorst R, Koch K. Extended daily veno-venous high-flux hemodialysis in patients with acute renal failure and multiple organ dysfunction syndrome using a single batch dialysis system. Nephrol Dial Transplant. 2000;15:1189–93.
14. Schwenger V, Weigand M, Hoffmann O, et al. Sustained low efficiency dialysis using a single-pass batch system in acute kidney injury – a randomized interventional trial: the Renal Replacement Therapy Study in Intensive Care Unit PatiEnts. Crit Care. 2012;1:R14.
15. Tu & Ahmad, Dialysis & Transplantation. Citrate dialysate in advanced liver failure (Abstr); 2000.
16. Sinha R, Sethi S, Bunchman T, Lobo V & Raina R. Prolonged intermittent renal replacement therapy in children. Pediatr Nephrol. 2017.
17. Wu V, Huang T, Shiao C, NSARF Group. The hemodynamic effects during sustained low-efficiency dialysis versus continuous veno-venous hemofiltration for uremic patients with brain hemorrhage: a crossover study. J Neurosurg. 2013;119:1288–95.
18. Fieghen H, Friedrich J, Burns K, et al. The hemodynamic tolerability and feasibility of sustained low efficiencydialysis in the management of critically ill patients with acute kidney injury. BMC Nephrol. 2010;11(1):32.
19. Albino B, Balbi A, Ponce D. Dialysis complications in AKI patients treated with extended daily dialysis: is the duration of therapy important? Biomed Res Int. 2014;2014:9. Article ID 153626
20. Dhondt A, Vanholder R, De Smet R, et al. Studies on dialysate mixing in the Genius_ single-pass batch system for hemodialysis therapy. Kidney Int. 2003;63:1540–7.
21. Chia-Ying L, Yeh H, Lin C-Y. Treatment of critically ill children with kidney injury by sustained low-efficiency daily diafiltration. Pediatr Nephrol. 2012;27:2301–9.
22. Kitchlu A, Adhikari N, , Burns K et al. Outcomes of sustained low efficiency dialysis versus continuous renal replacement therapy in critically ill adults with acute kidney injury: a cohort study; BMC Nephrol (2015) 16:127 – 134.
23. Marshall M, Creamer J, Foster M, et al. Mortality rate comparison after switching from continuous to prolonged intermittent renal replacement for acute kidney injury in three intensive care units from different countries. Nephrol Dial Transplant. 2011;26:2169–75.
24. Kovacs B, Sullivan K, Hiremath S, Patel R. Effect of sustained low efficient dialysis versus continuous renal replacement therapy on renal recovery after acute kidney injury in the intensive care unit: a systematic review and meta-analysis. Nephrology. 2017;22:343–53.
25. Zhang L, Yang J, Eastwood G, et al. Extended daily dialysis versus continuous renal replacement therapy for acute kidney injury: a meta-analysis. Am J Kidney Dis. 2015;66(2):322–30.
26. Deshpande P, Chen J, Gofran A, Murea M, Golestaneh L. Meropenem removal in critically ill patients undergoing sustained low-efficiency dialysis (SLED). Nephrol Dial Transplant. 2010;25(8):2632–6.
27. Ledebo I. On-line preparation of solutions for dialysis: practicalaspects versus safety and regulations. J Am Soc Nephrol. 2002;13(Suppl 1):S78–83.
28. Vaslaki L, Karátson A, Vörös P, Major L, Pethö F, Ladányi E, Weber C, Mitteregger R, Falkenhagen D. Can sterile and pyrogen-free on-line substitution fluid be routinely delivered? A multicentric study on the microbiological safety of on-line haemodiafiltration. Nephrol Dial Transplant. 2000;15(Suppl 1):74–8.
29. Holt BG, White JJ, Kuthiala A, Fall P, Szerlip HM. Sustained low-efficiency daily dialysis with hemofiltration for acute kidney injury in the presence of sepsis. Clin Nephrol. 2008;69(1):40–6.
30. Darío J, Manuel G, Ana A, et al. Intermittent hemodialysis low intensity vs. on line Hemodiafiltration in critically ill patients with sepsis and acute kidney injury. Choosing the best treatment in a developing country. J Nephrol Ther. 2017;7:4–8.

# Peritoneal Dialysis in Critically Ill Children

# 20

Hui-Kim Yap and Lourdes Paula R. Resontoc

**Case**

A male infant was born full term via emergency cesarean section with a birth weight of 2.3 kg. Echocardiogram showed transposition of the great arteries with a hypoplastic interrupted aortic arch, large patent ductus arteriosus, and ventricular septal defect. His oxygen saturation ranged from 93 to 98%. On day 9 he underwent open-heart surgery. Postoperatively, he had persistent hypotension and frequent dysarryhthmias requiring continuous cardiac pacing, fluid boluses, blood products, and multiple inotropic support. He also developed pulmonary hypertension and was treated with inhaled nitric oxide. His condition remained critical and he developed pulmonary edema with oxygen saturation decreasing to 80% on postoperative day 30, requiring high ventilatory pressures. The next day he was noted to be progressively oliguric and edematous. Acute Peritoneal Dialysis (PD) was subsequently initiated. His clinical progress is shown in Fig. 20.1.

H.-K. Yap (✉) · L. P. R. Resontoc
Department of Paediatrics, Yong Loo Lin School of Medicine, National University of Singapore, Singapore, Singapore

Division of Paediatric Nephrology, Dialysis and Renal Transplantation, Khoo Teck Puat-National University Children's Medical Institute, National University Health System, Singapore, Singapore
e-mail: hui_kim_yap@nuhs.edu.sg



A. Deep, S. L. Goldstein (eds.), *Critical Care Nephrology and Renal Replacement Therapy in Children*, https://doi.org/10.1007/978-3-319-90281-4_20

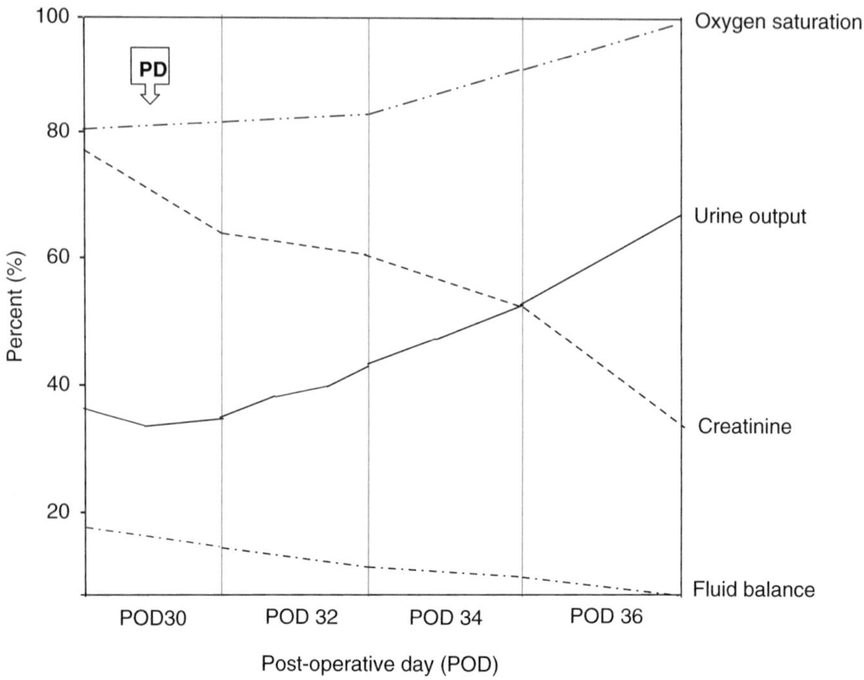


**Fig. 20.1** Clinical course showing clinical and laboratory improvement while on acute peritoneal dialysis

## 20.1 Introduction

With technological advances and the current availability of various forms of extracorporeal blood purification techniques, PD is becoming less popular in the management of critically ill infants and children. A survey among pediatric nephrologists in North America and Europe revealed the preferential use of continuous renal replacement therapies (CRRT) and intermittent hemodialysis (IHD) over PD as a form of renal replacement therapies (RRT) in the intensive care unit (ICU) [1]. Various improvements and refinements such as the development of machines with low circuit priming volume, miniaturized roller pumps, and accurate ultrafiltration control via calibrated scales, coupled with vascular catheters that can be used in the smallest of patients, have enabled CRRT to become the standard of care in many pediatric ICUs.

## 20.2 Indications and Limitations of PD in Critically Ill Children

In critically ill children where coagulopathy, difficult vascular access, cardiovascular and hemodynamic instability are common, acute PD is an option, especially when no other form of renal replacement therapy is available. Acute PD has been used extensively following cardiopulmonary bypass procedures among neonates [2]. A single-center study has reported that early initiation of PD in neonates and infants with acute kidney injury (AKI) following cardiac surgery is associated with significant decrease in mortality [3]. PD is also an important modality of dialysis in critically ill newborns weighing less than 1000 g [4–7].

In low-resource settings, acute PD is the most widely used modality, and is deemed safe, useful, and effective [8–10]. Compared with other modalities, PD requires less technological expertise, resource allocation, and is more cost-effective. Quick and safe access to PD allows for rapid institution of therapy. PD provides gradual, continuous solute and water clearance through diffusion and ultrafiltration obviating the complication of dialysis dysequilibrium, although the ability to separate these components is somewhat limited. Additionally, provision of glucose from the dialysate fluid is an advantage in infants who are prone to hypoglycemia when fluid is restricted.

PD is not the most efficient therapy for urgent fluid removal, rapid reversal of symptomatic hyperkalemia, clearance of dialyzable toxins and other higher molecular weight solutes. PD is therefore not suited for severe metabolic disturbances such as hyperammonemia except as an interim measure prior to transfer to a facility where HD or CRRT is available.

PD is contraindicated in patients with diaphragmatic defects, recent intra-abdominal surgery, intra-abdominal sepsis, lack of an adequate peritoneal surface, intra-abdominal malignancy, AKI secondary to HUS, and necrotizing enterocolitis [9]. Relative contraindications for PD include ventriculo-peritoneal shunts, prune belly syndrome, and previous abdominal surgeries. These situations may present some technical challenges for catheter placement as well as a higher risk of catheter dysfunction. PD may also be difficult in critically ill children on high-frequency oscillatory ventilation and in newborns with severe pulmonary disease where the respiratory status may worsen during the dialysis procedure [11].

## 20.3 Technical Considerations in Acute PD

A reliable PD access is crucial for effective PD. An important aspect of a good access is the selection of a reliable catheter type and the method of inserting the catheter, that is percutaneous or surgical (laparoscopy vs. laparotomy).

In the early days of acute PD, rigid peritoneal stylet catheters were widely used. These catheters are cheap and easy to insert, but the limited space of the peritoneal cavity poses a high risk of damage to the viscus. Several substitute catheters have been tried, including suction catheters, French 16 plastic catheters, G 14 or 16 IV cannulas, angiocaths, chest drains, JP drains, and nasogastric tubes [12–16]. However problems such as catheter dysfunction, poor dialysate flow, and pericatheter leaks may preclude successful dialysis in the critically ill child. Therefore the creation of an acute PD catheter that provides adequate inflow and outflow, absence of leakage, minimal catheter movement at exit site, and low incidence of catheter-related infections is imperative. An example would be the Cook Teflon non-cuffed flexible acute catheters (CTCs; Cook Inc., Bloomington, IN). This type of catheter offers the advantage of being able to be placed percutaneously at the bedside using the Seldinger technique under local anesthesia, and is a viable option in unstable patients [17]. Unfortunately, these catheters may leak after 5–7 days. On the other hand, the use of soft and flexible Tenckhoff catheters fabricated from silicone polymers of methylsilicate (Silastic®) with single or double Dacron cuffs (Quinton peritoneal catheters; Kendall Co, Mansfield, MA) will allow for placement longer than a week without leakage. Its subcutaneous or tunnelled placement, and the presence of one or two Dacron cuffs (DuPont, Wilmington, DE) reduces the risk of such complications as leakage, infection, and catheter migration [17]. Percutaneous insertion of the Tenckhoff catheter with a peel-away sheath allows for insertion in the unstable child in the pediatric intensive care unit.

Acute catheters can be inserted into the peritoneum centrally through the linea alba or paramedially through the rectus lateralis. The exit site should face downwards to reduce the risk of exit-site infection [18]. The direction of the catheter exit site is a special consideration for neonates, infants with stomas, and those with abdominal wall weakness. Presternal placement has been recommended in infants in order to avoid the diaper area, gastrostomy tubes, and vesicostomies [18, 19]. Another common problem following acute catheter insertion in children is catheter blockage by omentum. Partial omentectomy or omental tagging to epigastrium or lateral abdominal wall have been found to be beneficial to alleviate this problem, although these procedures are seldom performed in critically ill children who have other comorbidities, in particular coagulopathy [10]. A surgically inserted Tenckhoff catheter is therefore the current recommendation for initiation of acute PD in children [20].

Acute PD can be delivered manually or through an automated PD cycler. Manual exchange systems are gravity-based, and require a buretrol or a microset in neonates and small children for accurate measurement of inflow volumes, as well as a urometer for accurate measurement of outflow volumes (Fig. 20.2). Acute manual PD is

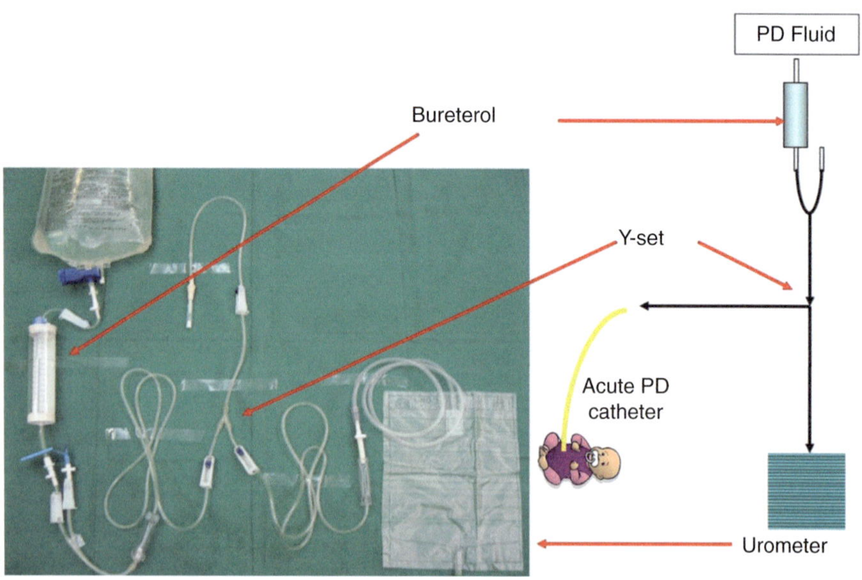


**Fig. 20.2** Components of the manual PD set

labor-intensive requiring constant supervision to ensure accurate delivery of dwell volume and measurement of net ultrafiltration. In comparison, the use of the automated device requires less manpower because the machines can be programmed to deliver the dialysis prescription. Automated PD cyclers however may not be feasible for use in neonates due to tubing "dead space" and unavailability of cyclers that allow for a very small fill volume.

## 20.4 Prescription

The elements of acute PD prescription include dialysate composition, fill volume, inflow and outflow times, dwell time, number of exchanges, dialysate additives, and volume of ultrafiltration.

### 20.4.1 Dialysate Composition

Commercially available PD solutions are defined by the osmolality, osmotic agent, buffer used, and electrolyte content. Solutions available in the market include the conventional dextrose-based solutions and the biocompatible PD solutions (Table 20.1). Solutions containing dextrose in varying concentrations to create an osmotic gradient to drive ultrafiltration and convective solute removal are commonly used. These solutions usually use lactate as buffer. The dextrose present in the dialysate can provide an extra source of carbohydrate nutrition and calories but it can also lead to hyperglycemia necessitating insulin administration [21–23]. Biocompatible PD solution has a neutral pH and lower content of glucose-degradation products. It has dual chambers within the bags to allow for separation of dextrose from the rest of the PD solution components in order to maintain the pH of the dextrose during heat sterilization to reduce the formation of glucose-degradation products (GDP). Use of biocompatible solutions with bicarbonate as buffer and lower lactate concentration in critically ill children with multiorgan failure and progressive lactic acidosis may be advantageous. In the absence of commercially prepared PD solutions, customized PD solutions can be prepared by

**Table 20.1** Composition of commercially available PD solutions

| | Dianeal® | Stay safe® | Physioneal® | Balance® |
|---|---|---|---|---|
| Sodium (mmol/L) | 132 | 132 | 132 | 134 |
| Chloride (mmol/L) | 95 | 102 | 95 | 100.5 |
| Calcium (mmol/L) | 1.25/1.75 | 3.5 | 1.25/1.75 | 1.25/1.75 |
| Magnesium (mmol/L) | 0.25 | 0.5/1.5 | 0.25 | 0.5 |
| Glucose (%) | 1.5/2.5/4.25 | 1.5/2.5/4.25 | 1.36/2.27/3.86 | 1.5/2.3/4.25 |
| Osmolarity (mOsm/L) | 344/395/483 | 347/398/486 | 344/395/483 | 356/399/509 |
| Lactate (mmol/L) | 40 | 35/40 | 15 | 35 |
| Bicarbonate (mmol/L) | 0 | 0 | 25 | 0 |
| pH | 5.5 | 5.5 | 7.0 | 7.0 |

hospital pharmacies to provide temporary renal replacement when there are no other options, although prescription errors pose a significant risk to patient safety. Other PD solutions such as icodextrin and amino acid-containing solutions have very little utility in the acute setting.

Patients requiring more rapid removal of fluid can be initiated using a PD solution containing 2.27–2.5% dextrose. However, in hemodynamically unstable patients and those with moderate fluid overload, a solution with 1.5% dextrose employing more frequent hourly exchanges may be more appropriate to achieve an ultrafiltration rate of up to 2 mL/kg/h. Dialysate solutions should be warmed to body temperature prior to infusion to avoid discomfort and to enhance solute transport.

### 20.4.2 Fill Volume

A low initial fill volume following insertion of the peritoneal catheter is required to minimize pericatheter dialysate leakage. The minimum allowable volume per exchange is 300 mL/m$^2$ for children and adolescents and 200 mL/m$^2$ (10 mL/kg) for infants. This volume can be slowly increased, observing for leakage and avoiding lung compression that can compromise ventilation. The maximum allowable volume per exchange for children and adolescents is about 1100 mL/m$^2$ and for infants 800 mL/m$^2$ (50 mL/kg) [20].

### 20.4.3 Dwell Time, Inflow and Outflow Times, and Number of Exchanges

Whereas prescription in chronic PD is guided by the results of peritoneal equilibration test (PET), PET-guided prescription in acute PD is not possible. The prescription should be individualized based on the patient's clinical status and underlying disease [20].

Inflow time is the time required to instill the dialysate into the peritoneal cavity. It usually lasts from 10 to 15 min. This is the shortest phase of the PD prescription and should be kept to a minimum to maximize the efficiency of the dialysis. This phase is dependent upon the volume of the dialysate, the height of the PD solution relative to the patient's abdomen as this process is driven by gravity (in cases where cycler is not available), the presence or absence of inflow resistance as determined by the size of the PD catheter, any kinking of the catheter or reduced bowel motility.

The dwell time is the period from end of the inflow to the beginning of the drain period. This is an important phase of acute PD, as it is a major determinant of the amount of ultrafiltration, solute clearance, and ultimately the patient's response to therapy. It usually lasts from 30 to 90 min, but shorter dwell times of 15–30 min have been recommended in smaller children and neonates, especially when low fill volumes are used in order to minimize glucose absorption that would limit ultrafiltration [15].

Outflow time is defined as the time required to drain the effluent from the peritoneal cavity. It is dependent on the dialysate volume to be drained, outflow resistance from the catheter, bowel motility, and the presence of fibrin. As the rate of fluid draining from the peritoneal cavity is gravity-dependent, the height difference between the patient and the drain bag must be considered. The outflow time is the rate-limiting step of the dialysis prescription, and times between 20 and 30 min are acceptable. If the outflow time is prolonged for more than 30 min, the dwell time and the number of exchanges per day affect the quality of fluid and solute removal. With the exception of tidal PD, complete drainage of the effluent at every cycle is important to prevent accumulation of dialysate in the peritoneal cavity, leading to abdominal discomfort and respiratory insufficiency.

The number of exchanges is dependent upon the requirement for solute and fluid removal, and usually ranges from 16 to 20 exchanges in a day with hourly dwell. In the presence of severe life-threatening hyperkalemia, shorter dwells of 15–30 min are useful at PD initiation for 5–10 cycles, until the serum potassium levels are lowered sufficiently. Reducing the dwell time in hypercatabolic patients increases dialysate flow, thus increasing the efficiency of solute clearance [24].

### 20.4.4 Additives

To prevent fibrin clot formation following acute catheter insertion, heparin at a dose of 250–1000 units per liter of dialysate should be added. If the effluent is very bloody initially, then in-out exchanges should be performed until the effluent is clearer. Intraperitoneal antibiotics should be prophylactically administered unless the child is already on appropriate systemic antibiotic cover. In order to maintain homeostasis in the critically ill child who is on continuous dialysis, electrolytes, in particular potassium (3–4 mmol/L), may need to be added to the dialysate.

### 20.4.5 Monitoring

Accurate monitoring of input and output and net ultrafiltration is an essential aspect of the acute PD prescription (Table 20.2). The following should be included in the recording: exchange number, dialysate glucose concentration, volume of exchange, medications added, amount of effluent obtained, if drained, appearance of effluent, and patient's weight. Blood glucose, electrolytes, blood urea nitrogen, and creatinine should be performed at least on a daily basis.

## 20.5 Strategies to Improve Dialysis Efficiency in Acute PD

The appropriate dose for acute PD in critically ill infant and children is poorly defined. Clinical parameters such as ability to wean off inotropes suggesting improvement in the hemodynamic status, resolution of edema indicating

**Table 20.2** Monitoring sheet for acute peritoneal dialysis

| Date/ time | Weight (kg) | PD fluid dextrose (%) | Number of exchanges | Fill volume (mL) | Dwell time | Ultrafiltrate volume (mL) | Appearance of effluent | Capillary blood glucose level | Additives |
|---|---|---|---|---|---|---|---|---|---|
| | | | | | | | | | |
| | | | | | | | | | |
| | | | | | | | | | |
| | | | | | | | | | |

improvement in volume overload, ultrafiltration adequate to provide sufficient nutrition without the risk of volume overload, and improvement in the metabolic parameters are, in principle, proof of efficient acute PD.

Urea kinetic modelling, which is used to define dialysis adequacy in end-stage renal disease (ESRD) and is expressed as a $Kt/V_{urea}$ measurement (urea clearance over time where: $K$ = volume of dialysate drained multiplied by dialysate/plasma urea concentration, $t$ = the duration of the dialysis, $V$ = the volume of distribution of urea), has not been validated for AKI. Interpretation of $Kt/V_{urea}$ in these patients is difficult as these critically ill infants and children are not in a steady state as they often have multiorgan failure with frequent changes in volume status, and are hypercatabolic. Most of the studies looking at dose of dialysis have been conducted in adult patients on hemodialysis [25, 26]. A large randomized controlled trial conducted by the Acute Renal Failure Trial Network comparing low dose (standardized $Kt/V_{urea}$ 2.1) versus high dose (standardized $Kt/V_{urea}$ 3.88) in adult patients with acute kidney injury on hemodialysis did not demonstrate any difference in mortality rate [26]. Therefore a minimum target of $Kt/V_{urea}$ of 2.1 has been proposed for adult patients with AKI [27]. Moreover, extrapolation from the chronic kidney failure setting has influenced recommendations for the acute setting and have been advanced by the International Society for Peritoneal Dialysis (ISPD) [28]. The recommended minimum target for small-solute clearance (e.g., urea) is a standardized weekly $Kt/V$ of 2.1 or 0.3 daily if performed 7 days/week [20]. An increase in the PD dose did not show any definite outcome advantage from the recommended minimum PD dose [29]. Due to the hypercatabolic state in critically ill children, the target for adequate solute clearance should be higher, unfortunately, there are currently no good studies examining this issue in children on acute PD. Studies have shown that a standard PD can provide $Kt/V_{urea}$ values of greater than 2.1 for most infants who underwent cardiac-bypass surgery [30].

Several techniques and modifications in the standard acute PD prescription have been employed to overcome the issues of inefficient solute clearance and inadequate ultrafiltration. The goal of acute dialysis, especially in the critically ill child with multiorgan failure, is to aim for maximum possible clearance with continuous exchanges to compensate for catabolic stress [9], and also to be able to achieve adequate ultrafiltration reliably, as mortality in these children has been associated with fluid overload [31, 32]. These strategies, adapted primarily from chronic PD prescriptions, include continuous equilibration PD (CEPD), tidal PD, high volume PD (HVPD), and continuous flow PD (CFPD) (Fig. 20.3). Tidal PD and continuous flow PD (CFPD) have been proven to increase acute PD efficiency.

### 20.5.1 Continuous Equilibration PD

CEPD involves the use of larger fill volumes of 40–45 mL/kg or 1200 mL/m$^2$ with longer dwells of 4–6 h by a cycler or manually, similar to but often more intensive than continuous ambulatory peritoneal dialysis [33]. This modality is associated with higher middle molecule clearance, although small molecule clearance is

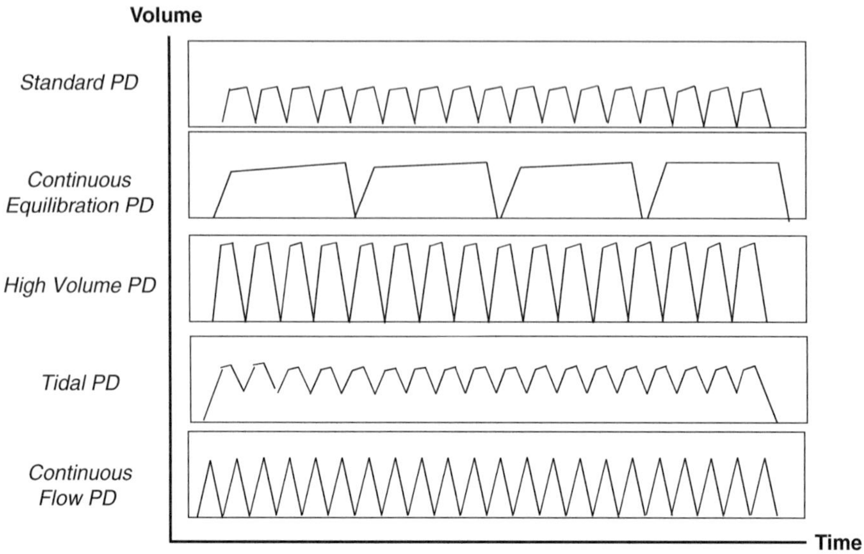


**Fig. 20.3** Strategies to improve PD efficiency

probably similar to acute intermittent PD. The limitation of CEPD is the possibility of leakage due to the higher fill volumes in the presence of a newly inserted peritoneal catheter, especially non-cuffed catheter.

## 20.5.2 High Volume PD

HVPD involves large fill volumes of 40–45 mL/kg or 1200 mL/m$^2$ with 18–24 frequent exchanges over a 24-h period in order to achieve high small solute clearances, but unfortunately does not address middle molecule clearance. HVPD has been shown to provide a dialysis dose approaching that of high dose continuous renal replacement therapies or daily hemodialysis in adults [34]. In both these modalities, metabolic control, infectious and mechanical complications, mortality rate, and renal function recovery were similar between HVPD and daily hemodialysis, whereas HVPD was associated with a significantly shorter time to the recovery of renal function. This is likely to be due to better cardiovascular tolerance with fewer episodes of hypotension and consequent renal ischemia compared to HD. Again, because of the high peritoneal fill volumes involved, this predisposes to leakage especially with immediate dialysis following peritoneal catheter insertion.

## 20.5.3 Tidal Peritoneal Dialysis

Tidal PD involves leaving a large volume of dialysis solution (at least 30% of the fill volume) in the peritoneal cavity throughout the dialysis session in order to optimize solute clearance. Tidal PD always employs the use of a cycler. An initial infusion of dialysis solution into the peritoneal cavity is followed by only partial drainage (usually 10–70%) of the peritoneal volume during each exchange. As a result, an intra-abdominal volume of dialysate is retained at the end of each exchange, and the constant contact between dialysis solution and the peritoneal membrane contributes to the increase in dialysis efficiency. The partial drain volumes are replaced by fresh dialysate to restore the initial intra-infusion volume with each cycle. By increasing the number of tidal volumes, small solute clearance can be increased, and because of the longer duration of contact between dialysate and peritoneum, dialysis efficiency is improved further in terms of middle molecule clearance. In a study among adults in hypercatabolic state, more efficient clearance of small molecules was observed in Tidal PD than in CEPD. Tidal PD was also found to be superior to CEPD in the removal of potassium, phosphates and in generating ultrafiltrate, in part related to the lesser degree of dextrose absorption [35, 36]. Although there are no studies in critically ill children, the smaller volumes required makes Tidal PD an attractive option.

### 20.5.4 Continuous Flow Peritoneal Dialysis (CFPD)

With the limited capacity of the current acute PD prescription, there is renewed interest for CFPD which, more than 50 years ago, has been shown to be more efficient than the standard PD prescription [37]. CFPD is a modality that combines PD with HD technology in which continuous circulation of PD fluid is maintained at a high flow rate (Fig. 20.4a). The peritoneal fluid effluent is transported to a twin coil dialyzer, dialyzed, regenerated, and sent back to the second catheter [37]. In addition, gravity-assisted CFPD with no fixed intraperitoneal volume has also been described [38] (Fig. 20.4b).

CFPD uses a fixed intraperitoneal volume and fast, synchronized continuous movement of dialysate into and out of the peritoneal cavity at a high flow rate up to 100–300 mL/min corrected for body surface area. The dialysate fluid from commercially available bags can be delivered using an adapted continuous venovenous hemofiltration machine (single-pass CFPD). The sterile dialysate could also be regenerated using an external dialyzer [39].

For peritoneal access, two peritoneal catheters, one for inflow and the other for outflow of dialysate, are required, the first is placed in the midline 1 cm below the umbilicus and oriented towards the pelvis, while the second is placed midway between the superior iliac crest and umbilicus oriented towards the diaphragm (Fig. 20.5) [40]. Ideally, the pelvic catheter should have a coiled tip and a preformed bend to produce an exit site below the insertion site. For minimal recirculation or streaming, the orientation of the catheter tip should be placed as far apart from each other as possible. An efficient dual lumen catheter with minimal intraperitoneal recirculation can also be used.

In children admitted to the intensive care unit with acute kidney injury, CFPD has been shown to be ninefold more effective than conventional PD for ultrafiltration and at least three- to fivefold more effective for urea and creatinine clearance [40, 41]. Because the PD solution is delivered continuously, there is less glucose

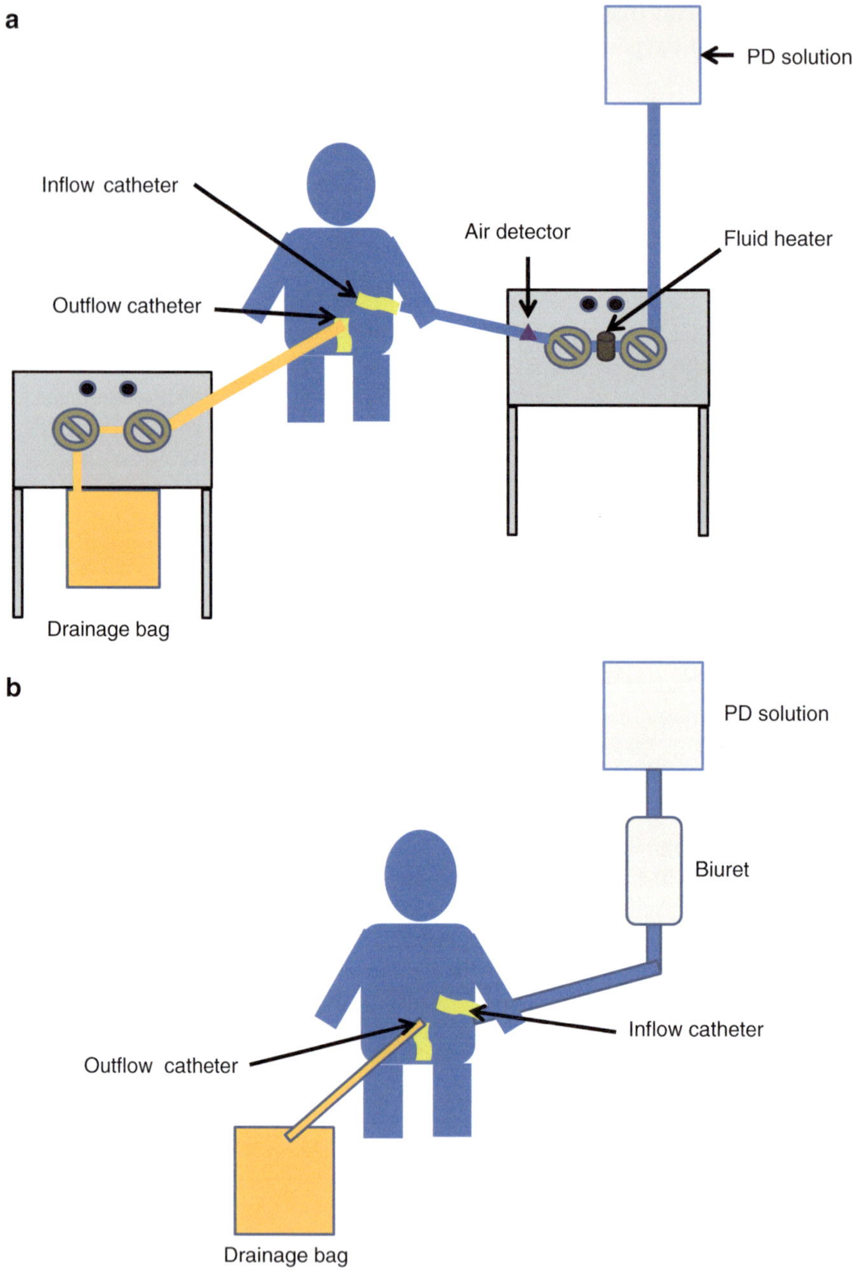


**Fig. 20.4** (**a**) A CFPD circuit that combines PD and HD technology. (**b**) Gravity-assisted CFPD

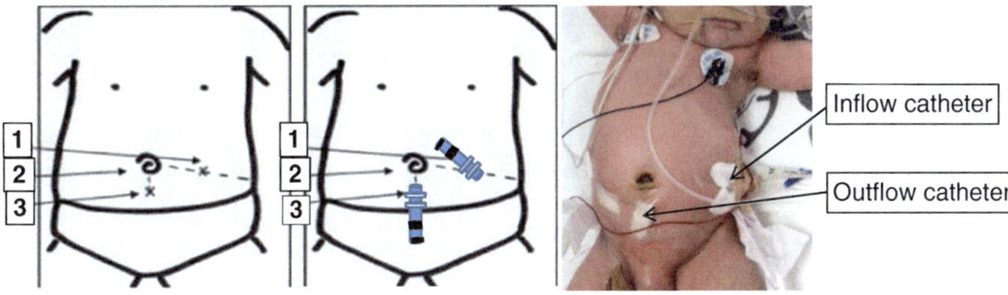


**Fig. 20.5** Catheter placement for CFPD. (1) Lateral catheter (dedicated to inflow). (2) Umbilicus. (3) Midline catheter (dedicated to outflow)

absorption and perhaps less GDP exposure. It also provides higher solute clearance and ultrafiltration rates than the standard regimens due to maintenance of the highest possible plasma to dialysate concentration and minimal exchanges during the procedure, both of which maximize the dialysis time. On the other hand, it can lead to excessive protein losses, and hypernatremia, because of continued glucose gradient and sodium sieving. Other drawbacks of this technique include increased intra-abdominal pressure especially if ultrafiltration and intraperitoneal fluid volume is not well monitored.

## 20.6 Complications

### 20.6.1 Noninfectious Complications

Mechanical complications as a result of increased intraperitoneal pressure include hernias, leaks (hydrothorax or pleuroperitoneal leaks), local edema, and back pain. Increasing abdominal girth, weight gain in the absence of generalized edema with decreased peritoneal fluid drainage volume, scrotal, labial or pericatheter swelling are clues to the diagnosis of local edema due to seepage of peritoneal fluid. CT scan with PD fluid-contrast materials infused in the abdomen or radioisotope scintigraphy may be useful in diagnosing local tissue edema resulting from PD fluid leak.

Malfunction of the PD catheter can present as inflow, outflow, or a "two-way" obstruction. Inflow obstruction may be due to mechanical blockage such as clamps or kinks in transfer set, tubing or catheter, including the segment under the dressing [14, 16]. Outflow obstruction may be due to mechanical blockage of transfer set or catheter, constipation, extrinsic bladder compression due to urinary retention, catheter tip migration out of pelvis and catheter entrapment by an omental wrap, epiploic appendices of colon, fallopian tubes or adhesions [14, 16]. "Two-way" obstruction is a potentially serious complication of PD. It can be due to intraluminal obstruction (by fibrin strands or blood clots) and extraluminal obstruction (by omental wrapping or adhesions) [14, 16]. The first step in the treatment of mechanical obstruction is to ascertain the cause. A radiograph of the abdomen to visualize the catheter position should be performed. In certain conditions, a lateral view may be necessary to identify a subcutaneous and intraperitoneal catheter kink. The next step is done in a noninvasive or conservative manner which includes elimination of kinks or removing clamps on transfer set, tubing and catheter. If the obstruction is due to intraluminal or extraluminal blockage by an omental wrap, epiploic appendices of colon, fallopian tubes or adhesions, the block can be dislodged by injecting dialysate or normal saline through the catheter using a 50 mL syringe under moderate pressure in a "push and pull" maneuver. The procedure is discontinued if the patient complains of pain or cramping. If the obstruction is due to constipation, measures to correct the constipation should be undertaken. In case of fibrin-related obstruction, heparin (500–1000 U/L), urokinase (5000–10,000 IU in equal volume of normal saline) or recombinant tissue plasminogen activator (tPA) (1–8 mg in equal amount of sterile water in a concentration of 1 mg/mL) is added to each dialysate exchange [14]. If noninvasive measures fail to resolve the obstruction, surgical readjustment or a catheter change may be necessary.

### 20.6.2 Infectious Complications

PD-related infections include catheter exit-site or tunnel infections and peritonitis. The most common organisms implicated in exit-site or tunnel infection are *Staphylococcus aureus* and *Pseudomonas aeruginosa*. PD-related peritonitis is the second most common infectious complication of PD. Measures to prevent peritonitis include the use of prophylactic antibiotics at the time of catheter placement and proper hand hygiene. Peritonitis should be considered in a patient presenting with cloudy peritoneal effluent, with or without fever and abdominal pain. An effluent WBC >100/mL with at least 50% polymorphonuclear leukocytes is presumptive of the diagnosis, and should be treated empirically with antibiotics, until antibiotic sensitivity patterns are available [18]. Current pediatric guidelines recommend the use of either intraperitoneal cefipime monotherapy or a first generation cephalosporin such as cefazolin combined with ceftazidime or an aminoglycoside as empiric therapy [18]. In centers where the rate of methicillin resistant *Staphylococcus aureus* exceeds 10%, the addition of an intraperitoneal glycopeptide to cefepime or ceftazidime is recommended.

**Conclusion**

Despite the ready availability of extracorporeal modalities of continuous renal replacement therapies in many pediatric intensive care units today, PD still has a role in the treatment of critically ill children, especially those with cardiovascular instability as it provides gradual solute clearance and ultrafiltration. There are still many centers especially in resource-poor countries where CRRT is not available and PD still forms the mainstay of renal support in these children. In the absence of clear evidence-based guidelines as to the modality that best impacts patient outcomes, local expertise and resources will often dictate choice of dialytic modality in these patients. Innovative strategies to improve dialysis efficiency in critically ill children with lactic acidosis and severe fluid overload will still need to be evaluated to determine their applicability in the different clinical settings. There is a need for multi-center randomized controlled trials comparing PD with other modalities of acute dialysis in patients with similar stages of acute kidney injury, stratified according to their clinical severity [9].

**Key Learning Points**

- Peritoneal dialysis is safe and useful for critically ill infants and children with cardiac and hemodynamic instability, newborns less than 1000 g with difficult vascular access and in low-resource settings.
- Reliable access is crucial for the success of PD. Current guidelines recommend surgical insertion of a Tenckhoff catheter.
- Appropriate dose and dialysis adequacy based on urea kinetic modelling ($Kt/V_{urea}$) is poorly defined in acute PD.
- HVPD, CEPD, Tidal PD, and CFPD can overcome the traditional limitations of the standard PD prescription.
- Mechanical complications and infections are common complications of acute PD.

## References


1. Warady BA, Bunchman T. Dialysis therapy for children with acute renal failure: survey results. Pediatr Nephrol. 2000;15(1–2):11–3.
2. Kwiatkowski DM, Menon S, Krawczeski CD, Goldstein SL, Morales DL, Phillips A, et al. Improved outcomes with peritoneal dialysis catheter placement after cardiopulmonary bypass in infants. J Thorac Cardiovasc Surg. 2015;149(1):230–6.
3. Bojan M, Gioanni S, Vouhe PR, Journois D, Pouard P. Early initiation of peritoneal dialysis in neonates and infants with acute kidney injury following cardiac surgery is associated with a significant decrease in mortality. Kidney Int. 2012;82(4):474–81.
4. Alparslan C, Yavascan O, Bal A, Kanik A, Kose E, Demir BK, et al. The performance of acute peritoneal dialysis treatment in neonatal period. Ren Fail. 2012;34(8):1015–20.
5. Rainey KE, DiGeronimo RJ, Pascual-Baralt J. Successful long-term peritoneal dialysis in a very low birth weight infant with renal failure secondary to feto-fetal transfusion syndrome. Pediatrics. 2000;2000:106.
6. Yokoyama S, Nukada T, Ikeda Y, Hara S, Yoshida A. Successful peritoneal dialysis using a percutaneous tube for peritoneal drainage in an extremely low birth weight infant: a case report. Surg Case Rep. 2017;3(1):115.
7. Yu JE, Park MS, Pai KS. Acute peritoneal dialysis in very low birth weight neonates using a vascular catheter. Pediatr Nephrol. 2010;25(2):367–71.
8. Goldstein SL. Overview of pediatric renal replacement therapy in acute renal failure. Artif Organs. 2003;27(9):781–5.
9. Walters S, Porter C, Brophy PD. Dialysis and pediatric acute kidney injury: choice of renal support modality. Pediatr Nephrol. 2009;24(1):37–48.
10. Flynn JT. Choice of dialysis modality for management of pediatric acute renal failure. Pediatr Nephrol. 2002;17:61.

11. Mahale AS, Katyal A, Khanna R. Complications of peritoneal dialysis related to increased intra-abdominal pressure. Adv Perit Dial. 2003;19:130–5.
12. Rath B, Gopalan S, Gupta S, Puri RK, Talukdar B. Simpler tools for peritoneal dialysis of term newborns and young infants. Indian Pediatr. 1994;31(9):1131–2.
13. Segar WE, Gibson RK, Rhamy R. Peritoneal dialysis in infants and small children. Pediatrics. 1961;27:603–13.
14. Steele BT, Vigneux A, Blatz S, Flavin M, Paes B. Acute peritoneal dialysis in infants weighing less than 1500 g. J Pediatr. 1987;110(1):126–9.
15. Swan H and Gordon HH. Peritoneal lavage in the treatment of anuria in children. Pediatrics. 1949;4.
16. Mizrahia SBM, Lunskia I. Simple technique for bedside peritoneal dialysis in neonates. Nephron. 1988;48(3):258.
17. Auron A, Warady BA, Simon S, Blowey DL, Srivastava T, Musharaf G, et al. Use of the multipurpose drainage catheter for the provision of acute peritoneal dialysis in infants and children. Am J Kidney Dis. 2007;49(5):650–5.
18. Warady BA, Bakkaloglu S, Newland J, Cantwell M, Verrina E, Neu A, et al. Consensus guidelines for the prevention and treatment of catheter-related infections and peritonitis in pediatric patients receiving peritoneal dialysis: 2012 update. Perit Dial Int. 2012;32(Suppl 2):S32–86.
19. Warchol S, Roszkowska-Blaim M, Latoszynska J, Jarmolinski T, Zachwieja J. Experience using presternal catheter for peritoneal dialysis in Poland: a multicenter pediatric survey. Perit Dial Int. 2003;23:242.
20. Cullis B, Abdelraheem M, Abrahams G, Balbi A, Cruz DN, Frishberg Y, et al. Peritoneal dialysis for acute kidney injury. Perit Dial Int. 2014;34(5):494–517.
21. Grodstein GP, Blumenkrantz MJ, Kopple JD, Moran JK, Coburn JW. Glucose absorption during continuous ambulatory peritoneal dialysis. Kidney Int. 1981;19(4):564–7.
22. Podel J, Hodelin-Wetzel R, Saha DC, Burns G. Glucose absorption in acute peritoneal dialysis. J Ren Nutr. 2000;10(2):93–7.
23. Reznik VM, Griswold WR, Peterson BM, Rodarte A, Ferris ME, Mendoza SA. Peritoneal dialysis for acute renal failure in children. Pediatr Nephrol. 1991;5(6):715–7.
24. Vasudevan A, Phadke K, Yap HK. Peritoneal dialysis for the management of pediatric patients with acute kidney injury. Pediatr Nephrol. 2017;32(7):1145–56.
25. Kellum JA. Renal replacement therapy in critically ill patients with acute renal failure: does a greater dose improve survival? Nat Clin Pract Nephrol. 2007;3(3):128–9.
26. VA/NIH Acute Renal Failure Trial Network, Palevsky PM, Zhang JH, O'Connor TZ, Chertow GM, Crowley ST, Choudhury D, Finkel K, Kellum JA, Paganini E, Schein RM, Smith MW, Swanson KM, Thompson BT, Vijayan A, Watnick S, Star RA, Peduzzi P. Intensity of renal support in critically ill patients with acute kidney injury. N Engl J Med. 2008;359(1):7.
27. Paganini EP, Tapolyai M, Goormastic M, Halstenberg W, Kozlowski L, Leblanc M, Lee JC, Moreno L, Sakai K. Establishing a dialysis therapy/patient outcome link in intensive care unit acute dialysis for patients with acute renal failure.
28. Chionh CY, Ronco C, Finkelstein FO, Soni SS, Cruz DN. Acute peritoneal dialysis: what is the 'adequate' dose for acute kidney injury? Nephrol Dial Transplant. 2010;25(10):3155–60.
29. Parapiboon W, Jamratpan T. Intensive versus minimal standard dosage for peritoneal dialysis in acute kidney injury: a randomized pilot study. Perit Dial Int. 2017;37(5):523–8.
30. McNiece KL, Ellis EE, Drummond-Webb JJ, Fontenot EE, O'Grady CM, Blaszak RT. Adequacy of peritoneal dialysis in children following cardiopulmonary bypass surgery. Pediatr Nephrol. 2005;20(7):972–6.
31. Sutherland SM, Zappitelli M, Alexander SR, Chua AN, Brophy PD, Bunchman TE, et al. Fluid overload and mortality in children receiving continuous renal replacement therapy: the prospective pediatric continuous renal replacement therapy registry. Am J Kidney Dis. 2010;55(2):316–25.
32. Goldstein SL, Somers MJ, Baum MA, Symons JM, Brophy PD, Blowey D, et al. Pediatric patients with multi-organ dysfunction syndrome receiving continuous renal replacement therapy. Kidney Int. 2005;67(2):653–8.

33. Passadakis PS, Oreopoulos DG. Peritoneal dialysis in patients with acute renal failure. Adv Perit Dial. 2007;23:7–16.
34. Gabriel DP, Caramori JT, Martim LC, Barretti P, Balbi AL. High volume peritoneal dialysis vs daily hemodialysis: a randomized, controlled trial in patients with acute kidney injury. Kidney Int Suppl. 2008;108:S87–93.
35. Jiang L, Zeng R, Yang K, Mi DH, Tian JH, Ma B, et al. Tidal versus other forms of peritoneal dialysis for acute kidney injury. Cochrane Database Syst Rev. 2012;6:CD007016.
36. Chitalia VC, Almeida AF, Rai H, Bapat M, Chitalia KV, Acharya VN, et al. Is peritoneal dialysis adequate for hypercatabolic acute renal failure in developing countries? Kidney Int. 2002;61(2):747–57.
37. Shinaberger JH, Shear L, Barry KG. Increasing efficiency of peritoneal dialysis: experience with peritoneal-extracorporeal recirculation dialysis. Trans Am Soc Artif Intern Organs. 1965;11:76–82.
38. Sagy M, Silver P. Continuous flow peritoneal dialysis as a method to treat severe anasarca in children with acute respiratory distress syndrome. Crit Care Med. 1999;27(11):2532.
39. Diaz-Buxo JA. Evolution of continuous flow peritoneal dialysis and the current state of the art. Semin Dial. 2001;15(5):373.
40. Nourse P, Sinclair G, Gajjar P, du Plessis M, Argent AC. Continuous flow peritoneal dialysis (CFPD) improves ultrafiltration in children with acute kidney injury on conventional PD using a 4.25% dextrose solution. Pediatr Nephrol. 2016;31(7):1137–43.
41. Raaijmakers R, Schroder CH, Gajjar P, Argent A, Nourse P. Continuous flow peritoneal dialysis: first experience in children with acute renal failure. Clin J Am Soc Nephrol. 2011;6(2):311–8.

# Plasmapheresis and Total Plasma Exchange in the PICU

21

Stuart L. Goldstein

**Case Presentation**

A 5-year-old male presents to a tertiary medical center emergency department following a 20 min generalized tonic-clonic seizure. In the ED, he was found to be afebrile, have a heart rate of 86/min, a respiratory rate of 32/min and a blood pressure of 160/100 mmHg. The boy had a 7-day history of painless gross hematuria that was described as "cola-colored." His primary pediatrician was concerned about a urinary tract infection, obtained a clean catch urine culture and initiated trimethoprim-sulfamethoxazole empirically. Past medical history was negative for trauma or recent infections. His family history was also negative for relevant kidney disease including chronic kidney disease, end-stage kidney disease, and nephrolithiasis.

In the ED, the patient was postictal, and was assessed to be pale with periorbital edema and 3+ edema to the pretibial level. The remainder of the physical examination was unremarkable, with relevant negative findings for skin rashes, purpura, petechiae, or joint swelling. Laboratory findings included the following: white blood cell count 15,500 per mcL, hemoglobin 9.8 g/dL, hematocrit 31%, platelet count 175,000 per mcL, serum sodium 134 meq/L, potassium 5.4 meq/L, chloride 105 meq/L, total carbon dioxide 19 meq/L, blood urea nitrogen 75 mg/dL, serum creatinine 1.9 mg/dL, glucose 254 mg/dL, calcium 8.9 mg/dL, phosphorus 5.7 mg/dL, and serum albumin 2.8 g/dL.

S. L. Goldstein
Center for Acute Care Nephrology, Cincinnati Children's Hospital Medical Center, Cincinnati, OH, USA

Pheresis Service, Cincinnati Children's Hospital Medical Center, Cincinnati, OH, USA
e-mail: stuart.goldstein@cchmc.org



A. Deep, S. L. Goldstein (eds.), *Critical Care Nephrology and Renal Replacement Therapy in Children*, https://doi.org/10.1007/978-3-319-90281-4_21

He was transferred to the intensive care unit where he was started on a continuous infusion of nicardipine and twice daily intermittent furosemide with a resultant improvement in blood pressure to 125/85 and urine output of 1.5 L over the first day of admission. On ICU day 2, his serum creatinine had increased to 2.9 mg/dL. He then received an empiric pulse dose of methylprednisolone, and a renal biopsy with the initial light microscopy reading of 50% of the glomeruli containing cellular crescents. The immunofluorescence and electron microscopy results won't be available until the next day. That evening, he develops hemoptysis, worsening respiratory status requiring intubation and invasive mechanical ventilation. His hemoglobin decreases to 5.4 g/dL, necessitating pack red blood cell transfusion. You are called to evaluate for the indications for therapeutic plasma exchange (TPE) and provide recommendations regarding the TPE prescription and course.

## 21.1 Introduction

The term "apheresis" is derived from a Greek word meaning "removal." In its most general sense, apheresis refers to techniques for large-scale removal of selected components of the blood. "Plasmapheresis" refers to removal of plasma, "erythrocytapheresis" to removal of red blood cells, and "leukapheresis" to removal of white blood cells. This chapter will focus solely on plasmapheresis therapeutic procedures.

The rationale for provision of therapeutic apheresis in children is challenged by the lack of studies with adequate sample size or design to make evidence-based inferences regarding benefit. Nearly all pediatric apheresis applications and protocols are extrapolated from adult patient studies, which are limited by sample size as well [1]. In addition, the critically ill child develops his or her maximal number of failed organs and illness severity very rapidly compared to adult patients [2–4]. As a result, aggressive intervention is often chosen to provide maximal support early [5] without the benefit of confirmatory tests or conservative management to determine if the underlying disease will remit spontaneously, since diseases which may be amenable to apheresis have rapid and often catastrophic consequences.

Provision of apheresis procedures to children is also challenged by a number of technical considerations. Apheresis is feasible regardless of the size of the child, as long as adequate vascular access can be established. However, apheresis procedures in young children must be customized to the situation and to the size of the patient since apheresis equipment and the software that controls it are, in general, designed for use in adults. The aim of this chapter is to describe the technical pediatric specific considerations and typical indications for apheresis provision for children seen in the pediatric intensive care unit setting.

## 21.2 Automated Apheresis Technology

### 21.2.1 Principle of Separation

Since apheresis technology is based on the use of automated cell separators, it is helpful to understand how these instruments work. The basic task of automated cell separators is to separate red blood cells, buffy coat, and plasma while maintaining sterility such that one or more of the components can be returned to the patient. In most instruments, this separation is accomplished by mechanical centrifugation. It is also possible to separate plasma from cells by filtration across a membrane, but these machines can only be used for plasmapheresis [6]. Centrifugal devices separate whole blood into components on the basis of density differences, while membrane separators work on the basis of differences in particle size.

### 21.2.2 Quantification of Removal

Plasmapheresis is the most commonly indicated apheresis treatment in the pediatric intensive care unit. The general rationale for plasmapheresis is to remove soluble substances in the plasma that might play a role in the patient's disease process, for example, the pathogenic anti-glomerular basement membrane antibody in patients with anti-glomerular basement membrane antibody (Goodpasture) syndrome. As plasma is removed from the patient, a replacement fluid must be given to maintain intravascular volume and oncotic pressure, which becomes admixed with the patient's plasma, and some of it is subsequently removed as the plasmapheresis proceeds. At the start of a plasmapheresis, most of what is removed is the patient's plasma, whereas at the end of the plasmapheresis, much of what is removed is replacement fluid. The amount of plasma removed (expressed as multiples of the patient's plasma volume) in a plasmapheresis treatment is related to the fraction of the original plasma remaining in the patient [7]. A plasmapheresis procedure that removes a volume equal to the patient's plasma volume (a "1.0 Volume Exchange") will achieve about 63% removal of the original plasma, with 37% remaining in the patient. Removal of twice the patient's plasma volume will remove 86% of the original plasma. Thus, it is apparent that the additional benefit of prolonging a plasmapheresis past two volumes is marginal. Finally, the overall efficiency of a single plasmapheresis procedure or of a series of treatments is also affected by the distribution between intra- and extravascular compartments of the targeted substance and on other metabolic characteristics such as rate of resynthesis and degradation [7].

### 21.2.3 Anticoagulation

An anticoagulant must be added to the blood as it enters the extracorporeal circuit in order to prevent clotting in the machine's tubing. Sodium citrate is the most commonly used anticoagulant for apheresis. Sodium citrate chelates calcium to prevent in vitro activation of the clotting cascade. When infused into the patient, the citrate may cause transient hypocalcemia in the patient. The severity of this side effect depends on the rate of citrate infusion, the capacity for hepatic metabolism of citrate, and the patient's state of calcium homeostasis (i.e., baseline hypocalcemia or hypoparathyroidism). In many apheresis protocols, the rate of citrate infusion to the patient is the limiting safety factor in determining how rapidly blood can be drawn and returned, and ultimately how long the procedure will last.

The symptoms of reduced ionized calcium related to citrate [8] are usually referred to as "citrate toxicity" or "citrate lock." The mildest and most common symptoms are peri-oral or hand and foot tingling and paresthesias. Some patients experience nausea, an unusual taste in the mouth or lightheadedness. More severe hypocalcemia may lead to tremors, twitching, muscular spasm, tetany, seizures, arrhythmias, and hypotension related to myocardial dysfunction [9–11]. In the intensive care unit setting, patients undergoing apheresis should be monitored for early signs of citrate toxicity by measurement of ionized calcium levels. In small children or sedated or unconscious patients, frequent vital sign measurement including blood pressure and EKG monitoring are necessary. Prevention of hypocalcemia can also be achieved using a regional anticoagulation protocol, adapted from continuous renal replacement therapy protocols [12], in which a calcium chloride (8 g per 1 L of normal saline) is infused in the return line at 1.5–2 times the blood pump rate in ml/hour. For example, if the blood pump rate is 60 mL/min, the calcium chloride rate would be 90 mL/h. In general, mild symptoms can be relieved by reducing the rate of citrate infusion or by stopping the procedure temporarily until symptoms subside.

## 21.3 The Plasmapheresis Procedure

### 21.3.1 Plasmapheresis

Plasmapheresis involves separation of the plasma from the cellular elements of blood, collecting the patient's plasma into a waste bag, and returning to the patient his own cells mixed with a fluid to replace the discarded plasma. The replacement fluid must contain colloid to maintain the patient's intravascular oncotic pressure. When 5% albumin is used as the only replacement fluid, the plasmapheresis procedure can be performed with minimal concern for transfusion-transmitted infectious disease or transfusion-associated acute lung injury (TRALI) [13]. Removal of plasma and replacement with 5% albumin will result in depletion of most plasma proteins including immunoglobulins and the components of the coagulation cascade. Plasmapheresis of one plasma volume will reduce the levels of coagulation proteins by about 63%, which can be associated with a fibrinogen level below 100 mg/dl and prolongation of the PT and aPPT but not usually with clinical bleeding. If the rate of hepatic regeneration of these lost coagulation factors is normal, a schedule of plasmapheresis procedures every other day generally does not require exogenous replacement with fresh frozen plasma (FFP). However, if daily plasmapheresis is necessary or if the patient has a concomitant coagulopathy, the replacement fluids must include FFP. If the pre-plasmapheresis fibrinogen level is less than 100 mg/dL, FFP should also be included as part of the replacement fluids. If FFP is used as the replacement fluid, the patient's plasma proteins and coagulation parameters will remain within normal limits.

## 21.4 Technical Pediatric Issues

Use of apheresis in children is feasible regardless of the size of the patient, as long as an adequate vascular access can be established. However, apheresis procedures in young children must be customized to the situation and to the size of the patient because apheresis equipment and the software that controls it are, in general, designed for use in adults.

### 21.4.1 Access

Successful pheresis provision depends on a well-functioning venous access. The access for drawing blood into the cell separator is the most critical, and critically ill children will usually require a double lumen venous catheter designed for hemodialysis to permit adequate flow of 2 mL/kg/min; Table 21.1 provides a guide to match access and patient size [14]. The softer single and double lumen catheters, such as the Broviac™ catheter, commonly used in oncology patients and in intensive care units, are not suitable for apheresis procedures. It is preferable to draw from the proximal ports and reinfuse at the distal point to minimize recirculation although in practice the better functioning port is usually chosen for the drawing access. The length, gauge, and positioning of the tip of the catheter will depend on the child's size. However, the wall of the catheter must be resilient enough to withstand the negative pressure generated during the apheresis procedure.

### 21.4.2 Volume

Extracorporeal volume is the most important consideration in adapting apheresis instruments designed for adults to use in children. The extracorporeal volume ECV for cell separators in clinical use varies from 200 to 400 mL depending on the

**Table 21.1** Patient and catheter size guide

| Patient size | Catheter size |
|---|---|
| NEONATE | Dual-lumen 7.0 French |
| 3–6 kg | Dual-lumen 7.0 French |
| 6–12 kg | Dual-lumen 8.0 French |
| >12–20 kg | Dual-lumen 9.0 French |
| >20–30 kg | Dual-lumen 10.0 French |
| >30 kg | Triple-lumen 11 or 12 French |

machine and the procedure to be performed. Unless specific measures are taken to compensate for this volume, the patient's blood volume will be depleted by this amount during the apheresis procedure. While an adult may easily tolerate the temporary loss of 200–400 mL of whole blood, this ECV may be too much for a small child. As a general guideline, modification of the procedure in the interest of patient safety is required if the ECV exceeds 15% of the patient's total blood volume (TBV) and should be considered if the ECV exceeds 10% of the TBV.

The ECV for an apheresis procedure is a fixed specification of the instrument and tubing, and can be determined precisely. The patient's TBV, however, must be estimated in order to plan the apheresis procedure. The TBV estimate is a basic parameter for the algorithms that control the pumps on an automated apheresis instrument. The traditional formula used by most pediatricians to estimate TBV is 70–75 cc/kg. More complex, empirically derived formulae [15] for blood volume estimation that take into account gender, weight and height are available. These formulae are programmed into the software of some automated apheresis instruments, while these formulae may be more accurate than a weight-based TBV estimate in adults, they may yield overestimates of TBV in children, especially prepubertal males.

### 21.4.3 Blood Priming

In addition to the ECV, there is an obligate extra-circulatory red cell mass (ECRCM), a volume of packed red blood cells which must be held in the apheresis instrument in order to achieve the separation of plasma from red cells. Two decisions arise with respect to this ECRCM. First, can the patient tolerate the temporary loss of this red cell mass during the procedure? The answer to this question depends not only on the patient's total blood volume, but also on the patient's hematocrit and cardiovascular and pulmonary reserve. Second, can the patient tolerate the bolus of fluid which is associated with returning the red cells, or "rinsing back" the red cells from the machine to the patient at the end of the apheresis procedure? The answer to this question also depends on a clinical assessment of the patient's blood volume cardiopulmonary reserve and kidney function.

The procedure modifications that compensate for the ECV and ECRCM for young children undergoing apheresis are often referred to as "priming." While it is possible to prime the apheresis instrument by filling all of the tubing with red blood cells at a predetermined hematocrit before starting, priming is usually accomplished by infusing additional red cells or fluids at the start of the procedure during the time that the machine is filling with blood from the patient. With proper planning, it is possible to perform an apheresis procedure in a small child with no change in the patient's blood volume or red cell mass during the procedure.

In general, the method of priming for an apheresis procedure affects the patient's blood volume during the procedure and also the final amount of fluid administered at the end of the procedure. The patient's ability to tolerate volume depletion, loss of red cell mass, and volume overload must be assessed as part of the planning before the procedure is started. For children weighing <20 kg or for patients who are anemic or hemodynamicaly unstable, red cell priming is usually indicated.

### 21.4.4 Hypothermia

Children and adults experience some degree of hypothermia during apheresis procedures because of cooling of blood in the extracorporeal circuit. This side effect may be more pronounced in younger children since the flow rate per kilogram is higher than for adults, as discussed above. A blood warmer is commonly incorporated into the return line in most pediatric apheresis procedures. Depending on the model used, the warmer increases the ECV by 20–50 cc.

## 21.5 Disease Specific Indications

The evidence that demonstrates the clinical efficacy of apheresis-based treatments is compelling in some disease states and marginal in others. For this reason, the Journal of Clinical Apheresis has published, most recently in 2016 [1], a categorized listing of the indications for therapeutic apheresis. The indications are placed into one of four categories, as shown in Table 21.2, based on the strength of evidence that therapeutic apheresis is effective for that disease process. Although this system of categories is imperfect, it is helpful in guiding clinical decisions about the use of apheresis. When therapeutic apheresis is applied to diseases seen in the ICU either plasmapheresis or plasma exchange is most commonly indicated. The pediatric critical care nephrology diseases for which therapeutic apheresis may be indicated are shown in Table 21.3, along with commonly used treatment schedules. Of course, these schedules must be individualized based on the patient's clinical condition. It is important to establish at the start of a course of apheresis how the success or failure of the therapy will be monitored and judged. This is often difficult to determine with certainty, because many diseases do not have a discrete identifiable marker to follow clinical response to treatment.

**Table 21.2** Indication categories of the American Society of Apheresis [1]

| Category | Description |
|---|---|
| I | Disorders for which apheresis is accepted as first-line therapy, either as a primary standalone treatment or in conjunction with other modes of treatment. |
| II | Disorders for which apheresis is accepted as second-line therapy, either as a standalone treatment or in conjunction with other modes of treatment. |
| III | Optimum role of apheresis therapy is not established.<br>Decision making should be individualized. |
| IV | Disorders in which published evidence demonstrates or suggests apheresis to be ineffective or harmful. IRB approval is desirable if apheresis treatment is undertaken in these circumstances. |

**Table 21.3** Application of plasmapheresis for diseases seen in children [1]

| Diagnosis | ASFA category | Typical treatment plans | | |
|---|---|---|---|---|
| | | Volume treated | Frequency | Duration/endpoint |
| TTP [16] | I | 1–1.5 FFP or cryopoor plasma | Daily | Normalized LDH and platelet count |
| Thrombotic microangiopathy, complement mediated [17–19] | I (anti-factor H antibody)<br>III (complement factor gene mutations)<br>III (MCP mutations | 1–1.5 FFP or cryopoor plasma | Daily | Normalized LDH and platelet count |
| Thrombotic microangiopathy, Shiga toxin related [20, 21] | III (severe neurologic symptoms)<br>III (Streptococcus pneumoniae)<br>IV (absence of severe neurologic symptoms) | 1–1.5<br>Albumin (S. pneumoniae) or FFP<br>STEC-HUS) | Daily | Normalized LDH and platelet count |
| Anti-glomerular basement membrane disease [22, 23] | I | 1–1.5<br>5% albumin | Daily or every other day for 2 weeks | Reduction in anti-GBM antibody/cessation of pulmonary hemorrhage |
| ANCA associated rapidly progressive glomerulonephritis [24, 25] | I | 1–1.5<br>5% albumin<br>FFP when pulmonary hemorrhage is present | Daily or every other day | 6–9 procedures |
| Lupus [26, 27] | II<br>(CNS disease) | 1–1.5<br>5% albumin | Daily or every other day | 3–6 treatments |
| Lupus nephritis [28] | IV | 1–1.5<br>5% albumin | Three times a week | 3–6 treatments |
| Recurrent FSGS [29, 30] | I | 1–1.5%<br>Albumin/FFP | Daily × 3 then every other day | Minimum 9 treatments until resolution/ improvement or resolution of proteinuria, taper treatments on individual basis |

**Table 21.3** (continued)

| | | Typical treatment plans | | |
|---|---|---|---|---|
| Diagnosis | ASFA category | Volume treated | Frequency | Duration/endpoint |
| Solid organ allograft rejection (antibody-mediated) [31, 32] | I–II | 1–1.5<br>5% albumin | Daily or every other day | 6 treatments minimum, consider more if donor specific antibodies still elevated |
| Thrombocytopenia-Associated multi-organ Failure (TAMOF), sepsis [6, 33] | III | 1–1.5<br>5% albumin/plasma | Daily or every other day | 2–14, assess for resolution of MOF, improvement in platelet count |

*TTP* Thrombotic Thrombocytopenic Purpura, *ASFA* American Society for Apheresis, *HUS* Hemolytic Uremic Syndrome, *FFP* Fresh Frozen Plasma, *LDH* Lactate Dehydrogenase, *FSGS* Focal Segmental Glomerulosclerosis, *GBM* Glomerular Basement Membrane, *ANCA* Anti-Neutrophil Cytoplasmic Antibody, *SLE* Systemic Lupus Erythematosus, *CNS* Central Nervous System, *MOF* Multi-Organ Failure

For many native immunological diseases and antibody-mediated solid organ transplant rejection, corticosteroids, other immunosuppressive agents, and intravenous immunoglobulin are commonly used in conjunction with plasmapheresis. In addition, critically ill children requiring apheresis are often receiving multiple organ support therapy including CRRT, extracorporeal membrane oxygenation and/or left-ventricular assist devices [5]. The apheresis machine can be connected in-line with many of these devices in order to obviate the need for separate dual lumen venous access or interruption of CRRT [5]. A number of technical issues require careful consideration when providing tandem therapies, which include matching the blood pump flow rates of each machine when possible, close attention to pressure and flow changes and most importantly, prevention of recirculation by ensuring the direction of blood flow is the same between the apheresis equipment and other extracorporeal device.

### 21.5.1 Apheresis and ACE Inhibitors

One unusual interaction of medications with apheresis therapy is relevant to the care of patients with kidney disease. Antihypertensive agents of the angiotensin converting enzyme (ACE) inhibitor class have been associated with an atypical and potentially severe reaction occurring shortly after the start of apheresis procedures. The symptoms include flushing and hypotension in most patients, and abdominal cramping, diarrhea, nausea, and diaphoresis in some. The reactions were first reported in patients taking ACE inhibitors who underwent staphylococcal protein A column therapy, but have been associated with plasmapheresis [34] and other therapies involving extracorporeal circuits. The postulated mechanism of these reactions is that during an apheresis procedure elevated levels of bradykinin are generated. In most apheresis patients this is inconsequential because of rapid degradation of bradykinin by kininase II. However, if the patient is receiving ACE inhibitors, the degradation mechanism may be blocked by the drug and the vasodilatory and gastrointestinal effects of bradykinin give rise to the symptoms. Many ACE inhibitor drugs have been implicated, and it is recommended that ACE inhibitors be withheld at least 24 h before an apheresis procedure.

## References

1. Schwartz J, Padmanabhan A, Aqui N, Balogun RA, Connelly-Smith L, Delaney M, et al. Guidelines on the use of therapeutic apheresis in clinical practice-evidence-based approach from the writing committee of the American society for apheresis: the seventh special issue. J Clin Apher. 2016;31(3):149–62.
2. Akcan-Arikan A, Zappitelli M, Loftis LL, Washburn KK, Jefferson LS, Goldstein SL. Modified RIFLE criteria in critically ill children with acute kidney injury. Kidney Int. 2007;71(10):1028–35.
3. Proulx F, Fayon M, Farrell CA, Lacroix J, Gauthier M. Epidemiology of sepsis and multiple organ dysfunction syndrome in children. Chest. 1996;109(4):1033–7.
4. Proulx F, Gauthier M, Nadeau D, Lacroix J, Farrell CA. Timing and predictors of death in pediatric patients with multiple organ system failure. Crit Care Med. 1994;22(6):1025–31.
5. Bunchman TE. Plasmapheresis and renal replacement therapy in children. Curr Opin Pediatr. 2002;14(3):310–4.
6. Nguyen TC, Han YY, Kiss JE, Hall MW, Hassett AC, Jaffe R, et al. Intensive plasma exchange increases a disintegrin and metalloprotease with thrombospondin motifs-13 activity and reverses organ dysfunction in children with thrombocytopenia-associated multiple organ failure. Crit Care Med. 2008;36(10):2878–87.
7. Chopek M, McCullough J. Protein and biochemical changes during plasma exchange. Washington: AABB Press; 1980.
8. Strauss R, McLeod B. Adverse reactions to therapeutic apheresis. Bethesda, MD: AABB Press; 1996.
9. Dzik WH, Kirkley SA. Citrate toxicity during massive blood transfusion. Transfus Med Rev. 1988;2(2):76–94.
10. Olson PR, Cox C, McCullough J. Laboratory and clinical effects of the infusion of ACD solution during plateletpheresis. Vox Sang. 1977;33(2):79–87.
11. Szymanski IO. Ionized calcium during plateletpheresis. Transfusion. 1978;18(6):701–8.
12. Bunchman TE, Maxvold NJ, Barnett J, Hutchings A, Benfield MR. Pediatric hemofiltration: normocarb dialysate solution with citrate anticoagulation. Pediatr Nephrol. 2002;17(3):150–4.
13. Mair DC, Hirschler N, Eastlund T. Blood donor and component management strategies to prevent transfusion-related acute lung injury (TRALI). Crit Care Med. 2006;34(5 Suppl):S137–43.
14. Bunchman TE, Brophy PD, Goldstein SL. Technical considerations for renal replacement therapy in children. Semin Nephrol. 2008;28(5):488–92.
15. Nadler S, Hidalgo J, Bloch T. Prediction of blood volume in normal human adults. Surgery. 1962;51(2):224–32.
16. Rock GA, Shumak KH, Buskard NA, Blanchette VS, Kelton JG, Nair RC, et al. Comparison of plasma exchange with plasma infusion in the treatment of thrombotic thrombocytopenic purpura. Canadian apheresis study group. N Engl J Med. 1991;325(6):393–7.
17. Caprioli J, Noris M, Brioschi S, Pianetti G, Castelletti F, Bettinaglio P, et al. Genetics of HUS: the impact of MCP, CFH, and IF mutations on clinical presentation, response to treatment, and outcome. Blood. 2006;108(4):1267–79.
18. Ariceta G, Besbas N, Johnson S, Karpman D, Landau D, Licht C, et al. Guideline for the investigation and initial therapy of diarrhea-negative hemolytic uremic syndrome. Pediatr Nephrol. 2009;24(4):687–96.

19. Zimmerhackl LB, Besbas N, Jungraithmayr T, van de Kar N, Karch H, Karpman D, et al. Epidemiology, clinical presentation, and pathophysiology of atypical and recurrent hemolytic uremic syndrome. Semin Thromb Hemost. 2006;32(2):113–20.
20. Colic E, Dieperink H, Titlestad K, Tepel M. Management of an acute outbreak of diarrhoea-associated haemolytic uraemic syndrome with early plasma exchange in adults from southern Denmark: an observational study. Lancet. 2011;378(9796):1089–93.
21. Spinale JM, Ruebner RL, Kaplan BS, Copelovitch L. Update on Streptococcus pneumoniae associated hemolytic uremic syndrome. Curr Opin Pediatr. 2013;25(2):203–8.
22. Levy JB, Turner AN, Rees AJ, Pusey CD. Long-term outcome of anti-glomerular basement membrane antibody disease treated with plasma exchange and immunosuppression. Ann Intern Med. 2001;134(11):1033–42.
23. Simpson IJ, Doak PB, Williams LC, Blacklock HA, Hill RS, Teague CA, et al. Plasma exchange in Goodpasture's syndrome. Am J Nephrol. 1982;2(6):301–11.
24. de Lind van Wijngaarden RA, Hauer HA, Wolterbeek R, Jayne DR, Gaskin G, Rasmussen N, et al. Clinical and histologic determinants of renal outcome in ANCA-associated vasculitis: a prospective analysis of 100 patients with severe renal involvement. J Am Soc Nephrol. 2006;17(8):2264–74.
25. Stegmayr BG, Almroth G, Berlin G, Fehrman I, Kurkus J, Norda R, et al. Plasma exchange or immunoadsorption in patients with rapidly progressive crescentic glomerulonephritis. A Swedish multi-center study. Int J Artif Organs. 1999;22(2):81–7.
26. Bambauer R, Schwarze U, Schiel R. Cyclosporin a and therapeutic plasma exchange in the treatment of severe systemic lupus erythematosus. Artif Organs. 2000;24(11):852–6.
27. Neuwelt CM. The role of plasmapheresis in the treatment of severe central nervous system neuropsychiatric systemic lupus erythematosus. Ther Apher Dial. 2003;7(2):173–82.
28. Lewis EJ, Hunsicker LG, Lan SP, Rohde RD, Lachin JM. A controlled trial of plasmapheresis therapy in severe lupus nephritis. The lupus nephritis collaborative study group. N Engl J Med. 1992;326(21):1373–9.
29. Savin VJ, Sharma R, Sharma M, McCarthy ET, Swan SK, Ellis E, et al. Circulating factor associated with increased glomerular permeability to albumin in recurrent focal segmental glomerulosclerosis. N Engl J Med. 1996;334(14):878–83.
30. Davenport RD. Apheresis treatment of recurrent focal segmental glomerulosclerosis after kidney transplantation: re-analysis of published case-reports and case-series. J Clin Apher. 2001;16(4):175–8.
31. Loupy A, Suberbielle-Boissel C, Zuber J, Anglicheau D, Timsit MO, Martinez F, et al. Combined posttransplant prophylactic IVIg/anti-CD 20/plasmapheresis in kidney recipients with preformed donor-specific antibodies: a pilot study. Transplantation. 2010;89(11):1403–10.
32. Lefaucheur C, Nochy D, Andrade J, Verine J, Gautreau C, Charron D, et al. Comparison of combination Plasmapheresis/IVIg/anti-CD20 versus high-dose IVIg in the treatment of antibody-mediated rejection. Am J Transplant. 2009;9(5):1099–107.
33. Busund R, Koukline V, Utrobin U, Nedashkovsky E. Plasmapheresis in severe sepsis and septic shock: a prospective, randomised, controlled trial. Intensive Care Med. 2002;28(10):1434–9.
34. Owen HG, Brecher ME. Atypical reactions associated with use of angiotensin-converting enzyme inhibitors and apheresis. Transfusion. 1994;34(10):891–4.

# 22 Tandem Therapies in Extracorporeal Support

Rachel Sirignano, Meral Patel, and Matthew L. Paden

**Case Vignette**

A 4-year-old (17 kg) previously healthy female presents to your hospital in acute respiratory failure due to pulmonary hemorrhage. She is intubated and brought to your intensive care unit requiring high conventional ventilator settings to maintain oxygenation and lung nodules are noted on chest X-ray. Initial labs obtained in the emergency department demonstrate anemia and hematuria. The patient has persistent hypoxia despite maximum ventilator support and she is cannulated onto veno-venous extracorporeal membrane oxygenation (VV-ECMO). Over the following day she is noted to have worsening fluid overload, and rising creatinine requiring CRRT to be started. Her anticoagulation for ECMO puts her at higher risk for line placement related bleeding complications, so the decision is made to run the CRRT hemofilter in line with your ECMO circuit. She continues to clot off hemofilters and membrane oxygenators requiring a change out of the full extracorporeal circuit. Autoimmune workup was sent, and on Day 3 of VV-ECMO the patient comes back positive for cytoplasmic staining anti-neutrophil cytoplasm antibodies (C-ANCA) confirming the diagnosis of granulomatosis with polyangiitis. After discussion with your apheresis physicians, you decide she meets criteria for therapeutic plasma exchange (TPE) due to severe renal vasculitis and a 7 day course is ordered.

R. Sirignano · M. Patel · M. L. Paden (✉)
Division of Pediatric Critical Care, Emory University, Atlanta, GA, USA
e-mail: Matthew.paden@choa.org



A. Deep, S. L. Goldstein (eds.), *Critical Care Nephrology and Renal Replacement Therapy in Children*, https://doi.org/10.1007/978-3-319-90281-4_22

## 22.1 Tandem Extracorporeal Therapies

Patient acuity in the pediatric intensive care unit (PICU) is increasing. This has been attributed to multiple factors, including, but not limited to, improved survival of extreme premature infants, increased rates of technology dependent patients, and improved technology leading to longer hospital stays. While improved survival of many diseases is to be celebrated, many of these survivors have long term comorbidities associated with their initial disease or treatment of it. This has created a new population of pediatric patients who have chronic co-morbidities, and have increased utilization of the PICU. In addition to this increasing chronic population of patients, standardized management of acute life threatening diseases such as sepsis and septic shock have led to improved survival of patients who just a few years before were "certain to die." This combination has dramatically increased the number of patients with multiple organ failure who need to be supported in the PICU. Using individual extracorporeal therapies as a means for supporting individual organs have been a mainstay of PICU care for the last two decades. Using these techniques, we have seen improved survival (compared to historical controls) in patients supported with extracorporeal membrane oxygenation (ECMO), ventricular assist devices (VAD), and continuous renal replacement therapies (CRRT). For many of these therapies, the presence of multiple organ failure has been considered a contraindication for use. However, over in the last decade, centers have been willing to challenge that dogma, and have started using combinations of extracorporeal therapies to manage multiple organ failure patients and provide extracorporeal life support (ECLS).

This chapter will review the current state of the art of tandem use of multiple extracorporeal therapies for patients with multiple organ failure from the aspect of a patient who is already supported on ECMO. With that aim, several caveats should be stated. Progress in this field has been slow and difficult, because of multiple factors. From a very practical standpoint, these independent devices were never engineered or designed to work together and just achieving forward flow of blood in them can be a significant hurdle. Additionally, when looking at this problem worldwide, due to country specific regulations, there is a wide variety of devices that may or may not be available to any individual center. This vastly increases the number of permutations of choices that can be made when designing your multiple organ therapy platform, and makes a discrete review of all possibilities difficult. In this chapter, we will thus focus on the engineering, physics, and physiology that are commonly seen in currently available devices. We will leave it to the reader to determine how best to balance those factors based on the choices of devices that they have locally. Another important caveat to understand is that this field and these techniques are very young. There is little substantial medical literature that has been published, and what has been published tends to be from a small number of single centers, has been published in the last 5 years, and has small numbers of patients supported. Expert opinion remains a common source of information. Multiple clinical trials need to be conducted to evaluate optimal design aspects, as well as clinical outcomes and complications.

## 22.2 Acute Kidney Injury (AKI) During ECMO

AKI is commonly seen and has been demonstrated as a risk factor for death in critically ill patients of all ages in the ICU. As noted throughout previous chapters in this textbook, multiple assessments for this topic have spanned across neonatal, pediatric, and adult ICU patients [1–3]. Historically, AKI definitions have been highly variable, but now multiple standardized scoring systems exist which utilize both urine output and serum creatinine to allow classification of AKI [4–6]. Similar to variability in definitions, AKI during ECLS is highly variable and dependent on age, type of ECLS, and classification for AKI. Reports have demonstrated AKI in 19–71% of neonates, 20–72% of pediatrics, and up to >70% of adult ECMO patients [7–11]. Many of these studies show a correlation between AKI and mortality for ECMO patients. Kidney injury can be demonstrated beyond traditional definitions of urine output and serum creatinine through the concept of fluid overload (FO). The systemic deleterious effects of FO have been demonstrated through an increased mortality for ECMO patients with FO, impaired oxygenation and increased duration of extracorporeal support [12–20]. As both AKI and FO negatively affect outcomes, focus has shifted to treating these comorbidities as a goal to improve ECMO outcomes.

Both AKI and fluid overload have been treated in ECMO patients by the standard renal replacement therapies (acute intermittent hemodialysis, slow continuous ultrafiltration, peritoneal dialysis, etc.). However, the most common way that AKI and fluid overload is treated in ECMO patients is by adding CRRT to the ECMO circuit. The timing and indication for CRRT to treat AKI and FO are not well established in ECMO. Recent consensus guidelines were published by the Acute Dialysis Quality Initiative (ADQI) on pharmacological and mechanical fluid removal [21, 22] and these principles are, in general, followed for ECMO patients. The Extracorporeal Life Support Organization (ELSO) also publishes a series guidelines (found at https://www.elso.org/Resources/Guidelines.aspx) to assist providers in ECMO treatment. These guidelines discuss the importance of fluid management in order to reach a homeostasis similar to the patient's normal (dry weight) extracellular fluid volume. For ECMO patients, indications for CRRT are broadly divided into removal of drugs/toxins, FO, AKI and electrolyte imbalances refractory to medical therapy, with usage varying among institutions [12, 23]. The most comprehensive and up-to-date evidence-based review of tandem CRRT and ECMO use can be found in Chen et al. [24].

## 22.3 Technical Aspects of CRRT During ECMO

Three main methods exist for providing CRRT to an ECMO patient [25, 26]. The first method involves a second vascular access point which utilizes a commercially available CRRT device without any connection to the ECLS circuit. This approach is the simplest method of simultaneous CRRT and ECMO, but is limited to those patients with vascular access prior to cannulation, as placing a new vascular access catheter for dialysis has an elevated severe bleeding risk once systemic ECMO anticoagulation has begun. Using this method, CRRT is run similar to non-ECMO patients, with the notable exception that systemic anticoagulation for ECMO precludes the need for local CRRT circuit anticoagulation.

The second method for CRRT on ECMO patients involves creating a shunt of blood post-pump from the ECMO circuit which flows through an isolated hemofilter. The pressure created by the extracorporeal pump drives blood through the hemofilter creating ultrafiltrate. The amount of ultrafiltrate produced is limited by using a standard intravenous (IV) pump programmed for the number of mL/h of ultrafiltrate desired and then this volume is measured with a bedside urimeter. The ultrafiltrate can be discarded to provide slow continuous ultrafiltrate (SCUF), or a replacement fluid with an appropriate electrolyte composition can be delivered back into the circuit via an additional standard IV pump to provide continuous veno-venous hemofiltration (CVVH). The now processed blood is returned to the ECLS circuit pre-pump (Fig. 22.1a). This method of "in-line" hemofiltration was the earliest form of tandem extracorporeal support therapies and is advantageous due to ease of use, simplicity for all ECMO specialists, and low cost of supplies. However, many disadvantages were noted with the use of this method. Notably, the creation of the shunt returning blood pre-pump creates a discrepancy between the blood flow listed on the ECMO pump and what is actually being delivered to the patient. The difference between ECMO pump flow and patient delivered flow must be monitored and represents the flow through the hemofilter circuit. Patient flow rates are now more accurately measured in the distal arterial limb of the ECMO circuit just prior to entry back into the patient. Additionally, the delivery of the blood exiting the hemofilter back pre-pump makes the CVVH less efficient due to recirculation of the already processed blood back through the hemofilter circuit. While this is a theoretical concern, clinically, the ECMO flow rates greatly exceed the hemofilter circuit flow rates, making clinically significant recirculation negligible. Also, using this method to provide SCUF for smaller children may create multiple electrolyte disturbances and is not recommended. The "in-line" circuit often has no pressure monitoring, which makes identifying hemofilter malfunction, thrombosis, or rupture more challenging. The most important disadvantage to "in-line" hemofiltration of CRRT during ECMO relates to inaccuracy of fluid balance. The IV pumps being used for control of ultrafiltrate and replacement fluid were not engineered for this therapy and truly function as flow restrictors (and not pumps), having an inherent error rate (~12.5%) when used in this setting [27]. An in vitro setup of "in-line" CRRT with ECMO, demonstrated a measured versus prescribed flow error of up to 34 mL/h (>800 mL/day), which in a small patient (5 kg) could equal their daily fluid goals (~150 mL/kg/day) [28]. Careful monitoring of the replacement fluid volume as well as ultrafiltrate volumes is essential to the ECMO specialist duties when providing these therapies concomitantly. This can be done either via volume measure (mL) or based off highly accurate scales (±1 g). The need for hourly monitoring increases ECMO specialist workload and is contributing to a reduction of use of this "in-line" technique.

The third and preferred method for CRRT on ECMO patients is via introduction of a commercially available CRRT device into the ECMO circuit. Multiple factors contribute to determining the optimal method to connect these separate extracorporeal support devices including, but not limited to, type and placement of pressure monitors, CRRT device software limitations for variables such as pressure and flow, type of ECMO pump, and ECMO circuit design. In general, the roller head pump driven ECMO circuit has more positive pressures in the venous limb, allowing for pre-pump venous limb placement and return of the CRRT device (Fig. 22.1b). The sole driving pressure for the CRRT circuit is based off

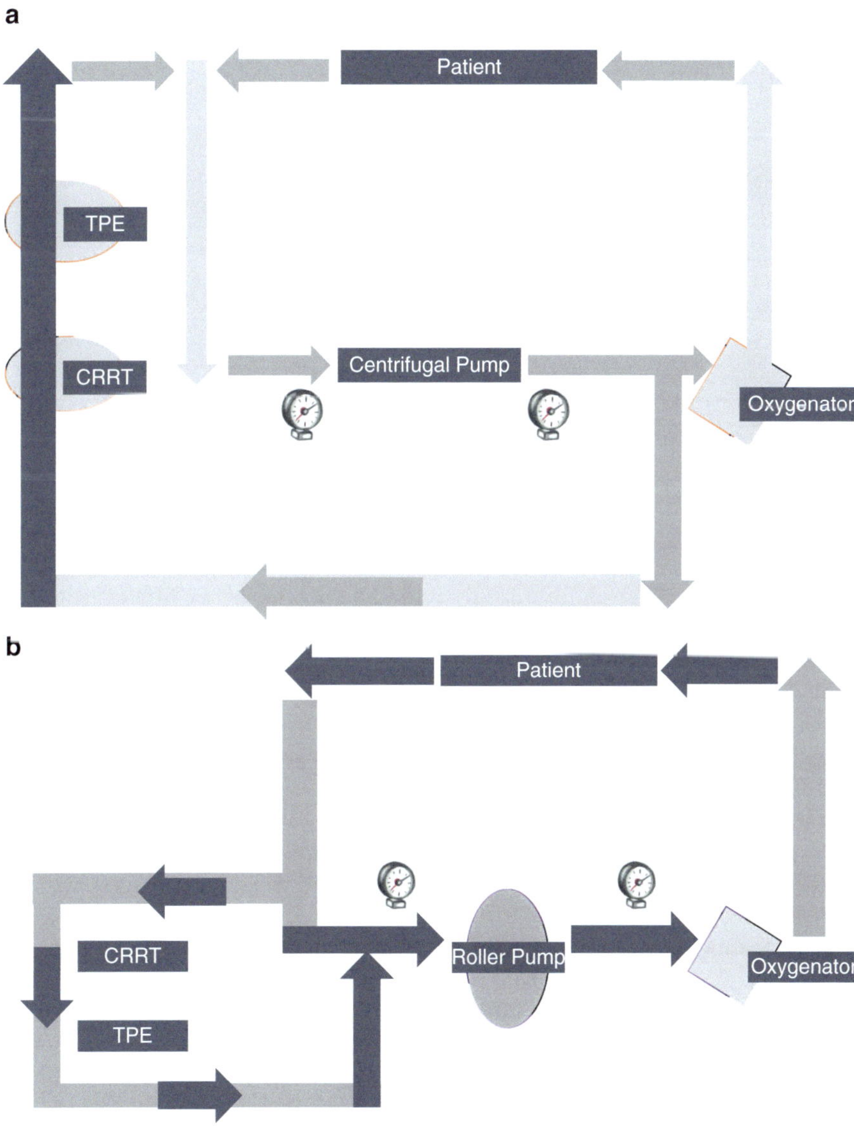


**Fig. 22.1** Representative schematic diagram of multi-tandem extracorporeal procedures: ECMO, TPE and CRRT. *ECMO* extracorporeal membrane oxygenation, *TPE* therapeutic plasma exchange, *CRRT* continuous renal replacement therapy. ECMO, 3 way stopcock valve. Note: ECMO flow rates: 250 mL–5000 mL/min; TPE flow rates: 30 mL/min–70 mL/min; CRRT flow rates: 50 mL/min–150 mL/min

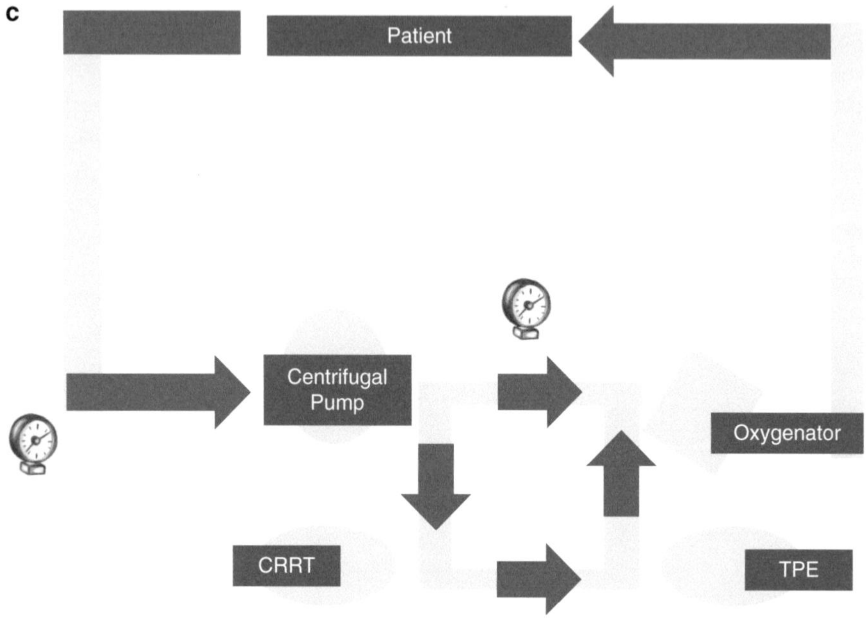


**Fig. 22.1** (continued)

the CRRT device pump generating a negative pressure to pull blood from the ECMO circuit and then creating a positive displacement and pressure to drive it through the hemofilter and ultimately return it back to the ECMO circuit. The pressures in the venous limb of a roller head circuit are not very negative and are similar to what would be expected in a well-functioning dialysis catheter, thus allowing the CRRT device software to function in a normal fashion. Alternately, a centrifugal pump driven ECMO circuit has a much larger negative venous limb pressure, and so an alternative configuration is often required. A common issue is that the CRRT device's software pressure limits will typically not allow it to function with the magnitude of negative pressures seen on the pre-pump venous limb of a centrifugal circuit. Additionally, when making the physical connections of the CRRT device to the ECMO circuit in this highly negative pressure environment the risk of air entrainment is large. For a centrifugal ECMO system, recommendations include placing the CRRT device post-pump, but pre-oxygenator, to both move the CRRT device to a region of positive pressure where it is more likely to function more consistently, as well as decrease the risk of air entrainment (Fig. 22.1c). In this third configuration, the blood is returned from the CRRT device to the ECMO circuit post pump venous limb, just prior to the membrane oxygenator. Having both the CRRT drain and return post-pump but pre-oxygenator is optimal because this configuration allows the oxygenator to act as a clot and air trap, and decreases the amount of recirculation through the CRRT circuit. When compared to the "in-line" method, this third method allows for more accurate fluid balance, a longer hemofilter life, standard pressure and flow monitoring of the CRRT circuit and the ability to use a CRRT device has been engineered for the purpose of providing CRRT [28–30]. It should be noted that all commercially available CRRT devices are not specifically approved or designed for use in ECMO patients. This method has the disadvantages of higher cost and additional training for the user.

## 22.4 Outcomes of CRRT During ECLS

Although theoretical advantages and disadvantages of differing methods for providing simultaneous CRRT and ECLS exist, very little outcome data are available to compare methods. Prior studies which looked at "in-line," commercial CRRT devices and stand alone, found all methods to be adequate for fluid and electrolyte control. Although, data have shown increased fluid accuracy when using commercially available devices compared to an "in-line" system, and a decreased duration of use [29–31]. These studies also demonstrated a longer filter life when a CRRT device was incorporated into the ECLS circuit (138.4 h) compared to 36.8 h seen in non-ECLS children with stand-alone CRRT, and 27.2 h seen in CRRT during ECLS with citrate anticoagulation added [30, 31]. No difference was noted in intensive care unit (ICU) length of stay, hospital length of stay, or mortality.

Currently, the largest set of outcome data for concomitant CRRT on ECLS comes from the ELSO registry [32, 33]. "Renal Failure" is defined in the ELSO registry as a complication of ECLS, with three levels of injury coded: Creatinine (Cr) 1.5 3, Cr >3, and use of dialysis/hemofiltration/continuous arteriovenous hemodialysis. These definitions are very limited compared to modern scoring systems (e.g., KDIGO), and the registry only counts it once per run with no duration information available. This further complicates analysis of outcomes, because there is no way to differentiate a patient who, for example, received CRRT for their entire 14 day run versus someone who had it started 2 h before death. With those caveats, analysis of the ELSO registry demonstrates the presence of renal failure in each age category of respiratory failure has associated worse survival (Table 22.1) compared to the overall survivals of these categories (Neonatal 63%, Pediatric 58%, Adult 61%). Similar data is noted in the cardiac population. As coded in the ELSO registry, both kidney injury and the use of renal replacement therapy (RRT) are risk factors for increased mortality. A subset of six ELSO centers across North America came together and formed the Kidney Injury During Membrane Oxygenation (KIDMO) research network to further investigate relationships between RRT use, AKI, and survival in pediatric patients (<19 years old) [12, 23]. They evaluated a cohort of 835 ECLS patients at their centers from 2007 to 2011

**Table 22.1** Renal complications and survival from ELSO Registry International Report 2016

| Renal complication category | Neonatal respiratory failure n (% reported, % survival) | Pediatric respiratory failure n (% reported, % survival) | Adult respiratory failure n (% reported, % survival) |
|---|---|---|---|
| Creatinine 1.5–3 | 1927 (6, 50) | 702 (9, 35) | 1947 (16, 47) |
| Creatinine >3 | 378 (1, 37) | 327 (4, 34) | 1106 (9, 45) |
| Renal replacement therapy | 6387 (23, 50) | 3475 (43, 42) | 4661 (38, 49) |

Note: *ELSO* extracorporeal life support organization

using the modern KDIGO definition of AKI. The data showed that AKI affects the majority of pediatric ECLS patients (50–69%), it occurs early (99% within first 48 h) and it is associated with longer duration of ECLS (~48 h) and higher mortality (Odds Ratio = 2). There was a clear association in this data between increasing AKI stage being associated with increased risk of death. Fluid overload has also been assessed from this KIDMO cohort, and fluid overload of >10% is present in almost half (46.4%) and > 20% in almost one quarter (24.1%) of ECMO patients at the time of cannulation [34]. In this cohort, fluid overload was also found to worsen once a patient was placed onto ECMO. During extracorporeal membrane oxygenation, 84.8%, 67.2%, and 29% of patients had a peak fluid overload greater than or equal to 10%, 20%, and 50%, respectively. The magnitude of fluid overload was correlated with survival, with median peak fluid overload being lower in patients who survived to hospital discharge (24.8% vs. 43.3%; $p < 0.0001$). A multivariate model incorporating acute kidney injury score, pH at extracorporeal membrane oxygenation initiation, nonrenal complications, extracorporeal membrane oxygenation mode, support type, center and patient age, demonstrated that the degree of fluid overload at extracorporeal membrane oxygenation initiation, and the peak fluid overload on extracorporeal membrane oxygenation predicted duration of extracorporeal membrane oxygenation in survivors. Further analysis of this large KIDMO cohort is ongoing, with a focus on specific patient populations, such as the pediatric cardiac population. In previous work, five case series have reviewed CRRT during ECMO for the pediatric cardiac population. All but one showed statistically higher mortality when CRRT was used on ECMO, with a combined odds ratio of 6.19 [24].

## 22.5 Summary of Concomitant CRRT and ECMO

The ECMO community commonly uses CRRT for the treatment of AKI and FO in their population. Methods of providing these tandem extracorporeal support therapies are not standardized and no products are commercially designed for this use. In all critically ill patients, mortality of ECMO patients who develop AKI exceeds those patients without AKI. In contrast to previous thinking, it has now been demonstrated that the presence and degree of AKI is the risk factor for death, not the use of the CRRT device. Additionally, in this population fluid overload has also been shown to be correlated to higher mortality and longer ECMO duration. Both AKI and fluid overload remain potential clinical targets to improve mortality in ECMO patients. However, the details for optimal treatment of AKI and fluid overload for ECMO patients are not well defined and therefore vary among institutions. Additional multicenter data and trials with standardized protocols are needed to better guide AKI management in ECMO patients.

## 22.6 Apheresis During ECMO

Therapeutic apheresis (TA) involves separating and removing individual constituents of blood. This is a well-established technology and many apheresis procedures are provided in the outpatient setting. Newer to the apheresis world, is providing TA to a critically ill population of children, especially those requiring ECMO. ECMO has often been considered a contraindication to TA as the patients were deemed "too sick/unstable." As the use of multiple extracorporeal therapies has grown, physicians are more regularly using TA procedures on ECMO patients and may even place patients on ECMO to achieve cardio-pulmonary stability in order to perform TA procedures. Details for indications and modalities of therapeutic apheresis are beyond the scope which will be covered in this chapter. The information in this chapter serves as a review for patients in multi-organ failure who require multiple tandem extracorporeal support therapies (TA, CRRT, and ECMO) and as a guide for how to provide these tandem procedures together successfully.

One method of therapeutic apheresis is via therapeutic plasma exchange (TPE). TPE is the separation, removal, and replacement of plasma from the blood. The goal of TPE is removal of large molecular weight constituents (e.g., antibodies, cytokines) or highly protein bound molecules while restoring depleted coagulation factors, and proteins to return homeostasis needed for recovery [35]. This is the most common form of TA utilized in ECMO patients, although no specific ELSO guidelines exist for indications of apheresis procedures while on ECMO. Instead, the decision to proceed is based on evidence of effectiveness for underlying disease based on the general guidelines set forth by the American Society for Apheresis (ASFA). Periodically, a set of evidence based guidelines are published by ASFA, with the last being in 2016 [36]. These guidelines review all medical evidence for apheresis by disease, and present a one-page summary with highlighted prescribed recommendations.

Regardless of indication, an anticoagulant is required to avoid excessive thrombosis due to the activation of blood through an apheresis device and its extracorporeal circuit. Although most patients on ECMO have systemic anticoagulation and no longer need local anticoagulation of either the apheresis and/or CRRT devices via citrate or other regional anticoagulation techniques However, one must be aware the effects of citrate toxicity may still be seen. Large amounts of plasma (which contains citrate as an anticoagulant for storage) utilized in TPE potentially expose a patient to citrate toxicity, with depletion of free, ionized extracellular calcium. The ECLS patient's cardiac function (especially in the neonatal population) may be negatively affected by low ionized calcium. This could become a relative contraindication for TPE utilizing fresh frozen plasma replacement, and physicians may decide to utilize albumin replacement or forgo therapy altogether due to the hypocalcemia risks. Alternatively, either a continuous infusion of exogenous calcium or increasing veno-arterial ECMO flow rate during the procedure may mitigate these adverse effects of large citrate exposure.

## 22.7 Indications for TA with CRRT and ECLS

No ELSO guidelines currently exist for the use of therapeutic apheresis while on ECLS. Instead, the decision to proceed with TA should be made based on evidence of underlying disease and not based off ECLS and CRRT support for the patient. It should be understood that there is very little evidence presented in these guidelines for patients who are receiving ECMO. ECMO is only mentioned once in the 190 page guideline document, in the setting of describing a case series TPE use during ECMO of pediatric patients with sepsis-associated multiple organ failure. However, these guidelines remain the best summary of evidence for the effectiveness of therapeutic apheresis procedures to correct the underlying diseases that have caused the patient to need ECLS. As defined by the ASFA (7th Special Issue) Category I indications are for disorders where apheresis is first-line therapy either alone or in conjunction with other treatments. Category II indications are defined as second-line therapy either in conjunction with or as stand-alone treatment. Category III indications include disorders for which the optimum role of apheresis therapy is not established and decision making should be individualized. Category IV are considered harmful to the patient. As mentioned above, little data exist regarding the use of therapeutic apheresis in the setting of ECMO. In the largest cohort of 53 pediatric patients (<21 years old) receiving tandem TA with ECMO reported, Sirignano et al. found the vast majority of these 180 procedures were conducted for patients requiring solid organ transplant (51% cardiac, 13% renal) and sepsis induced thrombocytopenia-associated multiple organ failure (TAMOF) (26%) (Table 22.2) [37]. Other case series have similarly noted the use of TPE and CRRT during ECMO for the management of sepsis with multi-organ dysfunction syndrome (MODS) and TAMOF [35, 37].

As often occurs at the frontier of medical care, diseases and clinical scenarios will exist with either no or little evidence to support the use of therapeutic apheresis. Essentially all cases of multi-tandem extracorporeal support (TA, CRRT, and ECLS) fall into this category. Although guidance can be found through the ASFA guidelines, prior to starting any treatment for uncategorized diseases, the treatment clinicians should carefully document their reasoning behind a chosen apheresis procedure, provide a mechanism of action to address the current disease, how TA will improve the patient's condition, a proposed therapeutic plan and duration, and how the clinician will assess for efficacy of therapy.

**Table 22.2** ASFA (7th Special Issue) indications

| Indication category | # Patients (% of Total) | # Procedures |
|---|---|---|
| Category I | 8 (15) | 42 |
| Renal transplantation[a] | 7 | 35 |
| ANCA-associated RPGN | 1 | 7 |
| Category II | 22 (42) | 35 |
| Cardiac transplantation desensitization | 21 | 32 |
| Hyperleukocytosis (Leukostasis) | 1 | 3 |
| Category III | 23 (43) | 103 |
| Cardiac transplantation antibody mediated rejection | 6 | 30 |
| TAMOF | 14 | 60 |
| AIHA | 1 | 7 |
| Acute liver failure | 2 | 6 |

Note: *ASFA* American Society for Apheresis, *ANCA* anti-neutrophil cytoplasmic antibody, *RPGN* rapidly progressive glomerulonephritis, *TAMOF* thrombocytopenia-associated multiple organ failure, *AIHA* autoimmune hemolytic anemia

[a]Antibody-mediated rejection and desensitization

## 22.8 Technical Aspects of TPE During Concomitant CRRT and ECMO

Similar to the concomitant CRRT and ECMO methods described above, apheresis procedures can be provided as stand-alone therapy through a separate vascular access or provided through the ECMO circuit. As seen with CRRT on ECMO the risks of bleeding for patients already anticoagulated on ECLS drive more providers to use TPE in line with ECMO circuit. No evidence suggests superiority to either stand-alone or in circuit use.

The first method of stand-alone therapy involves utilizing a second vascular access point for therapeutic apheresis for patients on CRRT and ECMO. As TA often has lower flower rates than CRRT, this can be achieved through two large bore peripheral catheters, or a preexisting apheresis compatible subcutaneous port but preferentially is done through a double lumen central venous line. As with all extracorporeal therapies, consideration must be made to the extracorporeal volume in relation to the patient's total blood volume. This is especially important in pediatric apheresis, where there often are not pediatric sized extracorporeal circuits. First, the apheresis device's extracorporeal volume (often being ~350 mL) needs to be accounted for in patients <20 kg, and in these patients a blood prime is preferred over crystalloid to avoid dilutional anemia. Blood prime could also be used in larger patients with inadequate oxygen delivery or unstable hemodynamics. In this stand-alone therapy, attention should be made to the temperature of the products being delivered as significant hypothermia can occur in smaller patients (<10 kg). Warming of the apheresis circuit to meet ECMO targets may also be required. The need of a regional anticoagulant during a therapeutic apheresis through a separate vascular is controversial, and no evidence exists to guide decision making. There is wide practice variation, with some centers relying only on the ECMO systemic anticoagulation, others who always additionally provide regional anticoagulation, and those who assess each patient at the time of the procedure and determine a plan for that individual procedure only. As TPE is an intermittent procedure, when using a separate vascular access point, an anticoagulant solution should be used to lock the venous access points, per a center's usual policy, to avoid thrombosis.

The second method involves connecting the apheresis circuit to the ECMO circuit is done in a similar manner to CRRT as noted above (Fig. 22.1) [38]. Multiple configurations are possible, and dependent upon the type of ECMO pumping system. As with CRRT, none of the commercially available apheresis devices have been validated or designed for use concomitant with ECLS circuits. Similar to what is seen during CRRT during ECMO, a common complication includes a venous limb negative pressure alarm on the apheresis device. This can be ameliorated by adjustment of ECMO cannula position to improve drainage, reducing ECMO flow (if hemodynamically tolerable), changing parameters for alarms on the apheresis device, or altering the position of apheresis drainage from ECMO circuit (e.g., Fig. 22.1a, b). For patients already receiving concomitant ECMO and CRRT, a common configuration is that the apheresis device is placed in series to the CRRT device [26, 39]. Multiple three way stopcocks may be connected to the pigtail connection coming off the pre-pump venous limb of the ECLS circuit (Fig. 22.1b). During the procedure, the apheresis device pulls blood from the first stopcock and returns to the second one, where the blood then continues on into the CRRT circuit and ultimately back to the ECMO circuit (Fig. 22.2). In this configuration, it is important the

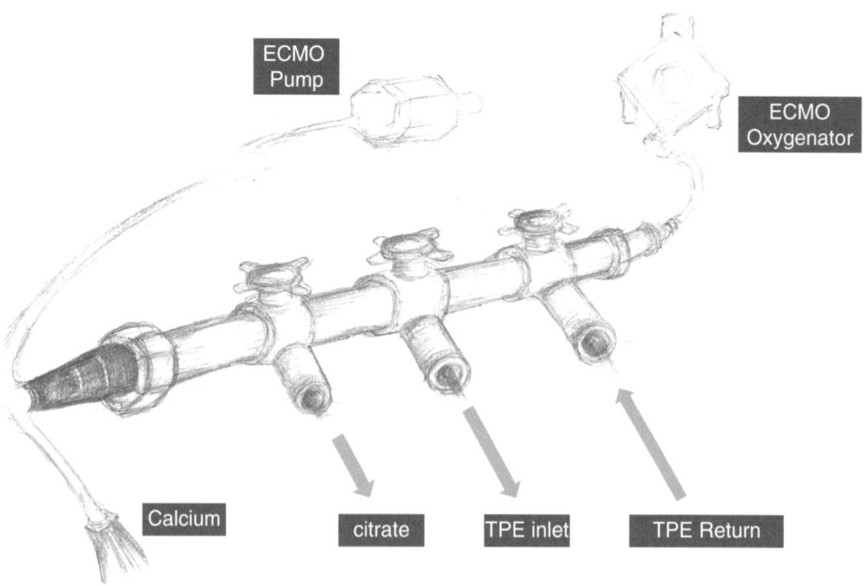


**Fig. 22.2** Representative standardized connectors to TPE and CRRT from ECLS circuit. *TPE* therapeutic plasma exchange, *CRRT* continuous renal replacement therapy, *ECLS* extracorporeal life support

apheresis device and CRRT devices which are run in series, have matching flow rates to avoid pressure alarms and recirculation.

ASFA guidelines help determine the indication, duration, and dose of therapy required for therapeutic plasma exchange, however certain alterations are required when doing in tandem to CRRT and ECMO circuits. According to guidelines, dosing is presented as based off a multiplier of "plasma volume" (PV) or "whole blood volume" [36]. Typically these volumes are based off equations calculating from weight or body surface area and standard hematocrit (Nadler's equation). However, these equations are not valid when concomitant to other extracorporeal support systems. During ECLS, you must calculate both the total blood volume of the patient as well as the total extracorporeal circuit(s) volume. The total extracorporeal circuit includes a sum of each individual circuit, in this case, CRRT + Apheresis + ECMO . Failure to account for these volumes will under calculate the plasma volume involved and provide inadequate dosing of TPE. For example, using the standard calculations our 17 kg case report would have a total blood and plasma volume of 1700 mL and 714 mL. But if we accounted for an ECLS volume of 400 mL, CRRT volume of 250 mL, and apheresis volume of 350 mL, with a recent hematocrit of 40%, the same child has a total blood and plasma volume of 2700 mL and 1755 mL. Not accounting for the volumes of each of the extracorporeal circuits would lead to 40% underdosing in this child.

Depending on the indication of TPE, the ASFA guidelines recommend processing of 1–1.5 PV, which are replaced with either fresh frozen plasma (FFP) or albumin [36]. Strict dosing by mL is not necessary, and it can be rounded to the nearest unit of product. This is because for a solely plasma based molecule removed by TPE, you remove 63.2% with 1 PV, 77.7% with 1.5 PV, and 95% with 3 PV. Recommendations do not call for a full removal of 3 PV on the first therapy because many of the targeted molecules are not solely confined to the blood compartment, and redistribute with time necessitating repeat therapies. When providing TPE, one must be mindful that although the removal target is removed, many other blood components are removed simultaneously. Drug dosing is particularly challenging with the use of multiple extracorporeal elimination methods such as ECMO, CRRT, and TA in tandem. While some pharmacokinetics data exists, much additional work is needed in this field and careful, repeated, clinical assessment of the effect of each prescribed drug is required to evaluate for signs of sub- or supra-therapeutic dosing [40, 41].

Similar to CRRT, local anticoagulation with citrate can be utilized of the apheresis circuit during ECMO, however complications of hypotension and hypocalcemia have been described in both adults and children [38] due to citrate toxicity. The systemic anticoagulation (e.g., heparin or direct thrombin inhibitors) required for ECMO is typically sufficient for anticoagulation of all extracorporeal support devices. Although, as discussed prior, pharmacokinetics can alter significantly pre- and post-therapeutic plasma exchange and close monitoring is recommended both during and immediately after TA. As these procedures are being performed as an "off label" use of these devices in a setting they were not designed for, complications can and do arise. For example, many commercially available apheresis devices are engineered to only work when an anticoagulant solution is hung and running. As systemic anticoagulation for ECLS precludes the need for local anticoagulation, a bag of crystalloid solution can be substituted for citrate allowing the apheresis device to function in the ECMO setting. Similarly, many of the commercially available apheresis devices utilize Nadler's formula to calculate the prescribed volumes required for TPE based off of inputted height and weight of patient. As noted above, much large volumes are required for patients on tandem extracorporeal circuits, and the devices will often alarm over concern that a very large exchange has been ordered. They may fail to run, or default to providing the procedure over extended periods of time (>8 h). In this scenario, the provider may choose to run therapy over an extended period, or more commonly, adjust the patient's weight programmed to reflect a patient with similar native (non-ECLS) blood volume. For example, our 17 kg patient was calculated to have 2700 mL of total blood volume (all circuits accounted) could be programmed as a 39 kg patient and this would allow processing of a similar volume of plasma over a shorter time course (~2 h). Whenever an institution is considering over-riding or altering a manufacturer's recommended practices, a formal written protocol should be established and closely followed, with multiple independent practitioners checking calculations and adherence to the protocol prior to initiating the procedure.

## 22.9 Use and Outcomes of Therapeutic Apheresis with CRRT During ECMO

Upon review of the current literature, the published experience is comprised of 67 patients across the world have received TPE simultaneous to CRRT and ECMO (Table 22.3). No randomized clinical trials have been published on disease process for the use of therapeutic apheresis on these extracorporeal support systems. All literature is currently based off individual case report and case series. The most common indications for use were sepsis with either thrombocytopenia-associated multi-organ failure (TAMOF) or multi-organ dysfunction syndrome [35, 37, 41, 43, 45, 47, 54]. Rationale for the use of TPE in this cohort of patients is best summarized by Nguyen et al., which includes removing ultra-large von Willebrand factor multimers, removal of antibodies to ADAMTS13, and replacement of ADAMTS13 with fresh frozen plasma [55]. The next most prevalent category is for antibody removal in active autoimmune diseases [26, 37, 42, 48–53, 55, 56] and organ transplantation [37]. Individual case reports exist for ingestions/poisonings [46] as well.

Significant heterogeneity exists in case reports for tandem extracorporeal supports due to the variety of rare diseases, differentiation in technique for TA, differences in technique for ECMO, and lack of severity of illness scoring. Together, these factors make commenting about complications and survival difficult. While center specific and regional registries exist, there is no international registry for these patients. As has been done with the ELSO registry for ECMO, capturing data about device related factors, therapy prescribed and patient related factors to an international database would allow for accrual of data which would be required to make definitions of best practices and improve outcomes for the patients with multiple extracorporeal therapy needs.

**Table 22.3** Case Reports of Therapeutic Plasma Exchange (TPE) and CRRT during ECLS

| Reference | n | Outcome Measure | Result | Year(s)/Center | Apheresis device | Anti coagulation | Apheresis complications |
|---|---|---|---|---|---|---|---|
| Sirignano et al. [37] | 30 pediatric<br>24 CRRT + ECLS<br>6 CRRT + TPE + ECLS<br>180 procedures | Survival | 79% survival | 2012–2015<br>USA—CHOA | Optia | ECLS heparin only | Air in line<br>Clot formation<br>Pump malfunction<br>Hypocalcemia |
| Kawai et al. [35] | 14 pediatric<br>12 CRRT + TPE + ECLS<br>2 TPE + ECLS<br>51 procedures | PICU survival<br>Organ failure index<br>Vasoactive score | 7[illegible]% survival<br>Improvement in organ failure and vasoactives | 2005–2013<br>USA—University of Michigan | If on CRRT, Prisma/ PrismaFlex<br>No CRRT, spectra or Optia | ECLS heparin<br>Apheresis citrate | Transient hypotension<br>New onset rash |
| Laverdure [26] | 5 adult<br>CRRT + TPE + ECLS<br>5 procedure | Hemofilter half life | Improved | 2017<br>France | Prismaflex | ECLS heparin | |
| Bridges et al. [40] | 3 pediatric<br>CRRT + TPE + ECLS<br>16 procedures | ADAMTS-13 level and platelet count before and after | Rise in ADAMTS-13 and platelet counts in all | 2012<br>USA—Vanderbilt | Spectra | ECLS heparin<br>Apheresis citrate | |
| Kolovos et al. [42] | 3 pediatric<br>CRRT + TPE + ECLS<br>? Procedures | Survival | Survived | 1991–2000<br>USA—Michigan | Spectra | ECLS heparin only | |
| Patel et al. [43] | 1 pediatric<br>CRRT + TPE + ECLS<br>3 procedures | Pediatric logistic organ dysfunction scores, $FiO_2$ and vasopressor requirements | Reduction in all 3 after two exchanges | 2009<br>USA—Shreveport, LA | Prisma | ECLS heparin only | |
| Tabbutt et al. [44] | 1 pediatric<br>CRRT + TPE + ECLS<br>2 procedures | CK and myoglobin levels | Reduction in CK and myoglobin | 2004<br>USA—CHOP | Spectra | | |

(continued)

**Table 22.3** (continued)

| Reference | n | Outcome Measure | Result | Year(s)/Center | Apheresis device | Anti coagulation | Apheresis complications |
|---|---|---|---|---|---|---|---|
| Mok et al. [45] | 1 pediatric<br>CRRT + TPE + ECLS<br>1 procedure | Survival | Survived | 1985–1992<br>Australia—Melbourne | | | |
| Maclaren et al. [46] | 1 adult<br>CRRT + TPE + ECLS<br>1 procedure | Survival | Survived | 2004<br>Australia—Melbourne | Spectra | | |
| Nasir et al. [47] | 1 adult<br>CRRT + TPE + ECLS<br>4 procedures | Survival | Died after 4 days | 2013<br>Turkey | | | |
| Hofenforst et al. [42] | 1 adult<br>CRRT + TPE + ECLS<br>25 procedures | Survival<br>Proteinase 3 titers | Survived<br>Titers were effectively reduced | 2011<br>Greece | | ECLS coated circuit and argatroban<br>Apheresis citrate | Heparin induced thrombocytopenia |
| Barnes et al. [48] | 1 adult<br>CRRT + TPE + ECLS<br>1 procedure | Survival | Survived | 2011<br>Australia | | | |
| Ahmed et al. [49] | 1 adult<br>CRRT + TPE + ECLS<br>5 procedures | Survival | Survived | 2004<br>USA—MUSC | | ECLS heparin | |
| Yusuff et al. [50] | 1 adult<br>CRRT + TPE + ECLS<br>8 procedures | Survival<br>PR3 levels | Survived<br>PR3 levels dropped | 2015<br>UK | | ECLS heparin only | |
| Joseph et al. [51] | 1 pediatric<br>CRRT + TPE + ECLS<br>5 procedures | Survival | Survived | 2011<br>USA—UNC | | ECLS heparin | |
| Di Maria et al. [52] | 1 pediatric<br>CRRT + TPE + ECLS<br>5 procedures | Resolution of pulmonary hemorrhage | Within 3 days | 2008<br>USA—Denver | | ECLS heparin<br>Apheresis citrate | |
| Dalabih et al. [53] | 1 pediatric<br>CRRT + TPE + ECLS<br>6 procedures | Survival | Survived | 2012<br>USA—Vanderbilt | | ECLS heparin<br>Apheresis citrate | |

## 22.10 Summary of TA During ECMO

Use of TA during ECMO technologically is feasible although is rarely used. Guidance related to the appropriateness of TA, timing, and prescribed therapy should be supported based on the underlying disease through the ASFA guidelines. When evidence is lacking, reliance on knowledge of the underlying pathophysiology of the disease is necessary to guide and support treatment options. Variation exists on how and when to perform TA during CRRT and ECLS, including variable anticoagulation strategies. A worldwide registry approach is needed to describe the potential harms and benefits of this rare combination of extracorporeal support.

**Box: Key Learning Points of Extracorporeal Tandem Therapies**

**Key Learning Points**

- A growing number of pediatric patients meet criteria for multiple extracorporeal support therapies (e.g., ECMO, CRRT, TPE).
- Multiple permutations exist to connect extracorporeal devices together. Knowledge of the pump flow and device pressure limitations can help guide optimal placement for each circuit.
- Size of patient and volume of extracorporeal circuits must be accounted for when calculating total body volume for therapeutic apheresis.
- The systemic anticoagulation required for ECLS can be utilized for CRRT and TPE, and supercedes the need for individual local circuit anticoagulation.

Note: *ECMO* extracorporeal membrane oxygenation, *CRRT* continuous renal replacement therapy, *TPE* therapeutic plasma exchange, *ECLS* extracorporeal life support

## References

1. Selewski DT, Charlton JR, Jetton JG, Guillet R, Mhanna MJ, Askenazi DJ, et al. Neonatal acute kidney injury. Pediatrics. 2015;136(2):e463–73.
2. Fortenberry JD, Paden ML, Goldstein SL. Acute kidney injury in children: an update on diagnosis and treatment. Pediatr Clin N Am. 2013;60(3):669–88.
3. Honore PM, Jacobs R, Hendrickx I, Bagshaw SM, Joannes-Boyau O, Boer W, et al. Prevention and treatment of sepsis-induced acute kidney injury: an update. Ann Intensive Care. 2015;5(1):51.
4. Bellomo R, Kellum JA, Ronco C. Defining and classifying acute renal failure: from advocacy to consensus and validation of the RIFLE criteria. Intensive Care Med. 2007;33(3):409–13.
5. Bellomo R, Ronco C, Kellum JA, Mehta RL, Palevsky P, Acute Dialysis Quality Initiative workgroup. Acute renal failure—definition, outcome measures, animal models, fluid therapy and information technology needs: the second international consensus conference of the acute dialysis quality initiative (ADQI) group. Crit Care. 2004;8(4):R204–12.
6. Mehta RL, Kellum JA, Shah SV, Molitoris BA, Ronco C, Warnock DG, et al. Acute kidney injury network: report of an initiative to improve outcomes in acute kidney injury. Crit Care. 2007;11(2):R31.

7. Askenazi DJ, Ambalavanan N, Hamilton K, Cutter G, Laney D, Kaslow R, et al. Acute kidney injury and renal replacement therapy independently predict mortality in neonatal and pediatric noncardiac patients on extracorporeal membrane oxygenation. Pediatr Crit Care Med. 2011;12(1):e1–6.
8. Smith AH, Hardison DC, Worden CR, Fleming GM, Taylor MB. Acute renal failure during extracorporeal support in the pediatric cardiac patient. ASAIO J. 2009;55(4):412–6.
9. Lou S, MacLaren G, Paul E, Best D, Delzoppo C, Butt W. Hemofiltration is not associated with increased mortality in children receiving extracorporeal membrane oxygenation. Pediatr Crit Care Med. 2015;16(2):161–6.
10. Gadepalli SK, Hirschl RB. Extracorporeal life support: updates and controversies. Semin Pediatr Surg. 2015;24(1):8–11.
11. Luo XJ, Wang W, Hu SS, Sun HS, Gao HW, Long C, et al. Extracorporeal membrane oxygenation for treatment of cardiac failure in adult patients. Interact Cardiovasc Thorac Surg. 2009;9(2):296–300.
12. Selewski DT, Askenazi DJ, Bridges BC, Cooper DS, Fleming GM, Paden ML, et al. The impact of fluid overload on outcomes in children treated with extracorporeal membrane oxygenation: a multicenter retrospective cohort study. Pediatr Crit Care Med. 2017;18(12):1126–35.
13. Arikan AA, Zappitelli M, Goldstein SL, Naipaul A, Jefferson LS, Loftis LL. Fluid overload is associated with impaired oxygenation and morbidity in critically ill children. Pediatr Crit Care Med. 2012;13(3):253–8.
14. Sutherland SM, Zappitelli M, Alexander SR, Chua AN, Brophy PD, Bunchman TE, et al. Fluid overload and mortality in children receiving continuous renal replacement therapy: the prospective pediatric continuous renal replacement therapy registry. Am J Kidney Dis. 2010;55(2):316–25.
15. Davison D, Basu RK, Goldstein SL, Chawla LS. Fluid management in adults and children: core curriculum 2014. Am J Kidney Dis. 2014;63(4):700–12.
16. Roy BJ, Cornish JD, Clark RH. Venovenous extracorporeal membrane oxygenation affects renal function. Pediatrics. 1995;95(4):573–8.
17. Swaniker F, Kolla S, Moler F, Custer J, Grams R, Barlett R, et al. Extracorporeal life support outcome for 128 pediatric patients with respiratory failure. J Pediatr Surg. 2000;35(2):197–202.
18. Weber TR, Kountzman B. Extracorporeal membrane oxygenation for nonneonatal pulmonary and multiple-organ failure. J Pediatr Surg. 1998;33(11):1605–9.
19. Kelly RE Jr, Phillips JD, Foglia RP, Bjerke HS, Barcliff LT, Petrus L, et al. Pulmonary edema and fluid mobilization as determinants of the duration of ECMO support. J Pediatr Surg. 1991;26(9):1016–22.
20. Selewski DT, Cornell TT, Blatt NB, Han YY, Mottes T, Kommareddi M, et al. Fluid overload and fluid removal in pediatric patients on extracorporeal membrane oxygenation requiring continuous renal replacement therapy. Crit Care Med. 2012;40(9):2694–9.
21. Goldstein S, Bagshaw S, Cecconi M, Okusa M, Wang H, Kellum J, et al. Pharmacological management of fluid overload. Br J Anaesth. 2014;113(5):756–63.
22. Rosner MH, Ostermann M, Murugan R, Prowle JR, Ronco C, Kellum JA, et al. Indications and management of mechanical fluid removal in critical illness. Br J Anaesth. 2014;113(5):764–71.
23. Fleming GM, Askenazi DJ, Bridges BC, Cooper DS, Paden ML, Selewski DT, et al. A multicenter international survey of renal supportive therapy during ECMO: the kidney intervention during extracorporeal membrane oxygenation (KIDMO) group. ASAIO J. 2012;58(4):407–14.
24. Chen H, Yu RG, Yin NN, Zhou JX. Combination of extracorporeal membrane oxygenation and continuous renal replacement therapy in critically ill patients: a systematic review. Crit Care. 2014;18(6):675.
25. Askenazi DJ, Selewski DT, Paden ML, Cooper DS, Bridges BC, Zappitelli M, et al. Renal replacement therapy in critically ill patients receiving extracorporeal membrane oxygenation. Clin J Am Soc Nephrol. 2012;7(8):1328–36.
26. Laverdure F, Masson L, Tachon G, Guihaire J, Stephan F. Connection of a renal replacement therapy or plasmapheresis device to the ECMO circuit. ASAIO J. 2017;64(1):122–5.

27. Jenkins R, Harrison H, Chen B, Arnold D, Funk J. Accuracy of intravenous infusion pumps in continuous renal replacement therapies. ASAIO J. 1992;38(4):808–10.
28. Sucosky P, Dasi LP, Paden ML, Fortenberry JD, Yoganathan AP. Assessment of current continuous hemofiltration systems and development of a novel accurate fluid management system for use in extracorporeal membrane oxygenation. J Med Dev, Transactions of the ASME. 2008;2(3):035002.
29. Symons JM, McMahon MW, Karamlou T, Parrish AR, McMullan DM. Continuous renal replacement therapy with an automated monitor is superior to a free-flow system during extracorporeal life support. Pediatr Crit Care Med. 2013;14(9):e404–8.
30. Santiago MJ, Sanchez A, Lopez-Herce J, Perez R, del Castillo J, Urbano J, et al. The use of continuous renal replacement therapy in series with extracorporeal membrane oxygenation. Kidney Int. 2009;76(12):1289–92.
31. Shum HP, Kwan AM, Chan KC, Yan WW. The use of regional citrate anticoagulation continuous venovenous hemofiltration in extracorporeal membrane oxygenation. ASAIO J. 2014;60(4):413–8.
32. Barbaro RP, Paden ML, Guner YS, Raman L, Ryerson LM, Alexander P, et al. Pediatric extracorporeal life support organization registry international report 2016. ASAIO J. 2017;63(4):456–63.
33. Thiagarajan RR, Barbaro RP, Rycus PT, McMullan DM, Conrad SA, Fortenberry JD, et al. Extracorporeal life support organization registry international report 2016. ASAIO J. 2017;63(1):60–7.
34. Selewski DT, Askenazi DJ, Bridges BC, Cooper DS, Fleming GM, Paden ML, Verway M, Sahay R, King E, Zappitelli M. The impact of fluid overload on outcome of children treated with extracorporeal membrane oxygenation: a multicenter retrospective cohort study. Pediatr Crit Care Med. 2017;18(12):1126–35.
35. Kawai Y, Cornell TT, Cooley EG, Beckman CN, Baldridge PK, Mottes TA, et al. Therapeutic plasma exchange may improve hemodynamics and organ failure among children with sepsis-induced multiple organ dysfunction syndrome receiving extracorporeal life support. Pediatr Crit Care Med. 2015;16(4):366–74.
36. Schwartz J, Padmanabhan A, Aqui N, Balogun RA, Connelly-Smith L, Delaney M, et al. Guidelines on the use of therapeutic apheresis in clinical practice-evidence-based approach from the writing committee of the American society for apheresis: the seventh special issue. J Clin Apher. 2016;31(3):149–62.
37. Sirignano RM, Meyer EK, Fasano R, Paden ML. Pediatric tandem therapeutic apheresis: a multidisciplinary approach. ASAIO J. 2017. https://doi.org/10.1097/MAT.0000000000000641.
38. Nguyen TC, Cruz MA, Carcillo JA. Thrombocytopenia-associated multiple organ failure and acute kidney injury. Crit Care Clin. 2015;31(4):661–74.
39. Dyer M, Neal MD, Rollins-Raval MA, Raval JS. Simultaneous extracorporeal membrane oxygenation and therapeutic plasma exchange procedures are tolerable in both pediatric and adult patients. Transfusion. 2014;54(4):1158–65.
40. Bridges BC, Hardison D, Pietsch J. A case series of the successful use of ECMO, continuous renal replacement therapy, and plasma exchange for thrombocytopenia-associated multiple organ failure. J Pediatr Surg. 2013;48(5):1114–7.
41. Jamal JA, Economou CJ, Lipman J, Roberts JA. Improving antibiotic dosing in special situations in the ICU: burns, renal replacement therapy and extracorporeal membrane oxygenation. Curr Opin Crit Care. 2012;18(5):460–71.
42. Hohenforst-Schmidt W, Petermann A, Visouli A, Zarogoulidis P, Darwiche K, Kougioumtzi I, et al. Successful application of extracorporeal membrane oxygenation due to pulmonary hemorrhage secondary to granulomatosis with polyangiitis. Drug Des Devel Ther. 2013;7:627–33.
43. Patel P, Nandwani V, Vanchiere J, Conrad SA, Scott LK. Use of therapeutic plasma exchange as a rescue therapy in 2009 pH1N1 influenza A--an associated respiratory failure and hemodynamic shock. Pediatr Crit Care Med. 2011;12(2):e87–9.
44. Tabbutt S, Leonard M, Godinez RI, Sebert M, Cullen J, Spray TL, et al. Severe influenza B myocarditis and myositis. Pediatr Crit Care Med. 2004;5(4):403–6.

45. Mok Q, Butt W. The outcome of children admitted to intensive care with meningococcal septicaemia. Intensive Care Med. 1996;22(3):259–63.
46. Maclaren G, Butt W, Cameron P, Preovolos A, McEgan R, Marasco S. Treatment of polypharmacy overdose with multimodality extracorporeal life support. Anaesth Intensive Care. 2005;33(1):120–3.
47. Nasir S, Kilic YA, Karaaltin MV, Erdem Y. Lessons learned from the first quadruple extremity transplantation in the world. Ann Plast Surg. 2014;73(3):336–40.
48. Barnes SL, Naughton M, Douglass J, Murphy D. Extracorporeal membrane oxygenation with plasma exchange in a patient with alveolar haemorrhage secondary to Wegener's granulomatosis. Intern Med J. 2012;42(3):341–2.
49. Ahmed SH, Aziz T, Cochran J, Highland K. Use of extracorporeal membrane oxygenation in a patient with diffuse alveolar hemorrhage. Chest. 2004;126(1):305–9.
50. Yusuff H, Malagon I, Robson K, Parmar J, Hamilton P, Falter F. Extracorporeal membrane oxygenation for life-threatening ANCA-positive pulmonary capillaritis. A review of UK experience. Heart Lung Vessel. 2015;7(2):159–67.
51. Joseph M, Charles AG. Early extracorporeal life support as rescue for Wegener granulomatosis with diffuse alveolar hemorrhage and acute respiratory distress syndrome: a case report and literature review. Pediatr Emerg Care. 2011;27(12):1163–6.
52. Di Maria MV, Hollister R, Kaufman J. Case report: severe microscopic polyangiitis successfully treated with extracorporeal membrane oxygenation and immunosuppression in a pediatric patient. Curr Opin Pediatr. 2008;20(6):740–2.
53. Dalabih A, Pietsch J, Jabs K, Hardison D, Bridges BC. Extracorporeal membrane oxygenation as a platform for recovery: a case report of a child with pulmonary hemorrhage, refractory hypoxemic respiratory failure, and new onset goodpasture syndrome. J Extra Corpor Technol. 2012;44(2):75–7.
54. Hites M, Dell'Anna AM, Scolletta S, Taccone FS. The challenges of multiple organ dysfunction syndrome and extra-corporeal circuits for drug delivery in critically ill patients. Adv Drug Deliv Rev. 2014;77:12–21.
55. Nguyen TC, Han YY, Kiss JE, Hall MW, Hassett AC, Jaffe R, et al. Intensive plasma exchange increases a disintegrin and metalloprotease with thrombospondin motifs-13 activity and reverses organ dysfunction in children with thrombocytopenia-associated multiple organ failure. Crit Care Med. 2008;36(10):2878–87.
56. Kolovos NS, Schuerer DJ, Moler FW, Bratton SL, Swaniker F, Bartlett RH, et al. Extracorporal life support for pulmonary hemorrhage in children: a case series. Crit Care Med. 2002;30(3):577–80.

# 23 CRRT Program Development

Theresa A. Mottes

## 23.1 Organizational Infrastructure

Continuous renal replacement therapy (CRRT) is a complex procedural therapy provided to patients for management of acute kidney injury (AKI) [1]. The delivery of CRRT requires significant organizational planning, considerations, and coordination of care. The care of these complex patients necessitates an interdisciplinary team approach. The decision to embark on implementing a CRRT program is not limited to deciding about machinery and staff, but encompasses all facets of the delivering the therapy. Thoughtful planning with the essential parties provides the foundation for identifying and describing the numerous processes necessary for implementing and maintaining a CRRT program [2]. Identification and engagement of key stakeholders is the first step. Key stakeholders include, but are not limited to, the physicians, nurses, pharmacists, dietitians, biomedical personnel, billing administration, information technology departments, and supply chain departments. Each discipline or department has specific needs and interest that should be addressed early in the development of the program. Often, much attention is focused on the process of initiating CRRT, with little attention to the smaller details such as the ordering, distributing, and hanging of the CRRT solution. All processes, big and small, need to be adequately addressed and described prior to implementation. Successful implementation of a CRRT program requires early initiated planning, continuous assessment, and ongoing evaluation of the processes [54].

T. A. Mottes
Renal Services, Texas Children's Hospital, Houston, TX, USA
e-mail: tamottes@texaschildrens.org



A. Deep, S. L. Goldstein (eds.), *Critical Care Nephrology and Renal Replacement Therapy in Children*, https://doi.org/10.1007/978-3-319-90281-4_23

## 23.2 Care Delivery Models

Various CRRT care delivery models have been described in the literature [3–7]. The care delivery model an institution adopts is influenced by the available resources, as well as the provider and caregiver preferences [8]. Thus, an important step in deciding on a care delivery model is a thorough assessment of the facility's available resources, motivation and engagement of essential staff, and administrative support (see Table 23.1).

Investigating for resources, such as dialysis, apheresis, or extracorporeal membrane oxygenation (ECMO) programs, provides networking opportunities for sharing of policies, procedures, guidelines, and potentially personnel. The second step

**Table 23.1** Planning a CRRT program

| Process | Considerations |
|---|---|
| Identify key stakeholders | Physician, nursing, pharmacy, dietician, supply management, business director, biomedical staff, capital purchasing, |
| Resource assessment | Dialysis, ECMO, other extracorporeal programs |
| Care delivery model | Nursing workload and resources<br>Physician resources |
| Education | Physician and nursing initial courses<br>Ongoing and annual courses |
| Equipment selection | Evaluation and purchase of available equipment |
| Disposables | Filters, tubing, solutions, catheters<br>Purchasing and storing products |
| Polices | Staffing requirements and education<br>Location/units providing care<br>Solution preparation–Pharmacy procedures<br>Provider credentialing<br>Nursing: Patient ratios |
| Standard practice guidelines | Patient selection—All ages/size vs. only certain age/size<br>Indications for initiating CRRT<br>Vascular access recommendations<br>Initiation procedure recommendations<br>Modality/filter standards<br>Minimum CRRT prescription<br>CRRT solution selection<br>Anticoagulation standards<br>Fluid removal standards<br>Laboratory monitoring frequency<br>Documentation guidelines<br>Frequency of circuit/filter change |
| Procedures | Initiation procedures—Saline and blood priming<br>Discontinuation procedures<br>CRRT solution preparation<br>Anticoagulation protocol |
| Quality improvement | Select process and outcome measures<br>Determine frequency of reporting<br>Process for reporting |

is evaluating the level of nursing and physician engagement, identifying champions to design and execute the care delivery model.

Traditionally the literature describes two basic nursing models, single and collaborative (see Fig. 23.1). In the single care model, the critical care nurses are responsible for all aspects of the CRRT care. In theory, the single care model reduces role confusion, and errors associated with miscommunication [8]. Additionally, with one department performing all associated CRRT task, care delays related to coordinating with other departments are minimized. However, critical care nurses may lack the expertise in nephrology based therapies, which lends to an increase need in initial and ongoing training. In contrast, the collaborative model employs a sharing of responsibilities and tasks between at least two departments [5]. The common partnership is between dialysis programs and critical care units. Partnering with dialysis nurses who have expertise in both dialysis and extracorporeal therapies, bridges the knowledge gap of critical care nurses [4, 5]. Yet, coordinating care between multiple disciplines may be associated with increased cost. Recent literature reports several non-traditional models; such as collaboration between critical care and ECMO, the implementation of specialized CRRT teams, and collaboration between critical care units within an institution [7, 9].

| Chronology of Care | Responsibility | Collaborative Care Model | Critical Care Model |
|---|---|---|---|
| Continuous renal replacement therapy setup | Prepare machine | DN | CCN-I |
| | Obtain supplies | DN | CCN-I |
| | Schedule initiation time | DN | Coordinator |
| Initiate therapy | Prime machine | DN | CCN-I |
| | Obtain pre labs | DN | CCN-I |
| | Assess catheter function | DN | CCN-I |
| | Performs procedure | DN | CCN-I |
| | Monitors patient during procedure | CCN | CCN-U |
| Maintain therapy | Circuit monitoring | CCN | CCN-U |
| | Obtain ACG labs | CCN | CCN-U |
| | Fluid calculations | CCN | CCN-U |
| | Adjust ACG per protocol | CCN | CCN-U |
| | Bag changes | CCN | CCN-U |
| | Adjust rates per orders | CCN | CCN-U |
| | Catheter care | CCN | CCN-U |
| Troubleshooting and other procedures | First responder to alarms | CCN | CCN-U |
| | Second responder to alarms | DN | Coordinator/CCN-U |
| | Reverse lines | DN | Coordinator/CCN-U |
| | Recirculation procedure | DN | Coordinator/CCN-U |
| | Perform in OR | DN | Coordinator |
| | Reinitiation procedure | DN | Coordinator/CCN-U |
| Terminate therapy | Return blood (as necessary) | DN | CCN-I or CCN-U |
| | Discards filter set | DN | CCN-I or CCN-U |

DN = dialysis nurse, CCN-I = critical care nurse initiator, Coordinator = continuous renal replacement therapy program coordinator nurse, CCN = critical care nurse, CCN-U = critical care nurse user.

**Fig. 23.1** Collaborative vs. single care nursing model

While the advantages and disadvantages of care delivery models continue to be debated, the ultimate goal is to design a model that ensures the delivery of the highest quality CRRT care. The ideal care delivery model involves coalition of expertise (e.g., knowledge and technical skills), care delivery (e.g., standardized guidelines, minimize care interruptions), and cost (e.g., overtime and reimbursement).

## 23.3 Physical Facilities/Location

The delivery of CRRT is a complex, highly technical therapy and requires a well-trained competent staff. While there is consensus that CRRT must be delivered in the critical care environment, the decision to provide the therapy in a single unit within an institution or multiple units remains a matter of debate. The majority of pediatric institutions have adopted specialty critical care units, such as neonatal intensive care units (NICU), pediatric intensive care units (PICU), and cardiac intensive care units (CICU). Patient care providers in these specialized units have an expertise in a specialty to deliver the best care to that particular group of patients [10]. For example, CICU staff is specifically trained to care for patients with congenital heart diseases (CHD), including presurgical and postsurgical unique characteristics associated with CHD. Recent studies suggest care provided in a specialty unit with expert staff and providers is associated with improved patient outcomes [11, 12]. However, the delivery of safe effective CRRT requires additional expertise and proficiency in this complicated patient population [13]. Therefore, institutions must weigh the benefits of continuing care in a specialty unit with the staff's ability to develop and maintain competency of CRRT care.

The number and frequency of patients receiving CRRT at an institution is the most important factor in maintaining competent staff. Low volume pediatric CRRT programs, generally defined as caring for, less than ten patients and providing less than 100 days of CRRT annually, will likely benefit from one dedicated team of caregivers/units for patients receiving CRRT. In contrast, larger pediatric CRRT programs, such as those caring for greater than 30 patients and providing more than 350 CRRT days annually, may have the volume to support maintaining competency of a larger number of staff from multiple units.

The advantage of cohorting patients in one unit reduces the number of staff and dedicated hours for initial training and ongoing education. The staff have more opportunity to provide CRRT care, contributing to the development of the knowledge and technical skills associated with CRRT. The negative aspect of cohorting patients is the necessity to transfer patients from their primary critical care unit to a unit without the expertise in a particular disease or population, i.e., transferring a neonate requiring CRRT to the PICU. While the PICU staff may be competent in delivering CRRT, they often lack neonatal expertise. Successful cohort CRRT programs provide interdisciplinary care to ensure that experienced practitioners are involved to address the specific needs of the population as well as the skills and knowledge for the renal replacement therapy.

In contrast to cohorting, institutions may choose to provide CRRT across multiple units. The primary advantage in this model is preserving the continuity of care. Patients remain in the appropriate unit with disease expertise. However, delivering

CRRT in all units requires a larger number of CRRT trained staff. Each unit must have adequate number of trained staff available on all shifts to ensure CRRT can be delivered 24/7. An important consideration in delivering CRRT in multiple units is the frequency of therapy; specifically, is there ample opportunity for staff to care for CRRT to ensure a high level of competence and comfort delivering care? And, if the opportunities are limited, what strategies can be implemented to allow for staff to develop proficiency.

## 23.4 Equipment and Supplies

An important consideration in implementing a pediatric CRRT program is selecting equipment and supplies that best fit the patient population, modalities, and therapies being planned for at the program. The commercially available CRRT machines are designed with crucial safety features, including ease of use, air detector, blood leak detector, flow (blood and solution) sensors, and filter pressure measuring devices. The biggest variation in CRRT machines is the availability of modalities and therapies. Some CRRT machines have the ability to deliver a wide range of modalities and therapies (SCUF, CVVH, CVVHD, CVVHDF, TPE), while others may have limited modalities. However, it is important to note that the majority of commercially available CRRT machines are not specifically designed for the pediatric and neonatal population. The options for neonatal and pediatric machines are very limited and not available in all areas [14–16]. Therefore, a careful selection process with a thorough machine evaluation is essential. Key stakeholders should assess both usability and adaptability of the machine for the intended population. Overall, the selected CRRT machine must meet the needs of the providers and caregivers and deliver safe effective therapy.

The next consideration is choosing disposables: filters, tubing sets, and solutions. Often the CRRT machine has dedicated filter and tubing sets, limiting the available choices for programs. However, it is essential for programs to consider the availability of filter and tubing sets for the smallest and largest intended patient population, such as a low volume filter/tubing sets for neonate and adult filter/tubing set for an obese adolescent. The next disposable choice is determining what solutions will be used to deliver CRRT. In previous years, commercially available solutions were limited, causing many programs to used custom-made, in-house prepared solutions. However, there is literature reporting high medication errors and even death associated with the use of in-house prepared solution [17]. A wide variety of commercially prepared solutions are now available, eliminated the need for in-house preparation of solutions. Several factors must be considered in selecting solutions. Of these, anticoagulation and patient diagnosis will significantly influence the decision. Regional anticoagulation with citrate requires the use of calcium free CRRT solutions [18–20]. While, patients with severe acidosis may require a higher bicarbonate solution [21, 22]. CRRT programs should limit the available choices to three or four, allowing for patient variation yet, ensuring adherence to standard practices. Additionally, the in-house manipulation of the solutions should be limited to specific additives and doses with secondary validation step to reduce medication errors.

## 23.5 Education and Training

Many technical advances have been made in the CRRT delivery. Key developments include introduction of highly sensitive, integrated machines with multiple prescription options and improved fluid balance accuracy. As a continuous modality, optimal CRRT delivery relies on expert staff to prescribe therapy, troubleshoot technical issues, and ensure patient safety. This requires experienced providers to identify acute circuit and patient issues expeditiously then determine the cause and effectively resolve the problem. Patient issues tend to be more complex requiring the team to effectively communicate the ever-changing patient status and adjust therapy goals as needed. Therefore, the safe and effect CRRT care is rooted in the educational program. However, there is a lack of standards for the required educational objectives and requirements [8]. Institutions are challenged with developing and implementing education that is promotes the development of proficiency in CRRT care.

## 23.6 Education Standards

As previously highlighted, there are little published data to guide institutions during the development of educational requirements and standards. A survey conducted among nurses providing CRRT revealed significant variation in dedicated CRRT education with only 50% of responders receiving dedicated CRRT education and 45% developed CRRT knowledge and skills during the course of their work [4]. There is a lack of consensus regarding the minimum qualifications/experience, didactic requirements, and orientation hours for nurses and physicians to provide CRRT. However, the complexity of CRRT care necessitates that all providers and caregivers receive dedicated CRRT education. The education must reflect the specific roles and responsibilities of the staff. In a collaborative care model, the critical care staff are specifically responsible for the alarm and hourly fluid balance management. Therefore, the education sessions must focus on techniques for troubleshooting and procedures for adequately manage the patient's fluid status [23, 24]. In contrast, the education for staff in a critical care based model provide all aspects of care. Critical care nurses require additional educational content such as setup, priming, and initiation procedures [9, 24, 25]. While controversies exist regarding education, patients receiving CRRT deserve a well-educated, competent staff providing care.

## 23.7 Educational Strategies

The ultimate goal of education is to provide is healthcare providers and caregivers a method for skill acquisition moving them through the five level of nursing experience as described in Benner's Nursing Theory: Novice to Expert [26]. Several strategies can be used to achieve the knowledge and skills to safely care for patients receiving CRRT. The most common strategies described in the literature lecture-based educational sessions. Didactic training is best used to impart knowledge, specifically the concepts and principles associated with the various CRRT modalities such as diffusion and convection. Richardson & Whatmore articulately described the necessary components of an effective educational course: indications and mechanisms, technical, complications, and interruption prevention [13]. Didactic training is traditionally delivered in a classroom setting, however a recent study describes the successful use of online modules to increase CRRT knowledge, eliminating the need for structured classroom education [27]. Other published strategies include just-in-time training (JITT), in which key concepts are delivered to the providers and caregivers at the bedside when the knowledge or skill is needed [28]. JITT allows for healthcare providers to actively learn, apply concepts in real time, and receive immediate feedback. Didactic training methods, whether through traditional classroom setting, online modules, or JITT are valuable strategies for teaching institutional policies and the basic concepts of CRRT.

In contrast, simulation-based training is a more effective method for acquiring the technical and teamwork skills necessary to deliver safe CRRT care [29]. Staff often have difficulty applying technical information learned in a lecture, without hands on application. Human patient simulators are currently utilized in a number of medical settings. Anesthesia, critical care and trauma teams have employed simulation training with positive effects on procedural and cognitive skills in the simulated setting [30, 31]. Simulation training provides an opportunity for staff to develop and maintain technical proficiency in high-risk, low frequency events, such as blood priming procedures and catheter dysfunction, without the fear of harming real patients [32]. Low- and high-fidelity simulation can be used. Low fidelity is more appropriate for situation with minimal patient involvement, such as setup and priming. High-fidelity simulation is reserved for more complex issues. The simulation environment is set up to reflect an authentic, realistic setting, with the CRRT machine connected to the appropriate patient simulator (infant, child, or adult). Fluid balance management is an example of a complex issue. Fluid balance management requires frequent assessments, critical thinking and adequate communication. Mottes and colleagues described using simulation-based instruction for teaching troubleshooting techniques for catheter dysfunction and fluid removal errors, which resulted in improved CRRT filter life; 48.4–59.4 h ($p < 0.01$) and a trend towards a decrease in unplanned filter changes; 40.7% to 35.5% ($p = 0.12$) [9]. In addition to providing an environment to practice skills, high-fidelity simulation can be used to assess and evaluate knowledge, skills, and attitudes associated with the providing CRRT care [33].

## 23.8 Education Recommendations

Successful CRRT programs utilize a combination of educational strategies to ensure staff have attained and maintain CRRT competency. Prior to assuming the responsibility of patients on CRRT, providers and caregivers should complete a CRRT course that combines didactic (classroom or online modules) and hands on training (simulation-based training). Additionally, all staff providing CRRT care need to demonstrate continued technical competency via low- or high-fidelity simulation. While there is no evidence based standards for staff education, one well established program describes their education requirements; in order to join the CRRT team, nurses must have 6 months of critical care experience, complete a 4 h didactic session, 24 h of bedside orientation with a qualified preceptor, and complete an annual competency assessment [34].

## 23.9 Patient Care Delivery: Standards and Procedures

Since the landmark report by the Institute of Medicine *To Err is Human: Building a Safer Health System*, a significant amount of resources, both financial and personnel, have been dedicated to improve patient safety [35]. A central conclusion from the report indicated the root of medical errors was in part secondary to a high degree of practice variability and inconsistency. Since that time, practice variation among practitioners at the same level and across levels has become a focus of study in quality improvement [36, 37]. There are many reasons for practice variation in healthcare, including the lack of consistent data driven best practice guidelines and evidence, inconsistent policies within an institution, and provider bias and beliefs [38]. Reducing variation, many believe, will create a consistent standard for care and ultimately increase the quality and safety for patients. Significant practice variation has already been shown in multiple patient environments to be directly associated with poor patient outcome.

CRRT is a complex therapy delivered to the most critically ill patients. Applying standard practice guidelines to the processes behind CRRT delivery may be meaningful and directly related to patient outcome. Standard practice guidelines are minimum recommendations intended to optimize patient care that are informed by a systematic review of evidence [39]. CRRT standard practice guidelines outline the minimum prescriptive and care delivery standards for all patients receiving CRRT. Prescriptive guidelines should include the standard modality, minimum blood flow rate, minimum CRRT dose, initial fluid removal goals, standard anticoagulation method, filter selection, and CRRT solution recommendations. In the pediatric population, it crucial to establish blood priming criteria, as well as size based vascular access guidelines. Additionally, prescriptive standards address specific patient diagnosis or conditions that necessitate a deviation from the standard, e.g., infant in-born errors of metabolism [40]. The delivery (who, how, when) of CRRT care is describe in the process standards. Process guidelines include nursing qualifications, staff education requirements, frequency of monitoring and documentation, and required personnel presence at CRRT filter initiation procedures. Other process standards, may include expected time to initiation (time from decision to starting CRRT) or circuit recirculation recommendation (appropriate patient selection and procedure). The other essential element to standard practice guidelines are developing detailed CRRT procedures; specifically blood prime procedure, standard initiation procedure, and filter change procedure. The development and adherence to standard practice guidelines eliminates unnecessary practice variation while ensuring the highest quality of care for all patients receiving CRRT. However, standard practice guidelines are not meant to be strict protocols, but rather evidence based recommendations that can modified to patient's specific conditions [53].

## 23.10 Program Evaluation: Quality Improvement

Quality improvement is a dynamic, interdisciplinary process that strives to achieve the best outcomes for patients. The importance of measuring and monitoring healthcare quality is no longer in doubt. Even in the most complex situations, the application of a continuous quality improvement process to reduce practice variations and establish best practices has demonstrated improvement in care delivery as well as patient outcomes. One such example is the utilization of quality improvement strategies focusing on process measures to improve cardiac arrest outcomes. Survival from cardiac arrest is directly linked to prompt responses and quality of cardiopulmonary resuscitation [41]. Optimizing response times, quality of compressions, and team cohesion through enhanced training and applying systems improvement processes has significantly impacted survival [42]. Therefore, applying similar strategies with a focus on the delivery of care processes, in other complex medical situations such as CRRT care, may provide more meaningful information. The paucity of evidence based quality indicators is a hindrance for implementing a CRRT quality improvement program. A recent systematic review suggested a list of potential indicators: dose prescription and delivery, anticoagulation selection and monitoring, catheter complications, and treatment interruptions [8, 43]. Connors and colleagues describe similar indicators to ensure high quality CRRT care [44]. However, benchmark or recommendations for targets remain debated.

Quality improvement indicators central to adequately evaluating a program must reflect both patient outcomes and process outcomes. Patient outcomes consist of basic fluid overload, and survival. Analyzing patient outcomes, allows leaders to understand how the patient characteristics at the time of CRRT initiation, influence program outcomes. The existing pediatric literature, multicenter and single center is patient outcomes focused, allowing programs the opportunity to compare and contrast published patient characteristics and outcomes with the institution outcomes [1, 45–49].

While patient outcomes are important to measure and monitor, process outcomes provide a more detailed look at the practices and procedures that may positively or negatively impact patient outcomes measures [50, 51]. Process measures reflect adherence to the standardized steps and practices performed by healthcare staff members that are necessary to ensure high quality care is delivered to every patient [52]. Therefore, process measures are equally and may be more important to follow than outcomes measures in the delivery of CRRT. CRRT activity, defined as the number of days CRRT is delivered, is an indicator essential to evaluating CRRT processes. For example, if an increase in activity negatively impacts other indicators such as filter life, this may suggest the current processes and resources are not adequate to deliver quality care. Some well recognized process measures that are relatively easy to track and monitor are filter life (difference between filter start time and the filter end time), filter survival (filter survival hours over time), and delivered CRRT (total effluent measured during the CRRT hours) [43]. Each of these measures is multifactorial and reflect the delivery of care. Other potential process indicators include unplanned filter changes and daily fluid management [9]. Selecting the "right" process measures can be challenging. The measure must assess and evaluate the program design (i.e., care delivery model) and processes (i.e., procedures), highlighting the strength, latent threats, and program progression.

## 23.11 Summary

The implementation of a CRRT program requires meticulous assessment and planning to ensure pediatric patients are receiving the highest quality of care. Key components of a successful program include early and continued engagement of key stakeholders, identifying and aligning available resources, outlining and defining processes and procedures, and frequent assessment and evaluation of the program.

## References


1. Goldstein SL, et al. Pediatric patients with multi-organ dysfunction syndrome receiving continuous renal replacement therapy. Kidney Int. 2005;67(2):653–8.
2. Craig MA, et al. Implementing a continuous renal replacement therapies program. Adv Ren Replace Ther. 1996;3(4):348–50.
3. Baldwin I. Is there a need for a nurse emergency team for continuous renal replacement therapy? Contrib Nephrol. 2007;156:191–6.
4. Ricci Z, et al. Nursing procedures during continuous renal replacement therapies: a national survey. Heart Lung Vessel. 2015;7(3):224–30.
5. Martin RK. Who should manage continuous renal replacement in the intensive care setting? A nursing viewpoint. EDTNA ERCA J. 2002;53(Suppl 2):43–5.
6. Page M, et al. Impact of a program designed to improve continuous renal replacement therapy stability. Ann Fr Anesth Reanim. 2014;33(12):626–30.
7. Kee YK, et al. The effect of specialized continuous renal replacement therapy team in acute kidney injury patients treatment. Yonsei Med J. 2015;56(3):658–65.
8. Rewa O, Mottes T, Bagshaw SM. Quality measures for acute kidney injury and continuous renal replacement therapy. Curr Opin Crit Care. 2015;21(6):490–9.
9. Mottes T, et al. Improving delivery of continuous renal replacement therapy: impact of a simulation-based educational intervention. Pediatr Crit Care Med. 2013;14(8):747–54.
10. Burstein DS, et al. Care models and associated outcomes in congenital heart surgery. Pediatrics. 2011;127(6):e1482–9.
11. Stiller CA. Non-specialist units, clinical trials and survival from testicular cancer. Eur J Cancer. 1995;31A(3):289–91.
12. Govan L, et al. Does the prevention of complications explain the survival benefit of organized inpatient (stroke unit) care?: further analysis of a systematic review. Stroke. 2007;38(9):2536–40.
13. Richardson A, Whatmore J. Nursing essential principles: continuous renal replacement therapy. Nurs Crit Care. 2015;20(1):8–15.

14. Ronco C, et al. Continuous renal replacement therapy in neonates and small infants: development and first-in-human use of a miniaturised machine (CARPEDIEM). Lancet. 2014;383(9931):1807–13.
15. Coulthard MG, et al. Haemodialysing babies weighing <8 kg with the Newcastle infant dialysis and ultrafiltration system (Nidus): comparison with peritoneal and conventional haemodialysis. Pediatr Nephrol. 2014;29(10):1873–81.
16. Askenazi D, et al. Smaller circuits for smaller patients: improving renal support therapy with Aquadex. Pediatr Nephrol. 2016;31(5):853–60.
17. Barletta JF, et al. Medication errors and patient complications with continuous renal replacement therapy. Pediatr Nephrol. 2006;21(6):842–5.
18. Rodriguez K, et al. Regional citrate anticoagulation for continuous renal replacement therapy in pediatric patients with liver failure. PLoS One. 2017;12(8):e0182134.
19. Rico MP, et al. Regional citrate anticoagulation for continuous renal replacement therapy in children. Pediatr Nephrol. 2017;32(4):703–11.
20. Fernandez SN, et al. Citrate anticoagulation for CRRT in children: comparison with heparin. Biomed Res Int. 2014;2014:786301.
21. Sutherland SM, Alexander SR. Continuous renal replacement therapy in children. Pediatr Nephrol. 2012;27(11):2007–16.
22. Yessayan L, et al. Continuous renal replacement therapy for the management of acid-base and electrolyte imbalances in acute kidney injury. Adv Chronic Kidney Dis. 2016;23(3):203–10.
23. Baldwin I. Continuous renal replacement therapy. Keeping pace with changes in technology and technique. Blood Purif. 2002;20(3):269–74.
24. Baldwin IC. Training, management, and credentialing for CRRT in the ICU. Am J Kidney Dis. 1997;30(5 Suppl 4):S112–6.
25. Baldwin I, Fealy N. Nursing for renal replacement therapies in the intensive care unit: historical, educational, and protocol review. Blood Purif. 2009;27(2):174–81.
26. Benner P, Tanner C, Chesla C. From beginner to expert: gaining a differentiated clinical world in critical care nursing. ANS Adv Nurs Sci. 1992;14(3):13–28.
27. Windt K. Development of online learning modules as an adjunct to skills fairs and lectures to maintain nurses' competency and comfort level when caring for pediatric patients requiring continuous renal replacement therapy (CRRT). Nephrol Nurs J. 2016;43(1):39–46; quiz 47.
28. Nishisaki A, et al. Effect of just-in-time simulation training on tracheal intubation procedure safety in the pediatric intensive care unit. Anesthesiology. 2010;113(1):214–23.
29. Yaeger KA, et al. High-fidelity simulation-based training in neonatal nursing. Adv Neonatal Care. 2004;4(6):326–31.
30. Friedrich MJ. Practice makes perfect: risk-free medical training with patient simulators. JAMA. 2002;288(22):2808, 2811-2.
31. Vandrey CI, Whitman KM. Simulator training for novice critical care nurses: preparing providers to work with critically ill patients. AJN Am J Nurs. 2001;101(9):24GG–LL.
32. Burton KS, et al. Impact of simulation-based extracorporeal membrane oxygenation training in the simulation laboratory and clinical environment. Simul Healthc. 2011;6(5):284–91.
33. Przybyl H, Androwich I, Evans J. Using high-fidelity simulation to assess knowledge, skills, and attitudes in nurses performing CRRT. Nephrol Nurs J. 2015;42(2):135–47; quiz 148.
34. Graham P, Lischer E. Nursing issues in renal replacement therapy: organization, manpower assessment, competency evaluation and quality improvement processes. Semin Dial. 2011;24(2):183–7.
35. Kohn LT, Corrigan JM, Donaldson MS. To err is human:: building a safer health system, vol. Vol. 6. Washington, USA: National Academies Press; 2000.
36. Committee on Patient Safety and Quality Improvement. Committee opinion no. 629: clinical guidelines and standardization of practice to improve outcomes. Obstet Gynecol. 2015;125(4):1027–9.
37. Rozich JD, et al. Standardization as a mechanism to improve safety in health care. Jt Comm J Qual Saf. 2004;30(1):5–14.
38. James B. Quality improvement opportunities in health care.Making it easy to do it right. J Manag Care Pharm. 2002;8(5):394–9.

39. Rosenfeld RM, Shiffman RN. Clinical practice guideline development manual: a quality-driven approach for translating evidence into action. Otolaryngol Head Neck Surg. 2009;140(6 Suppl 1):S1–43.
40. Spinale JM, et al. High-dose continuous renal replacement therapy for neonatal hyperammonemia. Pediatr Nephrol. 2013;28(6):983–6.
41. Abella BS, et al. CPR quality improvement during in-hospital cardiac arrest using a real-time audiovisual feedback system. Resuscitation. 2007;73(1):54–61.
42. Meaney PA, et al. Cardiopulmonary resuscitation quality: [corrected] improving cardiac resuscitation outcomes both inside and outside the hospital: a consensus statement from the American Heart Association. Circulation. 2013;128(4):417–35.
43. Rewa OG, et al. Quality indicators of continuous renal replacement therapy (CRRT) care in critically ill patients: a systematic review. Intensive Care Med. 2017;43(6):750–63.
44. Connor MJ Jr, Karakala N. Continuous renal replacement therapy: reviewing current best practice to provide high-quality extracorporeal therapy to critically ill patients. Adv Chronic Kidney Dis. 2017;24(4):213–8.
45. Rajasekaran S, et al. Outcomes of hematopoietic stem cell transplant patients who received continuous renal replacement therapy in a pediatric oncology intensive care unit. Pediatr Crit Care Med. 2010;11(6):699–706.
46. Hayes LW, et al. Outcomes of critically ill children requiring continuous renal replacement therapy. J Crit Care. 2009;24(3):394–400.
47. Askenazi DJ, et al. Continuous renal replacement therapy for children </=10 kg: a report from the prospective pediatric continuous renal replacement therapy registry. J Pediatr. 2013;162(3):587–592 e3.
48. Flores FX, et al. Continuous renal replacement therapy (CRRT) after stem cell transplantation. A report from the prospective pediatric CRRT registry group. Pediatr Nephrol. 2008;23(4):625–30.
49. Symons JM, et al. Demographic characteristics of pediatric continuous renal replacement therapy: a report of the prospective pediatric continuous renal replacement therapy registry. Clin J Am Soc Nephrol. 2007;2(4):732–8.
50. Donabedian A. The quality of care. How can it be assessed? 1988. Arch Pathol Lab Med. 1997;121(11):1145–50.
51. Measuring and improving quality of care: a report from the American Heart Association/American College of Cardiology First Scientific Forum on assessment of healthcare quality in cardiovascular disease and stroke. Circulation. 2000;101(12):1483–93.
52. Werner RM, Bradlow ET, Asch DA. Does hospital performance on process measures directly measure high quality care or is it a marker of unmeasured care? Health Serv Res. 2008;43(5 Pt 1):1464–84.
53. Woolf S, et al. Potential benefits, limitations, and harms of clinical guidelines. BMJ. 1999;318(7182):527–30.
54. Magnezi R. Disease management programs: barriers and benefits. Am J Manag Care. 2013;19(4):e140–7.

# The Future of Pediatric CRRT

# 24

William R. Clark, Stuart L. Goldstein, Jeffrey Letteri, and Claudio Ronco

## 24.1 Introduction

Continuous renal replacement therapy (CRRT) was originally developed as an alternative for hemodynamically unstable acute renal failure (ARF) patients who could not tolerate conventional hemodialysis [1, 2]. The early application of CRRT to both adult and pediatric patients largely involved technology adapted from the maintenance dialysis setting and almost exclusively occurred as a salvage therapy, typically in hypercatabolic patients with severe, diuretic-resistant fluid overload. The development of dedicated CRRT machines has contributed substantially to the growth of the therapy over the past two decades in the critically ill adult population and it is now used as a first-line treatment for acute kidney injury (AKI) [3]. In fact, consensus statements now suggest its use, rather than conventional hemodialysis, for hemodynamically unstable patients [4].

The development of AKI in children is now recognized to be a common occurrence, especially among critically ill neonates and infants, and is associated with substantial morbidity and mortality [5]. With respect to dialytic management,

W. R. Clark (✉)
Davidson School of Chemical Engineering, Purdue University, West Lafayette, IN, USA
e-mail: clarkw@purdue.edu

S. L. Goldstein
Center for Acute Care Nephrology, Cincinnati Children's Hospital Medical Center, Cincinnati, OH, USA

J. Letteri
Medical Affairs, Baxter Healthcare Corporation, Deerfield, IL, USA

C. Ronco
International Renal Research Institute of Vicenza (IRRIV), San Bortolo Hospital, Vicenza, Italy

Department of Nephrology, San Bortolo Hospital, Vicenza, Italy



A. Deep, S. L. Goldstein (eds.), *Critical Care Nephrology and Renal Replacement Therapy in Children*, https://doi.org/10.1007/978-3-319-90281-4_24

continuous RRT (CRRT) has supplanted peritoneal dialysis as the preferred dialytic modality for critically ill pediatric AKI patients in many parts of the world, especially the United States [6]. However, these devices generally have not had specific indications for pediatric use due to limitations related to fluid accuracy and extracorporeal circuit volumes. The recent introduction of a pediatric-specific machines [7] obviates the need to provide CRRT "off-label" with adult-based CRRT devices to small pediatric patients. In this chapter, some of the clinical challenges associated with treating the complex critically ill AKI patient population are discussed and several important questions for the future are addressed [8]. Objectives of writing this chapter are as follows:

- Understand the potential ways in which the clinical management of pediatric AKI patients will change over the next decade.
- Understand the concept of precision CRRT and the need to personalize the prescription and delivery of CRRT.
- For CRRT dosing, describe potentially new approaches that provide more specific information related to solute clearance beyond normalized effluent rate.
- Describe the role that quality metrics and data analytics may play in the future management of pediatric AKI patients.
- Describe new CRRT machine developments which create the potential for safer and more effective delivery of therapy, especially to neonates and small infants.

## 24.2 The Future of Renal Support for Pediatric AKI

### 24.2.1 Adoption of Precision CRRT

A recent Acute Dialysis Quality Initiative (ADQI) consensus conference focused on the need for CRRT patient management to be adapted to personalized medicine. In this regard, the ADQI participants proposed the term "precision CRRT," calling for technology to be applied on an individualized basis in a "dynamic" manner such that treatment is adapted continuously to the current clinical status of the critically ill AKI patient [9, 10]. Dynamic CRRT has several established elements, including solute clearance, delivered/prescribed dose, effective treatment time, solute control indicators, circuit/filter pressure trends, fluid and hemodynamic management, and anticoagulation. Considerations for the future, to be discussed subsequently, include quality metrics, biofeedback, and data analytics [11–13].

### 24.2.2 Dosing of CRRT

Based on the landmark study performed by Ronco et al. [14] and other prospective trials [15, 16], the use of effluent-based dosing to guide CRRT prescription and delivery is established firmly in adult AKI clinical practice [17] with a target delivered dose range of 20–25 mL/kg/h. Whether normalized to body surface area or weight, pediatric CRRT dosing is also based on effluent rate. Ricci and colleagues have recently reported a very wide range of published pediatric CRRT doses, spanning from 1000–4000 mL/h/1.73 $m^2$ and 20–150 mL/kg/h [18]. Nevertheless, dose parameters based on effluent rate do not provide an accurate estimation of actual solute clearance and substantial differences between effluent dose and actual solute clearance may exist under many CRRT operating conditions [19].

Two recent publications provide a reappraisal of dose prescription and delivery for CRRT. Clark et al. [20] proposed an adaptation of a chronic dialysis parameter (standard Kt/V) [21] as a benchmark to supplement effluent-based dosing. This proposed approach allows for the target standard Kt/V to vary on a patient-to-patient basis according to clinical circumstances and can be modified in an individual patient, depending on the clinical course (e.g., a hypercatabolic, septic patient in need of higher dose to control azotemia). These dosage adjustments are entirely consistent with the concept of dynamic CRRT.

Ricci and colleagues [22] have also addressed recently the lack of solute-specific dose parameters for pediatric patients. In ten critically ill neonates (median age and weight: 3 days and 2.6 kg, respectively) treated with CRRT after cardiac surgery for congenital heart disease, these investigators estimated delivered dose to be 35 mL/kg/h and daily urea Kt/V to be 0.5 (both median values). They also reported a direct association between dose intensity (as measured by daily Kt/V) and decrease in serum creatinine. These two recent publications suggest urea-based CRRT dose measurements may be used more extensively in the near future for both adult and pediatric patients.

In the longer-term future, the incorporation of effluent urea nitrogen measurements, through clinical protocols [23] and CRRT machines equipped with online sensors [24], is likely to occur in pediatric clinical practice. In addition, machines will provide clinicians automated alerts when therapy trends suggest filter clotting, based on changes in effluent measurements or circuit pressures [25]. Finally, additional molecules having specific relevance to AKI pathophysiology [26, 27] may be useful as CRRT dose surrogates for pediatric patients with AKI and other disorders.

### 24.2.3 Timing of CRRT Initiation

In the adult AKI population, recent RCTs have demonstrated conflicting results regarding the timing of RRT initiation [28, 29] and a global RCT evaluating this issue is ongoing in this patient population [30]. For both the adult and pediatric AKI populations, the concept of demand/capacity imbalance, proposed recently by Mehta and colleagues [31, 32], may also be a useful parameter guiding decisions about CRRT initiation in the future. The components of renal demand include AKI disease burden, solute load, and fluid load. A significant imbalance between this demand and diminished renal function in AKI patients should prompt serious consideration of RRT initiation.

The concept of demand/capacity balance will also be useful to guide decisions about renal recovery and RRT cessation. The ADQI group has recommended explicitly that RRT should be discontinued if kidney function has recovered sufficiently to reduce the demand–capacity imbalance (current and expected) to acceptable levels [32]. The preliminary work defining the important considerations with respect to renal recovery [33, 34] most likely will be refined over the next several years, allowing clinicians to make more informed decisions about RRT termination.

While awaiting the results from clinical trials, further progress likely will be made during the coming years in the clinical application of biomarkers [35–37], for the identification of pediatric patients at risk of AKI, the diagnosis of AKI itself, and decisions about CRRT initiation and termination. Within the next decade, these technologies will be used routinely in conjunction with established clinical criteria, especially the extent of fluid overload [38–40], to guide CRRT initiation. Likewise, these technologies will be useful in decisions about CRRT discontinuation or transition to another modality.

### 24.2.4 Drug Dosing in AKI

As is the case with adults, the prevalence of sepsis-associated severe AKI is likely to increase over the next several years, resulting in the need for antibiotic therapy in an increasingly greater percentage of AKI patients, particularly those requiring CRRT [41, 42]. Recent studies have focused on the potentially causative role that antibiotics play in the development of pediatric AKI [43, 44]. Moreover, the lack of reliable clinical data to guide antibiotic use and the associated risk of under-dosing for those patients requiring CRRT have been identified as major problems in both the adult and pediatric populations—dosing continues to be done largely on an empiric basis [45–47]. It is likely that multiple clinical trials evaluating the antibiotics most commonly prescribed to pediatric CRRT patients will be performed over the next several years. The typical range of CRRT flow parameters will be evaluated in these trials, along with commonly used filters, so that the contributions of diffusive, convective, and adsorptive clearance can be ascertained. These trials will provide relatively precise dosing recommendations for a series of widely used antibiotics, leading to the routine incorporation of this information into the CRRT prescription by pediatric clinicians.

As the clinical magnitude of drug-related nephrotoxicity is now being recognized [48], the focus will increasingly turn toward influencing the pediatrician's mindset about the use of potential nephrotoxins, with a particular emphasis on prevention [49]. As recently reported by Goldstein and colleagues [50], quality improvement initiatives should also support future efforts by institutions to mitigate this problem.

### 24.2.5 Quality Metrics

One of the current factors potentially limiting outcome improvements and further dissemination of the therapy is the lack of standardization for CRRT. A specific limitation that contributes to this lack of standardization is an insufficient evidence base. However, another major factor limiting therapy standardization is the lack of consensus CRRT quality metrics. Rewa and colleagues are currently evaluating what aspects of CRRT prescription and delivery should be targets for quality metric development, namely dose (including treatment downtime), anticoagulation, vascular access, and circuit-related issues [11]. As is the case in maintenance dialysis, a number of these quality metrics will be established by consensus initiatives and be part of routine clinical practice over the next decade [51]. Another recent development which will support therapy standardization is the use of simulation-based CRRT training, which has demonstrated tangible improvements in the delivery of CRRT specifically in the pediatric population [52].

It is worthwhile to note that CRRT practices in general are more standardized in children than adults. One explanation for this finding is the more collaborative clinical research approaches afforded by the smaller size of the pediatric clinical community. This aspect was in full display during operation of the American Prospective Pediatric CRRT (ppCRRT) Registry [38, 53–56]. In a short period of time, this initiative established CRRT as the primary therapy for critically ill children with AKI in the US and led to general clinical consensus on a number of aspects of pediatric CRRT, including anticoagulation, vascular access, and fluid management. Similar initiatives in the coming years should lead to further standardization of pediatric CRRT.

### 24.2.6 CRRT Data Analytics and Biofeedback

The technical limitations of current CRRT machines make efficient management of patient and treatment data difficult in some respects [13]. As opposed to the automated, real-time data capture that characterizes many interventions in the ICU, CRRT machine data are collected and analyzed manually at present. This is a laborious, time-consuming process that frequently delays necessary treatment intervention and is a barrier to providing dynamic CRRT. A desired technical aspect of dynamic CRRT is the availability of real-time CRRT machine data as part of a biofeedback system. While any prescription changes needed to close a biofeedback loop have to be made manually by the clinical team at present, such changes will be made automatically by the CRRT machine in the future [57] (Fig. 24.1). This will be accomplished by the incorporation of online tools for continuous, real-time measurement of dose delivery and fluid overload. Moreover, in addition to treatment data from the CRRT machine, patient-level data from the electronic medical record (EMR) will play a critical role in these biofeedback loops [58].

A dynamic CRRT program also implies the ability to use information technology beyond the real-time phase for longer-term purposes. At present, CRRT machine data are not routinely stored in an accessible warehouse, rendering impossible the systematic generation of reports for review by the clinical team. Within the next decade, clinicians will routinely be able to assess historical trends on a facility-level basis, especially those related to the basic quality metrics mentioned above, or to use these data for quality assurance purposes. Moreover, these data will facilitate design and implementation of pragmatic trials, including registries. Again, patient-level data from the EMR will supplement technical data here.

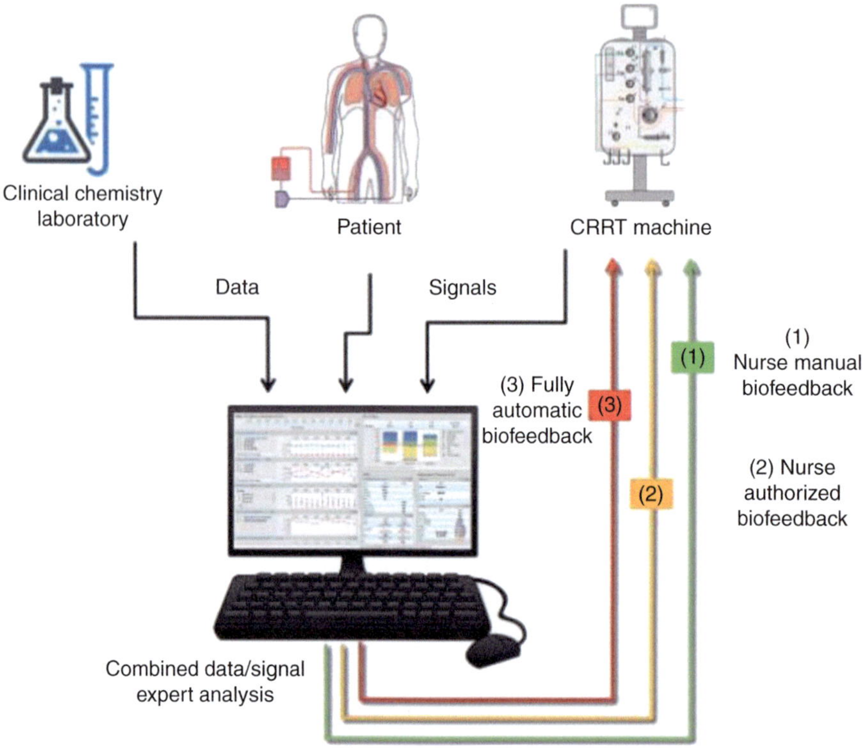


**Fig. 24.1** Various approaches for biofeedback in CRRT. Reprinted with permission from www.adqi.net [57]

### 24.2.7 Miniaturization of Technology

#### 24.2.7.1 Implantable/Wearable Devices for the Treatment of Renal Failure

As is the case with data analytics and information management, CRRT is lagging behind many other therapies with respect to technology "down-sizing." The incorporation of microfluidics, micromechanics, and nanotechnology is driven by the desire not only to decrease the physical footprint of medical technologies (thus enhancing portability) but also to extend their applicability to greater numbers and subsets of patients [59]. The enhanced portability of future devices should allow for a set of similar devices to be used over the entire RRT spectrum (ICU, ward, and even home) in a given patient. In turn, this will allow for more seamless transitions in care, leading to increased simplicity and possibly lower costs.

One clear example of this trend within the renal replacement field is the development of wearable dialysis and ultrafiltration devices, on which several investigative groups have made significant progress during the past decade [60, 61]. While the initial application of these devices has largely been focused on ESRD patients, they may yet prove to be useful in the management of fluid overload, especially in the setting of heart failure. Another potential application in the future is their use for severe AKI survivors who need supplementation of kidney function in the recovery phase.

#### 24.2.7.2 CARPEDIEM: The First Pediatric-Specific CRRT System

The recent development of a CRRT device specifically designed to treat pediatric AKI patients is a more immediate-term example of technology miniaturization. While treatment of pediatric AKI with CRRT has grown substantially over the past decade [62], pediatricians have been forced to use equipment designed primarily for adult patients, as noted previously. The design features of traditional CRRT equipment, especially with regard to fluid accuracy of the machine and extracorporeal blood volume of the circuit, have rendered pediatric treatments problematic—this is especially true for neonatal patients.

Ronco and colleagues have provided detailed reports of the technical aspects of the CARPEDIEM machine (Bellco/Medtronic; Mirondola, Italy) along with its first clinical application in a three-day-old neonate with AKI and severe fluid overload [7, 63]. The machine (Fig. 24.2) is specifically designed for patients less than 10 kg, particularly neonates and premature infants. The extracorporeal volume of the

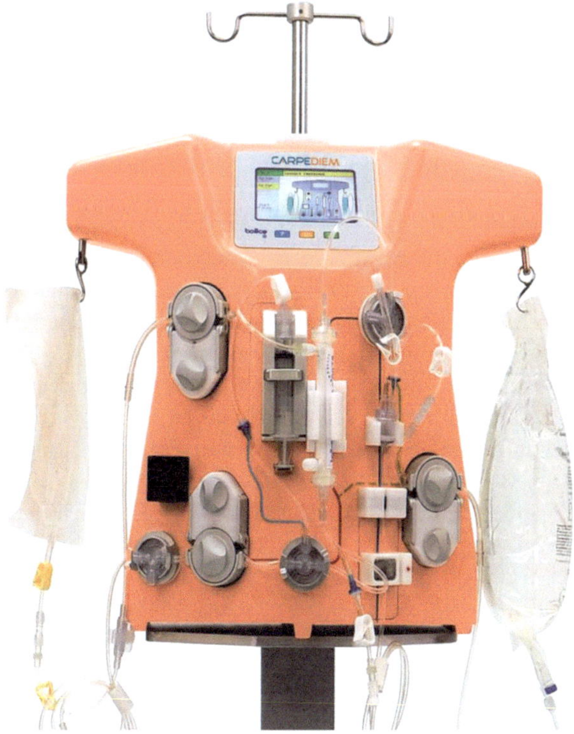


**Fig. 24.2** CARPEDIEM device. *Photo provided courtesy of Bellco/Medtronic*

circuit (including the filter) is only that 27 mL (versus approximately 90 mL or greater for adult sets). Blood is delivered at a rate of 5–50 mL/min via a miniaturized roller pump while fluid pumps (ultrafiltrate and replacement) operate at 0–10 mL/min in conjunction with precision scales having an accuracy up to 1 g. A neonatal patient (body weight at birth, 2.9 kg) with profound anasarca (63% fluid overload) in association with hemorrhagic shock was the first patient treated with the system in 2013. After 25 days of stable treatment, the patient was weaned off CRRT, with diuretics subsequently able to control her fluid overload.

While primarily developing devices with the adult patient in mind, other CRRT machine manufacturers are nevertheless in the process of incorporating features specifically addressing the needs of pediatric patients, especially from a fluid balance perspective. For example, the recently developed Prismax device (Baxter Healthcare; Deerfield, IL, USA) includes software that limits the net ultrafiltration (patient fluid removal) rate to a maximum of 20% of the estimated plasma flow rate or 2 mL/h per kg patient body weight, whichever is smaller [64]. This device also has features creating the potential for safer and more effective delivery of citrate anticoagulation to children. These features include low pre-blood pump infusion rate capability (for hypertonic citrate solutions), a citrate/blood line connection designed for optimized mixing, and prescription software accounting for calcium mass balance in the system.

Based on the introduction of CARPEDIEM and the pediatric-related adaptations being made in other devices, it can be expected the adoption of CRRT for children will accelerate, especially as CARPEDIEM becomes available for use around the world. Moreover, the technology advances that made possible the CARPEDIEM device will likely to accelerate the application of miniaturization principles to other aspects of both pediatric and adult CRRT.

In 1995, the Newcastle group from the UK designed a novel HD circuit, which operated on different principles. It was driven by syringes, and uncoupled the baby's blood flow capacity from the requirements of the dialysis filter. In 2005, the group reported the results of automating this as a miniaturized machine (circuit volume 13 mL), with which they treated four babies weighing between 800 g and 3.4 kg, using a single-lumen access line, and without the need for blood-priming. They have subsequently developed this device into the Newcastle infant dialysis and ultrafiltration system (NIDUS). This syringe-driven machine repeatedly withdraws 5–12.5 mL aliquots of blood from a single-lumen central venous line, passes and returns it across a dialysis filter, and then back to the baby. At a blood flow rate of 20 mL/min, this processes 5 mL of blood each minute. Ultrafiltration from 0 to 60 mL/h is precisely controlled in 3.2 μL steps by differential syringe movements. The pressure-control pattern and exact circuit position are displayed on a touch-screen, which also informs the operator about warning and stop-alarm states. If the line is poor, the NIDUS instantly slows its rate of blood withdrawal from the baby and informs the operator. It records its precise operating status and syringe positions every one-tenth of a second, and has battery backup. The circuits have been designed for up to 24 h of continuous use. A clinical trial evaluating the safety and efficacy of this machine will be initiated soon in the U.K.

### 24.2.8 Non-dialytic Management of AKI

The need for efficient processing of data in the management of critically ill AKI patients has been highlighted during a recent ADQI conference focused on the implications of "big data" for this population [65]. While the ability to utilize data efficiently is a challenge during CRRT, limitations also exist upstream with regard to AKI diagnosis. Moreover, recent adult data also demonstrate post-discharge management of patients (who have had an AKI episode) is fragmented and unpredictable [66, 67]. While earlier studies evaluating "sniffers" and alerts designed to facilitate the diagnosis of AKI have provided conflicting results [68], their utility will be demonstrated conclusively in prospective trials and they will become part of standard clinical practice over the next decade [69, 70]. Likewise, web-based algorithms will be developed to triage post-AKI follow-up to nephrologists or other medical specialties according to AKI severity, extent of CKD, and comorbidities. These algorithms will be used routinely in clinical practice to minimize the risk of progression to ESRD.

**Conclusion**

As the utilization of CRRT for pediatric AKI patients increases, it will be imperative that critical care clinicians are knowledgeable about the therapy and competent in prescribing it. In this chapter, some of the clinical challenges associated with treating the complex critically ill AKI patient population have been discussed and several important questions for the future are addressed. In addition to CRRT technology, the topics of therapy dosing, timing of initiation and termination, fluid management, anticoagulation, drug dosing, and data analytics have been discussed, with emphasis on anticipated developments over the next decade. While several problems and open questions currently exist, the future of CRRT for critically ill pediatric patients is very bright and its use in this patient population will continue to grow.

## References

1. Kramer P, Schrader J, Bohnsack W, Grieben G, Grone HJ, Scheler F. Continuous arteriovenous haemofiltration. A new kidney replacement therapy. Proc Eur Dial Transplant Assoc. 1981;18:743–9.
2. Ronco C, Brendolan A, Bragantini L, et al. Arteriovenous hemodiafiltration associated with continuous arteriovenous hemofiltration: a combined therapy for acute renal failure in the hypercatabolic patient. Blood Purif. 1987;5(1):33–40.
3. Ricci Z, Bonello M, Salvatori G, et al. Continuous renal replacement technology: from adaptive technology and early dedicated machines towards flexible multipurpose machine platforms. Blood Purif. 2004;22(3):269–76.
4. KDIGO clinical practice guideline for acute kidney injury: modality of renal replacement therapy in AKI. Kidney Int. 2012;2(1):107–10.
5. Kaddourah A, Basu RK, Bagshaw SM, Goldstein SL, AWARE Investigators. Epidemiology of acute kidney injury in critically ill children and young adults. N Engl J Med. 2017;376(1):11–20.

6. Warady BA, Bunchman T. Dialysis therapy for children with acute renal failure: survey results. Ped Nephrol. 2000;15:11–3.
7. Ronco C, Garzotto F, Brendolan A, et al. Continuous renal replacement therapy in neonates and small infants: development and first-in-human use of a miniaturised machine (CARPEDIEM). Lancet. 2014;383:1807–13.
8. Clark WR, Neri M, Garzotto F, Goldstein SL, Ricci Z, Ronco C. The future of critical care: renal support in 2027. Crit Care. 2017;21:92.
9. Kellum JA, Ronco C. The 17th acute disease quality initiative international consensus conference: introducing precision continuous renal replacement therapy. Blood Purif. 2016;42(3):221–3.
10. Bagshaw SM, Chakravarthi MR, Ricci Z, et al on behalf of the ADQI Consensus Group. Precision continuous renal replacement therapy: solute control in continuous renal replacement therapy. Blood Purif. 2016;42(3):238–47.
11. Rewa OG, Villeneuve PM, Eurich DT, et al. Quality indicators of continuous renal replacement therapy (CRRT) care in critically ill patients: protocol for a systematic review. Syst Rev. 2015;4:102.
12. Cruz D, Bellomo R, Kellum JA, de Cal M, Ronco C. The future of extracorporeal support. Crit Care Med. 2008;36(4 Suppl):S243–52.
13. Clark WR, Garzotto F, Neri M, Lorenzin A, Zaccaria M, Ronco C. Data analytics for continuous renal replacement therapy: historical limitations and recent technology advances. Int J Artif Organs. 2016;39(8):399–406.
14. Ronco C, Bellomo R, Homel P, et al. Effects of different doses in continuous veno-venous haemofiltration on outcomes of acute renal failure: a prospective randomised trial. Lancet. 2000;356(9223):26–30.
15. VA/NIH Acute Renal Failure Trial Network, Palevsky PM, Zhang JH, O'Connor TZ, et al. Intensity of renal support in critically ill patients with acute kidney injury. N Engl J Med. 2008;359(1):7–20.
16. RENAL Replacement Therapy Study Investigators, Bellomo R, Cass A, Cole L, et al. Intensity of continuous renal-replacement therapy in critically ill patients. N Engl J Med. 2009;361(17):1627–38.
17. KDIGO clinical practice guideline for acute kidney injury: dose of renal replacement therapy in AKI. Kidney Int. 2012;2(1):113–5.
18. Ricci Z, Guzzi F, Tuccinardi G, et al. Dialytic dose in pediatric continuous renal replacement therapy patients. Minerva Pediatr. 2016;68:366–73.
19. Huang Z, Letteri JJ, Clark WR, Ronco C. Operational characteristics of continuous renal replacement therapy modalities used for critically ill patients with acute kidney injury. Int J Artif Organs. 2008;31:525–34.
20. Clark WR, Leblanc M, Ricci Z, Ronco C. Quantification and dosing of renal replacement therapy in acute kidney injury: a reappraisal. Blood Purif. 2017;44:140–55.
21. Gotch FA. The current place of urea kinetic modelling with respect to different dialysis modalities. Nephrol Dial Transplant. 1998;13(Suppl 6):10–4.
22. Ricci Z, Guzzi F, Tuccinardi G, et al. Dose prescription and delivery in neonates with congenital heart diseases treated with continuous veno-venous hemofiltration. Ped Crit Care Med. 2017;18(7):623–9.
23. Claure-Del Granado R, Macedo E, Chertow GM, et al. Effluent volume in continuous renal replacement therapy overestimates the delivered dose of dialysis. Clin J Am Soc Nephrol. 2011;6(3):467–75.
24. Cruz D, Bobek I, Lentini P, Soni S, Chionh CY, Ronco C. Machines for continuous renal replacement therapy. Semin Dial. 2009;22(2):123–32.
25. Kakajiwala A, Jemielita T, Hughes JZ, et al. Membrane pressures predict clotting of pediatric continuous renal replacement therapy circuits. Pediatric Nephrol. 2017;32:1251–61.
26. Doi K. Role of kidney injury in sepsis. J Intensive Care. 2016;4:17.
27. Kellum JA, Gómez H, Gómez A, Murray P, Ronco C. ADQI XIV workgroup: XIV sepsis phenotypes and targets for blood purification in sepsis: the Bogota consensus. Shock. 2016;45(3):242–8.

28. Zarbock A, Kellum JA, Schmidt C, et al. Effect of early vs delayed initiation of renal replacement therapy on mortality in critically ill patients with acute kidney injury: the ELAIN randomized clinical trial. JAMA. 2016;315(20):2190–9.
29. Gaudry S, Hajage D, Schortgen F, et al. AKIKI study group: initiation strategies for renal-replacement therapy in the intensive care unit. N Engl J Med. 2016;375(2):122–33.
30. Wald R, Adhikari NK, Smith OM, Canadian Critical Care Trials Group, et al. Comparison of standard and accelerated initiation of renal replacement therapy in acute kidney injury. Kidney Int. 2015;88(4):897–904.
31. Macedo E, Mehta RL. When should renal replacement therapy be initiated for acute kidney injury. Semin Dial. 2011;24:132–7.
32. Ostermann M, Joannidis M, Pani A, Acute Disease Quality Initiative (ADQI) Consensus Group, et al. Patient selection and timing of continuous renal replacement therapy. Blood Purif. 2016;42(3):224–37.
33. Kellum JA. How can we define recovery after acute kidney injury? Considerations from epidemiology and clinical trial design. Nephron Clin Pract. 2014;127:81–8.
34. Kellum JA, Sileanu FE, Bihorac A, Hoste EA, Chawla LS. Recovery after acute kidney injury. Am J Respir Crit Care Med. 2017;195(6):784–91.
35. Gist KM, Goldstein SL, Wrona J, et al. Kinetics of the cell cycle arrest biomarkers (TIMP-2*IGFBP-7) for prediction of acute kidney injury in infants after cardiac surgery. Pediatr Nephrol. 2017;32(9):1611–9. https://doi.org/10.1007/s00467-017-3655-y.
36. Menon S, Goldstein SL, Mottes T, et al. Urinary biomarker incorporation into the renal angina index early in intensive care unit admission optimizes acute kidney injury prediction in critically ill children: a prospective cohort study. Nephrol Dial Transplant. 2016;31(4):586–94.
37. Basu RK, Wong HR, Krawczeski CD, et al. Combining functional and tubular damage biomarkers improves diagnostic precision for acute kidney injury after cardiac surgery. J Am Coll Cardiol. 2014;64(25):2753–62.
38. Sutherland SM, Zappitelli M, Alexander SR, et al. Fluid overload and mortality in children receiving continuous renal replacement therapy: the prospective pediatric continuous renal replacement therapy registry. Am J Kidney Dis. 2010;55(2):316–25.
39. Goldstein SL. Fluid management in acute kidney injury. J Intensive Care Med. 2014;29:183–9.
40. Garzotto F, Ostermann M, Martin-Langerwerf D, et al. The dose response multicentre investigation on fluid assessment (DoReMIFA) in critically ill patients. Crit Care. 2016;20:196.
41. Honore PM, Jacobs R, Hendrickx I, et al. Prevention and treatment of sepsis-induced acute kidney injury: an update. Ann Intensive Care. 2015;5(1):51.
42. Alobaidi R, Basu RK, Goldstein SL, Bagshaw SM. Sepsis-associated acute kidney injury. Semin Nephrol. 2015;35(1):2–11.
43. Downes KJ, Cowden C, Laskin BL, et al. Association of acute kidney injury with concomitant vancomycin and piperacillin/tazobactam treatment among hospitalized children. JAMA Pediatr. 2017;171(12):e173219. https://doi.org/10.1001/jamapediatrics.2017.3219.
44. Goldstein SL. Medication-induced acute kidney injury. Curr Opin Crit Care. 2016;22(6):542–5.
45. Nolin TD, Aronoff GR, Fissell WH, Kidney Health Initiative, et al. Pharmacokinetic assessment in patients receiving continuous RRT: perspectives from the kidney health initiative. Clin J Am Soc Nephrol. 2015;10(1):159–64.
46. Shaw AR, Mueller BA. Antibiotic dosing in continuous renal replacement therapy. Adv Chronic Kidney Dis. 2017;24(4):219–27.
47. Nehus EJ, Mizuno T, Cox S, Goldstein SL, Vinks AA. Pharmacokinetics of meropenem in children receiving continuous renal replacement therapy: validation of clinical trial simulations. J Clin Pharmacol. 2016;56(3):291–7.
48. Ostermann M, Chawla LS, Forni LG, et al. Drug management in acute kidney disease—report of the ADQI XVI meeting. Br J Clin Pharmacol. 2018;84(2):396–403. https://doi.org/10.1111/bcp.13449.
49. Kane-Gill SL, Goldstein SL. Drug-induced acute kidney injury: a focus on risk assessment for prevention. Crit Care Clin. 2015;31(4):675–84.
50. Goldstein SL, Mottes T, Simpson K, et al. A sustained quality improvement program reduces nephrotoxic medication-associated acute kidney injury. Kidney Int. 2016;90(1):212–21.

51. Heung M, Bagshaw SM, House AA, Juncos LA, Piazza R, Goldstein SL. CRRTnet: a prospective, multi-national, observational study of continuous renal replacement therapy practices. BMC Nephrol. 2017;18(1):222.
52. Mottes T, Owens T, Niedner M, Juno J, Shanley TP, Heung M. Improving delivery of continuous renal replacement therapy: impact of a simulation-based educational intervention. Pediatr Crit Care Med. 2013;14(8):747–54.
53. Symons JM, Chua AN, Somers MJ, et al. Demographic characteristics of pediatric continuous renal replacement therapy: a report of the prospective pediatric continuous renal replacement therapy registry. Clin J Am Soc Nephrol. 2007;2(4):732–8.
54. Goldstein SL, Somers MJ, Baum MA, et al. Pediatric patients with multi-organ dysfunction syndrome receiving continuous renal replacement therapy. Kidney Int. 2005;67(2):653–8.
55. Flores FX, Brophy PD, Symons JM, et al. Continuous renal replacement therapy (CRRT) after stem cell transplantation. A report from the prospective pediatric CRRT registry group. Pediatr Nephrol. 2008;23(4):625–30.
56. Askenazi DJ, Goldstein SL, Koralkar R, et al. Continuous renal replacement therapy for children ≤10 kg: a report from the prospective pediatric continuous renal replacement therapy registry. J Pediatr. 2013;162(3):587–92.
57. Cerda J, Baldwin I, Honore PM, Villa G, Kellum JA, Ronco C, ADQI Consensus Group. Role of technology in continuous renal replacement therapy for the management of critically ill patients: from adoptive technology to precision continuous renal replacement therapy. Blood Purif. 2016;42:248–65.
58. Kashani K, Herasevich V. Utilities of electronic medical records to improve quality of care for acute kidney injury: past, present, and future. Nephron Clin Prac. 2015;131:92–6.
59. Ronco C, Davenport A, Gura V. The future of the artificial kidney: moving towards wearable and miniaturized devices. Nefrologia. 2011;31:9–16.
60. Gura V, Rivera MB, Bieber S, et al. A wearable artificial kidney for patients with end-stage renal disease. JCI Insight. 2016;1(8). pii: e86397.
61. Fissell WH, Roy S, Davenport A. Achieving more frequent and longer dialysis for the majority: wearable dialysis and implantable artificial kidney devices. Kidney Int. 2013;84(2):256–64.
62. Ricci Z, Goldstein SL. Pediatric continuous renal replacement therapy. Contrib Nephrol. 2016;187:121–30.
63. Ronco C, Garzotto F, Ricci Z. CARPEDIEM (cardio-renal pediatric dialysis emergency machine): evolution of continuous renal replacement therapies in infants. A personal journey. Pediatr Nephrol. 2012;27:1203–11.
64. PrisMax Operator's Manual (AW6005, Rev. F) 2017, pages 29,127, Baxter Healthcare, Deerfield, IL USA.
65. Bagshaw SM, Goldstein SL, Ronco C, Kellum JA. ADQI 15 consensus group acute kidney injury in the era of big data: the 15(th) consensus conference of the acute dialysis quality initiative (ADQI). Can J Kidney Health Dis. 2016;3:5.
66. Siew ED, Peterson JF, Eden SK, et al. Outpatient nephrology referral rates after acute kidney injury. J Am Soc Nephrol. 2012;23:305–12.
67. Silver SA, Goldstein SL, Harel Z, et al. Ambulatory care after acute kidney injury: an opportunity to improve patient outcomes. Can J Kidney Health Dis. 2015;2:36.
68. Hoste EA, Kashani K, Gibney N, on behalf of the 15 ADQI Consensus Group, et al. Impact of electronic-alerting of acute kidney injury: workgroup statements from the 15$^{th}$ ADQI consensus conference. Can J Kidney Health Dis. 2016;3:10.
69. Kirkendall ES, Spires WL, Mottes TA, Schaffzin JK, Barclay C, Goldstein SL. Development and performance of electronic acute kidney injury triggers to identify pediatric patients at risk for nephrotoxic medication-associated harm. Appl Clin Inform. 2014;5(2):313–33.
70. Goldstein SL. Automated/integrated real-time clinical decision support in acute kidney injury. Curr Opin Crit Care. 2015;21(6):485–9.

# Part III

# CRRT in Specific Disease States

# CRRT in a Child in Cardiac ICU

# 25

Cristiana Garisto and Zaccaria Ricci

## 25.1 Introduction

Acute kidney injury (AKI) has a significant impact on morbidity and mortality among children admitted to the Cardiac Intensive Care Unit (CICU), whether they undergo cardiac surgery for correction or palliation of congenital heart disease (CHD) or they are hospitalized for the management of heart failure (secondary to residual heart defects or cardiomyopathies). In this population, the incidence of postoperative AKI is variable with values between 9% and 40% [1, 2], and the associated mortality is up to 79% [3]. Moreover, the onset of AKI is related to a prolonged length of CICU and hospital stay [4].

Given the limited therapeutic options for the treatment of AKI, priority should be given to the identification of patients at risk in order to prevent its early onset. Assuming that pathogenesis of AKI is multifactorial, the risk factors that contribute to its determination can be related to the patient (age, type of cardiac disease, preoperative renal function), or they can be related to treatments to which the patient is subjected in CICU (nephrotoxic drugs, hemodynamic instability, fluid loading, ineffective surgery, etc.).

In this context, renal replacement therapy (RRT) is currently the only available treatment in case of severe AKI, especially in case of anuria or significant metabolic or electrolyte derangements.

In this chapter, the clinical courses of two patients affected by CHD undergoing surgical or interventional procedures will be described, in order to exemplify specific risk factors for renal failure and their potential treatments.

C. Garisto · Z. Ricci (✉)
Department of Cardiology and Cardiac Surgery, Pediatric Cardiac Intensive Care Unit, Bambino Gesù Children's Hospital, IRCCS, Rome, Italy
e-mail: zaccaria.ricci@opbg.net

 
A. Deep, S. L. Goldstein (eds.), *Critical Care Nephrology and Renal Replacement Therapy in Children*, https://doi.org/10.1007/978-3-319-90281-4_25

**Clinical Case 1: Cardiorenal Syndrome Is a Lifelong Inheritage of CHD Patients and Early RRT Should Be Considered in Specific Cases**

*A 17-year-old patient, affected at birth by hypoplastic left heart syndrome, had underwent multiple palliative surgeries: Norwood stage I, Glenn and Fontan operations. The palliation of CHD is centered in these patients on the only functioning ventricle, typically the right ventricle, which becomes the systemic one and, throughout the various palliative stages, is required to serve both pulmonary and systemic circulations. The patient, some 5 years after the Fontan procedure, progressively developed a state of terminal cardiac failure and his heart function, initially requiring support with diuretics and angiotensin converting inhibitors, worsened. He is admitted to the CICU in order to stabilize his hemodynamics and vasoactive drugs with intravenous diuretics are administered. Renal function indices (creatinine, creatinine clearance, blood nitrogen and urine output) still lie within normal limits. To obtain an accurate definition of pressures in pulmonary vessels and left ventricular end-diastolic pressure, the patient undergoes cardiac catheterization, which requires the administration of contrast media for the angiography. After catheterization, the patient is listed for urgent cardiac transplantation.*

*After 2 weeks of stable hemodynamic parameters, still receiving milrinone and low dose adrenaline, the patient undergoes cardiac transplantation. This type of surgery obviously requires anesthetics, antibiotics, a prolonged time on cardiopulmonary bypass (CPB), and cross clamp (graft ischemia). After transplantation, the patient is readmitted to the CICU. At this stage, patient is accumulating fluids (fluid overload was > 15%), his central venous pressure (CVP) appears increased likely due to right ventricular dysfunction and elevated pulmonary artery pressure. He is sedated and intubated and pulmonary parameters do not allow a fast track ventilator weaning, due to hypoxia and administration of inhaled nitric oxide. Renal function indices begin to deteriorate, with a progressive increase in creatinine, blood nitrogen and progressive reduction of creatinine clearance. Urinary output is maintained (2–2.5 mL/kg/h) but ethacryinic acid is administered at high doses (0.4 mg/kg/h) and the fluid balance keeps being positive.*

*Therefore, we decide to treat the patient with continuous renal replacement therapy (CRRT).*

The pathophysiology of single ventricle anatomy is strictly related, in patients who undergo serial palliations, to their renal function and AKI incidence [5]. In the first stage of Norwood palliation, pulmonary circulation is connected to systemic circulation by systemic-pulmonary shunt: a significant diastolic run-off may expose the splanchnic organs and kidneys (that require a normal mean arterial pressure to maintain their function) to significant under-perfusion. As a second palliation, the Glenn operation is performed by connecting superior cava vein to pulmonary arteries: this implies a phase lasting about 12 months, of significant arterial desaturation (averaging around 80%). The Fontan operation concludes the single ventricle palliation by subsequently connecting inferior vena cava to the pulmonary arteries. At this stage, the increased filling pressure in the systemic venous circulation, and consequently in the splanchnic system, causes venous congestion with CVP ranging between 10 and 18 mmHg. Furthermore, the fact that systemic circulation is served by a morphological right ventricle (therefore it has an inadequate conformation to serve systemic circulation), leads in most cases to progressive ventricular failure that ultimately leads to low cardiac output. When combined with low cardiac output and hypotension, elevated systemic venous pressure may result in decreased renal perfusion pressure (RPP) [5].

A prolonged use of diuretics, ACE-inhibitors, acetyl salicylic acid (the triple whammy), repeated surgery with CPB [6–15], the perioperative potential accumulation with fluid overload [16], the administration of antibiotics, may altogether impact renal function throughout the clinical history of these patients.

The need for intravascular injection of iodinated contrast to obtain accurate imaging of coronary and peripheral circulation, cardiac chambers, and great vessels is a further AKI risk factor. The administration of iodinated contrast imaging agents during cardiac catheterization can cause kidney damage with a mechanism linked to adenosine metabolism, perturbations of glomerular flow, endothelin and prostaglandin metabolism, and oxidative stress [17]. Iodinated contrast is water soluble; consequently, the damage induced on the kidneys by contrast administration can be reduced by administering isotonic crystalloid solutions to enhance renal elimination of contrast increasing renal filtration and tubular flow of urine into collecting ducts, into the ureters and bladder [18]. However, in these patients with cardiac risks, administration of high doses of crystalloids is not always possible because it can worsen fluid overload and promote pulmonary edema.

Immunosuppressive drugs have a potential nephrotoxicity that is the ultimate AKI risk factor for the described patient. The possible pathogenetic mechanism of calcineurin inhibitors are involved in both reversible alterations and irreversible damage to all compartments of the kidneys, including glomeruli, arterioles, and tubulo-interstitium. In particular, cyclosporin renal damage results from the release of reactive oxygen metabolites. In fact, the administration of cyclosporine A results in enhanced generation of hydrogen peroxide. The renal proximal tubules have a high dependence on oxidative phosphorylation for energy production, and thus may be susceptible to oxidant stress [6].

In the postoperative period of heart transplantation, right ventricle dysfunction occurs frequently. In fact, the transplanted organ has to interact with hemodynamic condition of recipient, often characterized by high pulmonary pressures, which are the consequence of prolonged cardiac failure. Also, the transplanted organ suffers from ischemia-reperfusion injury and surgical trauma. These conditions may result in increased CVP and venous congestion in systemic circulation with an increase in inferior caval pressure. Right ventricular dysfunction and increased CVP, even if transient, can lead to increased risk of renal failure.

### 25.1.1 Indications and Timing for Renal Replacement Therapy (RRT) in Cardiac Children

Indications for urgent RRT are: pulmonary edema unresponsive to diuretic therapy; progressive and intractable hyperkalemia; persistent acidosis; uremia and drug intoxications.

However, in clinical practice, a patient may develop renal injury (which appears to be a reduction in urinary output) that requires immediate treatment as it compromises the patient's hemodynamic state, acid-base and electrolytic equilibrium, phosphate-calcium balance and determines tissue edema.

In adult setting, there are several studies that associate early RRT initiation with improved outcomes in patients with AKI which develops as a consequence of cardiovascular surgery [7, 8], and as a part of multiorgan failure unassociated with cardiac surgery [9, 10].

In pediatric setting, it has been shown in recent literature that early initiation of RRT (within the first 24 postoperative hours), both peritoneal dialysis (PD) in neonates and continuous RRT (CRRT) in children, improves morbidity and mortality associated with AKI [11, 12].

However, there are no precise guidelines to treat AKI post cardiac surgery in children that define what kind of renal replacement therapy: (PD versus CRRT) should be preferred. In 1995, Fleming et al. [13] compared the use of PD versus CRRT in children affected by AKI and requiring renal replacement therapy after cardiac surgery evaluating the efficacy (fluid removal, caloric intake, clearance of urea and creatinine), complications, and outcome of the two methods. The authors concluded that the use of CRRT after cardiac surgery for congenital heart disease is more effective as compared to peritoneal dialysis and is associated with a decrease in the mortality rate observed in renal failure after cardiac surgery.

Some studies report an increase in mortality associated with CRRT in children [1, 14], but it should be noted that this occurs predominantly in patients undergoing CRRT when they present with multiorgan dysfunction and severe fluid overload [19]. Conversely, there might be a reduction in mortality when treatment with CRRT starts when AKI is not yet in the advanced stage [15, 20].

There is no specific laboratory parameter that can indicate the need for RRT. Serum creatinine (SCr) values, in children as in adult population, may reflect the glomerular filtration rate (GFR) in patients with almost normal renal function, but they underestimate the level of kidney dysfunction during the evolution of the dysfunction [21]. Other biomarkers are currently under evaluation but none has shown to be effective enough to be able to indicate when to initiate RRT [22–25].

The KDIGO group [26] in 2012 defined AKI as an increase in serum creatinine SCr level exceeding 0.3 mg/dL within 48 h, or an increase in SCr to 1.5 times the baseline value within 7 days, or urine output less than 0.5 mL/kg/h for 6 h. Based on this classification, patients requiring RRT are those included in stage 3 of the classification (see dedicated chapter) [27].

It has to be noted, however, that regardless of exact indications, timing of CRRT initiation is another important aspect to consider. Even if generally speaking an earlier intervention may be recommended [28], RRT timing is difficult to define and implies multidisciplinary clinical overview of each single case. The patient we are presenting is a typical example of this issue: he probably had unidentified type 2 cardiorenal syndrome [29], who had potentially lost his renal reserve [30], in an early postoperative, post CPB phase, who was accumulating fluids regardless of his actual KDIGO staging and who had several nephrotoxic drugs prescribed (immunosuppressants, high dose diuretics, vancomycin). Furthermore, high levels of CVP (due to right ventricular dysfunction, high mechanical ventilation pressures, tricuspid regurgitation, and high pulmonary resistance) have been repeatedly associated with worse renal and nonrenal outcomes [31–33]. In this light, proactive early RRT initiation was likely to be indicated in this patient, before routine renal indices (urine output and serum creatinine) worsened to significantly pathological levels (i.e., KDIGO stages 2 and 3).

### 25.1.2 Extracorporeal Dialysis: Continuous RRT (CRRT)

CRRT techniques include the use of biocompatible, high-flux filters of polyacrylonitrile, polysulphone, or polymethyl-methacrylate; these are filters with high porosity and variable surface area of hollow fibers that allow both diffusive and convective treatment [34].

Blood purification through CRRT is based on mechanism of diffusion and convection. Settings are described on Table 25.1.

*Diffusion* removes solutes based on several variables that are: gradient of solute concentration between the two sides of membrane, temperature, diffusivity coefficient, thickness, and surface area of the membrane.

In *convection*, water and solutes cross the semipermeable membrane through a pressure gradient between the two fiber sides, determining ultrafiltration. The ultrafiltrate contains plasma, water, urea, solutes with low and middle weight, but it does not contain solutes exceeding the membrane cutoff and, obviously, cells.

Various CRRT modalities include:

- Continuous arteriovenous hemofiltration (CAVH): the pressure gradient existing between arterial and venous circulation "pushes" blood flow into the circuit and determines a transmembrane pressure. The ultrafiltration column provides a negative pressure to the system that, together with the hydrostatic pressure gap in the filter, results in ultrafiltration. CAVH depends on patient's mean arterial pressure and cardiac output and it is currently exclusively used when a filter is inserted into the extracorporeal membrane oxygenation circuit (instead of using in series devices).
- Slow continuous ultrafiltration (SCUF): this technique is used to control fluid balance in patients with fluid overload; the blood is pushed through a filter with high permeability by a veno-venous extracorporeal circuit. The ultrafiltrate produced corresponds to net (circuit) fluid balance.

**Table 25.1** Proposed settings of a pediatric continuous renal replacement therapy (pCRRT)

| | Blood flow rate | Estimated urea clearance ($K_{CALC}$): | Comments | Prescription in mL/Kg/h | Prescription in mL/h/1.73 m$^2$ |
|---|---|---|---|---|---|
| CVVH Postdilution | Patient's weight ≤ 5 kg: Qb 10 mL/min/kg; Patient's weight 5–10 kg: Qb 5 mL/min/kg; Patient's weight > 20 kg: Qb > 50 mL/min | $K_{CALC}$ = Qrep | Always keep filtration fraction <20% (Qrep/Qb*100) | Qrep: 35 mL/kg/h (i.e., in a 10 kg patient: 350 mL/h) | 2000 mL/h/1.73 m$^2$ (i.e., in a 10 kg patient with 0.5 m$^2$ of BSA: 580 mL/h) |
| CVVH Predilution | As above | $K_{CALC}$ = Quf/[1 + (Qrep/Qb)] | Always keep filtration fraction <25% (Qb + Qrep/Qb*100) | Qrep: 40–50 mL/kg/h (i.e., in a 10 kg patient: 400–500 mL/h) | 2500–3500 mL/h/1.73 m$^2$ (i.e., in a 10 kg patient with 0.5 m$^2$ of BSA: 720–1000 mL/h) |
| CVVHD | As above | $K_{CALC}$ = Qd | Keep Qb at least thrice Qd (Qd/Qb*100 = 30) | Qd: 35–50 mL/kg/h (i.e., in a 10 kg patient: 350–400 mL/h) | 2000 mL/h/1.73 m$^2$ (i.e., in a 10 kg patient with 0.5 m$^2$ of BSA: 580 mL/h) |
| CVVHDF Postdilution (50% convective and diffusive K) | As above | $K_{CALC}$ = Qrep + Qd | Consider both notes of CVVH and CVVHD | Qrep: 20 mL/kg/h + Qd: 20 mL/kg/h (i.e., in a 10 kg patient: Qrep 200 mL/h + Qd 200 mL/h) | 2000 mL/h/1.73 m$^2$ (i.e., in a 10 kg patient with 0.5 m$^2$ of BSA: Qrep 300 mL/h + Qd 300 mL/h) |

Blood flow (Qb) rate obviously depends on vascular access performance. Regardless of the prescribed dose, this table intends to depict the important relationship existing between treatment flows (Qrep: replacement solution flow rate; Qd: dialysate solution flow rate) and Qb. Furthermore, currently, two alternative prescription modalities are generally utilized: mL/kg/h or mL/h/1.73 m$^2$ of body surface area (BSA). In both cases the prescription of a general "one size fits all" dose (35 mL/kg/h vs. 2000 mL/Kg/1.73 m$^2$) has been described, although no evidence exists about the association between a specific dialytic dose and outcomes in children. However, it has to be highlighted that the two methods ultimately lead to very different operational flows (for example, a 10 kg, 0.5 m$^2$ BSA patient). Finally, the prescriptions proposed in the table theoretically aim to deliver similar $K_{CALC}$ among different modalities: this is another important aspect to consider when Qb, Qrep and Qd are set (predilution hemofiltration and hemodialysis are theoretically slightly less efficient than postdilution hemofiltration and may require higher Qrep and Qd, respectively)

This table does not include the net ultrafiltration (the water removed by the machine in the time unit): during pCRRT this is another important parameter to set according to patient's needs

Prescription of pCRRT in cardiac surgery patients should take into account several aspects (solute control, electrolyte derangements, unwanted clearance of antibiotics and amino acids) even probably fluid balance is one of the most important

*CVVH* continuous veno-venous hemofiltration, *CVVHD* continuous veno-venous hemodialysis, *CVVHDF* continuous veno-venous hemodiafiltration

- Continuous veno-venous hemofiltration (CVVH); this technique is based on mechanism of convection: the transmembrane pressure gradient determines the formation of an ultrafiltrate by passing the plasma water from the blood through the membrane. Plasma water removed "drags" the solutes-solvent across the membrane. A reinfusion balanced solution is then administered to compensate for the ultrafiltrate produced and ultimately complete the convective purification process. Filtration fraction is the rate of plasma water that is removed from blood during ultrafiltration. It is a value expressed as % and it must be maintained <20% to avoid excessive hemoconcentration during ultrafiltration. Reinfusion or replacement fluid can be administered before filter (predilution hemofiltration) or after filter (postdilution hemofiltration). The prefilter administration of substitution solution allows for a longer life of the filter; the postfilter administration allows a greater clearing efficiency. During hemofiltration, the net ultrafiltration is the difference between the volume of plasma water removed in ultrafiltrate and the volume of substitution solution administered during reinfusion.
- Continuous veno-venous hemodialysis (CVVHD); this technique is based on mechanism of diffusion: with the blood and dialysate fluid flowing in counter current directions in the filter. The solutes cross from blood to dialytic solution depending on the concentration of the solutes in the two compartments.
- Continuous veno-venous hemodiafiltration (CVVHDF); diffusion and convection mechanisms are delivered simultaneously in order to increase dialytic dose and efficacy.

*Anticoagulation*: the need to keep the circuit used for CRRT patent and to prevent thrombus formation in the extracorporeal circuit and decrease the downtimes for treatment, an anticoagulation is required but the need must always be evaluated in relation to patient's coagulation disorders. The most common anticoagulation methods used in clinical practice are:

- Unfractionated heparin (UFH) as a continuous infusion, starting with a low dose of 10 U/kg/h and titrating it to obtain systemic aPTT around 40–50 s. The advantage of this anticoagulation method is the availability of antidote (protamine) in case of excessive anticoagulation and the possibility to monitor anticoagulation by aPTT or bedside ACT; UFH can also be used pre-filter into the circuit and hence a regional anticoagulant. This reduces the risk of systemic anticoagulation and reduces the chance of patient bleeding.
- Low molecular weight heparin: the advantage of this drug is the better bioavailability with respect to UFH
- Citrate: the advantage is that it is a regional (not systemic) anticoagulation method. However, it can induce hypocalcemia because calcium is chelated in the filter.

These anticoagulation aspects are better detailed in Chap. 17: however, some peculiar characteristics of cardiac surgery children should be taken into account. Patients who require extracorporeal CRRT in a postoperative phase, due to the post-CPB coagulation derangements and potentially problematic intraoperative hemostasis, are generally managed without any anticoagulation or low heparin doses. Furthermore, citrate-induced calcium derangements, although never systematically described in the pediatric cardiac population, may have potentially detrimental hemodynamic consequences, due to the poor intra-myocardial calcium storage of these patients. A recent report of 15 cardiac surgery patients and 59 circuits described a relatively low incidence of hypocalcemia (8%), with a fair duration of CRRT sessions (43 h) but hemodynamic aspects were not described in the paper [35].

*CRRT complications and outcomes in cardiac surgery children*: possible complications of CRRT are thrombocytopenia, filter clotting, bleeding due to excessive anticoagulation (from the gastrointestinal tract, from the airways or from the insertion points of the catheters), hypotension especially at the beginning of the procedure, and hypothermia.

Excessive removal of nutritional elements, brain natriuretic peptide, and antibiotics has been described in cardiac patients [36, 37].

The outcome of post-cardiac surgery patients undergoing RRT is mostly affected by patient's clinical condition namely, the need for vasoactive drugs, hemodynamic stability during the CRRT treatments, and the degree of multi-organ dysfunction. A prospective observational study reported a mortality of 43%. Factors associated with mortality were age less than 12 months, weight less than 10 kg, higher Pediatric Risk of Mortality Score, hypotension (particularly at CRRT initiation), lower urea and creatinine on starting CRRT, and use of hemofiltration [38]. None of these variables except for hypotension remained significantly associated with mortality at multivariable analysis. As a matter of fact, the high mortality rate observed in RRT patients in cardiac surgery patients is heavily influenced by the residual heart defects existing after surgery and by cardiorespiratory function of patients with other systemic complications (i.e., sepsis or pulmonary hypertension), with mortality peaking in selected population (high risk neonates) to 80% [39].

## 25.2 Dedicated Pediatric CRRT Technology

The most challenging cardiac children requiring CRRT are neonates. The authors of this chapter achieved clinical experience by applying a dedicated dialysis equipment to selected neonates with severe complications, the Cardio-Renal, Pediatric Dialysis Emergency Machine (CARPEDIEM). This device was conceived in order to reduce circuit's priming volumes to a minimum level (ranging from 25 to 50 mL) and roller pumps have been engineered to run at slow speeds (from 1 to 50 mL/min), maintaining a good level of accuracy together with the possibility of warranting integrity of lines (small roller pumps running small tubes are expected to cause a quick decline in their performance) [40]. Fluid balance accuracy warrants a resolution of 1 g of error. Further studies on dedicated devices are warranted in order to verify if a significant outcome improvement for neonates with severe AKI requiring RRT may be expected by these innovations.

The ideal pediatric CRRT machine has been depicted in Fig. 25.1: unfortunately, such equipment is currently not existing.

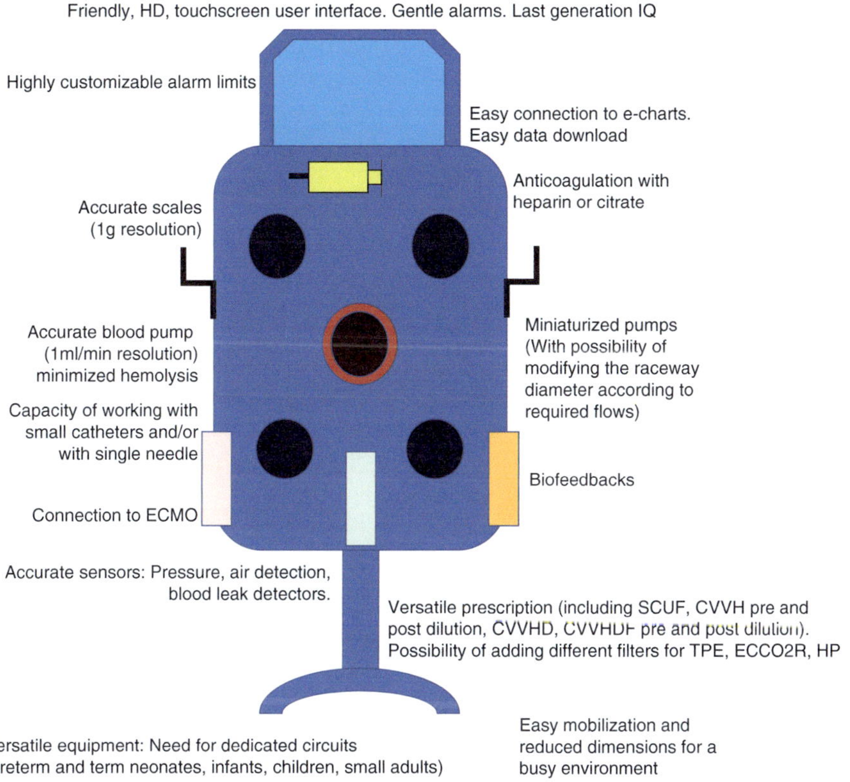


**Fig. 25.1** The main characteristics of the "ideal pediatric continuous renal replacement machine" are described here. All of these qualities are particularly important in the cardiac children, due to the peculiar clinical aspects of these patients: widely ranging weight and age of these patients, need to carefully treat a hemodynamic unstable patient, strict requirement for high accuracy of scales and sensors. A particular mention should be given to the concept of "biofeedback": the ideal machine should be able to interact with some patient's clinical aspects. That is, reducing flows (especially net ultrafiltration) in case of blood pressure decrease, controlling patient's hematocrit in order to adequately target fluid removal, or modify settings (according to strict protocols) in case some target solutes changed their blood levels. Legend: *HD* high definition, *IQ* intelligence quotient, *ECMO* extracorporeal membrane oxygenation, *SCUF* slow continuous ultrafiltration, *CVVH* continuous veno-venous hemofiltration, *CVVHD* continuous veno-venous hemodialysis, *CVVHDF* continuous veno-venous hemodiafiltration

### 25.2.1 Pediatric CRRT Dose

No published recommendations for RRT dose prescription in cardiac children currently exist and only observational data appear in the literature in the general pediatric population [41]. In a recent systematic review including studies published after the year 2000 and excluding patients treated for inborn errors of metabolism, pediatric dose prescriptions ranging from less than 1000 to more than 4000 mL/h/1.73 $m^2$ and from 20 to 150 mL/kg/h have been reported [42].

Theoretically, infants and neonates might require a relatively higher dialytic dose in comparison to adult patients, when dose prescription is indexed to body surface area: due to the relatively higher volume of distribution of solutes, in order to achieve the same level of blood purification (i.e., serum creatinine concentration) treatment intensity for neonates and infants should be 1.5–3 times greater than that of an adult patient. Consequently, the most commonly proposed pediatric dose of 2 L/h/1.73 $m^2$ [41, 42] corresponds approximately to 80 mL/kg/h for a newborn patient but to 35 mL/kg/h for a 16-year-old young man weighting 70 kg with a body surface area of 2 $m^2$.

Peculiar aspects of cardiac children are related to the fact that, generally, metabolic requirements during extracorporeal blood purification are not particularly demanding and that solutes (urea and creatinine) do not require high CRRT doses to achieve adequate control [43]. Furthermore, in cardiac surgery patients, an aggressive, effective, and accurate correction of fluid overload is particularly important in these patients, even if prospective evaluation of the effects of fluid "downloading" on children's mortality are currently lacking.

**Clinical Case 2: Neonates with CHD Requiring Dialysis Are the Most Challenging Cases**

*A newborn affected by pulmonary atresia with intact interventricular septum is admitted to the CICU after birth. Prostaglandin E2 is administered as continuous infusion for ductal patency. On the second day of life, he undergoes transcatheter radiofrequency perforation of pulmonary valve. After the procedure, echocardiography detects a moderate pulmonary regurgitation that is associated with severe tricuspid regurgitation due to sudden right ventricular dilatation. The clinical progress post-procedure is complicated by the onset of desaturation, oligo-anuria, hypotension, and diffuse edema. A circular shunt is suspected (retrograde flow from ductus arteriosus to pulmonary artery back to right ventricle and again into right atrium, shunting to left atrium, and then directed to left ventricle, aorta and again into ductus arteriosus) causing significant low cardiac output syndrome. Continuous infusion of diuretic is started. Fenoldopam is administered in the attempt of decreasing systemic vascular resistances (in order to reduce circular shunt) and adrenaline is infused to sustain the right ventricle. Because of the persistence of generalized edema, oligo-anuria, significant ascites accumulation in the abdomen and respiratory distress, a peritoneal catheter is placed and peritoneal dialysis is started. After initiation of peritoneal dialysis, negative fluid balance is achieved and abdomen ascites is drained, diuresis achieved to obtain further negativity of fluid balance and tissue edema is reduced. Once adequate clinical conditions have been obtained (stable hemodynamic parameters, adequate urinary output), the patient undergoes a cardiac surgical operation of outflow patch, systemic-pulmonary shunt and arterial duct closure. At this stage, after body fluids homeostasis is re-gained and surgery has optimized patient's cardiac output, the patient is easily weaned from PD and from mechanical ventilation.*

Because of the improvement in pediatric cardiac surgery techniques and increase in short-term survival of CHD children, intensivists working in CICU often have to treat more and more sick patients, particularly neonates with very complex anatomies. Therefore, the therapeutic strategy has to be adapted to the individual patient on a case-by-case basis, searching for the optimal treatment in each clinical situation. The same concepts apply to AKI management, interventions vary according to the severity of renal damage, clinical conditions, and patient's age.

In case of right ventricular failure, one of the most commonly occurring complications is ascites. In fact, poor ventricular compliance results in increasing filling pressure and venous congestion of inferior vena cava and hepatic veins. In addition, neonates have elevated permeability of vascular endothelium that, in conditions of hypoalbuminemia and cardiac output, can lead to tissue edema and capillary leak syndrome. Abdominal compartment syndrome in neonatal patients is a component of reduced venous return to the failing right ventricle and is a significant cause of post-renal AKI.

*Peritoneal catheter placement* in neonates or infants is often useful to drain ascites accumulated and to decompress the abdominal organs. Indeed, in some institutions, peritoneal catheter placement at the end of cardiac surgery is considered regardless of the need for PD, to obtain negativity of fluid balance and to prevent increase in intra-abdominal pressure [44].

The possible complications related to peritoneal catheter placement are generally mechanical: catheter dysfunction, hemoperitoneum, hydrothorax, bowel perforation, increased risk of peritonitis [13].

*Indications for PD*: with respect to CRRT, PD has the advantage, especially in younger patients, not to require a dedicated vascular access and systemic anticoagulation. For this reason, PD is currently considered as first line treatment of AKI especially in neonates [45, 46].

*Mechanism of PD*: an osmotic solution is administered into the abdomen; peritoneum is used as a semipermeable membrane and allows the passage of solutes and water ultrafiltration.

*Indications of PD:* as for CRRT, there are no specific guidelines on the indications and timing of PD post cardiac surgery in children. The most commonly used criteria to start PD in cardiac children are the need to manage the intraoperative fluid accumulation in the postoperative phase. An inadequate urinary output to maintain a negative fluid balance, or < 1 mL/kg/h for >4 h, unresponsive to fluid challenge or to increase in diuretic dose, can be considered a parameter to start PD [13]. Dwell cycles are intermittently performed with a dialysate fluid (0.36% or 2.27% of dextrose concentration). The cycle volume amount in cardiac patients is generally around 10–15 mL/kg in order to avoid excessive intra-abdominal pressure rise which may cause hemodynamic instability. The duration of stay of the fluid in peritoneum ranges from 10 min to 1 h depending on the need for more or less aggressive solute control. Ultrafiltration rate averages around 5–10 mL per cycle, allowing a fair amount to be removed to optimize fluid balance control, even if with less capacity of precisely adapting to patients' needs as during extracorporeal CRRT.

In our second case, Peritoneal Dialysis (PD) was delivered as a bridge to optimize the patient's condition for cardiac surgery with better hemodynamic conditions and reduced fluid overload. The discontinuation of dialysis treatment occurred when he recovered renal function to maintain adequate urine output and adequate negative fluid balance.

**Conclusions**

Severe AKI requiring RRT in cardiac children is a severe clinical condition burdened by death in more than 40% of treated patients: to dialyze critically ill children is further complicated by several technical issues. Early diagnosis, timely management, and novel technology are all part of a multidimensional approach to adequately dialyze critically ill children. The outcomes may vary significantly depending on the underlying disease, the severity of illness, the time of intervention, and the institutional expertise and practice. Long-term outcomes of survivors, especially those who do not completely recover baseline function and patients with palliative surgery, are potentially hampered by the threat of chronic renal dysfunction. In this scenario, new technological advances such as miniaturized circuits and membranes, accurate CRRT machines and effective prescription schedules promise to help the clinician in improving quality of treatment and possibly overall outcomes.

## References


1. Jander A, Tkaczyk M, Pagowska-Klimek I, et al. Continuous veno-venous hemodiafiltration in children after cardiac surgery. Eur J Cardiothorac Surg. 2007;31(6):1022–8.
2. Webb TN, Goldstein SL. Congenital heart surgery and acute kidney injury. Curr Opin Anaesthesiol. 2017;30(1):105–12.
3. Cooper DS, Basu RK, Price JF, et al. The kidney in critical cardiac disease: proceedings from the 10th international conference of the pediatric cardiac Intensive Care Society. World J Pediatr Congenit Heart Surg. 2016;7(2):152–63.
4. Sanchez-de-Toledo J, Perez-Ortiz A, Gil L, et al. Early initiation of renal replacement therapy in pediatric heart surgery is associated with lower mortality. Pediatr Cardiol. 2016;37(4):623–8.
5. Patterson T, Hehir DA, Buelow M, et al. Hemodynamic profile of acute kidney injury following the fontan procedure: impact of renal perfusion pressure. World J Pediatr Congenit Heart Surg. 2017;8(3):367–75.
6. Baliga R, Ueda N, Walker PD, et al. Oxidant mechanisms in toxic acute renal failure. Am J Kidney Dis. 1997;29(3):465–77.
7. Elahi MM, Lim MY, Joseph RN, et al. Early hemofiltration improves survival in post-cardiotomy patients with acute renal failure. Eur J Cardiothorac Surg. 2004;26(5):1027–31.
8. Zou H, Hong Q, Xu G, et al. Early versus late initiation of renal replacement therapy impacts mortality in patients with acute kidney injury post cardiac surgery: a meta-analysis. Crit Care. 2017;21(1):150.
9. Bagshaw SM, Uchino S, Bellomo R, et al. Beginning and ending supportive therapy for the kidney (BEST kidney) investigators: timing of renal replacement therapy and clinical outcomes in critically ill patients with severe acute kidney injury. J Crit Care. 2009;24(1):129–40.

10. Bouman CS, Oudemans-Van Straaten HM, Tijssen JG, et al. Effects of early high-volume continuous venovenous hemofiltration on survival and recovery of renal function in intensive care patients with acute renal failure: a prospective, randomized trial. Crit Care Med. 2002;30(10):2205–11.
11. Ronco C, Ricci Z, Goldstein SL. (R)evolution in the management of acute kidney injury in newborns. Am J Kidney Dis. 2015;66(2):206–11.
12. Bojan M, Gioanni S, Vouhé PR, et al. Early initiation of peritoneal dialysis in neonates and infants with acute kidney injury following cardiac surgery is associated with a significant decrease in mortality. Kidney Int. 2012;82(4):474–81.
13. Fleming F, Bohn D, Edwards H, et al. Renal replacement therapy after repair of congenital heart disease in children. A comparison of hemofiltration and peritoneal dialysis. J Thorac Cardiovasc Surg. 1995;109(2):322–31.
14. Santiago MJ, López-Herce J, Urbano J. Evolution and mortality risk factors in children with continuous renal replacement therapy after cardiac surgery. Rev Esp Cardiol (Engl Ed). 2012;65(9):795–800.
15. Foland JA, Fortenberry JD, Warshaw BL, et al. Fluid overload before continuous hemofiltration and survival in critically ill children: a retrospective analysis. Crit Care Med. 2004;32(8):1771–6.
16. Hazle MA, Gajarski RJ, Yu S, et al. Fluid overload in infants following congenital heart surgery. Pediatr Crit Care Med. 2013;14(1):44–9.
17. Rihal CS, Textor SC, Grill DE, et al. Incidence and prognostic importance of acute renal failure after percutaneous coronary intervention. Circulation. 2002;105(19):2259–64.
18. McCullough PA, Choi JP, Feghali GA, et al. Contrast-induced acute kidney injury. J Am Coll Cardiol. 2016;68(13):1165 73.
19. Selewski DT, Goldstein SL. The role of fluid overload in the prediction of outcome in acute kidney injury. Pediatr Nephrol. 2018;33(1):13–24.
20. Goldstein SL, Somers MJ, Baum MA, et al. Pediatric patients with multi-organ dysfunction syndrome receiving continuous renal replacement therapy. Kidney Int. 2005;67(2):653–8.
21. Bellomo R, Kellum JA, Ronco C. Defining acute renal failure: physiological principles. Intensive Care Med. 2004;30(1):33–7.
22. Bucholz EM, Whitlock RP, Zappitelli M, et al. TRIBE-AKI consortium: cardiac biomarkers and acute kidney injury after cardiac surgery. Pediatrics. 2015;135(4):e945–56.
23. Hornik CP, Krawczeski CD, Zappitelli M, et al. Serum brain natriuretic peptide and risk of acute kidney injury after cardiac operations in children. Ann Thorac Surg. 2014;97(6):2142–7.
24. Toda Y, Sugimoto K. AKI after pediatric cardiac surgery for congenital heart diseases-recent developments in diagnostic criteria and early diagnosis by biomarkers. J Intensive Care. 2017;5:49.
25. Belley-Côté EP, Parikh CR. Shortt CR, et al;TRIBE-AKI consortium: association of cardiac biomarkers with acute kidney injury after cardiac surgery: a multicenter cohort study. J Thorac Cardiovasc Surg. 2016;152(1):245–51.
26. Kidney Disease Improving Global Outcomes (KDIGO) Acute Kidney Injury Work Group. KDIGO clinical practice guideline for acute kidney injury. Kidney Int Suppl. 2012;2:1–138.
27. Tsai TY, Chien H, Tsai FC, et al. Comparison of RIFLE, AKIN, and KDIGO classifications for assessing prognosis of patients on extracorporeal membrane oxygenation. J Formos Med Assoc. 2017;116(11):844–51.
28. Modem V, Thompson M, Gollhofer D, et al. Timing of continuous renal replacement therapy and mortality in critically ill children. Crit Care Med. 2014;42(4):943–53.
29. Ronco C, Di Lullo L. Cardiorenal syndrome. Heart Fail Clin. 2014;10(2):251–80.
30. Ronco C, Bellomo R, Kellum J. Understanding renal functional reserve. Intensive Care Med. 2017;43:917–20.
31. Damman K, Deursen v, Navis G, et al. Increased central venous pressure is associated with impaired renal function and mortality in a broad spectrum of patients with cardiovascular disease. J Am Coll Cardiol. 2009;53:582–8.

32. Damman K, Voors AA, Hillege HL, CIBIS-2 Investigators and Committees, et al. Congestion in chronic systolic heart failure is related to renal dysfunction and increased mortality. Eur J Heart Fail. 2010;12:974–82.
33. Guglin M, Rivero A, Matar F, et al. Renal dysfunction in heart failure is due to congestion but not low output. Clin Cardiol. 2011;34:113–36.
34. Ricci Z, Romagnoli S, Ronco C: Renal Replacement Therapy. F1000Res. 2016 Jan 25;5. pii: F1000 Faculty Rev-103.
35. Musielak A, Warzywoda A, Wojtalik M, et al. Outcomes of continuous renal replacement therapy with regional citrate anticoagulation in small children after cardiac surgery: experience and protocol from a single center. Ther Apher Dial. 2016;20(6):639–44.
36. Ricci Z, Garisto C, Morelli S, et al. Brain natriuretic peptide is removed by continuous veno-venous hemofiltration in pediatric patients. Interact Cardiovasc Thorac Surg. 2009;9(1):33–6.
37. Ricci Z, Carotti A, Parisi F, et al. Extracorporeal membrane oxygenation and high-dose continuous veno-venous hemodiafiltration in a young child as a successful bridge to heart transplant for management of combined heart and kidney failure: a case report. Blood Purif. 2010;29(1):23–6.
38. Santiago MJ, López-Herce J, Urbano J, et al. Continuous renal replacement therapy in children after cardiac surgery. J Thorac Cardiovasc Surg. 2013;146(2):448–54.
39. Ricci Z, Guzzi F, Tuccinardi G, et al. Dose prescription and delivery in neonates with congenital heart diseases treated with continuous veno-venous hemofiltration. Pediatr Crit Care Med. 2017;18(7):623–9.
40. Ronco C, Garzotto F, Ricci Z. CA.R.PE.DI.E.M. (cardio-renal pediatric dialysis emergency machine): evolution of continuous renal replacement therapies in infants. A personal journey. Pediatr Nephrol. 2012;27(8):1203–11.
41. Ricci Z, Guzzi F, Tuccinardi G, et al. Dialytic dose in pediatric continuous renal replacement therapy patients. Minerva Pediatr. 2016;68(5):366–73.
42. Clark WR, Leblanc M, Ricci Z, et al. Quantification and dosing of renal replacement therapy in acute kidney injury: a reappraisal. Blood Purif. 2017;44(2):140–55.
43. Askenazi D, Ingram D, White S, et al. Smaller circuits for smaller patients: improving renal support therapy with Aquadex™. Pediatr Nephrol. 2016;31(5):853–60.
44. Kwiatkowski DM, Menon S, Krawczeski CD, et al. Improved outcomes with peritoneal dialysis catheter placement after cardiopulmonary bypass in infants. J Thorac Cardiovasc Surg. 2015;149(1):230–6.
45. Baskin E, Gulleroglu KS, Saygili A, et al. Peritoneal dialysis requirements following open-heart surgery in children with congenital heart disease. Ren Fail. 2010;32(7):784–7.
46. Ronco C, Ricci Z. Pediatric continuous renal replacement: 20 years later. Intensive Care Med. 2015;41(6):985–93.

# CRRT in the Septic Patient

# 26

Matthew L. Paden

**Case Vignette**

A 12-year-old (48 kg) previously healthy male presents to your hospital in acute respiratory failure and overwhelming suspected septic shock. He is intubated in the emergency department, received broad spectrum antibiotics (vancomycin and ceftriaxone), fluid resuscitated with 4 L of normal saline, placed on an epinephrine infusion and titrated to 0.4 mcg/kg/min, and brought to your intensive care unit. Initial labs obtained in the emergency department demonstrate thrombocytopenia, anion gap metabolic acidosis, transaminitis (AST 650, ALT 525), and an elevated creatinine at 2.5 mg/dL. He is febrile at 40.1, and has had no urine output in the 2 h since his arrival in the emergency department. He is given another 2 L of normal saline, loaded with steroids for vasopressor refractory shock, and given two additional anti-staphylococcal drugs. He is becoming increasingly hypoxic, requiring increases in ventilator settings, with a pattern consistent with pulmonary edema seen on a repeat chest radiograph. Echocardiogram demonstrates poor cardiac contractility, and in consultation with pediatric surgery, nephrology, and blood bank, the decision is made to place the patient on ECMO to gain stability to provide CRRT and plasma exchange.

Infections and their complications are the number one cause of pediatric mortality worldwide. Accordingly, sepsis and septic shock are two common reasons why children are admitted to the pediatric intensive care unit (PICU). While in adults, the mortality associated with septic shock is between 30 and 40%, in children it has been thought to be much lower (in the 5–10% range) based on previous studies [1, 2].

M. L. Paden
Division of Pediatric Critical Care, Emory University, Atlanta, GA, USA
e-mail: Matthew.Paden@choa.org



A. Deep, S. L. Goldstein (eds.), *Critical Care Nephrology and Renal Replacement Therapy in Children*, https://doi.org/10.1007/978-3-319-90281-4_26

However, a recent point prevalence study of pediatric severe sepsis over 128 sites in 26 countries demonstrated a prevalence of 8.2% of 6925 patients with 25% mortality [3]. One potential reason for the higher mortality in this study was the frequent presence of multiple organ dysfunction syndrome (MODS), which from previous work we know is associated with higher mortality rates [4]. MODS was present in 67% of the patients on the day of sepsis recognition and 30% of those with MODS went on to have additional organ failures. With the progress in medical science, there are very few diseases in the pediatric population which have such high mortality rates, and thus pediatric sepsis is a common target for attempting to reduce childhood mortality. Attempts at improving sepsis outcomes over the last decade have targeted prevention (immunization), early recognition (sepsis scoring systems, community pediatrician and family education, etc.), and standardized practice (sepsis bundles, mandated antibiotic choices, etc.). Many have met with some degree of success, however this remains a pressing public heath focus.

At the bedside in the PICU, one must acknowledge that caring for the patient with sepsis not only involves treatment of the causative infection, but also managing the multiple other organ dysfunctions that are common in pediatric sepsis. With advanced technologies, such as continuous renal replacement therapy (CRRT), we have available to provide organ support and replacement. As a result, the outcome for a septic child is less related to the ability to eradicate the inciting infection, and more dependent on the clinician's ability to support the patient's other organ failures until they recover. This chapter will review the use of one of those therapies, CRRT, during sepsis. Chapter 22 in this textbook covers the use of multiple extracorporeal therapies together to support a patient with multiple organ failure. An important notation is that while the last decade has provided us with some evidence on how best to perform CRRT, many questions remain and there is a lack of evidence to answer them conclusively. Pediatric specific evidence will be covered if available, and if not, I will present data from adult trials and leave it to the reader to balance whether that data is applicable to the pediatric population. As we described in Chap. 22, in this field, expert opinion remains a common source of information and additional clinical trials are needed in order to best define the optimal practice of CRRT in pediatric sepsis patients.

## 26.1 Septic Acute Kidney Injury

Acute kidney injury (AKI) is a common manifestation of injury seen in both adult and pediatric critically ill patients in the intensive care unit and occurs from a variety of pathologic insults. While AKI is commonly recognized at the bedside, consistent definitions have limited research into this important topic in the past. Over the last decade, advances have been made in this area and other chapters in this text cover comprehensively the intricacies of the diagnosis, consensus definitions, severity scoring systems, and outcomes associated with AKI. In a similar manner, sepsis has had the same problems—a disease easily recognizable at the bedside, but suffering from a lack of consistent formal definitions that would facilitate worldwide research. Over the last decade, the sepsis community has collaborated and developed consensus definitions for both adult and pediatric patients [5, 6]. The copresence of AKI during an episode of sepsis defines the condition known as septic AKI. Estimates of the prevalence of septic AKI have been published in the adult population and range from 22 to 53% depending on the method of the study and definitions used [7, 8]. In pediatrics, a subanalysis of the SPROUT study demonstrated a 21% prevalence of septic AKI [9].

The pathophysiology of septic AKI is not completely understood, but the pathways involved appear to be quite different from traditional renal insults due to drug induced, hypoxic/ischemia mechanisms, and rhabdomyolysis induced injuries. Previously, the major theories surrounding the causes of septic AKI revolved around changes in blood flow to the kidney during times of either low global blood pressure or due to the renal perfusion effects of the vasopressors used to support the global blood pressure, and that these changes in perfusion led to acute tubular necrosis. There is increasing evidence, both on the bench and at bedside, that this model is partially incorrect. A combination of studies have demonstrated acute tubular necrosis plays a lesser role in septic AKI injury, and that renal perfusion is much more dynamic during sepsis than first thought, and may actually be increased during certain phases of sepsis. Increasing understanding of the immune and coagulation systems during the body's response to sepsis have allowed further insight into the both the AKI, as well as led to some observations which may explain the higher levels of chronic kidney disease in AKI survivors. The implication of the immune and coagulation systems in septic AKI also provides plausible pathophysiologic pathways that could be involved in the injury of other organs and subsequent development of MODS. While some two organ dysfunction syndromes, such as hepato-renal, are established, new models of organ cross talk, such as cardio-renal syndrome, have been proposed based on this new paradigm [10]. A thorough understanding of these pathways is important, especially for those caring for the septic pediatric patient, who as described above, is most likely to present with established MODS. Detailed reviews of the underlying pathways implicated in septic AKI have been published, and they are covered more extensively in Chap. 6 [11–13].

Similar to AKI, fluid overload (FO) is common during sepsis, from a combination of resuscitation fluids given empirically to support blood pressure, as well as to provide adequate oncotic pressure (and thus intravascular volume) during periods of vascular leak that are commonly seen in sepsis. Fluid overload has been associated with mortality in multiple clinical conditions in the pediatric population, in both single and multiple center studies. The association of fluid overload with poor outcomes in a multitude of conditions resulting in pediatric critical illness has been reviewed elsewhere in this textbook, however, it is worth reviewing a few newer examples of the evidence specifically in pediatric sepsis. While the original work on fluid overload and outcomes in children receiving CRRT came from the United States in the 2000s, more recent work has replicated the findings in other settings. In Venezuela, Naveda recently retrospectively reviewed 149 pediatric patients with an average age of 6 years, with 60% having sepsis as the etiology for their shock. In this septic group, the overall mortality was 25.5%, and fluid overload was identified as an independent risk factor (OR 1.5, CI = 1.2–4.9) for the development of kidney failure [14]. Similarly, in China, Chen evaluated 202 children with severe sepsis, finding a 30.2% mortality rate and a 23% rate of fluid overload [15]. They found the previously described correlation between increasing degree of fluid overload and increasing mortality risk. While this correlation usually has been reported as starting at >10% FO, they evaluated a novel concept of early fluid overload being defined as >5% FO in the first 24 h of ICU admission. This test predicted mortality with a sensitivity of 67% and specificity of 80% (ROC 0.74, CI 0.65–0.82). In both of these studies, a significant portion of the fluids given were due to fluid boluses. No discussion of fluid boluses in the treatment of sepsis would be complete without mentioning the findings of the FEAST trial. While fluid overload was not specifically calculated, the FEAST trial is one of the largest pediatric sepsis trials, having evaluated 3141 children with sepsis in limited resource settings in Africa. It found that saline fluid boluses at the time of admission to the hospital were associated with a significant increase in mortality at 48 h (10.5% saline, 7.3% control, RR 1.44, CI 1.09–1.9) [16]. While one must determine if the results of this study are generalizable to the patient population and diseases that you care for at your center, it certainly has introduced controversy into a mainstay of pediatric sepsis care. Fluid overload, especially in sepsis, remains a potentially modifiable risk factor for poor outcome and thus is a tempting target for intervention.

## 26.2 Why CRRT During Sepsis?

AKI and FO are both common during sepsis, and renal replacement therapy is often needed to mitigate the consequences of the renal injuries. When evaluating options for providing renal replacement therapies, the three most common options in pediatrics are intermittent hemodialysis (IHD), CRRT, and peritoneal dialysis (PD). Looking at the epidemiology of which therapy is chosen, we often see a predominance for CRRT use in the pediatric population. For example, Westrope recently reviewed the Pediatric Intensive Care Audit Network (PICANet) database which collects data on all children <16 years old who receive care in a PICU in the United Kingdom [17]. They found that 2.9% of PICU admissions received renal replacement therapy, and that about 50% received CRRT only, 45% received PD, and 4% received IHD. Similar findings have been seen in other countries, and for the sickest population of patients—those on ECMO—CRRT use is >90% [18]. With these varying options for providing renal replacement therapy, why is CRRT often the predominant form used?

Increased rates of hemodynamic instability with the use of IHD in septic patients are a common reason given for the primary use of CRRT. In the pediatric population, there are very little data comparing hemodynamic parameters between these two groups. In adults, John examined 30 septic AKI patients who were randomized to CRRT or IHD and found patients treated with CRRT had increased blood pressure and decreased HR at 2 h and an increased systemic vascular resistance at 24 h compared to those who received IHD [19]. Avoiding the need for systemic anticoagulation, usually with heparin, is another frequent reason cited for choosing CRRT over IHD in the septic population, since many regional anticoagulation strategies have been published (see Chap. 17). With the increased prevalence of disseminated intravascular coagulation and thrombocytopenia that often coexist in septic shock patients, this concern of bleeding complications is certainly warranted. Similarly, this concern of hemorrhagic complications with catheter placement often is cited as a reason to not perform acute PD in the septic patient. Seen more commonly in the smaller pediatric patients, the diaphragmatic loading associated with infusion of PD fluids into the abdominal cavity leads to a reduction in functional residual capacity and may make adequate oxygenation and ventilation more difficult. Other experts share concerns that clearance may be inadequate when using PD due to increased metabolic demands seen during sepsis. It should be pointed out that while CRRT use predominates, many centers are able to use IHD and PD successfully in septic patients, and that while each of these above concerns are valid in general, since there is no convincing evidence of superiority that choice of renal replacement modality should be individualized to meet the needs of each patient best utilizing the skills and equipment available at a particular center.

Advocates for using CRRT for septic AKI generally point to several key advantages of using a continuous therapy modality. The first is that in sepsis, cellular metabolism is greatly increased and rapidly changes throughout the day with increases in fever, dosing of anti-infectives, and blood products. Use of a continuous renal replacement therapy allows a slow, but steady correction of acidosis and electrolyte abnormalities back to their prescribed baseline and provide a more normal homeostasis when compared to the saw tooth shaped clearance of IHD or to a lesser degree PD. Increased clearance of middle-sized molecules, including cytokines, chemokines, and other immune-derived molecules has been another proposed benefit of the use of continuous renal replacement therapies. Understanding that the underlying pathophysiology of septic AKI is likely to be related to a dysregulation of host immune response, has led to the desire to use continuous therapies in order to blunt the agents causing the dysregulation. In the early 2000s, Ronco proposed the "peak concentration hypothesis" that states that high levels of both inflammatory and anti-inflammatory mediators are associated with both the end-organ damage seen in MODS as well as the increased mortality rates [20]. This has led to the introduction of "blood purification" techniques that attempt to lower the peak levels of such mediators and regain the usual immunologic homeostasis. To achieve this goal, continuous therapies are favored over intermittent ones, and CRRT was the first of these therapies to be used. Clearance of the mediators of sepsis have been described in multiple studies, however the exact amounts and types of mediators cleared varies by dose of CRRT, filter variables (pore size, surface coatings, material, frequency of replacement, etc.), and timing of initiation. For those wishing to follow this path, Honore et al. provide a recent pragmatic review of the variables involved and a strategy for choosing equipment and dosing for patients with septic AKI [21]. In addition to CRRT-based clearance, hemoperfusion columns are also available that can remove mediators and are added to a CRRT system. The polymyxin B-based systems are the most commonly used (>100,000 cases in Japan alone) in both adult and pediatric patients. Shimizu provides a recent review of this technology and application [22]. When used in combination with CRRT, it can further reduce mediators of sepsis. Among others using this combined approach, Zheng recently reported significant reductions in high mobility group box protein 1 (HMGB1) levels and improved 30 days survival in an adult population of septic AKI [23].

## 26.3 Practical Issues with CRRT During Sepsis

Using CRRT in the septic patient is not without potential risks and issues. The first question in prescribing CRRT is to determine when the patient should receive this therapy. The timing of CRRT initiation is a complicated subject, and remains the subject of research investigation. There are proponents in the medical literature from the extremes of initiating CRRT only once the "traditional" indications of dialysis (acidosis/pulmonary edema/hyperkalemia/etc. that have failed medical management and are life threatening) have been met to the other extreme of initiating it in certain populations, such as extracorporeal membrane oxygenation, empirically on all patients even in the absence of evidence of renal injury in an attempt to prevent fluid overload and other electrolyte complications. It should be mentioned that the current KDIGO guidelines recommend a global assessment of the patient's current condition and trend of changes, and not relying on absolute numbers to trigger CRRT initiation. While a few studies have been attempted to evaluate issues of "early" versus "late" initiation of CRRT, their interpretation for the pediatric community are complicated by being done prior to the consensus definitions of AKI, differing in definitions of "early" and "late" between studies, and mostly involving adult patients with disease processes that differ from what is seen in children. Two new studies, IDEAL-ICU and STARRT-AKI, will address the issue of timing in the adult population. Additional studies in pediatrics are now being developed to better define optimal care for this important question.

Once to the decision has been made to initiate CRRT, the question of optimal prescription is the next to be addressed. Other chapters in this textbook address in other clinical settings the different modes of CRRT that can be used (continuous veno-venous hemofiltration, continuous veno-venous dialysis, and continuous veno-venous hemodiafiltration) and the potential associated benefits and issues. This information is applicable to sepsis patients as well, with some expert opinion favoring convective modalities of clearance. Many centers standardize on one mode and utilize one type of filter for all CRRT procedures regardless of indication, since there is little substantial evidence of outcome benefit demonstrated for tailoring this therapy more specifically. While not an evidence-based statement, the concept of doing one thing and doing it well will likely serve the patient better (by reducing interruptions in therapy due to complications, and maximizing the delivered dose) than introducing new modes or filters in these unstable sepsis patients. The dose of therapy has been a controversial topic, for both adults and children.

Ronco performed the first randomized trial with dosing divided between 20, 35, and 45 mL/kg/h and demonstrated improved survival with 35 mL/kg/h compared to 20, but no difference in mortality between the 35 mL/kg/h and 45 mL/kg/h groups [24]. Later subgroup analyses of the septic AKI patients in the ATN and RENAL trials also showed no difference in dose [25, 26]. Based on this study, the "standard" dose for all patients has been 20–30 mL/kg/h. Several other adult trials have attempted "high dose" (~70–100 mL/kg/h) CRRT in the setting of sepsis, attempting to maximize the mediator clearance with some demonstrated success in that outcome, but with no difference seen in mortality [27, 28]. It is important to note that in many of these studies, increased clearance of antibiotics is also demonstrated, which raises particular concern in the septic patient. Clearance, both of anti-infectives, but also nutrition must be taken into consideration in the patient on CRRT, and frequent drug and nutritional monitoring must be performed to ensure optimal dosing. Guidelines and best practice reviews have been published to aid with appropriate anti-infective and nutrition prescribing and monitoring for the patient with septic AKI [29, 30]. Finally, choosing an anticoagulation strategy is important for the septic patient. While it can be performed safely, considering the coagulopathy and disseminated intravascular coagulation that often coexists during septic shock, there are advantages to avoiding heparin-based strategies that require both the patient and the CRRT circuit to be anticoagulated in order to reduce bleeding complications. Regional anticoagulation techniques, for example with citrate, have been reviewed in other chapters and are ideal for use in septic AKI patients. Frequent monitoring of, and avoiding low patient ionized calcium levels is necessary in these sepsis patients, so as not to impair cardiac function. This occurs more prominently in the youngest pediatric patients whose immature myocardium is more dependent on extracellular calcium concentrations to promote contractility. A more novel approach for these septic children is to use low dose prostacyclin infusions to provide short duration, localized platelet inhibition within the CRRT circuit as a source of anticoagulation [31]. Potential benefits of this approach in septic AKI are avoiding hypocalcemia induced hypotension or dysrhythmias as well as citrate lock.

As seen above, while many patients' hemodynamics improve in the first few hours after initiating CRRT, the first few minutes after connection can often be more precarious. First described during intermittent hemodialysis, the correlation between bradykinin release and subsequent vasodilatory induced hypotension with exposure of blood to membranes has also been described in CRRT use. While often attributed to only AN69 membranes, the phenomenon has also been described in patients with polysulfone membranes [32, 33]. Various techniques have been described to mitigate this problem, and should be considered in patients on high amounts of cardiovascular support or who are already unstable at CRRT initiation. During CRRT, circuit and filter life is variable and not predictable in patients with sepsis. Similarly, the total duration of CRRT needed for septic AKI remains variable, and clinical criteria of when to stop in order to evaluate for recovery of native renal function are poorly defined.

## 26.4 Outcomes in Septic AKI

As has been discussed, there are many different approaches to prescribing CRRT for the septic AKI population. There is an increasing amount of outcome data, mostly from large adult trials, however many of the basic components of optimal renal replacement therapy remain incompletely defined. A brief review of some of the major controversies in renal replacement therapy during sepsis follows.

With regard to choice of therapy, adult trials demonstrate similar mortality, renal recovery, and complication rates when using IHD, slow low-efficiency dialysis (SLED), and CRRT [34, 35]. Similarly, in total, there appear to be similar outcomes when evaluating convective versus diffusive clearance modes [35]. The mode of CRRT has been found to change outcome in one, single-center, randomized prospective study, published in 2006 which demonstrated improved 90 day survival with CVVHDF as compared to CVVH (hazard ratio 0.59, CI 0.40–0.87) [36]. No subsequent prospective study has evaluated this specifically. Two retrospective studies, from Canada and Croatia (which specifically evaluated septic AKI) have been subsequently published demonstrating no difference in survival between these modes [37, 38]. Timing of CRRT initiation was addressed in the recently published AKIKI study, which involved 31 adult ICUs in France [39]. The study randomized patients to CRRT initiation within 6 h of meeting stage 3 AKI or using a set of "standard" indications for CRRT. There was no difference in mortality between the two groups, and interestingly almost half of the "standard" indication patients never received CRRT. There was an additional single-center trial, that was able to demonstrate a mortality difference (39.3% vs. 54.7%, hazard ratio 0.66, CI 0.45–0.97) with randomization within 8 h of meeting stage 2 AKI versus within 12 h of meeting stage 3 AKI [40].

Anticoagulation during CRRT is always a controversial topic, and potential benefits and harms are frequently reviewed in the medical literature. Many of the more recent reviews make statements such as, "regional citrate anticoagulation can be recommended as the therapy of choice for the majority of critically ill patients requiring CRRT" [41]. While avoiding heparin anticoagulation for CRRT in septic AKI has some potential benefits, at least in the adult population, it is important to remember that there is data suggesting that using IHD or CRRT with systemic heparin anticoagulation in septic patients can have low complication rates. In a subanalysis to the CONVINT study which randomized patients between IHD and CRRT and had a 66% rate of septic AKI, there was a low rate of death from bleeding complications (3.6%) and no complication rate difference between IHD and CRRT [42].

Considering the dose of CRRT, the current KDIGO guidelines recommend 20–25 mL/kg/h based on the finding of Grade 1A evidence in the medical literature. As discussed earlier, in the realm of septic AKI, other investigators have attempted higher dosing in an attempt to alter outcomes. Park et al. randomized 212 adult patients with septic AKI between 40 mL/kg/h and 80 mL/kg/h and evaluated the effect on mortality and cytokine levels [28]. They found no difference in 28 day mortality between the two groups. While the higher dose CRRT group significantly reduced multiple pro- and anti-inflammatory mediators, the standard dose did not.

This and other studies demonstrate that while you can clear these mediators via high dose CRRT, that the end effect may not be enough to change clinical outcomes such as survival.

We briefly examined the potential role of polymyxin B-based hemoperfusion columns in septic AKI when used in conjunction with CRRT. Previous smaller studies have been promising and the results of the much larger and now recently completed EUPHRATES randomized trial of polymyxin B hemoperfusion columns in septic shock have not been formally reported yet, but a press release stated that there was a reduction in mortality between groups (36.9% and 31.9% with the device) that did not reach statistical significance. There are some interesting subgroup analyses that are ongoing looking at the sickest population with MODS, where a post hoc analysis demonstrated a 10.7% reduction in mortality was seen [43]. Further evaluation and publication of the entire clinical trial data and outcomes will be necessary in order to fully understand these findings.

## 26.5 Role of Multiple Organ Support Therapies in Sepsis

Understanding the pathophysiology of the development of MODS as described above, it is becoming increasingly common in the ICU to be supporting patients with 4–5 organ failures. It is interesting that the pathophysiology of MODS appears to be a common end pathway to many different inciting injuries. With 66% of septic pediatric patients presenting with MODS, it is not unusual for the intensivist to be taking care of a patient for the first few days with no clearly defined diagnosis of the underlying disease that got the patient there. For the sickest of patients, organ support therapies provide a lifesaving bridge to give time to figure out the underlying cause, give time for therapies such as antibiotics or immune suppression to work, or allow surgeries to obtain source control of infections that would otherwise be lethal. Extracorporeal therapies, such as ECMO, CRRT, and plasma exchange, play major roles in supporting these patients. While Chap. 22 discusses the practical side of getting these various devices to work together from a clinical and biomedical engineering standpoint, a brief focus on the framework of how we use these devices at our center to provide multiple organ support is warranted.

The patient presented at the beginning of this chapter represents a common scenario that is seen in the pediatric ICU. In summary, the patient shows up with overwhelming shock that is thought to be septic in nature, but no definitive organism has been identified yet. As is seen with many septic patients, this patient presents in four organ MODS, with respiratory, cardiac, hepatic, and hematologic organ dysfunctions. He is rapidly declining since his admission to the ED and initial efforts at support are failing to meet goals of adequate oxygen delivery and organ support. This is a patient that not so long ago, would have been treated by escalating inotrope/vasopressor infusions and ventilator settings until they have reached center-based "maximum" doses and often resulted in complications from therapy (pneumothorax, dysrhythmias, etc.) and death within the first 24 h of therapy. While diagnostic labs were sent, often the results would return post-mortem.

Currently, these unstable and rapidly decompensating patients are managed at our center by a multidisciplinary team that can bring organ support therapies to the bedside and initiate them in a short period of time (<1 h goal). The underlying pathophysiology that these patients have in common is often an initial insult that leads to organ damage, and then through the immunologic and coagulation pathways described above leads to damage of other organs and the rapid progression into MODS. Many of the traditional therapies that are used (mechanical ventilation, high dose inotropes/vasopressors, diuretics, blood products, etc.) cause injury to the very organs they are being used to support, and often lead to increasing other organ damage due to these "cross talk" pathways, and the vicious cycle of increasing multiple organ damage escalates eventually ending in death. A detailed review of the problems associated with our traditional therapies are out of the scope of this chapter, but are derived from evaluating the advances that cardiac intensivists and surgeons have made with the introduction of early mechanical support for heart failure over traditional therapies and the long held understanding of the negative effects of mechanical ventilation (currently >8000 articles in PubMed).

A cornerstone of our approach is acknowledging that breaking this cycle of traditional therapy induced injuries is vital. This starts with evaluation of the cardiorespiratory system. ECMO is commonly used as a platform to gain control over the cardiorespiratory system and gain enough stability to be able to provide the other organ support and medical therapies. While veno-arterial (VA) ECMO, which provides both cardiac and respiratory support, would at first thought be the ideal modality in this situation, it has significant issues associated with it, including, but not limited to, need for carotid cannulation, higher risk of embolic stroke and cerebral hemorrhage, and ineffectiveness in high output cardiac failure often seen in vasodilatory septic shock. The benefit of it is that it provides excellent forward blood flow when a replacement for cardiac failure is needed in a classic cold shock setting. Our approach is to try venovenous (VV) ECMO first to avoid the complications associated with VA ECMO, with an understanding that this will not be effective for all patients. A review of the outcomes of septic, noncardiac, pediatric patients in the Extracorporeal Life Support Organization's (ELSO) registry demonstrated improved outcomes with VV ECMO [44]. From a surgical standpoint, the surgeons open the neck and isolate and control both the internal jugular and carotid artery. We then proceed with venovenous (VV) cannulation and turn down the ventilator to minimal levels. Often the adequate supply of oxygen from the ECMO circuit combined with the ability to reduce the intrathoracic pressures caused by high ventilator settings (which have substantial cardio-pulmonary interactions with respect to venous return and transmural pressure) are sufficient to allow both gas exchange and a rapid weaning of various inotropes/vasopressors. It is not unusual for patients to be on 2–3 high dose inotropes/vasopressors prior to VV ECMO, and be completely off of them within the first 15–30 min of ECMO. During that time, the surgeons and the intensivists remain at bedside and if rapid improvement is not seen, then cannulation of the carotid artery occurs and the patient is transitioned to veno-arterial ECMO. Now that cardiorespiratory stability has been achieved, either natively on VV or mechanically via VA ECMO we move to adding additional organ support.

Over the last decade at our center in the PICU, our approach has been that CRRT is provided for all ECMO patients at the time of ECMO initiation. From a practical standpoint, it is usually started within 0.5–1 h of cannulation immediately after cannulas have been confirmed in an appropriate position and secured. A review of the reasons behind this is discussed in Chap. 22, as well as the KIDMO series of papers that are cited there. In brief, essentially all of these septic patients meet criteria for >10% fluid overload and > 50% of them have > stage 2 AKI, and we wish to both prevent that fluid overload from worsening, as well as to correct it when hemodynamically improved, providing renal replacement therapy for electrolyte and acidosis control, and allowing improved nutrition [45]. The previously mentioned KIDMO data has demonstrated that the risk of mortality is best associated with stage of AKI and not solely the use of CRRT. Considering the degree of acidosis often present in these patients, we often initially start with a replacement fluid with a higher base concentration to more rapidly correct the acidosis which will help improve cardiac function. Initial fluid balance prescription is usually to be fluid neutral including insensible losses. In this setting, one also needs to consider water losses from the oxygenator which will be related to the amount of sweep gas flow used across the oxygenator. A reasonable estimate of oxygenator water losses for the adult Quadrox D™ membrane is 50–60 mL/day per liter of sweep gas [46, 47]. Diuretics are not used in these patients after CRRT initiation, even in the absence of urine output. Anuria is commonly seen and may persist for the duration of CRRT, however renal recovery of survivors is not affected by this in children. Using this approach, our center's survival and renal recovery rates are similar to the overall worldwide ELSO data [48].

Having addressed the respiratory, cardiac, and renal systems rapidly, we turn to the hematologic and hepatic systems. At this point, it is important to try to figure out the underlying cause of the patient's shock. Rapid diagnostics, such as infectious PCR-based methods, echocardiography, and labs that can be run at your center are often helpful in providing a provisional diagnosis. Carcillo has recently published a mental framework for classifying these MODS children, which can lead to the next therapeutic options for supporting the remaining organ systems [49].

In brief, often patients fall into three clinical and laboratory syndromes. An "immunoparalysis syndrome" is described which is characterized by persistent and new infections that are difficult to clear with traditional therapy, with prolonged lymphopenia and decreased response of leukocytes to stimulators such as tumor necrosis factor alpha or endotoxin. These patients may benefit from immunomodulation techniques, reduction of immunosuppressants (if used), and addition of granulocyte macrophage colony stimulating factor (GM-CSF). The second syndrome describes patients with "TAMOF" (thrombocytopenia associated multiple organ failure). These patients are characterized by having a thrombotic microangiopathy due to failure to clear von Willebrand factor after endothelial injury due to reduced ADAMSTS13 levels. Excessive inflammation in these patients is also associated with complement activation and has similarities in pathophysiology to disseminated intravascular coagulation, thrombotic thrombocytopenic purpura, and atypical hemolytic uremic syndrome. These patients benefit from aggressive and immediate plasma exchange to both replace missing ADAMSTS13 and to remove any autoantibodies to ADAMSTS13. This procedure also corrects the coagulopathy that is commonly seen in sepsis, helping restore both hematologic and hepatic homeostasis. Like the case presentation patient, approximately 75% of our rapidly decompensating previously healthy children with new onset MODS have the TAMOF syndrome. The final syndrome is described as "SMOF" or sequential multiple organ failure with new hepatobiliary dysfunction. This syndrome is clinically seen with patients who usually start out with respiratory failure and then develop rapid onset of hepatic and then other organ failures. Massive increases in inflammation are often present, leading to extremes of cardiac instability associated with lab findings of severe liver failure, hyperferritinemia, cellular hypoxia, and inability to clear viral infections. Diseases such as hemophagocytic lymphohisticytosis, post-transplant lymphoproliferative disorder, and macrophage activation syndrome are examples of conditions that often carry the SMOF phenotype. Immune modulation in this group can be useful, and anti-inflammatory cytokine-based strategies such as anakinra (IL-1 receptor antagonist) has shown potential for benefit in small studies.

While these syndromes of multiple organ failure do not identify a specific disease, taking this approach to classification and empiric therapy along with total organ support provide adequate stability for the underlying diagnosis to be identified and specific therapy initiated prior to death. Serial evaluations of underlying organ function and disease status is important during multiple organ support therapy, because patients who present as hyperinflammatory may revert to the immunosuppressed phenotype later in their course and changes in approach will be necessary. Trading traditional approaches to life support to an extracorporeal-based system is not without its own set of complications, and the team must be fastidious in care for each of these systems to prevent complications. Although this approach is being performed in a few high volume centers in the United States with reasonable results, additional work is needed with multicenter studies to see if these techniques can ultimately improve outcomes of this most unstable group of patients.

## 26.6 Summary of CRRT During Sepsis

Septic AKI is a commonly encountered problem for the pediatric intensivist and nephrologist. Our understanding of the underlying pathophysiology of septic AKI has changed over the last decade, and is beginning to influence the way we approach, diagnose, and treat this disease. As our technology improves, we are being faced with sicker and more complicated patients than ever before. We have an increasing amount of both pediatric and adult literature to guide some of the decision-making surrounding renal replacement for these patients. Use of multiple extracorporeal organ support therapies during sepsis is occurring successfully at several large pediatric centers. However, controversies and much work remains, with many questions about how to provide optimal care for this complex, unstable, and heterogeneous population.

**Key Learning Points**

- Septic acute kidney injury is common in the pediatric population.
- CRRT, with changes in technique, can be used to support these patients to recovery.
- Multiple extracorporeal support therapies can be used together to support patients with multiple organ dysfunction syndrome.

## References


1. Hartman ME, Linde-Zwirble WT, Angus DC, Watson RS. Trends in the epidemiology of pediatric severe sepsis. Pediatr Crit Care Med. 2013;14:686–93.
2. Watson RS, Carcillo JA, Linde-Zwirble WT, Clermont G, Lidicker J, Angus DC. The epidemiology of severe sepsis in children in the United States. Am J Respir Crit Care Med. 2003;167:695–701.
3. Weiss SL, Fitzgeral JC, Pappachan J, Wheeler D, et al. Global epidemiology of pediatric severe sepsis: the sepsis prevalence, outcomes, and therapies study. Am J Respir Crit Care Med. 2015;191(10):1147–57.
4. Kutko MC, Calarco MP, Flaherty MB, Helmrich RF, Ushay HM, Pon S, Greenwald BM. Mortality rates in pediatric septic shock with and without multiple organ system failure. Pediatr Crit Care Med. 2003;4:333–7.
5. Singer M, Deutschman CS, Seymour CW, et al. The third international consensus defnitions for sepsis and septic shock (Sepsis-3). JAMA. 2016;315:801–10.
6. Goldstein B, Giroir B, Randolph A, et al. International pediatric sepsis consensus conference: definitions for sepsis and organ dysfunction in pediatrics. Pediatr Crit Care Med. 2005;6:2–8.
7. Angus DC, Linde Zwirble WT, Lidicker J, et al. Epidemiology of severe sepsis in the United States: analysis of incidence, outcome, and associated costs of care. Crit Care Med. 2001;29:1303–10.
8. Poukkanen M, Vaara ST, Pettila V, et al. Acute kidney injury in patients with severe sepsis in finiish intensive care units. Acta Anaesthesiol Scand. 2013;57:863–72.
9. Fitzgerald JC, Basu R, Arkcan-Arikan A, et al. Acute kidney injury in pediatric severe sepsis, an independent risk factor for death and new disability. Crit Care Med. 2016;44(12):2241–50.
10. Cooper DS, Kwiatkowski DM, Goldstein SL, Krawczeski CD. Acute kidney injury and cardiorenal syndromes in pediatric cardiac intensive care. Pediatr Crit Care Med. 2016;17(8 Suppl 1):S250–6.
11. Fani F, Regolisti G, Delsante M, et al. Recent advances in the pathogenetic mechanisms of sepsis-associated acute kidney injury. J Nephrol. 2017. https://doi.org/10.1007/s40620-017-0452-4.
12. Schrier RW, Wang W. Acute renal failure and sepsis. N Engl J Med. 2004;351(2):159–69.
13. Bellomo R, Kellum JA, Ronco C, Wald R, et al. Acute kidney injury in sepsis. Inten Care Med. 2017;43:816–28.
14. Naveda-Romero OE, Naveda-Melendez AF. Fluid overload and kidney failure in children with severe sepsis and septic shock. Arch Argent Pediatr. 2017;115(2):118–24.
15. Chen J, Li X, Bai Z, Fang F, et al. Association of fluid accumulation with clinical outcomes in critically ill children with severe sepsis. PLoS One. 2016;11(7):e0160093.
16. Maitland K, Kiguli S, Opoka RO, et al. Mortality after fluid bolus in African children with severe infection. NEJM. 2011;264:2483–95.
17. Westrope CA, Fleming S, Kapetanstrataki M, et al. Renal replacement therapy in the critically ill child. Pediatr Crit Care Med. 2018;19(3):210–7.
18. Fleming GM, Askenazi DJ, Bridges BC, et al. A multicenter international survey of renal supportive therapy during ECMO: the kidney intervention during extracorporeal membrane oxygenation (KIDMO) group. ASAIO J. 2012;58(4):407–14.

19. John S, Griesbach D, Baumgartel M, et al. Effects of continuous haemofiltration vs. intermittent haemodialysis on systemic haemodynamics and splanchnic regional perfusion in septic shock patients: a prospective, randomized trial. Nephrol Dial Transplant. 2001;16(2):320–7.
20. Ronco C, Bonello M, Bordoni V, et al. Extracorporeal therapies in non-renal disease: treatment of sepsis and the peak concentration hypothesis. Blood Purif. 2004;22(1):164–74.
21. Honore PM, Jacobs R, Joannes-Boyau O, et al. Newly designed CRRT membranes for sepsis and SIRS—a pragmatic approach for bedside intensivists summarizing the more recent advances: a systematic structured review. ASAIO J. 2013;59(2):99–106.
22. Shimizu T, Miyake T, Kitamura N, et al. Endotoxin adsorption: direct hemoperfusion with the polymixin B immobilized fiber column (PMX). Tranfus Apher Sci. 2017;56(5):682–8.
23. Zheng S, Weng Q, Wu W, Ding G. Blood purification treatment initiated at the time of sepsis diagnosis effectively attenuates serum HMGB1 upregulation and improves patient prognosis. Exp Ther Med. 2017;14(4):3029–35.
24. Ronco C, Bellomo R, Homel P, et al. Effects of different doses in continuous veno-venous haemofiltration on outcomes of acute renal failure: a prospective randomised trial. Lancet. 2000;356:26–30.
25. Palevsky PM, Zhang JH, O'Conner TZ, et al. Intensity of renal support in critically ill patients with acute kidney injury. NEJM. 2008;359:7–20.
26. Bellomo R, Cass A, Cole L, et al. Intensity of continuous renal replacement therapy in critically ill patients. NEJM. 2009;361:1627–38.
27. Joannes-Boyau O, Honore PM, Perez P, et al. High-volume versus standard volume haemofiltration for septic shock patients with acute kidney injury (IVOIRE study): a multicenter randomized controlled trial. Intensive Care Med. 2013;39:1535–46.
28. Park JT, Lee H, Kee YK, et al. High-dose versus conventional dose continuous venovenous hemodiafiltration and patient and kidney survival and cytokine removal in sepsis-associated acute kidney injury: a randomized controlled trial. Am J Kidney Dis. 2016;68:599–608.
29. Wong WT, Choi G, Gomersall CD, Lipman J. To increase or decrease dosage of antimicrobials in septic patients during continuous renal replacement therapy: the eternal doubt. Curr Opin Pharmacol. 2015;24:68–78.
30. Sethi SK, Maxvold N, Bunchman T, et al. Nutritional management in the critically ill child with acute kidney injury: a review. Pediatr Nephrol. 2017;32(4):589–601.
31. Deep A, Zoha M, Dutta Kukreja P. Prostacyclin as an anticoagulant for continuous renal replacement therapy in children. Blood Purif. 2017;43(4):279–89.
32. Jones CH, Goutcher E, Newstead CG, et al. Hemodynamics and survival of patients with acute renal failure treated by continuous dialysis with two synthetic membranes. Artif Organs. 1998;22(8):638–43.
33. Stoves J, Goode NP, Visvanathan R, et al. The bradykinin response and early hypotension at the introduction of continuous renal replacement therapy in the intensive care unit. Artif Organs. 2001;25(1):1009–13.
34. Friedrich JO, Wald R, Bagshaw SW, Burns KE, Adhikari NK. Hemofiltration compared to hemodialysis for acute kidney injury: systematic review and meta-analysis. Crit Care. 2012;16(4):R146.
35. Kovacs B, Sullivan KJ, Hiremath S, et al. Effect of sustained low efficiency dialysis versus continuous renal replacement therapy on renal recovery after acute kidney injury in the intensive care unit: a systematic review and meta-analysis. Neprhology. 2017;22(5):343–53.
36. Saudan P, Niederberger M, De Seigneux S, et al. Adding a dialysis dose to continous hemofiltration increases survival in patients with acute renal failure. Kidney Int. 2006;70(7):1312–7.
37. Al Enezi F, Al Hazzani W, Ma J, et al. Continuous venovenous hemofiltration versus continuous venovenous hemodiafiltration in critically ill patients: a retrospective cohort study from a Canadian tertiary Centre. Can Respir J. 2014;21(3):176–80.
38. Premuzic V, Basic-Jukic N, Jelakovic B, Kes P. Differences in CVVH vs. CVVHDF in the management of sepsis-induced acute kidney injury in critically ill patients. J Artif Organs. 2017;20:326–34.

39. Gaudry S, Hajage D, Schortgen F, et al. Initiation strategies for renal replacement therapy in the intensive care unit. NEJM. 2016;375(2):122–33.
40. Zarbock A, Kellum JA, Schmidt C, et al. Effect of early vs. delayed initation of renal replacement therapy on mortality in critically ill patients with acute kidney injury: the ELAIN randomized clinical trial. JAMA. 2016;315(20):2190–9.
41. Brandenburger T, Dimski T, Slowinski T, Kindgen-Milles D. Renal replacement therapy and anticoagulation. Best Pract Res Clin Anaesthesiol. 2017;31(3):387–401.
42. Pschowski R, Briegel S, Von Haehling S, et al. Effects of dialysis modality on blood loss, bleeding complications and transfusion requirements in critically ill patients with dialysis-dependent acute renal failure. Anaesth Intensive Care. 2015;43(6):764–70.
43. Iba T, Fowler L. Is polymyxin B immobilized fiber column ineffective for septic shock? A discussion on the press release for EUPHRATES trial. J Intensive Care. 2017;5:40.
44. Skinner SC, Iocono JA, Ballard HO, Turner MD, Ward AN, Davenport DL, Paden ML, Zwischenberger JB. Improved survival in venovenous vs. venoarterial extracorporeal membrane oxygenation for pediatric noncardiac sepsis patients: a study of the extracorporeal life support organization registry. J Pediatr Surg. 2012;47(1):63–7.
45. Hoover NG, Heard M, Reid C, Wagoner S, Rogers K, Foland J, Paden ML, Fortenberry JD. Enhanced fluid management with continuous venovenous hemofiltration in pediatric respiratory failure patients receiving extracorporeal membrane oxygenation support. Intensive Care Med. 2008;34(12):2241–7.
46. Lawson DS, Holt D. Insensible water loss from the Jostra Quadrox D oxygenator: an in vitro study. Perfusion. 2007;22(6):407–10.
47. Li L, Oi Yan T, Ming Chit Arthur K, Hoi Ping S, et al. Insensible water loss through adult extracorporeal membrane oxygenation circuit: an in vitro study. ASAIO J. 2014;60(4).508–12.
48. Paden ML, Warshaw BL, Heard ML, Fortenberry JD. Recovery of renal function and survival after continuous renal replacement therapy during extracorporeal membrane oxygenation. Pediatr Crit Care Med. 2011;12(2):153–8.
49. Carcillo JA, Halstead ES, Hall MW, Nguyen TC, et al. Three hypothetical inflammation pathobiology phenotypes and pediatric sepsis induced multiple organ failure outcome. Pediatr Crit Care Med. 2017;18(6):513–23.

# Hyperammonaemia and IEM

# 27

Roshni Vara and Andrew Durward

> **Clinical Scenario**
> A 2-day-old male infant presents with a 24 h history of poor feeding, not waking for feeds and increased respiratory rate. The initial blood gas shows a respiratory alkalosis (pH 7.41, pCO2 3.1, HCO3 19 and base excess −4.2) with a normal lactate and blood sugar. The plasma ammonia returns as 550 μmol/L. What are the initial differential diagnoses and initial management?

## 27.1 Ammonia Metabolism and the Urea Cycle

Ammonia, $NH_3$, is an important source of nitrogen for protein synthesis, amino acid metabolism and pH homeostasis. Ammonia dissolves in water and at physiological pH ammonia exists predominantly in its ionized form, ammonium, $NH_4^+$. The normal concentration of ammonium in plasma is between 11 and 50 μmol/L. Ammonia is continuously produced and consumed during cellular metabolism and arises from breakdown of purine and pyrimidine products and deamination of several amino acids including glutamine, asparagine, serine, threonine, glycine, proline and lysine [1]. In mammals, the urea cycle is the main pathway of ammonia detoxification. The complete urea cycle is only expressed in the liver and proximal parts are expressed in the gastrointestinal tract and kidney [2]. Periportal hepatocytes receive the high nitrogen load of portal blood arriving from the intestine. The urea cycle consists of

R. Vara (✉)
Department of Paediatric Inherited Metabolic Disease, Evelina London Children's Hospital, London, UK
e-mail: Roshni.Vara@gstt.nhs.uk

A. Durward
Paediatric Intensive Care Unit, Evelina London Children's Hospital, London, UK



A. Deep, S. L. Goldstein (eds.), *Critical Care Nephrology and Renal Replacement Therapy in Children*, https://doi.org/10.1007/978-3-319-90281-4_27

six enzymatic steps; the proximal part within the mitochondria and distal part in the cytoplasm (Fig. 27.1). The first step of the urea cycle involves the conversion of ammonia and bicarbonate into carbamoylphosphate by carbamoylphosphate synthetase 1 (CPS1). The urea cycle, i.e. CPS1 requires allosteric activation by N-acetylglutamate (NAG) which is synthesized by N-acetylglutamate synthetase (NAGS). Inherited deficiency of this enzyme is extremely rare, moreover toxic metabolites can lead to a secondary hyperammonaemia via impairment of NAGS activity.

The second step in the urea cycle involves the condensation of carbamoylphosphate with ornithine to form citrulline, a reaction catalysed by ornithine transcarbamoyltransferase (OTC), the only X-linked urea cycle defect. The following three reactions involving argininosuccinate synthetase (ASS), argininosuccinate lyase (ASL) and arginase (AR1) take place in the cytoplasm. The final step hydrolyses arginine into ornithine and urea, and ornithine is regenerated for another rotation of the cycle. Hence transporters are required to transfer the urea cycle intermediates across the mitochondrial membrane in both directions; ornithine-citrulline antiporter (ORTN1) and aspartate-glutamate antiporter (citrin). Deficiencies of citrin, carbonic anhydrase Va (CAVA) and Δ [3]-pyrroline-5-carboxylate synthetase (P5CS) can also cause hyperammonaemia by restriction of the supply of asparate, bicarbonate and ornithine, respectively, to the urea cycle. The main focus of this

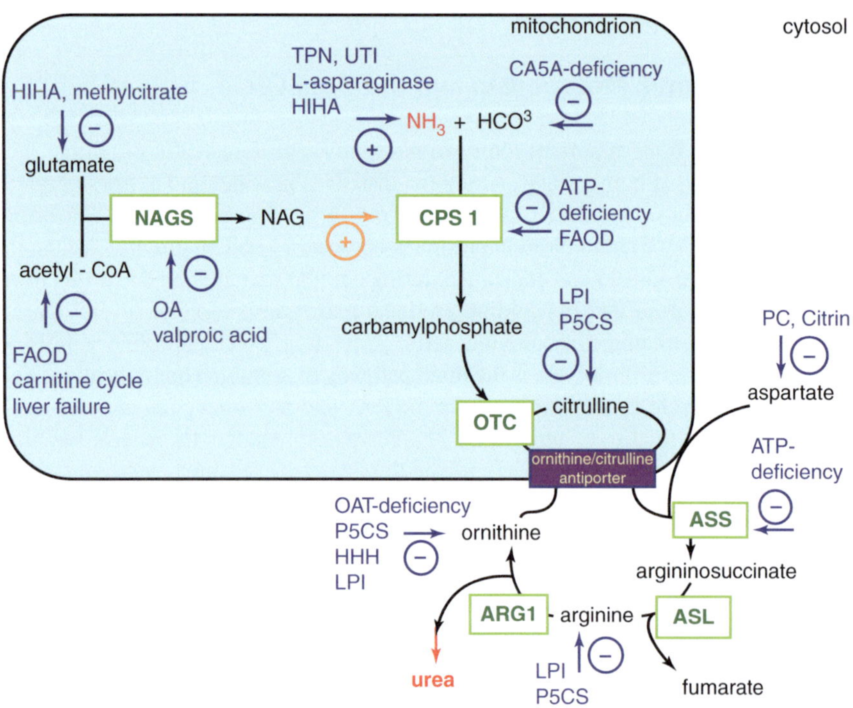


**Fig. 27.1** The urea cycle (J Haberle 2013)

chapter will be the main primary hyperammonaemic disorders, their manifestations and management. Table 27.1 shows primary and secondary causes of hyperammonaemia to be considered.

## 27.2 Clinical Manifestations of Hyperammonaemia

Clinically, hyperammonaemia presents with signs of encephalopathy. In the neonatal period, there may be a short symptom-free period and subsequent vomiting, poor feeding, increased sleepiness, irritability, muscular hypotonia, seizures, hyper- or hypoventilation and coma. In infants and older children there is commonly an intercurrent illness or other catabolic stress, e.g. fasting, post-surgery (and post-partum), rapid weight loss, treatment with steroids/chemotherapy or followed by a high-protein containing meal or load. Some children can display a history of self-selecting a low protein diet. A more chronic presentation in some may be reported with cyclical or chronic vomiting, developmental delay, faltering growth, neurocognitive and behavioural impairment. These symptoms in older children and adults can often be mistaken for encephalitis, drug or alcohol intoxication or a space occupying lesion. Hence investigations in any child or adult with unexplained reduced level of consciousness should include an ammonia measurement [4–6].

**Table 27.1** Causes of hyperammonaemia

| |
|---|
| *Primary* |
| Urea cycle defects (NAGS, CPS1, OTC, ASS, ASL, AR1 deficiencies) |
| Urea cycle transporter defects<br>– Hyperammonaemia-hyperornithinaemia-homocitrullinaemia (ORN1 deficiency)<br>– Citrin deficiency |
| Urea cycle substrate deficiencies<br>– Lysinuric protein intolerance<br>– Pyrroline-5-carboylate synthetase deficiency<br>– Pyruvate carboxylase deficiency<br>– Ornithine aminotransferase deficiency<br>– Carbonic anhydrase Va deficiency |
| Organic acidaemias |
| Fatty acid oxidation defects |
| Hyperinsulinisim-hyperammonaemia syndrome |
| Mitochondrial disorders |
| Glutamine synthetase deficiency |
| *Secondary* |
| Acute or chronic liver failure |
| Valproic acid treatment (NAGS inhibition) |
| L-Asparaginase treatment (increased ammonia production due to hydrolysis of asparagine) |
| Urease-producing organisms |
| Total parenteral nutrition (relative arginine deficiency) |
| Post-lung/bone marrow transplantation (reduced glutamine synthetase activity) |
| Vascular malformations (portosystemic shunting) |
| Transient hyperammonaemia of the newborn |

## 27.3 Diagnostic Tests

Accurate plasma ammonia measurement requires a free-flowing venous or arterial sample, capillary samples are not recommended to avoid spurious results as haemolysis causes positive interference. The sample should be collected into an ammonia-free specimen tube and transported immediately to the laboratory on ice, the sample needs to be separated within 15 min of collection [7]. Generally ammonia levels more than 500 μmol/L suggest an underlying IEM, however, this is not the rule. In UCDs there is often the absence of hypoglycaemia, lactic acidosis or ketosis in contrast to organic acidaemias for example, where ketosis and metabolic acidosis predominates. Ammonia is a respiratory stimulant and respiratory alkalosis is frequently present, particularly in the neonate.

Plasma amino acids can show characteristic patterns with elevation of glutamine and alanine indicating hyperammonaemia and low or high citrulline and arginine indicting specific UCDs. In OTC and ASS deficiency there is an elevation of orotic acid in the urine due to excess carbamolyphoshate, whilst this is absent in NAGS or CPS1 deficiency (Fig. 27.2).

Acylcarnitine profiles and urine organic acids can detect specific fatty acid oxidation defects or organic acidaemias.

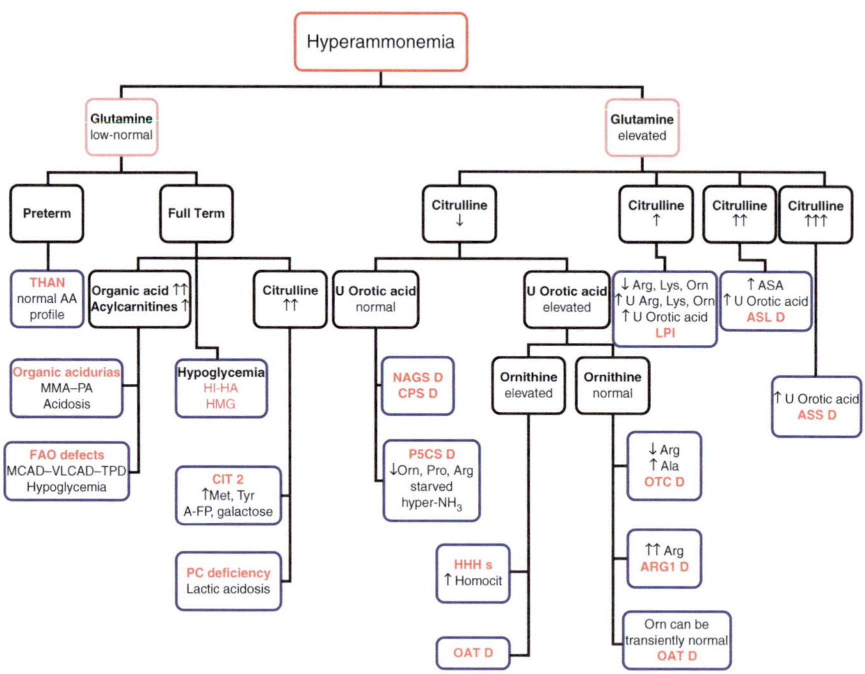


**Fig. 27.2** Diagnostic algorithm (Orphanet J Rare Dis 2012)

Mutation analysis is the gold standard for diagnosis. The majority of disorders are autosomal recessive excluding OTC deficiency which is X-linked, where mutation detection has at least 80% sensitivity [8]. The use of next generation sequencing of multiple genes simultaneously is increasingly being used [9]. In deceased patients or when blood DNA is not available, some diagnoses can be made from frozen liver tissue or cultured fibroblasts. Genetic diagnosis allows appropriate counselling, prenatal diagnosis and appropriate family screening.

## 27.4 Urea Cycle Defects (UCDs)

UCDs result from loss of function of any of the enzymatic steps within the mitochondrial or cytosolic part of the urea cycle. The overall frequency is quoted as 1 in 35,000 [10].

*Clinical manifestations*: The classical UCDs can all lead to severe hyperammonaemia and can present at any age. The most common UCD is OTC deficiency followed by ASS deficiency. NAGS and CPS1 deficiency are extremely rare.

Classical presentation in the neonate is typically within the first few days of life with poor feeding, lethargy, vomiting and hyperammonaemic encephalopathy. Hypoglycaemia, lactic acidosis and ketosis may or may not be present. Clinical presentation outside the neonatal period is variable and often triggered by intercurrent illness, fasting and/or ingestion of a high protein containing meal or protein supplements, post-partum, treatment with steroids or chemotherapy. Older children and adults can present acutely with unexplained reduced level of consciousness and/or neurological signs (tremor, irritability, seizures) which can be mistaken for encephalitis or drug intoxication. Hence the importance of measuring plasma ammonia in patients of any age with unexplained reduced level of consciousness.

Female carriers of OTC deficiency can manifest clinical and biochemical signs which are variable due to X-inactivation (lyonization), ranging from asymptomatic to recurrent episodes of hyperammonaemia.

Children with UCDs can have ongoing episodes of hyperammonaemia triggered by intercurrent illness or fasting. Those with ASL deficiency are less prone to recurrent hyperammonaemia but can still develop neurocognitive difficulties, seizures and chronic liver disease. Hypertension is frequent in adolescent and adults with ASL deficiency and brittle hair (trichorrhexis nodosa) secondary to arginine deficiency is a pathognomonic finding. In contrast the clinical manifestations of AR1 deficiency are characterized by developmental delay, neurocognitive impairment, seizures and spastic tetra- or diplegia.

*Diagnostic tests:* Plasma amino acids and urine organic acids are first line tests which can distinguish between some of the UCDs. CPS1 and NAGS deficiency are biochemically indistinguishable. Enzyme assays in cultured fibroblasts or liver tissue are available in selective laboratories, however, these are recently superseded by genetic analysis. Mutation analysis can then be made available for prenatal testing.

### 27.4.1 Treatment

1. Emergency management in acute hyperammonaemia must be commenced immediately. The main principles of treatment are:
   (a) Stop protein intake
   (b) Promote anabolism with adequate calorie intake from glucose (8–10 mg/kg/min) and lipid (1–2 g/kg/day)
   (c) Alternate pathway medications to lower ammonia (sodium benzoate and sodium phenylbutyrate) with supplementation of arginine and/or citrulline depending on the type of UCD. Carbaglutamic acid or N-carbamyl-L-glutamate, a synthetic analogue of NAG is the treatment for NAGS deficiency and CPS1 deficiency can sometimes respond to therapy.
   (d) Use of acute dialysis to reduce ammonia levels depending on the expertise of the centre (see CRRT section)

It is important to provide sufficient calories with glucose and lipid until the ammonia is lowered and protein can gradually be reintroduced. The mechanism of action of drugs is described later in the chapter and dosing is shown in Table 27.2.

2. Maintenance treatment involves a carefully supervised protein-restricted diet, ammonia-lowering agents and supplementation of essential amino acids. Regular metabolic follow-up is required with monitoring of growth and development, plasma amino acid levels, vitamins, minerals and trace elements.
3. Liver transplantation is curative for the proximal urea cycle defects and is a viable treatment option to prevent hyperammonaemic episodes, further neurological injury and improve quality of life. Hepatocyte transplantation has been used a 'bridge' to liver transplantation in the male neonate with OTC deficiency [11–13].

**Table 27.2** Intravenous medications (bimdg.org.uk—undiagnosed hyperammonaemia management)

| Drug | Loading dose over 90 min (mg/kg) | Followed by maintenance dose over 24 h (mg/kg) | Maximum daily dose (every 24 h thereafter) (mg/kg) | Sodium content of daily maintenance dose (mmol/kg/d) |
|---|---|---|---|---|
| Sodium benzoate | 250 | 250 | 500 | 3.5 |
| Sodium phenylbutyrate | 250 | 250 | 600 | 2.8 |
| Arginine | 150 | 300 | 500 | Nil |
| Carnitine | 100 | 100 | 300 | Nil |
| *See important note below | | | | |

IMPORTANT NOTE: Carnitine should NOT be given if there is evidence of cardiomyopathy, any cardiac arrhythmia or if a long chain fatty acid oxidation disorder is suspected

### 27.4.2 Prognosis

Urgent recognition and management of hyperammonaemia is vital. The impact on neurological outcome can be catastrophic if treatment is delayed. Mortality in neonatal onset OTCD is reported at 24% and 11% in late onset cases [14]. For UCDs collectively the mortality remains 60% for early onset OTCD in males and of the collective group 52% had developmental delay [15].

Age at onset and peak ammonia concentration at presentation (>500 µmol/L) best predict neurological outcome [16]. Prognosis is considered very poor if: hyperammonaemic coma has lasted more than 3 days, intracranial pressure is clearly increased and ammonia peaked at >1000 µmol/L (although impact of this level on prognosis depends on the duration of hyperammonaemia) [17].

## 27.5 Other IEMs Causing Hyperammonaemia

### 27.5.1 Organic Acidaemias

These are disorders of branched chain amino acid metabolism. Classical organic acidaemias associated with hyperammonaemia are propionic acidaemia, methylmalonic acidaemia, isovaleric acidaemia and maple syrup urine disease. Presentation is commonly in the neonatal period with metabolic acidosis, lactic acidosis, ketosis and hyperammonaemia. The metabolic acidosis often distinguishes this group of disorders from UCDs. The hyperammonaemia is thought to arise from a secondary inhibition of NAGS and CPS1 function and is often responsive to the addition of carbaglutamic acid in emergency management. Organic acids can cause bone marrow suppression and pancytopenia can be a feature. Diagnosis is established with urine organic acids, acylcarnitine profile and genetic confirmation. Management is aimed at restriction of natural protein, carnitine supplementation, ammonia-lowering agents as required and emergency regimens in the acute situation [18].

### 27.5.2 Fatty Acid Oxidation and Carnitine Cycle Defects

Fatty acid oxidation is a mitochondrial process and clinical presentation is variable. Medium chain acyl CoA dehydrogenase (MCAD) deficiency is the most common defect and is part of the UK newborn screening programme. Clinical presentation of other defects (e.g. Very long chain acyl CoA dehydrogenase (VLCAD) deficiency, long chain hydroxyl acyl CoA dehydrogenase (LCHAD) deficiency, carnitine-acylcarnitine translocase (CACT) deficiency) tend to exhibit hypoketotic hypoglycaemia, liver dysfunction, mild–moderate hyperammonaemia, cardiomyopathy and rhabdomyolysis. End organ effects occur due to accumulation of medium- or long-chain acylcarnitines, depending on the enzymatic deficiency. The hyperammonaemia results from lack of acetyl-CoA and subsequent urea cycle dysfunction. Urine organic acids and acylcarnitines will aid initial diagnosis and confirmatory testing is with DNA analysis and/or cultured fibroblast fatty acid oxidation studies. Treatment aims to limit fasting periods, emergency regimen in the acute situation and the use of fat restriction and medium chain triglycerides in certain defects [19].

### 27.5.3 Lysinuric Protein Intolerance (LPI)

LPI is due to a defect in the transport of dibasic amino acids (lysine, ornithine and arginine) at the basolateral intestinal membrane and renal tubular epithelium. The defect leads to impaired absorption and loss, respectively, of the dibasic amino acids. Urine and plasma amino acids can be diagnostic with genetic confirmation. This is a multisystemic disease with clinical features, including faltering growth, short stature, interstitial lung disease, chronic renal disease, osteopenia, hepatosplenomegaly and immune dysfunction [20]. Mild to moderate hyperammonaemia results from lack of substrates and subsequent impairment of the urea cycle.

### 27.5.4 Hyperornithinemia-Hyperammonemia-Homocitrullinuria (HHH Syndrome)

HHH is a rare IEM of the urea cycle which has a variable phenotype ranging from mild form with learning difficulties and neurological involvement to severe form with lethargy, hepatic failure and seizures. The defect is in the protein ORC1, which is a transporter of ornithine, lysine and arginine into the mitochondrial matrix. The presence of homocitrulline is a hallmark of the disease and is detected in the urine. Hyperammonaemia is variable and often moderate [21].

### 27.5.5 Hyperinsulinism-Hyperammonaemia (HIHA) Syndrome

HIHA tends to cause mild hyperammonaemia. The disorder results from a gain of function mutation in the gene encoding glutamate dehydrogenase (GDH1). This protein is expressed in the liver, kidney, brain and pancreatic β-cells. Neonates tend to present with profound hypoketotic hypoglycaemia and mild hyperammonaemia. They have an increased risk of seizures and learning difficulties. The hypoglycaemia usually responds to diazoxide and the hyperammonaemia often does not require intervention [22].

### 27.5.6 Mitochondrial Disorders

This is a large and heterogeneous group of disorders involving energy metabolism. The resulting ATP deficiency from impaired mitochondrial oxidative phosphorylation is thought to impair urea cycle function as some of the enzymes are ATP-dependent. A specific mitochondrial condition with mutations in *TMEM70* gene (which encodes a transmembrane protein involved in ATP synthase activity) tends to present in the neonatal period with hyperammonaemia and lactic acidosis [23, 24].

### 27.5.7 Carbonic Anhydrase Va Deficiency (CAVA)

This is a recently described cause of early onset hyperammonaemia with hypoglycaemia, hyperlactataemia, ketosis and metabolic acidosis. Defective hepatic bicarbonate production leads to this unique combination of biochemical findings. Diagnosis is confirmed by genetic confirmation. The hyperammonaemia responds to carbaglutamic acid and may reach levels which require haemofiltration. Outcomes in reported cases appear good in the short-term [25].

## 27.6 Intravenous Medications Used in Hyperammonaemia

Ammonia-lowering or scavenging agents commonly used are sodium benzoate and sodium phenylbutyrate, both conjugate specific amino acids within the liver and require co-enzyme A. Table 27.2 shows recommended drug doses. Loading doses followed by the maintenance infusions are used in the emergency setting, advice should always be sought from a metabolic specialist.

Sodium benzoate combines with glycine to form hippurate, which is excreted in the urine and thus removal of a nitrogen source. Adverse effects from intravenous infusion include metabolic acidosis, hypernatraemia, hyperbilirubinaemia due to displacement of bilirubin from albumin and in view of its caustic nature, protection from extravasation injury is important.

Sodium phenylbutyrate combines with glutamine to form phenylacetylglutamine, which is also excreted in the urine. Potassium can become depleted and hence should be monitored.

Arginine becomes an essential amino acid in certain defects and often requires supplementation intravenously. In large doses, resulting nitric oxide accumulation can lead to systemic hypotension.

Plasma amino acids should be monitored during treatment and doses adjusted accordingly with advice from metabolic specialists [26, 27].

## 27.7 The Role of Dialysis in Hyperammonaemia

At physiologic pH, 1–2% of plasma ammonia exists in the form of NH3, which readily permeates across cellular membranes (pK = 9.0) [28]. The process is pH dependent with a significantly higher accumulation of cerebral ammonia at alkaline pH [29].

Glutamate is converted in the astrocyte cytosol in an equimolar ratio into glutamine via glutamine synthetase. In hyperammonaemia, there is dysfunction of the astrocytes with shrinkage and secondary hyperactivation of the NMDA receptors which leads to disruption of cerebral metabolism and neuronal and glial injury [30]. Although the pathway is well described, there is no clear and consistent threshold or duration of ammonia toxicity that correlate closely with clinical signs (seizures, encephalopathy and cerebral oedema) or that is predictive of permanent neurologic injury as many confounding factors such as hypoxia or hypotension may also be present especially in the shocked neonate.

In the largest published series of neonatal hyperammonaemia over a 25-year period (56 neonates), peak blood level > 1000μmol/L had poorest survival [31]. Uchino similarly concluded raised ammonia (peak levels >350 μmol/L) had poor survival or neurodevelopmental outcome in a study of 92 neonates with urea cycle disorder [32]. In a study of 26 neonates, Msall demonstrated duration of coma was associated with peak ammonia level [33].

In contrast Westrope ($n = 14$) and Picca ($n = 45$) failed to identify peak ammonia or duration of raised ammonia as outcome markers [34, 35].

This exemplifies the complexity of modelling outcomes for rare metabolic diseases where many confounding factors are present and sample size spans many years (sometimes decades) over which historical treatment strategies have changed and been refined.

### 27.7.1 Ammonia Removal by Dialysis

Ammonia (NH3) is a small water-soluble molecule (molecular mass 17 g/mol) with low protein binding. It therefore has a favourable profile for clearance via peritoneal or extracorporeal dialysis. Using best practice as a guide, the aim of dialytic therapy is to reduce brain ammonia toxicity as fast as possible into a "safe" zone below 100–200 μmol/L within the first 12–24 hours of therapy [31, 36, 37]. With effective dialysis, ammonia blood levels should halve in 2–4 h. There are no studies addressing the speed of ammonia reduction and if there are adverse consequences to this (e.g. osmolar shifts) versus ongoing toxicity if ammonia levels are reduced more gradually.

Dialysis should be considered if ammonia levels start increasing above 300 μmol/L despite medical therapy been optimized [31]. Effective extracorporeal dialysis requires securing a large bore central venous dual lumen catheter and having a period of effective trouble-free dialysis without circuit thrombosis or downtime. In the neonatal population, it is technically challenging with even experts experiencing complications and delays [28, 38, 39].

*Peritoneal dialysis* has been used widely in neonatal hyperammonaemia with the advantage of being quick to initiate and relatively easy to perform. Picca demonstrated the advantages of early initiation of PD sometimes at outlying non-tertiary hospitals with similar outcome to those treated primarily by extracorporeal dialysis (HD or CVVHD) in tertiary centres [35]. In some studies, ammonia clearance rates with PD were similar to hemofiltration [35, 36]. Peritoneal dialysis (PD), when applied early, can allow safe and relatively risk-free method to reduce plasma ammonia before extracorporeal dialysis [35]. Others have demonstrated a slower initial rate of ammonia reduction with PD (time to half the plasma ammonia level) relative to CVVHD ($n = 21$ neonates); however, both took a similar time to reach a "safe" zone within 24 h [37]. Typically acute PD is prescribed at 10–20 mL/kg volumes. Frequent cycles (<30 min) may maximize dialytic ammonia clearance rates when ammonia levels are very high.

### 27.7.2 Extracorporeal Dialysis

At maximal efficiency, all extracorporeal dialysis modes (intermittent haemodialysis, CVVH, CVVHD and CVVHDF) may provide excellent ammonia clearance [30, 35, 39, 40]. Historically, intermittent hemodialysis has had the reputation of having the highest ammonia clearance rates using blood flow rates of 5–10 mL/kg/min and dialysate flow rates of 500 mL/min (2000–4000 mL per 1.73 $m^2$ [38]. Ammonia extraction with these settings is above 95% [35].

McBryde demonstrated improved survival with HD as the primary therapy ($n = 18$) [38]. The main problems experienced are technical issues (adequate vascular access) and side effects such as hypotension which may limit the required blood flow rates. Typically, rebound hyperammonaemia may occur when the hemodialysis cycle has finished. For this reason, continuous high-dose renal replacement therapy has been proposed as an alternative [34, 37, 39, 41].

For CVVH or CVVHD, three key factors largely determine clearance of ammonia: blood flow rate, haemofilter surface area and ultrafiltration rate. For neonates, typically slightly larger filters relative to patient size are used (0.3–0.4 $m^2$). These are designed to operate at maximal efficiency at higher blood flow rates of around 150 ml/min. Using lower blood flow rates of 20–50 mL/min (5–15 mL/kg), which is more appropriate for neonates may result in ultrafiltration on the flow dependent part of the mass solute clearance curve (Fig. 27.3, point B). Large filtration gains can be achieved by increasing blood flow rate (if tolerated by the patient) as filtration is more efficient at the same transmembrane pressure (Fig. 27.3a, point A). This concept is well described by Clarke and Huang [42, 43].

Blood flow rates of 80 mL/min are achievable in neonates with well-placed 7–8 Fr internal jugular catheters (author's personal experience) with access pressures below 80 $cmH_20$. Small vascular access catheters (5Fr) should be avoided as blood flow is limited and circuit thrombosis is universal (100% by 60 h) [44]. Low flow rates of 20 mL/min for a 0.3 $m^2$ filter may be at the lower end of efficiency. Picca demonstrated ammonia extraction of just above 50% at these lower flows [35].

The second factor to consider in hemofiltration is dialysate flow rate. Troyanov compared CVVH versus CVVHD for ammonia clearance in adult patients and identified maximal efficiency with a dialysate flow rate of 4.5 L per hour (blood blow rate of 150 mL/min or 9 L/h) [45].

This is a ratio of dialysate to blood flow of 50%. In contrast, neonates may use a similar size filter (0.3–0.4 $m^2$) yet blood flow rates are as much as 10-fold lower

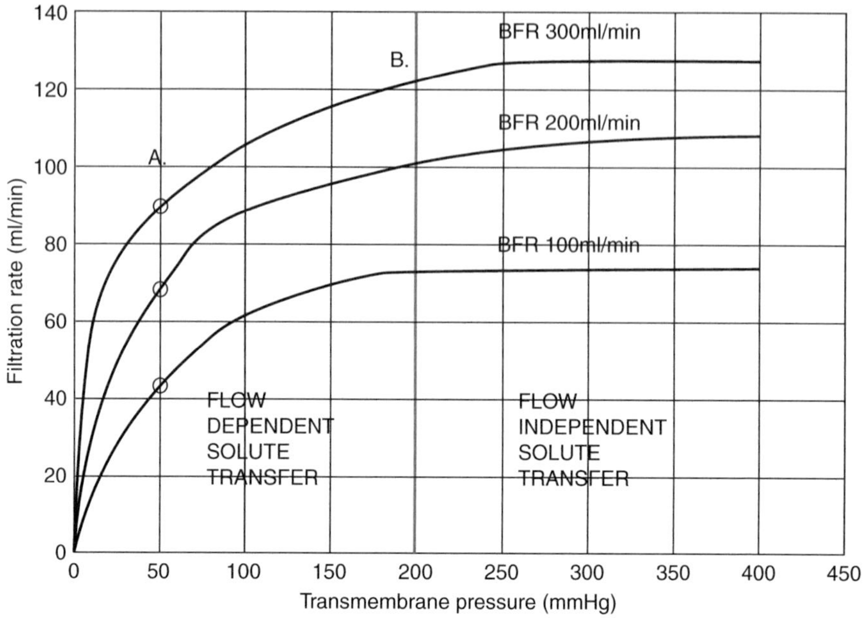


**Fig. 27.3** Mass transfer of solutes across a hypothetical haemofilter at three different blood flow rates (BFR). Red vertical line represents the point where maximal filter efficiency is achieved (point B). Ultrafiltration rate is higher at the same transmembrane pressure when blood flow rate is maximized (point A)

(20–50 mL/min). If dialysate flow rates are greater than the blood flow rate, no benefit is gained as only a fixed concentration of ammonia is presented to the filter over time. Figure 27.4 shows curves for dialysate flow rate (mls/h) in a 3.5 kg patient at different blood flow rates. It demonstrates the wide variations and dialysate flow rates for some published cases. For points B and C, ammonia extraction was just above 50%. This demonstrates that ammonia clearance can be maximized at higher blood flow rates (greater clearance at the same ratio of dialysate to blood flow rate). It also highlights that it is important to be aware of the relationship of blood flow rate and dialysis rate in neonates who are 3–5 kg in size. With CVVH, predilution affords a greater flow rate (30–60 mL/kg/h) but this is partially offset by a dilution effect and a loss of 40% efficiency especially if low blood flow rates are used [45].

### 27.7.3 Recirculation

In adult patients, femoral site vascular access demonstrates the highest recirculation rates using saline dilution technique of 26% compared to jugular venous access [46]. This is because there is less of blood reservoir around the femoral vein compared to the right atrium. Recirculation rate also increase significantly at higher flow. Unfortunately, recirculation rates have not been measured in paediatric dialysis, but are likely to be much higher around 50% as the distance between the proximal and distal lumen in paediatric dual lumen lines is very close, as little as 5–10 mm

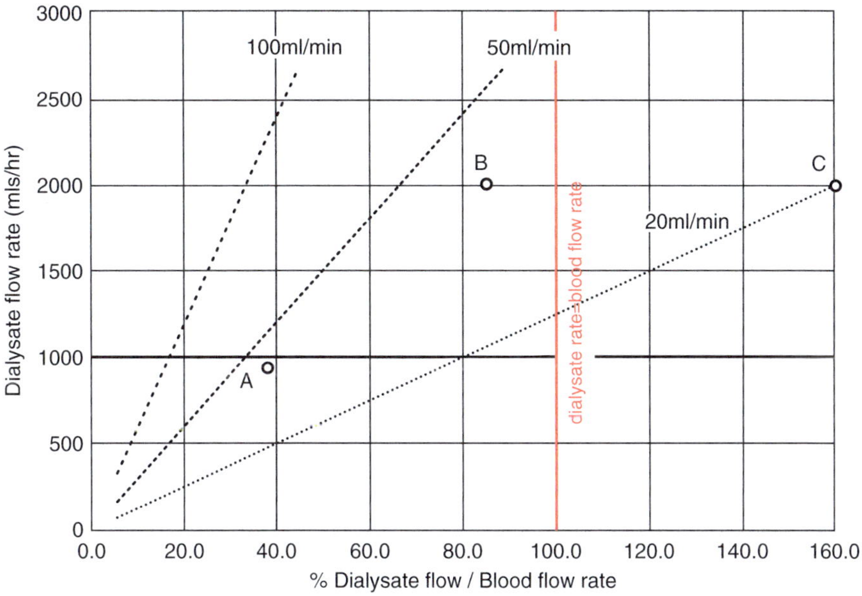


**Fig. 27.4** Absolute dialysate flow rate (mL/h) for a 3.5 kg neonate at three different blood flow rates. The x-axis is the ratio of dialysate to blood flow. The vertical red line is the point where dialysate flow equals blood flow rate. The horizontal line is the dialysate flow rate suggested by Spinale [11]. Point A represents a neonate on 40 mL/min blood flow rate [11], Point B and C are neonates from series by Picca et al (112). Point C, the neonate received 33.3 mL/min dialysate at 20 mL/min blood flow rate

apart. This is partly why efficiency of CVVH or CVVHD is only about 50% in neonates. The femoral vein is also significantly smaller in diameter in neonates and is more prone to catheter related complications and thrombosis.

The ideal site for vascular access is therefore the internal jugular vein, preferable the right as it has a more direct course to the right atrium.

### 27.7.4 Maximizing Efficiency of Dialysis

In some circumstances the ammonia levels fail to decline or even increase despite apparently adequate dialysis. Occasionally ammonia production will exceed even the most effective dialytic clearance. Important points to consider in this scenario are:

1. Minimize recirculation through the vascular access. Use the proximal and distal catheter drainage ports as the manufacturer intended. "Swapping" the lumens around, even if flow appears better only increases recirculation. Try using internal jugular access.
2. Optimize blood flow rate(BFR). BFR >40 mL/min enhances filtration but this is dependent on good vascular access. Recirculation will increase with higher blood flow rate if the catheter position is problematic.

3. Ensure adequate delivery of intravenous sodium benzoate and sodium phenylacetate. Both are small molecular weight molecules that are not protein bound and are freely diffusible [47]. Giving excessive doses may also precipitate neurologic deterioration [31].
4. Consider dual mode dialysis (peritoneal dialysis and hemofiltration or HD)
5. In hyperammonaemia due to organic acid disorders, larger organic acids may be more effectively cleared with convective hemofiltration as opposed to counter current haemodialysis or haemodiafiltration.
6. Alkalosis promotes ammonia entry into the brain. If pH >7.45, aim for normal $pCO_2$. If the patient is haemodynamically stable, mild to moderate acidosis could be tolerated to reduce cerebral ammonia uptake.

**Conclusion**

Hyperammonaemia secondary to IEM is a common neonatal/paediatric emergency. Measurement of ammonia levels should form a part of investigations for any collapsed newborn or in fact any child who presents with sudden onset of loss of consciousness. A very close liaison should always be sought between the treating intensive care team and metabolic specialist. Peritoneal dialysis is a good modality to lower serum ammonia levels awaiting transfer to tertiary centres for extracorporeal dialysis or even as the primary form of renal replacement therapy. There are no head to head studies comparing convective versus dialysis mode of renal replacement therapy. All efforts should be made to optimize CRRT including minimizing circuit downtimes. Prognosis depends on the type of inborn error of metabolism, peak ammonia levels and the duration of hyperammonaemic coma. Despite optimizing dialytic therapy, one might not be able to control ammonia levels if the rate of production of ammonia is higher than what the extracorporeal therapy can remove.

**Key Learning Points**

- Hyperammonaemia secondary to IEM can occur at any age
- Measure ammonia in any patient with unexplained reduced level of consciousness
- Age of onset and peak ammonia levels at presentation impact neurological outcome
- Consider dialysis to acutely lower blood ammonia levels above 300 μmol/L. Ideal target is to half ammonia in 2–4 h with a level below 150–200 μmol/L within 24 h.
- At maximal efficiency, all modes of dialysis including perineal dialysis can acutely lower blood ammonia levels. The mode and type of dialysis should be chosen according to the expertise of the clinical team or institution.
- For neonatal haemofiltration (CVVH or CVVHD), a large bore right internal jugular vascular access catheter (e.g. 7Fr) is preferable for optimal blood flow. Femoral catheters may have significant recirculation.

## References


1. Adeva MM, Souto G, Blanco N, Donapetry C. Ammonium metabolism in humans. Metabolism. 2012;61(11):1495–511.
2. Jackson MJ, Beaudet AL, O'Brien WE. Mammalian urea cycle enzymes. Annu Rev Genet. 1986;20:431–64.
3. Häberle J, Boddaert N, Burlina A, Chakrapani A, Dixon M, Huemer M, Karall D, Martinelli D, Crespo PS, Santer R, Servais A, Valayannopoulos V, Lindner M, Rubio V, Dionisi-Vici C. Suggested guidelines for the diagnosis and management of urea cycle disorders. Orphanet J Rare Dis. 2012;7:32.
4. Bowker R, Green A, Bonham JR. Guidelines for the investigation and management of a reduced level of consciousness in children: implications for clinical biochemistry laboratories. Ann Clin Biochem. 2007;44:506–11.
5. Smith W, Kishnani PS, Lee B, Singh RH, Rhead WJ, Sniderman King L, Smith M, Summar M. Urea cycle disorders: clinical presentation outside the newborn period. Crit Care Clin. 2005;21(4 Suppl):S9–17.
6. Saudubray JM, Nassogne MC, de Lonlay P, Touati G. Clinical approach to inherited metabolic disorders in neonates: an overview. Semin Neonatol. 2002;7(1):3–15.
7. Barsotti RJ. Measurement of ammonia in blood. J Pediatr. 2001;138(1 Suppl):S11–9.
8. Wertheim-Tysarowska K, Gos M, Sykut-Cegielska J. Bal J; genetic analysis in inherited metabolic disorders--from diagnosis to treatment. Own experience, current state of knowledge and perspectives. Dev Period Med. 2015;19(4):413–31.
9. Yamaguchi S, Brailey LL, Morizono H, Bale AE, Tuchman M. Mutations and polymorphisms in the human ornithine transcarbamylase (OTC) gene. Hum Mutat. 2006;27(7):626–32.
10. Summar ML, Koelker S, Freedenberg D, Le Mons C, Haberle J, Lee HS, Kirmse B. The incidence of urea cycle disorders. European registry and network for intoxication type metabolic diseases (E-IMD). Mol Genet Metab. 2013;110(1–2):179–80.
11. Legido-Quigley C, Cloarec O, Parker DA, Murphy GM, Holmes E, Lindon JC, Nicholson JK, Mitry RR, Vilca-Melendez H, Rela M, Dhawan A, Heaton N. First example of hepatocyte transplantation to alleviate ornithine transcarbamylase deficiency, monitored by NMR-based metabonomics. Bioanalysis. 2009;1(9):1527–35.
12. Kido J, Matsumoto S, Momosaki K, Sakamoto R, Mitsubuchi H, Endo F, Nakamura K. Liver transplantation may prevent neurodevelopmental deterioration in high-risk patients with urea cycle disorders. Pediatr Transplant. 2017;21(6)
13. Yu L, Rayhill SC, Hsu EK, Landis CS. Liver transplantation for urea cycle disorders: analysis of the united network for organ sharing database. Transplant Proc. 2015;47(8):2413–8.
14. Bachmann C. Outcome and survival of 88 patients with urea cycle disorders: a retrospective evaluation. Eur J Pediatr. 2003;162(6):410–6.
15. Batshaw ML, Tuchman M, Summar M, Seminara J, Members of the Urea Cycle Disorders Consortium. A longitudinal study of urea cycle disorders. Mol Genet Metab. 2014;113(1–2):127–3.
16. Burgard P, Kölker S, Haege G, Lindner M, Hoffmann GF. Neonatal mortality and outcome at the end of the first year of life in early onset urea cycle disorders—review and meta-analysis of observational studies published over more than 35 years. J Inherit Metab Dis. 2016;39(2):219–2.
17. Posset R, Garcia-Cazorla A, Valayannopoulos V, Teles EL, Dionisi-Vici C, Brassier A, Burlina AB, Burgard P, Cortès-Saladelafont E, Dobbelaere D, Couce ML, Sykut-Cegielska J, Häberle J, Lund AM, Chakrapani A, Schiff M, Walter JH, Zeman J, Vara R, Kölker S. Additional individual contributors of the E-IMD consortium; age at disease onset and peak ammonium level rather than interventional variables predict the neurological outcome in urea cycle disorders. J Inherit Metab Dis. 2016;39(5):661–72.
18. Fraser JL, Venditti CP. Methylmalonic and propionic acidemias: clinical management update. Curr Opin Pediatr. 2016;28(6):682–93.

19. Oplin SE. Pathophysiology of fatty acid oxidation disorders and resultant phenotypic variability. J Inherit Metab Dis. 2013;36(4):645–58.
20. Ogier de Baulny H, Schiff M, Dionisi-Vici C. Lysinuric protein intolerance (LPI): a multi organ disease by far more complex than a classic urea cycle disorder. Mol Genet Metab. 2012;106(1):12–7.
21. Martinelli D, Diodato D, Ponzi E, Monné M, Boenzi S, Bertini E, Fiermonte G, Dionisi-Vici C. The hyperornithinemia-hyperammonemia-homocitrullinuria syndrome. Orphanet J Rare Dis. 2015;10:29.
22. Palladino AA, Stanley CA. The hyperinsulinism/hyperammonemia syndrome. Rev Endocr Metab Disord. 2010;11(3):171–8.
23. Häberle J. Clinical and biochemical aspects of primary and secondary hyperammonemic disorders. Arch Biochem Biophys. 2013;536(2):101–8.
24. Magner M, Dvorakova V, Tesarova M, Mazurova S, Hansikova H, Zahorec M, Brennerova K, Bzduch V, Spiegel R, Horovitz Y, Mandel H, Eminoğlu FT, Mayr JA, Koch J, Martinelli D, Bertini E, Konstantopoulou V, Smet J, Rahman S, Broomfield A, Stojanović V, Dionisi-Vici C, van Coster R, Morava E, Sperl W, Zeman J, Honzik T. TMEM70 deficiency: long-term outcome of 48 patients. J Inherit Metab Dis. 2015;38(3):417–26.
25. Diez-Fernandez C, Rüfenacht V, Santra S, Lund AM, Santer R, Lindner M, Tangeraas T, Unsinn C, de Lonlay P, Burlina A, van Karnebeek CD, Häberle J. Defective hepatic bicarbonate production due to carbonic anhydrase VA deficiency leads to early-onset life-threatening metabolic crisis. Genet Med. 2016;18(10):991–1000.
26. Auron A, Brophy PD. Hyperammonemia in review: pathophysiology, diagnosis, and treatment. Pediatr Nephrol. 2012;27(2):207–22.
27. Häberle J. Clinical practice: the management of hyperammonemia. Eur J Pediatr. 2011;170(1):21–34.
28. Lang W, Blöck TM, Zander R. Solubility of NH3 and apparent pK of NH4+ in human plasma, isotonic salt solutions and water at 37 degrees C. Clin Chim Acta. 1998;273(1):43–58.
29. da Fonseca-Wollheim F, Heinze KG. Solubility of NH3 and apparent pK of NH4+ in human plasma, isotonic salt solutions and water at 37 degrees C. Eur J Clin Chem Clin Biochem. 1992;30(12):867–9.
30. Thrane V, Thrane A, Wang W, et al. Solubility of NH3 and apparent pK of NH4+ in human plasma, isotonic salt solutions and water at 37 degrees C. Nat Med. 2013;19(12):1643–8.
31. Berry E, Rhead S, Brusilow W, Hamosh S. Survival after treatment with phenyl acetate and benzoate for urea cycle disorders. NEJM. 2007;356:2282–92.
32. Uchino T, Endo F, Matsuda I. Neurodevelopmental outcome of long-term therapy of urea cycle disorders in Japan. J Inherit Metab Dis. 1998;21(Suppl 1):151–9.
33. Msall M, Batshaw ML, Suus R, Brusilow SW, Mellitis ED. Neurologic outcome in children with inborn errors of urea synthesis. Outcome of urea-cycle enzymopathies. N Engl J Med. 1984;310(23):1500–5.
34. Westrope C, Morris K, Burford D, Morrison G. Continuous hemofiltration in the control of neonatal hyperammonemia: a 10-year experience. Pediatr Nephrol. 2010;25(9):1725–30.
35. Picca S, Dionisi-Vici C, Bartuli A, De Palo T, Papadia F, Montini G, Materassi M, Donati MA, Verrina E, Schiaffino MC, Pecoraro C, Iaccarino E, Vidal E, Burlina A, Emma F. Short-term survival of hyperammonemic neonates treated with dialysis. Pediatr Nephrol. 2015;30:839–47.
36. Schaefer F, Straube E, Oh J, Mayatepeck E. Dialysis in neonates with inborn errors of metabolism. Nephrol Dial Transplant. 1999;14:910–8.
37. Arbeiter AK, Kranz B, Wingen AM, Bonzel KE, Dohna-Schwake C, Hanssler L, Neudorf U, Hoyer PF, Büscher R. Continuous venovenous haemodialysis (CVVHD) and continuous peritoneal dialysis (CPD) in the acute management of 21 children with inborn errors of metabolism. Nephrol Dial Transplant. 2010;25(4):1257–65.
38. McBryde KD, Kershaw DB, Bunchman TE, Maxvold NJ, Mottes TA, Kudelka TL, Brophy PD. Renal replacement therapy in the treatment of confirmed or suspected inborn errors of metabolism. J Pediatr. 2006;148:770–8.

39. Spinale JM, Laskin BL, Sondheimer N, Swartz SJ, Goldstein SL. High-dose continuous renal replacement therapy for neonatal hyperammonemia. Pediatr Nephrol. 2013;28:983–6.
40. Hackbarth R, Bunchman TE, Chua AN, et al. The effect of vascular access location and size on circuit survival in pediatric continuous renal replacement therapy: a report from the PPCRRT registry. Int J Artif Organs. 2007;30:1116–21.
41. Picca S, Dionisi-Vici C, Abeni D, Pastore A, Rizzo C, Orzalesi M, Sabetta G, Rizzoni G, Bartuli A. Extracorporeal dialysis in neonatal hyperammonemia: modalities and prognostic indicators. Pediatr Nephrol. 2001;16(11):862–7.
42. Lai Y-C, Huang H-P, Tsai I-J, Tsau Y-K. High-volume continuous venovenous hemofiltration as an effective therapy for acute management of inborn errors of metabolism in young children. Blood Purif. 2007;25:303–8.
43. Clark WR, Turk JE, Kraus MA, Gao D. Dose determinants in continuous renal replacement therapy. Int J Artif Organs. 2003;27:815–20.
44. Huang Z, Letteri J, Clark WJ, Ronco C, Gao D. Operational characteristics of continuous renal replacement modalities used for critically ill patients with acute kidney injury. Int J Artif Organs. 2008;31(6):525–34.
45. Troyanov S, Cardinal J, Geadah D, Parent D, Courteau S, et al. Solute clearances during continuous venovenous haemofiltration at various ultrafiltration flow rates using Multiflow-100 and HF1000 filters. Nephrol Dial Transplant. 2003;18:961–6.
46. Little MA, Conlon PJ, Walshe JJ. Access recirculation in temporary hemodialysis catheters as measured by the saline dilution technique. Am J Kidney Dis. 2000;6:1135–9.
47. Bunchman TE, Barletta GM, Winters JW, Gardner JJ, Crumb TL, McBryde KD. Phenylacetate and benzoate clearance in a hyperammonemic infant on sequential hemodialysis and haemofiltration. Pediatr Nephrol. 2007;22(7):1062–5.

# CRRT and Extracorporeal Techniques in Exogenous Intoxications

28

Irfan Khan and Patrick D. Brophy

**Case Vignette**

A 16-year female with a history of bipolar disorder presents to the Emergency Department (ED) comatose and hypotensive. A toxicology screen performed on her arrival to the ED (estimated to be 4–5 h post-ingestion) demonstrates a salicylate level of 100 mg/dL. Her radiographic and physical examination reveal acute pulmonary edema and prolonged QTc on electrocardiogram (EKG) assessment. As you are examining the patient she starts to have generalized seizures.

## 28.1 Introduction

In 2016 alone, the US poison control center reported about 2.2 million human exposures. The top five substance classes most frequently involved in all human exposures were analgesics (11.2%), household cleaning substances (7.54%), cosmetics/personal care products (7.20%), sedatives/hypnotics/antipsychotics (5.84%), and antidepressants (4.74%) [1].

I. Khan
Presbyterian Hospital, Albuquerque, NM, USA

P. D. Brophy (✉)
Department of Pediatrics, University of Rochester School of Medicine and Dentistry, Rochester, NY, USA

Golisano Children's Hospital at the University of Rochester Medical Center, Rochester, NY, USA
e-mail: Patrick_brophy@urmc.rochester.edu



A. Deep, S. L. Goldstein (eds.), *Critical Care Nephrology and Renal Replacement Therapy in Children*, https://doi.org/10.1007/978-3-319-90281-4_28

Intoxications are generally either accidental or intentional. Management of the poisoned patient includes [2]:

1. Having a high degree of suspicion that poisoning has occurred, and looking for toxidromes.
2. Assessment of the degree of severity of poisoning: availability of different drugs in the environment, timing, quantity, and type of drug ingested. Evidence of cellular level toxicity (such as elevated lactate). Specific organ or multi-organ involvement usually in cellular level toxin.
3. Attempts to prevent further absorption of toxin with charcoal administration or gastric lavage.
4. Laboratory data: including blood gases, electrolytes, serum and urine osmolality, EKG, serum and urine toxicology screens. Specific quantitative drug screens.
5. Decision to provide supportive care, including establishment of an airway, mechanical ventilation, fluids, use of vasopressors and or inotropes.
6. Provide a specific antidote if available.
7. Enhancing the elimination of the toxin using urinary alkalinization/acidification or extracorporeal methods (about 0.1% of the intoxications) [3].

The characteristics of an exogenous toxin that determine its absorption and clearance include:

1. Molecular weight, usually expressed in kilo Daltons.
2. Degree of protein binding, in turn affecting the amount of free drug available for clearance.
3. Volume of distribution, highly lipophilic xenobiotics (exogenous toxins) may take a longer time to clear.
4. Ability to cross the blood brain barrier.
5. Metabolism into other toxic byproducts.
6. Dependence on liver or kidney function for clearance.

## 28.2 Enhanced Elimination (Clearance) Techniques Include

### 28.2.1 Urinary Alkalinization

It is a treatment regimen that increases poison elimination by the administration of intravenous sodium bicarbonate to produce urine with a pH > or = 7.5. Mechanistically, it involves alteration in the urine pH to catalyze un-dissociated acid or base in the renal tubular lumen into its ionized form. Enhanced elimination occurs due to decreased diffusion of the charged particles from the renal tubular lumen back into the blood. Target urine pH is around 7.5–8.5 for maximal efficacy [2]. Phenobarbital and salicylate poisoned patients greatly benefit from this technique. In fact, in 2004, the AACT and EAPCCT published a joint statement supporting it as a first-line therapy for moderately severe salicylate ingestion patients who were not candidates for hemodialysis. Hypokalemia should be anticipated, as it is the most common complication but can be corrected by giving potassium supplements [4].

### 28.2.2 Urine Acidification

Although effective to enhance elimination of weak bases like amphetamine, amantadine, and quinidine, this technique is applied in a limited fashion due to the potential side effects of systemic metabolic acidosis. Generally, in such cases extracorporeal elimination is employed in order to better control electrolyte and acid base status.

### 28.2.3 Extracorporeal Elimination Methods

Extracorporeal elimination techniques (ECTR) are employed in approximately 0.1% of all intoxications treated in the U.S. [3]. ECTRs are considered to be more invasive, expensive, and generally require specially trained staff. The risk-to-benefit ratio must be ascertained before embarking on this path. Multiple extracorporeal techniques are available and include:

1. Hemodialysis (HD): one of the most commonly used techniques.
2. CRRT [continuous renal replacement therapy—including continuous venovenous hemofiltration (CVVH), continuous venovenous hemodialysis (CVVHD), or continuous venovenous hemodiafiltration (CVVHDF)]
3. Peritoneal dialysis (PD)
4. Hemoperfusion (HP
5. Exchange transfusion (ET)
6. Plasmapheresis (TPE)
7. Liver/albumin dialysis
8. Combined HD and CRRT.
9. SLED (Slow low efficiency dialysis)

There are no randomized controlled trials to support one therapy over the other. Most literature has been based on case series and case reports. Utilization of extracorporeal techniques can generally be justified if two key criteria are met. One is that the drug toxicity is severe and the other is that the use of ECTR results at least in an increase of total body elimination by 30% or more [5].

## 28.3 Hemodialysis

The principle of diffusion across a permeable membrane down a concentration gradient is utilized in this technique. Water solubility, low molecular weight (<2000 Da), low protein binding rates (<50%), and low volumes of distribution (<0.75 mL/kg) are favorable pharmacokinetic profiles [6].

HD has the ability to rapidly correct electrolyte and acid base disturbance as an additional benefit. It is useful in removal of even highly protein bound toxins if the dissociation constant to protein is small. Newer high flux membranes can remove even high molecular weight substances. Titration of the blood and dialysate flow rates can optimize the rates of diffusion and elimination. Even though it is considered the preferred modality for ECTR, it has some limitations. HD can be difficult to conduct in patients with hemodynamic instability. The chance of having rebound toxicity from redistribution of the toxin after completing treatment can occur necessitating ongoing multiple treatments or switching to an alternative modality.

## 28.4 Continuous Techniques

There is insufficient evidence to support the use of CRRT as a first-line modality in the removal of exogenous toxins. However, in some cases the use of high volume approaches (8000 mL/1.73 $m^2$/h. of Ultrafiltration) may result in sufficient removal of the toxin. CVVH and CVVHD are two techniques that are utilized for ECTR, especially in patients with hemodynamic instability and to minimize risks of rebound toxicity [7]. The continuous techniques are generally slower in clearance compared to HD due to lower ultrafiltrate flow rates, usually about 60–70 mL/min as compared to 500 mL/min, respectively. Although there are theoretical advantages to using CVVH to prevent hemodynamic instability, due to its lower efficacy it is really preferred in situations where intermittent HD is either unavailable or in situations where patients have hypotension and/or oligo-anuric acute kidney injury.

Other positive attributes of continuous techniques include prevention of delayed rebound from toxin redistribution from tissues to plasma after cessation of ECTR. In the case of IHD, monitoring toxin levels post IHD and repeating another round of IHD if toxicity recurs may be necessary. In some specific intoxications (i.e., lithium poisoning), the redistribution may not necessarily be a problem as the toxin transfers from the site of toxicity, the CNS, to an alternative compartment—the plasma, where it may not cause problems. One situation that may justify the use of CVVH is if the toxin has a prolonged absorption in which case, the prolonged use of CVVH can continuously remove the toxin in real time.

There are differences in the membrane permeability when it comes to CRRT vs. IHD. CRRT membranes may allow clearance of larger molecules up to 20,000–40,000 Da [8]. Larger molecules like vancomycin can be cleared using predominant convective modalities like CVVH.

CRRT usually requires continuous anticoagulation and in some cases might place the patient at risk for bleeding and electrolyte disturbances. It also limits the mobility of the patients. The correction of serious or life-threatening acid base imbalance can be done much faster with IHD as compared to CRRT. If there is any requirement for urgent removal of a toxin, then IHD is generally the preferred option.

IHD is often more readily available even in developing countries as opposed to CRRT, which requires more intensive involvement.

## 28.5 Peritoneal Dialysis

The use of peritoneal dialysis for ingestions/intoxications is quite limited. It may be used in situations where small molecular weight overdoses are present (i.e., Lithium), but its general efficacy does not lend itself to a first-line treatment modality except when it is the only modality available [9].

## 28.6 Albumin-Based Dialysis

A variety of technical options are available for the employment of albumin-based dialysis systems. Molecular adsorbent recirculating system (MARS), other extracorporeal liver assist devices (ELAD), and single pass albumin dialysis (SPAD) are ECTR techniques that provide intermittent, slow (similar to CRRT) options, that employ albumin as a supplement in the dialysate. Albumin binding to toxins is utilized in ECTR, by using an albumin impermeable membrane. The toxin binds to the albumin as the blood passes through the circuit and the albumin bound toxin is then sent to a secondary circuit (or discarded in the case of SPAD) where it is adsorbed and the albumin is recycled which is then infused back into the circuit. Similar to CRRT, this technique provides lower clearance rates with blood flow rates approaching 35–40 mL/min [10]. This technique is expensive and specialized and its role in ECTR is still unclear. Some toxins like carbamazepine and valproate can be removed reasonably efficiently with albumin dialysis [11].

In a worldwide survey on the availability and cost of ECTR, Bouchard et al. showed that the most available modality for ECTR was IHD followed by therapeutic plasma exchange (TPE), CRRT, ET, PD, and HP. IHD was found to be least expensive whereas CRRT was almost twice as expensive as IHD. Time to initiation (60 min) was similar for both IHD and CRRT [12].

## 28.7 The Extracorporeal Treatment in Poisoning (EXTRIP)

The EXTRIP workgroup has come up with specific recommendations for various toxins. Their recommendations are based on a systematic literature review and structured voting statements.

### 28.7.1 EXTRIP Workgroup Recommendations for Salicylate Ingestions

IHD is the preferred modality and hemoperfusion and CRRT are acceptable alternatives if IHD is unavailable. Indications for ECTR include altered mental status, ARDS requiring supplemental oxygen, and failure of standard therapy regardless of salicylate concentration. Salicylate levels >100 mg/dL: warrant ECTR regardless of signs and symptoms with lower threshold (>80–90 mg/dL) for patients with impaired kidney function [13].

### 28.7.2 EXTRIP Workgroup Recommendations for Lithium Ingestions

ECTR is recommended strongly in severe lithium ingestions (when [$Li^+$] are >3.5 mEq/L) and in presence of a decreased level of consciousness, seizures, or life-threatening dysrhythmias irrespective of the [$Li^+$]. Extracorporeal treatment is suggested if the [$Li^+$] is >5.0 mEq/L, significant confusion is present, or the expected time to reduce the [$Li^+$] to <1.0 mEq/L is >36 h (2D). Extracorporeal treatment should be continued until clinical improvement is apparent or [$Li^+$] is <1.0 mEq/L. Extracorporeal treatments should be continued for a minimum of 6 h if the [$Li^+$] is not readily measurable. Hemodialysis is the preferred extracorporeal treatment, but CRRT is an acceptable alternative [14].

### 28.7.3 EXTRIP Workgroup Recommendations for Carbamazepine Ingestions

ECTR is suggested in severe carbamazepine poisoning. ECTR is recommended if multiple seizures occur and are refractory to treatment, or if life-threatening dysrhythmias occur. ECTR is suggested if prolonged coma or respiratory depression requiring mechanical ventilation is present or if significant toxicity persists, particularly when carbamazepine concentrations rise or remain elevated, despite using multiple-dose activated charcoal (MDAC) and supportive measures. ECTR should be continued until clinical improvement is apparent or the serum carbamazepine concentration is below 10 mg/L (42 μmol/L). Intermittent hemodialysis is the preferred ECTR, but intermittent hemoperfusion or continuous renal replacement therapies are alternatives if hemodialysis is not available. MDAC therapy should be continued during ECTR [15].

### 28.7.4 EXTRIP Workgroup Recommendations for Valproate (VPA) Ingestions

ECTR is recommended in severe VPA poisoning; recommendations for ECTR include a VPA concentration > 1300 mg/L (9000 μmol/L), the presence of cerebral edema or shock; suggestions for ECTR include a VPA concentration > 900 mg/L (6250 μmol/L), coma or respiratory depression requiring mechanical ventilation, acute hyperammonemia, or pH ≤ 7.10 (2D). Cessation of ECTR is indicated when clinical improvement is apparent or the serum VPA concentration is between 50 and 100 mg/L (350–700 μmol/L). Intermittent hemodialysis is the preferred ECTR in VPA poisoning. If hemodialysis is not available, then intermittent hemoperfusion or continuous renal replacement therapy are acceptable alternatives [16].

### 28.7.5 EXTRIP Workgroup Recommendations for Phenytoin Ingestions

Phenytoin appears to be amenable to extracorporeal removal. However, because of the low incidence of irreversible tissue injury or death related to phenytoin poisoning and the relatively limited effect of ECTR on phenytoin removal, the workgroup proposed the use of ECTR only in very select patients with severe phenytoin poisoning with severe ataxia or prolonged coma [17].

### 28.7.6 EXTRIP Workgroup Recommendations for Acetaminophen (*APAP* or Acetyl-Para-Aminophenol) Ingestions

Given that APAP is dialyzable, the workgroup agreed that ECTR is suggested in patients with excessively large overdoses who display features of mitochondrial dysfunction. This is reflected by the early development of altered mental status and severe metabolic acidosis prior to the onset of hepatic failure. Specific recommendations for ECTR include an APAP concentration over 1000 mg/L if N-acetyl cysteine (NAC) is not administered, signs of mitochondrial dysfunction and an APAP concentration over 700 mg/L (4630 mmol/L) if NAC is not administered and signs of mitochondrial dysfunction and an APAP concentration over 900 mg/L (5960 mmol/L) if NAC is administered. Intermittent hemodialysis is the preferred ECTR modality in APAP poisoning [18].

### 28.7.7 EXTRIP Workgroup Recommendations for Metformin Ingestions

Extracorporeal treatment is recommended in severe metformin poisoning. Indications for extracorporeal treatment include lactate concentration greater than 20 mmol/L, pH less than or equal to 7.0, shock, failure of standard supportive measures, and decreased level of consciousness. Extracorporeal treatment should be continued until the lactate concentration is less than 3 mmol/L and pH greater than 7.35, at which time close monitoring is warranted to determine the need for additional courses of extracorporeal treatment. Intermittent hemodialysis is preferred initially, but continuous renal replacement therapies may be considered if hemodialysis is unavailable. Repeat extracorporeal treatment sessions may employ hemodialysis or continuous renal replacement therapy [19].

**Conclusion**

IHD is the preferred modality for most severe ingestions with toxins that are amenable to ECTR. Use of the EXTRIP recommendations helps clinicians practice evidence-based approaches to toxin management. CRRT should be used if severe hemodynamic instability precludes use of IHD and if prolonged absorption is an issue. A working knowledge of drug properties and membrane clearance-based properties of ECTR equipment is exceedingly important when employing these interventional therapies. Team-based collaborative approaches with emergency providers, toxicologists, intensivists, pharmacists, nephrologists, and other healthcare professionals using established practice guidelines can expedite patient care and reduce morbidity and mortality in the case of significant intoxications.

## References


1. Gummin DD, Mowry JB, Spyker DA, Brooks DE, Fraser MO, Banner W. 2016 Annual report of the American Association of Poison Control Centers' National Poison Data System (NPDS): 34th annual report. Clin Toxicol (Phila). 2017;55(10):1072–252. https://doi.org/10.1080/15563650.2017.1388087. Epub 2017 Nov 29.
2. Zimmerman JL. Poisonings and overdoses in the intensive care unit: general and specific management issues. Crit Care Med. 2003;31(12):2794–801.
3. Ouellet G, Bouchard J, Ghannoum M, Decker BS. Available extracorporeal treatments for poisoning: overview and limitations. Semin Dial. 2014;27(4):342–9. https://doi.org/10.1111/sdi.12238. Epub 2014 Apr 3.
4. Proudfoot AT, Krenzelok EP, Vale JA. Position paper on urine alkalinization. J Toxicol Clin Toxicol. 2004;42(1):1–26.
5. Maher JF, Schreiner GE. The dialysis of poisons and drugs. Trans Am Soc Artif Intern Organs. 1968;14:440–53.
6. Winchester JF, et al. Use of dialysis and hemoperfusion in treatment of poisoning. Handbook of dialysis. 4th ed. Philadelphia: Lippincott Williams & Wilkins; 2007. p. 300–22.
7. Feinfeld DA, Rosenberg JW, Winchester JF. Three controversial issues in extracorporeal toxin removal. Semin Dial. 2006;19:358–62.
8. Forni LG, Hilton PJ. Continuous hemofiltration in the treatment of acute renal failure. N Engl J Med. 1997;336(18):1303–9.
9. Walters S, Porter C, Brophy PD. Dialysis and pediatric acute kidney injury: choice of renal support modality. Pediatr Nephrol. 2009;24(1):37–48. https://doi.org/10.1007/s00467-008-0826-x.
10. Drexler K, Baustian C, Richter G, Ludwig J, Ramlow W, Mitzner S. Albumin dialysis molecular adsorbents recirculating system: impact of dialysate albumin concentration on detoxification efficacy. Ther Apher Dial. 2009;13(5):393–8. https://doi.org/10.1111/j.1744-9987.2009.00757.x.
11. Churchwell MD, Pasko DA, Smoyer WE, Mueller BA. Enhanced clearance of highly protein-bound drugs by albumin-supplemented dialysate during modeled continuous hemodialysis. Nephrol Dial Transplant. 2009;24(1):231–8. https://doi.org/10.1093/ndt/gfn467. Epub 2008 Aug 22.
12. Bouchard J, Lavergne V, Roberts DM, Cormier M, Morissette G, Ghannoum M. Availability and cost of extracorporeal treatments for poisonings and other emergency indications: a worldwide survey. Nephrol Dial Transplant. 2017;32(4):699–706. https://doi.org/10.1093/ndt/gfw456.
13. Juurlink DN, Gosselin S, Kielstein JT, Ghannoum M, Lavergne V, Nolin TD, Hoffman RS, EXTRIP Workgroup. Extracorporeal treatment for salicylate poisoning: systematic review and recommendations from the EXTRIP workgroup. Ann Emerg Med. 2015;66(2):165–81. https://doi.org/10.1016/j.annemergmed.2015.03.031. Epub 2015 May 15.
14. Decker BS, Goldfarb DS, Dargan PI, Friesen M, Gosselin S, Hoffman RS, Lavergne V, Nolin TD, Ghannoum M, EXTRIP Workgroup. Extracorporeal treatment for lithium poisoning: systematic review and recommendations from the EXTRIP workgroup. Clin J Am Soc Nephrol. 2015;10(5):875–87. https://doi.org/10.2215/CJN.10021014. Epub 2015 Jan 12.

15. Ghannoum M, Yates C, Galvao TF, Sowinski KM, Vo TH, Coogan A, Gosselin S, Lavergne V, Nolin TD, Hoffman RS, EXTRIP workgroup. Extracorporeal treatment for carbamazepine poisoning: systematic review and recommendations from the EXTRIP workgroup. Clin Toxicol (Phila). 2014;52(10):993–1004. https://doi.org/10.3109/15563650.2014.973572. Epub 2014 Oct 30.
16. Ghannoum M, Laliberté M, Nolin TD, MacTier R, Lavergne V, Hoffman RS, Gosselin S, Workgroup EXTRIP. Extracorporeal treatment for valproic acid poisoning: systematic review and recommendations from the EXTRIP workgroup. Clin Toxicol (Phila). 2015;53(5):454–65. https://doi.org/10.3109/15563650.2015.1035441.
17. Anseeuw K, Mowry JB, Burdmann EA, Ghannoum M, Hoffman RS, Gosselin S, Lavergne V, Nolin TD, EXTRIP Workgroup. Extracorporeal treatment in phenytoin poisoning: systematic review and recommendations from the EXTRIP (extracorporeal treatments in poisoning) workgroup. Am J Kidney Dis. 2016;67(2):187–97. https://doi.org/10.1053/j.ajkd.2015.08.031. Epub 2015 Nov 11.
18. Gosselin S, Juurlink DN, Kielstein JT, Ghannoum M, Lavergne V, Nolin TD, Hoffman RS, Workgroup E. Extracorporeal treatment for acetaminophen poisoning: recommendations from the EXTRIP workgroup. Clin Toxicol (Phila). 2014;52(8):856–67. https://doi.org/10.3109/15563650.2014.946994. Epub 2014 Aug 18.
19. Calello DP, Liu KD, Wiegand TJ, Roberts DM, Lavergne V, Gosselin S, Hoffman RS, Nolin TD, Ghannoum M, Extracorporeal Treatments in Poisoning Workgroup. Extracorporeal treatment for metformin poisoning: systematic review and recommendations from the extracorporeal treatments in poisoning workgroup. Crit Care Med. 2015;43(8):1716–30. https://doi.org/10.1097/CCM.0000000000001002.

# Continuous Renal Replacement Therapy (CRRT) in Liver Failure and Other Liver Assist Devices

29

Bogdana Sabina Zoica, Ayse Akcan-Arikan, and Akash Deep

## Abbreviations

| | |
|---|---|
| AC | Ammonia clearance |
| ALF | Acute liver failure |
| ACLF | Acute on chronic liver failure |
| AKI | Acute kidney injury |
| CE | Cerebral edema |
| CRRT | Continuous renal replacement therapy |
| CVVH | Continuous veno-venous hemofiltration |
| CVHD | Continuous veno-venous hemodialysis |
| CVVHDF | Continuous veno-venous hemodiafiltration |
| ECLD | Extracorporeal liver assist devices |
| FFP | Fresh frozen plasma |
| GFR | Glomerular filtration rate |
| HE | Hepatic encephalopathy |
| HRS | Hepatorenal syndrome |
| HVHF | High volume hemofiltration |
| ICP | Intracranial pressure |
| LF | Liver failure |
| MARS | Molecular absorbing recirculating system |
| OLT | Orthotopic liver transplantation |
| RCA | Regional citrate anticoagulation |
| SPAD | Single pass albumin dialysis |
| TPE | Total plasma exchange |

B. S. Zoica · A. Deep (✉)
Pediatric Intensive Care, King's College Hospital, London, UK
e-mail: akash.deep@nhs.net

A. Akcan-Arikan
Department of Pediatrics, Sections of Critical Care and Nephrology, Texas Children's Hospital, Houston, TX, USA

Critical Care Nephrology, Texas Children's Hospital, Houston, TX, USA



A. Deep, S. L. Goldstein (eds.), *Critical Care Nephrology and Renal Replacement Therapy in Children*, https://doi.org/10.1007/978-3-319-90281-4_29

**Clinical Vignette**

A previously fit and well 9-year-old girl with history of cough and cold 2 weeks prior, developed jaundice and lethargy and was taken to a hospital in Dublin, where investigations revealed acute liver failure (ALF). She was transferred to a quaternary center and progressively developed encephalopathy and renal impairment. She was intubated and ventilated for neuroprotection while awaiting OLT. CRRT was initiated for high ammonia levels (>250 μmol/L), management of fluid balance, and acute kidney injury. ICP was constantly 50 $cmH_2O$, measured by intracranial bolt. Full neuroprotective measures failed to bring the ICP down and an urgent hepatectomy was performed. Immediately after removal of the necrotic liver, the ICP normalized. Unfortunately, a liver donor was not available and for the next 8h she was anhepatic, supported by continuous renal replacement therapy (CRRT). Therefore, CRRT worked both as renal and liver support. A less than optimal cadaveric liver was offered and accepted as a bridge to another liver transplant. Following 72 h of neuroprotection and clinical stability the patient was extubated and had no neurologic deficits.

A month later she received a second liver transplant. Throughout this period her kidney function never recovered and she became dialysis dependent. Her bone marrow failed and she was listed for bone marrow transplantation. After 8 months of intensive care she developed systemic aspergillosis and unfortunately died.

This case highlights the various challenges encountered in the treatment of LF with regard to timing of initiation of CRRT, dose of CRRT, indications and impact of CRRT on survival including chronic kidney disease.

## 29.1 Introduction

ALF and ACLF present unique challenges in critical care hepatology; although survival has improved due to advances in medical technology, the only established treatment for LF, particularly chronic, is orthotopic liver transplantation (OLT). The clinical setting for appropriate management is dependent upon the clinical presentation which determines the level of monitoring and support the child requires but rapid referral to transplantation centers for triage and OLT evaluation is crucial.

Impaired detoxification in hepatic dysfunction leads to the accumulation of multiple water-soluble and protein-bound toxins which, together with the release of inflammatory cytokines, have been implicated in a cascade of events leading to multi-organ-system failure: hepatic encephalopathy (HE), cardiovascular collapse, renal failure, and a mortality of up to 80%.

The major comorbidities, HE, hepatic cardiomyopathy, hepatopulmonary syndrome (HPS), and hepatorenal syndrome (HRS), affect short- and long-term survival. Pediatric intensivists rely largely on data derived from adult studies for management of critical LF; however, adult LF is essentially a different disease due to unique etiologies and accompanying comorbidities.

HE is caused by accumulation of toxins in particular ammonia secondary to detoxification failure [1, 2]. Some degree of HE was present in 50% of pediatric ALF patients at admission and developed an additional 15% over the first week [3]. Recently, improved understanding of the pathophysiology of HE has revealed the role of inflammation in the onset of HE [4].

Ammonia, a by-product of nitrogen metabolism, is central in the pathogenesis of HE; blood ammonia levels predict HE and death [5]. Peak levels, persistence, and duration of hyperammonemia all correlate with development of cerebral edema (CE) and intracranial hypertension (ICH). A level > 100 μmol/L predicts the onset of severe HE with 70% accuracy, while ammonia levels >200 μmol/L are associated with development of ICH. Patients with persistent hyperammonemia are more likely to progress to advanced HE, have higher incidence of renal failure and infections [5]. Persistently elevated ammonia over 3 days of hospital stay is associated with complications and death in patients with ALF. Other toxins such as bile acids, aromatic amino acids, mediators of inflammation like cytokines, chemokines, and medium chain fatty acids have also been postulated to contribute to multi-organ dysfunction.

CE is reported in up to 80% of ALF [6, 7] though not as common in ACLF due to astrocyte adaptation. Neuroprotective measures to prevent secondary injury are crucial [7, 8]. Vasoactive infusions are used to maintain cerebral perfusion pressure, though an age-specific ideal target is not known. Mechanical ventilation and mild hypocapnea together with pharmacologically induced coma might be needed for refractory ICH. A strategy of "4 H therapy" (mild hyperventilation, hypernatremia, hypothermia, and hemofiltration) has been proposed to prevent onset of HE.

## 29.2 Role of Extracorporeal Liver Devices (ECLD) as Bridging Therapies

There are four categories of liver patients who could potentially benefit extracorporeal liver assist device therapy (ECLD)—ALF, sick cirrhotic patient, decompensated cirrhosis, and ACLF—in different ways (Table 29.1). The main culprit in ALF is raised intracranial pressure is hyperammonaemia and hence continuous renal replacement therapy (CRRT) is the most frequently used modality to adequately control ammonia levels without causing excessive fluid shifts. Early initiation of CRRT is thought to be beneficial, allowing tight control of hyperammonemia, fluid balance, and serum osmolality, and might assist in temperature control. The current recommendation is to aim for ammonia levels <100 μmol/L [7, 9]. High diffusive clearance or high volume hemofiltration (HVHF) might be necessary to control ammonia levels especially if the rate of production is high [10]. Hypertonic saline is utilized increasingly in CE management and provides a unique challenge in extracorporeal considerations as commencement of CRRT, specifically HVHF, will lead to rapid "normalization" of serum sodium levels. Addition of sodium to the

**Table 29.1** Aims for extracorporeal liver assist devices

| | |
|---|---|
| Acute liver failure | Control ICH/ fluid overload<br>Bridge to recovery or transplantation |
| Critically ill cirrhotic patient | Reversal of organ failure<br>Bridge to transplantation |
| Decompensated cirrhosis | Prevention of further deterioration—i.e., ACLF<br>Stability on transplant list:<br>• Decreased infections<br>• Decreased portal pressure<br>• Decreased variceal bleeding;<br>• Control of ascites |
| Acute on chronic liver disease | Reversal of type I HRS,<br>Stabilization type II HRS<br>Reversal of hepatic encephalopathy<br>Improved synthetic function/ nutritional status<br>Control pruritus |

dialysate and replacement fluids to a level of at least 155 μmol/L would prevent this occurrence and is the standard of care in certain institutions.

Coexisting and independent liver and renal dysfunction impact significantly on hospital and intensive care mortality in pediatric LF; superimposed renal failure has also been associated with reduced patient survival after transplantation [11, 12]. Traditionally, the most common acute kidney injury (AKI) in patients with LF are prerenal failure and acute tubular necrosis (also known as functional AKI and structural AKI). AKI can be missed as diagnosis is dependent on elevations in serum creatinine and endogenous creatinine production is decreased in LF. Use of novel biomarkers has revealed a higher incidence of intrinsic AKI in adults with LF. The etiology of AKI in ALF is multifactorial: hypovolemia, hypotension with severe vasoplegia, direct drug toxicity (paracetamol, NSAIDs), HRS, and intraabdominal hypertension secondary to abdominal compartment syndrome. RRT is indicated for severe AKI and adequate fluid management and is frequently required in ALF, acute decompensation of chronic liver disease, post-liver transplant renal failure, metabolic liver disease, and patients with liver disease who develop AKI as a part of multi-organ failure [13]. HRS is the classical renal involvement described in ACLF. Functional prerenal failure with relatively normal tubular function and bland histology unresponsive to volume expansion is described in 20% of hospitalized end stage liver disease. Cirrhotic cardiomyopathy and ongoing inflammation fueled by bacterial translocation from the gut contribute to HRS development. Discontinuation of diuretics, and introduction of vasoconstrictor agents (terlipressin or octreotide) and albumin loading is the key to treatment [14].

The spectrum of AKI in LF is not limited to HRS alone but also includes true intrinsic AKI, likely secondary to infectious/inflammatory insults which may not be readily reversible after OLT. Patients with ALF frequently develop renal dysfunction. Tujios [15] investigated the incidence of AKI among ALF patients, using defined criteria to identify risk factors and to evaluate its effect on overall outcomes in 1604 patients enrolled in the Acute Liver Failure Study Group; 70% of patients with ALF developed AKI, and 30% received RRT. Patients with severe AKI had higher international normalized ratio (INR) values and a higher proportion had advanced-grade coma or presented with hypotension requiring vasopressor therapy. A greater proportion of patients with acetaminophen-induced ALF had severe kidney injury than patients with other etiologies of ALF; 34% required RRT, compared with 25% of patients with ALF not associated with acetaminophen or ischemia. Although AKI reduced the overall survival time, more than 50% of patients with acetaminophen-associated or ischemic ALF survived without OLT, compared with 19% of patients with ALF attributed to other causes. Only 4% of patients requiring RRT became dialysis-dependent.

The reported incidence of HRS varies between 6 and 11% but is likely higher. Due to the diagnostic limitation of serum creatinine in LF, changes in GFR do not correlate well with changes in serum creatinine [11]. CRRT is commonly required in children awaiting OLT [14]. Kreuzer concluded that children with end stage LF have a high risk for dialysis-dependent AKI and that CRRT is associated with better efficacy and less mortality than peritoneal dialysis in 367 children listed for OLT [14]. Over 10 years, 30 children (8%) out of 367 listed for OLT required dialysis and 23 (77%) of them died. The most common cause of death was cardiovascular failure. None of the children died due to dialysis-related complications.

Despite significant advances in therapies it is still impossible to reproduce the unique and complex architectural function of the liver. The liver is the only solid organ in the body that can regenerate. Therefore, in an ideal world, all attempts should be made to create conditions to promote spontaneous regeneration and avoid liver transplantation associated with a lifelong requirement for immunosuppression. Therefore, an ideal artificial hepatic support should mimic all of the functions of a normal liver including metabolic, synthetic and detoxification functions, allowing time for recovery and regeneration of the host organ or for transplantation. However, it is almost impossible to predict which patients with ALF will spontaneously recover, the length of time required for regeneration versus which patients will require a transplant. An important ethical debate, especially when organs are scarce, with a fulminant disease process is whom *not* to transplant. The majority of children with acute, acute-on-chronic, and progressive chronic LF require OLT [16]. Extracorporeal liver support systems are increasingly applied to bridge the time to recovery or to transplantation. Multiple systems are currently in use but none have shown clear improvements in survival rates in end stage LF. As such, indications regarding the initiation of extracorporeal support, the type of support, and the technical logistics remain under debate and scrutiny [17].

## 29.3 Indications for Extracorporeal Replacement Therapy in Acute LF

Standard indications for initiating CRRT in critically ill non-LF children (hyperkalemia, rising blood urea nitrogen and creatinine, fluid overload, intractable metabolic acidosis) are also used in patients with LF. However, an ideal extracorporeal

**Table 29.2** Indications for initiation of CRRT in children with acute liver failure (ALF)

| | |
|---|---|
| 1. | Metabolic abnormalities |
| | Sodium <130 meq/L |
| | High/increasing lactate despite optimizing fluid therapy |
| | Metabolic acidosis resistant to fluid therapy |
| 2. | Hepatic encephalopathy grade 3–4 |
| 3. | Ammonia >150 µmol/L and uncontrolled, or an absolute value >200 µmol/L |
| | *Insert dual lumen venous catheter when serum ammonia reaches 100 µmol/L* |
| 4. | Renal dysfunction (oligo-anuria, hyperkalemia, fluid overload) |
| No indication is an absolute for initiation of CRRT | |
| Seek expert advice before deciding to start CRRT | |

therapy should also remove toxins responsible for HE and replace the functions of the failing liver. Table 29.2 summarizes the indications of initiating CRRT in children with liver failure.

## 29.4 Extracorporeal Replacement Therapies

The question of how to best support two interrelated systems—the liver and the kidney—both responsible of detoxification, when both are failing remains unanswered in full. An ideal extracorporeal system should be able to remove both water-soluble and protein-bound substances.

While conventional CRRT effectively removes water-soluble small molecules (urea, creatinine, and ammonia), highly protein-bound substances cannot be removed effectively necessitating augmented clearance with albumin-assisted dialysis or plasma filtration/adsorption. Single pass albumin dialysis (SPAD) consists of addition of albumin to conventional dialysate to enhance removal of protein-bound substances; after one countercurrent "pass" spent-dialysate is discarded. Plasma filtration/adsorption is separation of the colloid rich plasma from the cellular elements of the blood and either replacement by fresh plasma or "cleansing" via adsorption/hemoperfusion to provide blood purification.

The molecular adsorbent recirculating system (MARS™) is another albumin-augmented dialysis where blood is first dialyzed against an albumin containing solution and then the albumin solution in turn is dialyzed against a conventional dialysate. The difference from SPAD is the regeneration of albumin via passage through a charcoal column and an ion exchanger to cleanse off bound toxins and allow the same solution to be reused for the duration of the treatment. MARS™ clears protein-bound toxins, removes cytokines, and curbs the inflammatory pathway that is also implicated in the multiple organ failure of LF. Therapeutic plasma exchange (TPE) has the added advantage of treating coagulopathy effectively without exogenous protein or fluid load, and has been used as stand-alone, or in conjunction with CRRT or hemodialysis.

Studies in adults have demonstrated the effectiveness of these devices in decreasing ammonia and lactate, improving hemodynamics and multi-organ dysfunction but to date have failed to show a survival benefit. Pediatric data consist mostly of retrospective chart reviews and case presentations, and uncontrolled single-center studies.

Symons et al. [18] prospectively looked at survival rates of children included in the Prospective Pediatric CRRT (ppCRRT) registry, according to the diagnoses leading to the use of CRRT. The overall survival rate was 58%, but it varied widely depending on diagnosis, with the lowest survival rate found in children with liver diseases (31%).

### 29.4.1 Continuous Veno-Venous Hemofiltration (CVVH) and High Volume Hemofiltration (HVHF)

Used in LF over many decades, CVVH is the least complicated of all the modalities; it is relatively quick and easy to set up. Ammonia, metabolic acidosis, hyperkalemia, and high lactate levels are all efficiently cleared by CVVH. Optimizing fluid balance, nutrition and clearance of drugs are some of the other rationales for using CVVH as fluid overload, a well-known predictors of unfavorable outcome in the ICU, can rapidly develop in LF secondary to repeated FFP and albumin infusions to replace the synthetic failure of the liver, nutrition, and medications. In 1989 Davenport [19] reported successful use of continuous arteriovenous hemofiltration in a patient with HE and renal failure in one of the first studies on CRRT in ALF.

At King's College Hospital, London, a full analysis of all children admitted to the pediatric intensive care unit (PICU) with ALF between Jan 2002 and Dec 2013 analyzed the effect of CRRT on pediatric ALF. CRRT requirement was an independent risk factor for mortality. Children who required CRRT were sicker, with higher Liver Injury Unit scores; 26 (58%) survived; 19 were successfully bridged to OLT; and 7 spontaneously recovered. Among nonsurvivors, 31% died prior to transplant and the remaining following transplant, confirming that in children with LF, superimposed AKI is associated with reduced patient survival after transplantation [11, 12, 15]. Table 29.3 describes the CRRT protocol used at King's College Hospital, London.

**Dose of CRRT:** There is no evidence to suggest a particular dose in children with ALF. In 2002, Sadamori et al. [20] reported high flow hemodiafiltration with up to 9 L/h of turnover rate in conjunction with plasma exchange as successful bridge to OLT in a patient with hyperacute fulminant LF and CE.

**Table 29.3** Proposed CRRT protocol for ALF in children at King's College Hospital, London

| Weight of child | <5 kg | 5–15 kg | 15–30 kg | >30 kg |
|---|---|---|---|---|
| Vascath size | 6.5F | 8–10Fr | 11.5F | 11.5–13.5F |
| Length available | 75 mm | 90–120 mm | 125–160 mm | 160–195 mm |
| Blood flow rate | 50–80mls/min | 100mls/min | 150mls/min | 200mls/min |
| Pre-dilution rate | 60 mL/kg/h<br>4 L/1.73 $m^2$/h | 60 mL/kg/h<br>4 L/1.73 $m^2$/h | 60 mL/kg/h<br>4 L/1.73 $m^2$/h | 60 mL/kg/h<br>4 L/1.73 $m^2$/h |
| Anticoagulation | Prostacyclin<br>4–8 ng/kg/min | Prostacyclin<br>4–8 ng/kg/min | Prostacyclin<br>4–8 ng/kg/min | Prostacyclin<br>4–8 ng/kg/min |

For child <10 kg prime circuit with blood (except if immediately post-liver transplant, or those at risk of GVHD or hemolytic disease)

Blood flow should start at half desired blood flow rate and gradually reach the desired blood flow rate

Dose of CVVH can be increased to 8–10 L/1.73 $m^2$/h if ammonia is not controlled

Slack [9] from King's College looked at the effect of hemofiltration at different treatment intensities on ammonia clearance (AC) and arterial ammonia concentration in a prospective study of adult LF patients with arterial ammonia >100 μmol/L requiring CVVH. Arterial ammonia concentration and AC were measured at 1–24 h after initiation of low (35 mL/kg/h) or high (90 mL/kg/h) filtration volume. Clearance of urea and ammonia solutes correlated closely and clinically significant AC can be achieved in adult patients with hyperammonemia utilizing CVVH.

HVHF [21], with ultrafiltrate flow of more than 80 mL/kg/h, was shown to significantly improve hemodynamic stability and neurological status in children with ALF awaiting emergency OLT, with the rationale that LF is an inflammatory milieu, like sepsis, and physiopathology of ALF hemodynamic derangements is similar. After 48 h of treatment, improvement in mean arterial pressure, grade of HE, and serum creatinine was noted. Overall mortality was 45.4%.

**Anticoagulation:** Patients with ALF, despite high INR and prothrombin time, have a deficiency in both pro and anticoagulant factors. Some patients may have a paradoxical coagulation status in which they appear anticoagulated based on clotting times yet they tend to be hypercoagulable, partially due to depressed levels of anticlotting factors and a degree of intravascular coagulation. The risk of bleeding is impacted by the degree of thrombocytopenia and platelet functional status.

Habib [22] from King's College Hospital compared 30 patients with ALF with fully matched healthy controls and noted that pro-coagulant and anticoagulant factors were equally decreased leading to a fairly balanced coagulation profile. The endogenous thrombin potential ratio in ALF patients versus controls strongly points towards hypercoagulability. Thus, these patients need as much anticoagulation to keep their circuits running, as do the non-LF patients.

Goonasekara [23] studied 31 children in LF who underwent CRRT and concluded that circuits blocked despite deranged clotting parameters. Texas Children's Hospital, which utilizes regional citrate anticoagulation (RCA), found 33% of the filters were lost to clotting among148 filters in 15 children with LF over 12 months, most commonly due to access clotting.

The common options for anticoagulation are heparin, regional citrate anticoagulation (RCA), or anti-platelet agent prostacyclin. RCA in CRRT for LF, once considered contraindicated due to concerns about citrate accumulation, has recently been revisited. Citrate induces anticoagulation by chelating ionized calcium, a cofactor for multiple steps in the coagulation cascade. Bleeding is a relatively common complication in pediatric CRRT, particularly exacerbated by the requirement of a large bore catheter to achieve reliable flows. Bleeding complications in up to 30% children receiving CRRT regardless of anticoagulation has been reported. Citrate avoids systemic anticoagulation. A residual amount of citrate spills over into the circulation [24, 25] sparking concerns about toxicity in the setting of impaired metabolism in LF, with ongoing chelation of serum ionized calcium in vivo and metabolic acidosis as a direct result of circulatory citrate accumulation [26].

Shultheiss [17] reported a prospective observational study in medical ICU of 43 CVVHD runs with RCA in 28 critically ill patients with decompensated liver cirrhosis or ALF and concluded that despite substantial accumulation of citrate in serum, CVVHD with RCA seemed feasible in patients with severely LF. RCA is effective as an anticoagulant in pediatric extracorporeal therapies with longer filter lives and fewer incidences of clotting compared to heparin [27–30]. Texas Children's Hospital routinely uses RCA in all CRRT circuits regardless of the underlying pathology and coagulopathy profile. The RCA protocol is modified in LF patients to lower citrate flow rates and higher circuit calcium (up to 0.6) with 30–50% higher clearance dose that is adjusted for concerns of citrate accumulation, closely monitored by keeping total calcium/ionized calcium ratio < 2.5.

A large report demonstrated median filter life was 66 h in 223 filters in 51 patients with LF on almost 900 CRRT days [31]; more than 60% and 30% of filters lasted longer than 48–72 h, respectively, only 15% of filters lost due to clotting [31, 32]. Adverse events, defined as bleeding, hypotension or arrhythmia requiring intervention, were seen in 34/51 patients (92 events per 1000 CRRT days) and were not related to hypocalcemia or citrate accumulation. The timing of 29 events in 22 patients coincided with citrate accumulation, while the other 50 events did not. Forty percent of patients experienced at least one episode of bleeding, similar to other reports, and without relation to hypocalcemia or citrate accumulation. The acceptable adverse event profile suggests RCA might be a superior option, evidenced by long filter lives and low incidence of filter clotting, with adequate treatment delivery facilitating optimal filter life if used under close monitoring in centers with expertise. Regardless, anticoagulation use in LF can be a challenging balancing act. Early recognition of citrate accumulation may be facilitated with the use of standard criteria improving medical management and preventing treatment interruption. Other regional anticoagulation options such as prostacyclin deserve further exploration.

### 29.4.2 Therapeutic Plasma Exchange (TPE) with Hemofiltration

TPE has been used in patients with LF for more than half a century. Although it provides deficient essential factors such as clotting factors it has also been proven to lower blood hepatocyte growth factor levels [33]. A prospective, randomized, controlled, multicenter trial by Larsen [34] concluded that high volume plasma exchange (HVP) improves OLT-free survival in patients with ALF through attenuation of the innate immune activation and improvement of multi-organ failure. Patients treated with HVP had a 58.7% overall hospital survival compared to 47.8% in controls.

In a retrospective analysis of children with ALF, Singer [35] concluded that TPE is extremely effective in preventing life-threatening bleeding without beneficial effect on neurological complications of LF or on liver regeneration. In infants, receiving combined CVVHDF and TPE until OLT could take place, overall survival was 88%, 73% survived without neurological morbidities [36]. They concluded that their multidisciplinary approach had yielded favorable outcomes, which warrant further investigation.

Texas Children's Hospital utilizes TPE for medically refractory coagulopathy (Table 29.5) Patients are monitored every 15 minutes during tandem TPE. Despite no additional citrate use in the plasma exchange circuit and frequent monitoring of ionized calcium levels with corresponding titration of calcium infusion, hypocalcemia and acute citrate accumulation was twice as common in patients with LF who received tandem TPE, with 90% of the TPE patients having at least one measurement of total calcium/ionized calcium ratio > 2.5, compared to 55% in patients who did not receive TPE [31]. Added citrate load from the FFP is likely responsible for this observation as no additional citrate is used in tandem TPE. TPE use in pediatric patients with LF requires close attention to citrate accumulation and calcium levels.

### 29.4.3 Molecular Adsorbent Recirculating System (MARS™)

The MARS™ system consists of a unit connected to a conventional CRRT or hemodialysis machine. The filter is a high-flux dialyzer with deep surface crypts where albumin molecules adhere during the albumin priming, creating alternative binding sites for circulating protein-bound toxins. Toxins are theorized to bind to albumin in the filter and the albumin-dialysate. The albumin solution gets dialyzed in the CRRT or the HD machine for aqueous toxin removal. The MARS™ unit also contains an anion exchanger and a charcoal perfuser to "strip" the albumin of impurities to be reused in the countercurrent flow through the MARS™ filter. Multiple studies have demonstrated improvement in biochemical and hemodynamic parameters with MARS™ use in LF [37–39]. Despite improvement in HE no survival benefit has been demonstrated in adults [40]. A study aiming to test MARS™ in fulminant ALF was unsuccessful due to patients randomized to receive MARS™ getting transplanted before treatment could commence [41]. Bridge to spontaneous recovery or successful OLT due to toxic hepatopathy have been reported in pediatrics in single-center case series [42–44]. In 20 children with ALF listed for high urgency OLT, 33 MARS™ treatment sessions (average 1–2/patient) were given [43] at the discretion of the treatment team, 73% were transplanted with similar mortality to patients not requiring MARS™ despite higher LIU scores in the MARS™ group. Six patients were noted to have qualitative improvement in HE. 25% of the patients experienced serious bleeding complications; however, bleeding rate was similar in patients awaiting transplantation who did not receive MARS™.

In a single-center comparison between hemodialysis combined with TPE either simultaneous or sequentially with plasma exchange or MARS™, hemodialysis/TPE provided greater reduction in biomarkers of interest, but this result could have been confounded by sampling timing [42]. Interestingly, the decrease in serum ammonia with tandem PE/HD in children was inferior to that achieved by CRRT alone [45].

### 29.4.4 Single Pass Albumin Dialysis (SPAD)

Albumin-bound toxins such as bilirubin and bile acids that get accumulated in patients with ALF are not removed by CVVH. SPAD is a type of hemodiafiltration in which 20% albumin is run along with the dialysate solution countercurrent with the blood flow to eliminate albumin-bound toxins especially bile acids and bile salts. Thereafter, albumin is discarded. SPAD utilizes a standard hemodialysis or CVVHDF machine with no additional perfusion pump. Blood is pumped through a high-flux hollow fiber hemodiafilter. SPAD needs an albumin gradient for effective toxin removal. It's inexpensive, easy to set up, and technically less demanding than other modalities of treatment. The protocol for SPAD used in King's College Hospital is presented in Table 29.4.

Sauer showed in vitro clearance of bilirubin, ammonia, and bile acids using MARS™, SPAD, and CVVHDF. Clearance of bile acids was equal with MARS™ and SPAD but the clearance of bilirubin was much better with SPAD than with MARS™. There was no difference in ammonia clearance between MARS™, SPAD, and CVVHDF [16]. A recent prospective randomized cross-over study by Sponholz et al. [46] demonstrated that both MARS™ and SPAD are safe for temporary extracorporeal liver support and that they displayed comparable results for most parameters especially in light of bilirubin reduction. However, MARS™ provided an additional advantage in bile acid clearance and improving albumin binding capacity.

Ringe [47] has shown that treatment with SPAD was generally well tolerated on 9 children (aged 2–15 yrs) with ALF and seems to be effective in detoxification and improving blood pressure and may be beneficial in avoiding severe neurologic sequelae after ALF. Kortgen [48] described 163 albumin dialysis treatments, 126 with MARS™ and 37 with SPAD, in 57 adult patients comparing MARS™ and SPAD demonstrating equal efficacy, however the authors have recommended a prospective assessment to further define the role of SPAD.

SPAD is very effective in treating resistant pruritus after drugs and biliary drainage have failed. A major disadvantage is the need of large amounts of albumin in older children. A prospective randomized study on this relatively inexpensive modality of detoxification in LF will be highly beneficial.

Limited donors leading to long wait times on the transplant list have forced a search for leveraging of available modalities to offer continued support to viable transplant candidates. The indications for the use of CRRT, TPE, and MARS™ in ALF/ACLF should be protocolized in most institutions. Texas Children's Hospital has implemented a successful protocolized use of complex extracorporeal therapies in hybrid fashion, combining CRRT, TPE, and MARS™, for their respective benefits to bridge to transplantation with serial improvements in outcomes with the introduction of each additional therapy (Table 29.5). Over the last 3 years, 15/17 patients with ALF/ACLF (all CLIF-SOFA score > 12) were successfully bridged to transplantation with the hybrid treatment protocol; 90-day post-transplant survival was 100%.

**Table 29.4** King's College Hospital—SPAD Protocol

| | | |
|---|---|---|
| Indication | Clearance of protein-bound toxins<br>– Bile salts<br>– Copper<br>– Conjugated bilirubin | |
| Equipment required | Vascular access<br>CCVH set and filter<br>3 way tap<br>Pump + giving set | 1000 mL 0.9% saline bag<br>800 mls—20% HAS<br>5 L dialysate solution with or without K added depending on patient K |
| Tests before each treatment | – Full blood count<br>– Na, K, Ca, Mg, Cl<br>– AST, ALT, conjugated bilirubin, bile salts<br>– Take a sample of waste dialysate fluid after each treatment, labelled accordingly and send to lab for same as above | |
| Machine settings | Select CVVHD mode<br>Blood pump: 150 mL/min<br>Dialysate rate: 500 mls | Fluid loss rate: 130 mL/h<br>Total fluid loss: 780 mL<br>Temperature: 39°<br>HAS rate: 130 mL/h |
| Procedure | 1. Turn on machine, allow self test and select CVVHD mode<br>2. Attach effluent line at top of filter<br>3. Attach 3 way tap to bottom of filter for albumin and dialysate<br>4. Prime and recirculate for min 10 min<br>5. Run albumin through giving set then attach to 3 way tap on filter<br>6. Take blood samples, blood gas and ACT (activated clotting time)<br>7. ACT should guide anticoagulation as per your protocols<br>8. Attach patient using double connection<br>9. Start blood pump at 50 mL/h and increase over next 20 min<br>10. Start albumin pump when the patient's blood has reached the air bubble trap and dialysate has started<br>11. Run treatment for 6 h<br>12. Monitor $K^+$ 2 hourly using blood gases<br>13. When treatment complete dispose of circuit.<br>14. Send sample of waste dyalisate for bile salt analysis<br>15. Heplock (and label clearly) both lumens of vascath when not in use. | |
| Monitoring | Continuous ECG and $SaO_2$<br>Hourly blood pressure<br>Hourly neuromonitoring including pupils<br>Pruritus score before and after treatment | |
| Adverse effects | Thrombocytopenia<br>Air emboli | Thrombosis<br>Anemia |
| Treatment frequency | 5 cycles of SPAD each lasting for 6 h over a 5 day period | |

**Table 29.5** Protocol of various Liver Assist Devices used at Texas Children's Hospital

| Therapy | Indication | Technique/ Modality | Dose | Duration/frequency | Anticoagulation | Special monitoring |
|---|---|---|---|---|---|---|
| CRRT | Hyperammonemia[a]<br>Oliguric AKI<br>Fluid overload | CVVHDF | 3000 mL/1.73 $m^2$/h | Continuous | RCA | Keep circuit/iCal <2.5 |
| Total plasma exchange | Medically refractory coagulopathy[b]<br>Clinical life-threatening bleeding | Centrifugal TPE | 1.3–1.5 × plasma volume exchange volume with all FFP replacement | As needed | No additional | Q 15 min calcium monitoring, increased rate of calcium infusion |
| MARS | HE grade 3 or higher<br>HE grade 2 + MODS[c] | MARS in series with CRRT in CVVHDF mode | 3000 mL/1.73 $m^2$/h | **ACLF**:<br>Minimum 8 h session, at least 5 consecutive days, then as needed<br>**ALF**:<br>Daily minimum 8 h treatments until recovery | RCA | Maintain:<br>Platelets >50,000; fibrinogen >150 |

[a] >75 μmol/L or rapidly rising while on maximum medical therapy
[b] >30 mL/kg of fresh frozen plasma in 24 h
[c] 2 or more failing organ systems

**Conclusions**

The cornerstone of management of ALF is supportive treatment. We have good quality evidence to show that when compared to standard medical treatment patients awaiting liver transplantation benefit from renal replacement therapies. Combined extracorporeal therapy is often necessary to support the multiple organ failure associated with a failing liver as a bridge to spontaneous regeneration or successful liver transplantation.

**Key Learning Points**

- Management of critical LF is challenging for the intensivists and hepatologist alike and ideally done in liver transplant centers.
- Extracorporeal treatments are often necessary to provide support for the multiple organ failure of advanced liver disease and present unique challenges.
- Controversies exist around several aspects of renal replacement therapy (RRT) in liver failure—indications, timing of initiation, dose of CRRT used, anticoagulation, and when to stop RRT.
- An ideal liver assist device is the one which performs both the detoxification function and the synthetic function of the failing liver.
- Early aggressive treatment with a goal to bridge to transplantation or to native liver recovery seems beneficial.

## References

1. Gazzard BG, Weston MJ, Murray-Lyon IM, Flax H, Record CO, Williams R, et al. Charcoal haemoperfusion in the treatment of fulminant hepatic failure. Lancet. 1974;1(7870):1301–7.
2. Loening WE, Coovadia HM, Parent MA. Exchange transfusion in fulminant hepatic failure in children. S Afr Med J. 1974;48(4):128–30.
3. Squires RH Jr, Shneider BL, Bucuvalas J, Alonso E, Sokol RJ, Narkewicz MR, et al. Acute liver failure in children: the first 348 patients in the pediatric acute liver failure study group. J Pediatr. 2006;148(5):652–8.
4. Coltart I, Tranah TH, Shawcross DL. Inflammation and hepatic encephalopathy. Arch Biochem Biophys. 2013;536(2):189–96.
5. Bernal W, Hall C, Karvellas CJ, Auzinger G, Sizer E, Wendon J. Arterial ammonia and clinical risk factors for encephalopathy and intracranial hypertension in acute liver failure. Hepatology. 2007;46(6):1844–52.
6. Wendon J, Lee W. Encephalopathy and cerebral edema in the setting of acute liver failure: pathogenesis and management. Neurocrit Care. 2008;9(1):97–102.
7. Warrillow SJ. Predictions and outcomes for the critically ill patient with cirrhosis: is it time to settle on the SOFA and let jaundiced views on outcome MELD away? Crit Care Med. 2010;38(11):2259–60.
8. Larsen FS, Wendon J. Prevention and management of brain edema in patients with acute liver failure. Liver Transpl. 2008;14(Suppl 2(S2)):S90–6.
9. Slack AJ, Auzinger G, Willars C, Dew T, Musto R, Corsilli D, et al. Ammonia clearance with haemofiltration in adults with liver disease. Liver Int. 2013;34(1):42–8.

10. Spinale JM, Laskin BL, Sondheimer N, Swartz SJ, Goldstein SL. High-dose continuous renal replacement therapy for neonatal hyperammonemia. Pediatr Nephrol. 2013;28(6):983–6.
11. Ellis D, Avner ED, Starzl TE. Renal failure in children with hepatic failure undergoing liver transplantation. J Pediatr. 1986;108(3):393–8.
12. Bridges BC, Askenazi DJ, Smith J, Goldstein SL. Pediatric renal replacement therapy in the intensive care unit. Blood Purif. 2012;34(2):138–48.
13. Stange J. Extracorporeal liver support. Organogenesis. 2011;7(1):64–73.
14. Kreuzer M, Gähler D, Rakenius AC, Prüfe J, Jack T, Pfister E-D, et al. Dialysis-dependent acute kidney injury in children with end-stage liver disease: prevalence, dialysis modalities and outcome. Pediatr Nephrol. 2015;30(12):2199–206.
15. Tujios SR, Hynan LS, Vazquez MA, Larson AM, Seremba E, Sanders CM, et al. Risk factors and outcomes of acute kidney injury in patients with acute liver failure. Clin Gastroenterol Hepatol. 2015;13(2):352–9.
16. Sauer IM, Goetz M, Steffen I, Walter G, Kehr DC, Schwartlander R, et al. In vitro comparison of the molecular adsorbent recirculation system (MARS) and single-pass albumin dialysis (SPAD). Hepatology. 2004;39(5):1408–14.
17. Schultheiß C, Saugel B, Phillip V, Thies P, Noe S, Mayr U, et al. Continuous venovenous hemodialysis with regional citrate anticoagulation in patients with liver failure: a prospective observational study. Crit Care. 2012;16(4):R162.
18. Symons JM, Chua AN, Somers MJG, Baum MA, Bunchman TE, Benfield MR, et al. Demographic characteristics of pediatric continuous renal replacement therapy: a report of the prospective pediatric continuous renal replacement therapy registry. Clin J Am Soc Nephrol. 2007;2(4):732–8.
19. Davenport A, Will EJ, Davison AM, Swindells S, Cohen AT, Miloszewski KJ, et al. Changes in intracranial pressure during haemofiltration in oliguric patients with grade IV hepatic encephalopathy. Nephron. 1989;53(2):142–6.
20. Sadamori H, Yagi T, Inagaki M, Shima Y, Matsuda H, Tanaka N, et al. High-flow-rate haemodiafiltration as a brain-support therapy proceeding to liver transplantation for hyperacute fulminant hepatic failure. Eur J Gastroenterol Hepatol. 2002;14(4):435–9.
21. Chevret L, Durand P, Lambert J, Essouri S, Balu L, Devictor D, et al. High-volume hemofiltration in children with acute liver failure*. Pediatr Crit Care Med. 2014;15(7):e300–5.
22. Habib M, Roberts LN, Patel RK, Wendon J, Bernal W, Arya R. Evidence of rebalanced coagulation in acute liver injury and acute liver failure as measured by thrombin generation. Liver Int. 2014;34(5):672–8.
23. Goonasekera CD, Wang J, Bunchman TE, Deep A. Factors affecting circuit life during continuous renal replacement therapy in children with liver failure. Ther Apher Dial. 2014;19(1):16–22.
24. Chadha V, Garg U, Warady BA, Alon US. Citrate clearance in children receiving continuous venovenous renal replacement therapy. Pediatr Nephrol. 2002;17(10):819–24.
25. Elhanan N, Skippen P, Nuthall G, Krahn G, Seear M. Citrate anticoagulation in pediatric continuous venovenous hemofiltration. Pediatr Nephrol. 2004;19(2):208–12.
26. Musielak A, Warzywoda A, Wojtalik M, Kociński B, Kroll P, Ostalska-Nowicka D, et al. Outcomes of continuous renal replacement therapy with regional citrate anticoagulation in small children after cardiac surgery: experience and protocol from a single center. Ther Apher Dial. 2016;20(6):639–44.
27. Brophy PD, Somers MJG, Baum MA, Symons JM, McAfee N, Fortenberry JD, et al. Multi-Centre evaluation of anticoagulation in patients receiving continuous renal replacement therapy (CRRT). Nephrol Dial Transplant. 2005;20(7):1416–21.
28. MacLaren G, Butt W. Controversies in paediatric continuous renal replacement therapy. Intensive Care Med. 2009;35(4):596–602.
29. Jacobs R, Honoré PM, Bagshaw SM, Diltoer M, Spapen HD. Citrate formulation determines filter lifespan during continuous veno-venous hemofiltration: a prospective cohort study. Blood Purif. 2015;40(3):194–202.
30. Bai M, Zhou M, He L, Ma F, Li Y, Yu Y, et al. Citrate versus heparin anticoagulation for continuous renal replacement therapy: an updated meta-analysis of RCTs. Intensive Care Med. 2015;41(12):2098–110.

31. Rodriguez K, Srivaths PR, Tal L, Watson MN, Riley AA, Himes RW, et al. Regional citrate anticoagulation for continuous renal replacement therapy in pediatric patients with liver failure. PLoS One. 2017;12(8):e0182134.
32. Deep A, Stewart CE, Dhawan A, Douiri A. Effect of continuous renal replacement therapy on outcome in pediatric acute liver failure. Crit Care Med. 2016;44(10):1910–9.
33. Abe T, Kobata H, Hanba Y, Kitabata Y, Narukawa N, Hasegawa H, et al. Study of plasma exchange for liver failure: beneficial and harmful effects. Ther Apher Dial. 2004;8(3):180–4.
34. Larsen FS, Schmidt LE, Bernsmeier C, Rasmussen A, Isoniemi H, Patel VC, et al. High-volume plasma exchange in patients with acute liver failure: an open randomised controlled trial. J Hepatol. 2016;64(1):69–78.
35. Singer AL, Olthoff KM, Kim H, Rand E, Zamir G, Shaked A. Role of plasmapheresis in the management of acute hepatic failure in children. Ann Surg. 2001;234(3):418–24.
36. Ide K, Muguruma T, Shinohara M, Toida C, Enomoto Y, Matsumoto S, et al. Continuous veno-venous hemodiafiltration and plasma exchange in infantile acute liver failure. Pediatr Crit Care Med. 2015;16(8):e268–74.
37. Stefoni S, Colì L, Bolondi L, Ruggeri G, Feliciangeli G, Piscaglia F, et al. Molecular adsorbent recirculating system (MARS) application in liver failure: clinical and hemodepurative results in 22 patients. Int J Artif Organs. 2006;29(2):207–18.
38. Novelli G, Rossi M, Pretagostini R, Novelli L, Poli L, Ferretti G, et al. A 3-year experience with molecular adsorbent recirculating system (MARS): our results on 63 patients with hepatic failure and color Doppler US evaluation of cerebral perfusion. Liver Int. 2003;23(Suppl 3):10–5.
39. Donati G, La Manna G, Cianciolo G, Grandinetti V, Carretta E, Cappuccilli M, et al. Extracorporeal detoxification for hepatic failure using molecular adsorbent recirculating system: depurative efficiency and clinical results in a long-term follow-up. Artif Organs. 2013;38(2):125–34.
40. Bañares R, Nevens F, Larsen FS, Jalan R, Albillos A, Dollinger M, et al. Extracorporeal albumin dialysis with the molecular adsorbent recirculating system in acute-on-chronic liver failure: the RELIEF trial. Hepatology. 2013;57(3):1153–62.
41. Saliba F, Camus C, Durand F, Mathurin P, Letierce A, Delafosse B, et al. Albumin dialysis with a noncell artificial liver support device in patients with acute liver failure: a randomized, controlled trial. Ann Intern Med. 2013;159(8):522–31.
42. Schaefer B, Schaefer F, Engelmann G, Meyburg J, Heckert KH, Zorn M, et al. Comparison of molecular adsorbents recirculating system (MARS) dialysis with combined plasma exchange and haemodialysis in children with acute liver failure. Nephrol Dial Transplant. 2011;26(11):3633–9.
43. Lexmond WS, Van Dael CML, Scheenstra R, Goorhuis JF, Sieders E, Verkade HJ, et al. Experience with molecular adsorbent recirculating system treatment in 20 children listed for high-urgency liver transplantation. Liver Transpl. 2015;21(3):369–80.
44. Novelli G, Rossi M, Morabito V, Pugliese F, Ruberto F, Perrella SM, et al. Pediatric acute liver failure with molecular adsorbent recirculating system treatment. Transplant Proc. 2008;40(6):1921–4.
45. Schaefer B, Ujszaszi A, Schaefer S, Heckert KH, Schaefer F, Schmitt CP. Safety and efficacy of tandem hemodialysis and plasma exchange in children. Clin J Am Soc Nephrol. 2014;9(9):1563–70.
46. Sponholz C, Matthes K, Rupp D, Backaus W, Klammt S, Karailieva D, et al. Molecular adsorbent recirculating system and single-pass albumin dialysis in liver failure—a prospective, randomised crossover study. Crit Care. 2016;20(1):2.
47. Ringe H, Varnholt V, Zimmering M, Luck W, Gratopp A, König K, et al. Continuous veno-venous single-pass albumin hemodiafiltration in children with acute liver failure. Pediatr Crit Care Med. 2011;12(3):257–64.
48. Kortgen A, Rauchfuss F, Götz M, Settmacher U, Bauer M, Sponholz C. Albumin dialysis in liver failure: comparison of molecular adsorbent recirculating system and single pass albumin dialysis--a retrospective analysis. Ther Apher Dial. 2009;13(5):419–25.

MIX
Papier aus verantwortungsvollen Quellen
Paper from responsible sources
FSC® C105338

If you have any concerns about our products,
you can contact us on
**ProductSafety@springernature.com**

In case Publisher is established outside the EU,
the EU authorized representative is:
**Springer Nature Customer Service Center GmbH**
**Europaplatz 3, 69115 Heidelberg, Germany**

Printed by Libri Plureos GmbH
in Hamburg, Germany